Techniques in Wrist and Hand Arthroscopy

Techniques in Wrist and Hand Arthroscopy

David J. Slutsky, MD, FRCS[C]

Clinical Assistant Professor
UCLA
David Geffen School of Medicine
Chief of Reconstructive Hand Surgery
Harbor-UCLA
Torrance, California

Daniel J. Nagle, MD, FACS, FAAOS

Professor of Clinical Orthopedics
Northwestern Feinberg School of Medicine
Chicago, Illinois

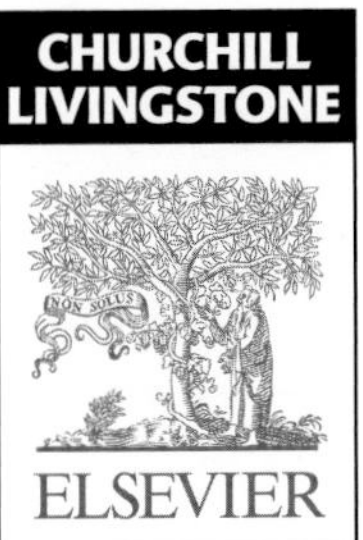

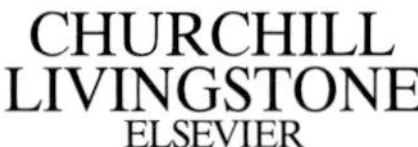

1600 John F. Kennedy Blvd.
Ste 1800
Philadelphia, PA 19103-2899

TECHNIQUES IN WRIST AND HAND ARTHROSCOPY ISBN: 978-0-443-06697-9

Library of Congress Cataloging-in-Publication Data

Techniques in wrist and hand arthroscopy / [edited by] David J. Slutsky, Daniel J. Nagle.—1st ed.
p. ; cm.
Includes bibliographical references.
ISBN 978-0-443-06697-9
1. Hand—Endoscopic surgery. 2. Wrist—Endoscopic surgery. 3. Arthroscopy. I. Slutsky, David J. II. Nagle, Daniel J.
[DNLM: 1. Wrist Joint—surgery. 2. Arthroscopy—methods. 3. Hand Joints—surgery. WE 830 T2565 2007] I. Title.

RD559. T438 2007
617.5'750597—dc22

2007026202

Acquisitions Editor: Emily Christie
Developmental Editor: Karen Lynn Carter
Project Manager: Mary B. Stermel
Design Direction: Gene Harris
Marketing Manager: Matt Latuchie

Printed in China
Last digit is the print number: 9 8 7 6 5 4 3 2 1

"To Brett and Jesse, whose love and laughter make life worth living"
David J. Slutsky

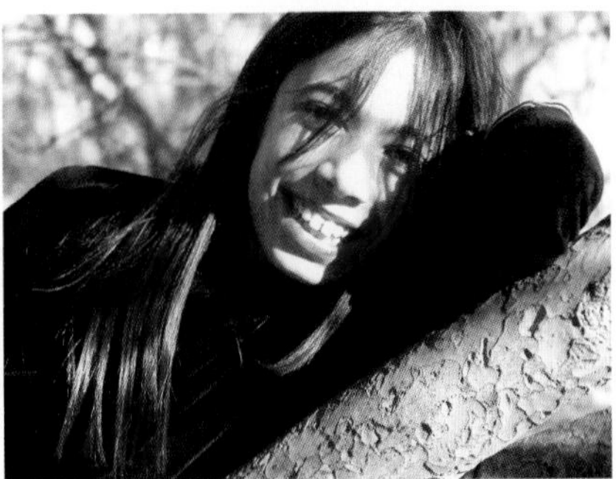

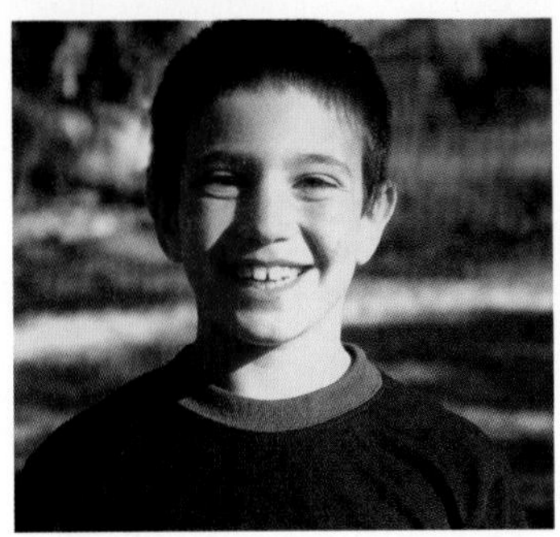

"To my mother and father"
Daniel J. Nagle

Contents

Preface

Arthroscopy of the wrist and hand has evolved from being a diagnostic modality to being a valuable and effective therapeutic tool. Arthroscopy has revolutionized the diagnosis and treatment of scapholunate and lunotriquetral ligament disorders as well as triangular fibrocartilage tears. Wrist arthroscopy is a useful adjunct in the reduction of intra-articular fractures of the distal radius as well as percutaneous screw fixation of scaphoid fractures. The staging of degenerative conditions is facilitated through the use of arthroscopy. Innovative surgeons have developed arthroscopic techniques for partial carpal resections, release of wrist contractures, synovectomies, and ganglionectomies.

This book features a compendium of procedures from some of the true leaders in this field. It is intended to serve as a user's manual for both the entry-level wrist arthroscopist and the experienced surgeon. The methodology and the practical aspects of each procedure are stressed along with myriad pearls and tips, oftentimes from the originators of the technique. The accompanying DVDs illustrate the techniques and provide a glimpse into the surgical anatomy in real time.

It was a real joy working with many of the pioneers and innovators in wrist and hand arthroscopy. We are indebted to our contributors, without whom this book would not exist. We appreciate the time, effort, and personal sacrifice they have put forth to educate their peers. We are also indebted to Kim Murphy, senior publishing director of Global Medicine at Elsevier, for allowing us to move forward with this project, as well as the associate editors who contributed their time and energy to this project, including Karen Carter, who moved mountains to complete this book, Elyse O'Grady, and Matthew Ray. Special thanks to Jenny Koleth, Emily Christie, and Michael Troy for their postproduction work as well as multimedia producer Bruce Robison and his team and Dave Sewel of Motion Video for their help with the video editing.

We hope that you will find this book useful as you tackle new arthroscopic techniques.

David J. Slutsky, MD, FRCS[C]
Daniel J. Nagle, MD, FACS, FAAOS

Contributors

Brian D. Adams, MD
Professor
Department of Orthopaedics
University of Iowa School of Medicine
Iowa City, Iowa

N. Ashwood, MD, FRCS(Orth)
University of Adelaide
Royal Adelaide Hospital
Modbury Public Hospital
North Adelaide, Australia

G.I. Bain, MD, FRACS
University of Adelaide
Royal Adelaide Hospital
Modbury Public Hospital
North Adelaide, Australia

Ferdinando Battistella, MD
Chief Surgeon
Center for Reconstructive Arthroscopic Shoulder Surgery
Istituto Ortopedico Galeazzi
Milan, Italy

Richard A. Berger, MD, PhD
Professor of Orthopedics
Department of Orthopedic Surgery and Anatomy
Mayo Clinic
Rochester, Minnesota

Randy R. Bindra, MD
Professor of Orthopaedics
Director of the Center for Hand and Upper Extremity Surgery
University of Arkansas for Health Sciences
Department of Orthopaedic Surgery
Little Rock, Arkansas

César J. Bruno
Clinical Assistant Professor of Orthopedic Surgery
University of Virginia
Charlottsville, Virginia
Co-Director Hand, Microvascular and Upper Extremity Division
Carilion Bone and Joint Center
Roanoke, Virginia

Robert E. Carroll, MD
Professor Emeritus of Hand Surgery
Department of Orthopaedic Surgery
Columbia University College of Physicians and Surgeons
New York, New York

Randall W. Culp, MD
Associate Professor of Orthopedic, Hand, and Microsurgery
Thomas Jefferson University
Philadelphia, Pennsylvania
The Philadelphia Hand Center, P.C.
King of Prussia, Pennsylvania

Francisco del Piñal, MD
Instituto de Cirugia Plastica y de la Mano
Hospital Mutua Montanesa and Clinica Mompia
Santander, Spain

Seth D. Dodds, MD
Assistant Professor, Hand and Upper Extremity Surgery
Department of Orthopaedics and Rehabilitation
Yale University School of Medicine
New Haven, Connecticut

William B. Geissler, MD
Professor and Chief, Division of Hand and Upper Extremity Surgery
Chief, Section of Arthroscopic Surgery and Sports Medicine
Director, Hand and Upper Extremity Fellowship
Department of Orthopaedic Surgery and Rehabilitation
University of Mississippi Medical Center
Jackson, Mississippi

Pau Golano, MD
Departamento Anatomía
Universidad de Barcelona
Barcelona, Spain

Steven H. Goldberg, MD
Hand Surgery Ltd.
Waukesha, Wisconsin

Jeffrey A. Greenberg, MD
Indiana Hand Center
Clinical Assistant Professor
Indiana University School of Medicine
Indianapolis, Indiana

Gregory J. Hanker, MD
Assistant Clinical Professor
Plastic and Reconstructive Surgery
University of Southern California
Southern California Orthopaedic Institute
Van Nuys, California

Brian J. Harley, MD, FRCS[C]
Associate Professor of Orthopedic Surgery
SUNY Health Science Center
Syracuse, New York

Michael R. Hausman, MD
Professor, Orthopaedics
Assistant Professor, Surgery
The Leni and Peter W. May Department of Orthopaedics
Mount Sinai School of Medicine
New York, New York

Ericka A. Lawler, MD
Visiting Assistant Professor
Department of Orthopaedic Surgery
University of Iowa
College of Medicine
Iowa City, Iowa

Jason W. Levine, MD
Fellow
Mississippi Sports Medicine and Orthopaedic Center
Jackson, Mississippi

David M. Lichtman, MD
Assistant Professor
Department of Orthopaedic Surgery
University of North Texas Health Science Center at Fort Worth
John Peter Smith Hospital
Fort Worth, Texas

Greg Merrell, MD
Department of Orthopaedics and Rehabilitation
Yale University School of Medicine
New Haven, Connecticut

Michael J. Moskal, MD
Shoulder and Elbow Center
Clinical Instructor, Department of Orthopaedic Surgery and Sports Medicine
University of Washington
Seattle, Washington
Clinical Instructor, Department of Orthopaedic Surgery
University of Louisville
Louisville, Kentucky

Daniel J. Nagle, MD, FACS, FAAOS
Professor of Clinical Orthopedics
Northwestern Feinberg School of Medicine
Chicago, Illinois

A. Lee Osterman, MD
Professor Hand Surgery
Philadelphia Hand Center
Thomas Jefferson University
Philadelphia, Pennsylvania

Andrew K. Palmer, MD
Professor of Orthopaedic Surgery
SUNY Health Science Center
Syracuse, New York

Kevin D. Plancher, MD
Associate Clinical Professor
Albert Einstein College of Medicine
New York, New York
Orthopaedic Foundation for Active Lifestyles
Greenwich, Connecticut

Kongkhet Riansuwan, MD
Postdoctoral Research Fellow
Department of Orthopedic Surgery
New York Presbyterian Hospital
Columbia University Medical Center
New York, New York

Melvin P. Rosenwasser, MD
Robert E. Carroll Professor of Surgery
Hand in the Department of Orthopaedic Surgery
New York Presbyterian Hospital
Columbia University Medical Center
New York, New York

Felix H. Savoie III, MD
Co-Director, Shoulder/Elbow Service
Mississippi Sports Medicine and Orthopaedic Center
Jackson, Mississippi

Joseph F. Slade III, MD
Associate Professor
Yale Orthopaedics
Director
Yale Hand and Upper Extremity Center
New Haven, Connecticut

David J. Slutsky, MD, FRCS[C]
Clinical Assistant Professor
UCLA
David Geffen School of Medicine
Chief of Reconstructive Hand Surgery
Harbor-UCLA
Torrance, California

Ettore Taverna, MD
Instituto Galleazi
Milan, Italy

Matthew M. Tomaino, MD
Professor and Chief
Division of Hand and Upper Extremity
University of Rochester Medical Center
Rochester, New York

Thomas E. Trumble, MD
Professor and Chief, Division of Hand and Microvascular Surgery
Department of Orthopaedic Surgery
University of Washington Medical Center
Seattle, Washington

Jennifer Weintraub, MD
Division of Plastic and Reconstructive Surgery
Stanford University Medical Center
Stanford, California

Eric S. Wroten, MD
Philadelphia Hand Center
King of Prussia, Pennsylvania

Jeffrey Yao, MD
Assistant Professor of Orthopaedic Surgery
Stanford University School of Medicine
Stanford University Medical Center
Stanford, California

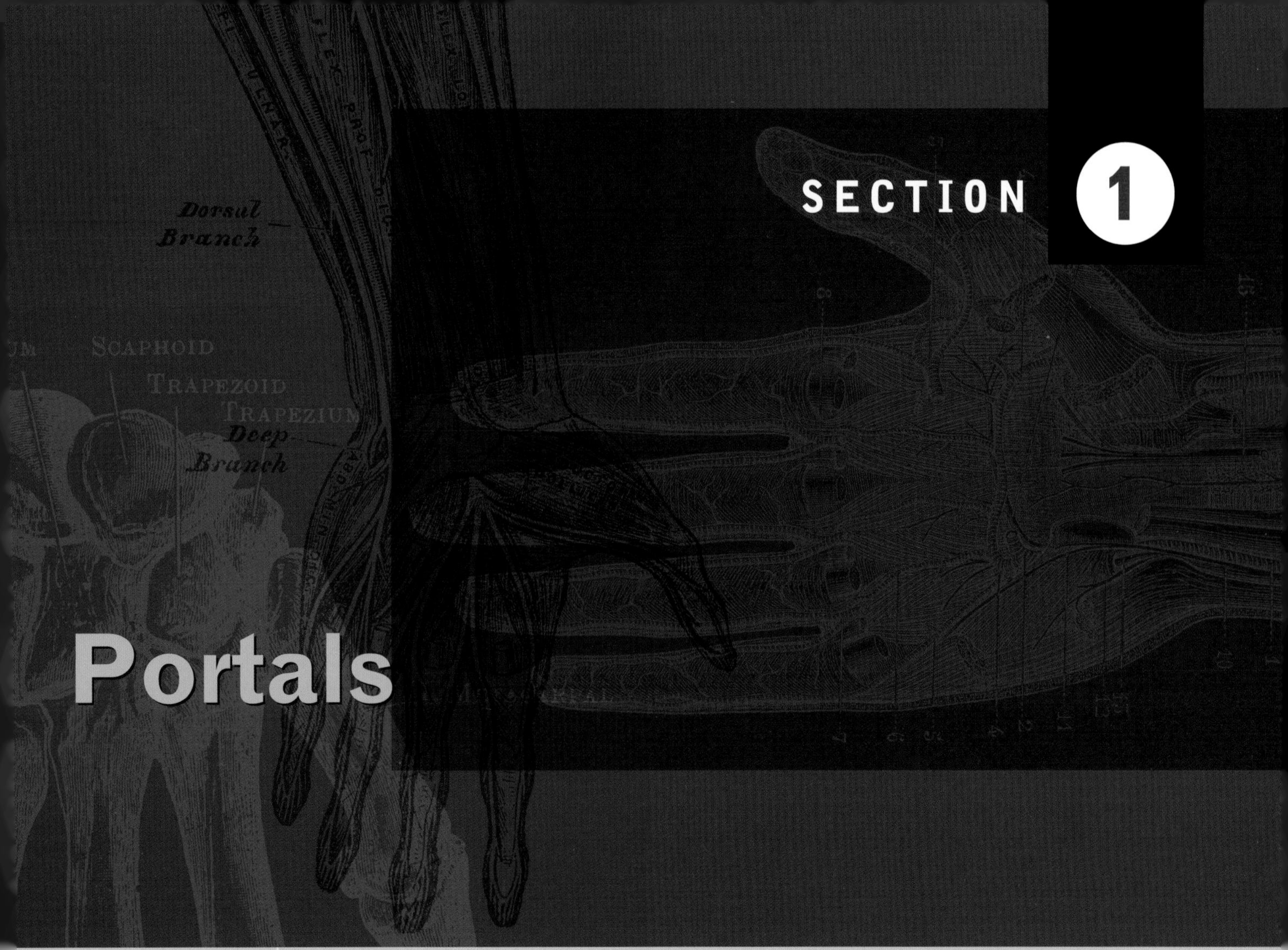

SECTION 1

Portals

David J. Slutsky

CHAPTER 1

Wrist Arthroscopy Portals

Introduction

Since its inception, wrist arthroscopy has continued to evolve. The initial emphasis on viewing the wrist from the dorsal aspect arose from the relative lack of neurovascular structures as well as the familiarity of most surgeons with dorsal approaches to the radiocarpal joint. Anatomical studies provided a better understanding of both the interosseous ligaments as well as carpal kinematics, which led to the development of midcarpal arthroscopy. Innovative surgeons continued to push the envelope through the development of techniques for treating intracarpal pathology, which in turn culminated in a plethora of new accessory portals. This chapter explores the standard arthroscopic portals, as well as some of the more recent and special-use portals.[1]

Indications

The indications for the use of the standard dorsal portals are intertwined with the indications for wrist arthroscopy and are largely dependent on the indication for surgery, in that this will vary considerably between arthroscopic fracture reduction compared to performing a diagnostic procedure for chronic wrist pain. These include variable combinations of the 3-/,4 portal, the 4-/,5 portal, and the 6 radial (6R) and 6 ulnar (6U) portals. Typically, the 3-/,4 and 4,/-5 portals are used interchangeably for visualizing the radiocarpal joint and for instrumentation. The 4-/,5 portal and the 6R portal are used to access the ulnocarpal joint. The 6U portal is typically used for outflow. However, with careful attention to surface landmarks any portal can be used for viewing or instrumentation.

Midcarpal arthroscopy is essential in making the diagnosis of scapholunate and lunotriquetral instability. The grading scale reported by Geissler et al.[2] provides a means of staging the degree of instability in order to provide an algorithm for treatment. Midcarpal arthroscopy is also useful for the assessment and treatment of chondral lesions of the proximal hamate.[3] The triquetro-hamate joint can also be accessed through another special-use midcarpal portal.[4]

The clinical utility of volar portals has been recently elucidated.[5–7] As kinematic and biomechanical studies have shed light on the role of the dorsal capsular structures and palmar subregions of the interosseous ligaments in maintaining carpal stability, it has become prudent to view the wrist from a palmar perspective. Volar portals for wrist arthroscopy have certain advantages over the standard dorsal portals for visualizing dorsal capsular structures as well as the palmar aspects of the carpal ligaments. The volar radial (VR) portal is relatively easy to use and is an ideal portal for evaluation of the dorsal radiocarpal ligament (DRCL) and the palmar subregion of the scapholunate interosseous ligament (SLIL). It facilitates the identification of and repair of DRCL tears.[8,9] The VR portal also facilitates arthroscopic reduction of intra-articular fractures of the distal radius fractures by providing a clear view of the dorsal rim fragments.[10]

The volar radial midcarpal (VRM) portal may be considered an occasional accessory portal for visualizing the palmar aspects of the capitate and hamate in cases of avascular necrosis or osteochondral fractures.[6] This portal facilitates visualization of the palmar aspect of the capitohamate interosseous ligament (CHIL), which is important in minimizing translational motion[11] and has an essential role in providing stability to the transverse carpal arch.[12]

The volar ulnar (VU) portal provides unparalleled views of the dorsal radioulnar ligament and the dorsal ulnar wrist capsule, which contains the extensor carpi ulnaris subsheath (ECUS). Establishing the VU portal is more technically demanding but has potential use in the arthroscopic diagnosis and treatment of patients with ulnar sided wrist pain and suspected injuries to the ulnar sling mechanism. It is especially useful for visualizing and debriding palmar tears of the lunotriquetral ligament.[13] It also aids in the repair or debridement of dorsally located TFC tears because the proximity of the 4/-,5 and 6R portals makes triangulation of the instruments difficult. The volar aspect of the distal radioulnar joint can be visualized through the VU portal to assess the foveal attachment of the triangular fibrocartilage in cases of suspected peripheral detachment of the TFC.[7]

Two dorsal DRUJ portals have been described. The dorsal DRUJ portals may be used to assess the status of the articular cartilage of the ulnar head and sigmoid notch. This information may be useful in cases of DRUJ instability, or when there is the suspicion of early osteoarthritis (in which case arthroscopy may differentiate between the need for DRUJ stabilization or ulnar head excision and arthroplasty. With inflammatory disorders such as rheumatoid arthritis DRUJ, an arthroscopic synovectomy may obviate the need for a capsular incision. The dorsal DRUJ portals are infrequently used as an adjunct to arthroscopic wafer resections of the ulnar head.

Contraindications

Contraindications to the use of dorsal or volar portals include any cause of marked swelling that distorts the topographic anatomy, large capsular tears that might lead to extravasation of irrigation fluid, neurovascular compromise, bleeding disorders, and infection. Unfamiliarity with the regional anatomy is a relative contraindication.

Relevant Anatomy

The standard portals for wrist arthroscopy are mostly dorsal (Figure 1.1a through c). This is in part due to the relative lack of neurovascular structures on the dorsum of the wrist as well as the initial emphasis on assessing the volar wrist ligaments. The dorsal portals, which allow access to the radiocarpal joint, are so named in relation to the tendons of the dorsal extensor compartments. For example, the 1-/,2 portal lies between the first extensor compartment tendons—which include the extensor pollicus brevis (EPB) and the abductor pollicus longus (APL)—and the second extensor compartment, which contains the extensor carpi radialis brevis and longus (ECRB/L).

The 3-/,4 portal is named for the interval between the third dorsal extensor compartment—which contains the extensor pollicus longus tendon (EPL)—and the fourth extensor compartment, which contains the extensor digitorum communis (EDC) tendons. In a similar vein, the 4-/,5 portal is located between the EDC and the extensor digiti minimi (EDM). The 6R portal is located on the radial side of the extensor carpi ulnaris (ECU) tendon, compared to the 6U portal (which is located on the ulnar side).

The midcarpal joint is assessed through two portals, which allows triangulation of the arthroscope and the instrumentation. The midcarpal radial portal (MCR) is located 1 cm distal to the 3-/,4 portal and is bounded radially by the ECRB and ulnarly by the EDC. The ulnar midcarpal portal (MCU) is similarly located 1 to 1.5 cm distal to the 4-/,5 portal and is bounded by the EDC and the EDM.

The relative safety of the portals has been studied by way of cadaver dissection. Although some artifact is inescapable due to the displacement of neurovascular structures postmortem, this research provides useful guidelines. In the clinical situation, distortion of the topographical anatomy due to fracture/dislocation or swelling as well as the use of intraoperative traction may increase the potential for harm. Hence, a standardized method for establishing each portal is useful.

Dorsal Cortals

Dorsal Radiocarpal Portals

Abrams and co-workers performed anatomical dissections on 23 unembalmed fresh cadaver extremities and measured the distances between the standard dorsal portals and the contiguous neurovascular structures.[14] The 1-/,2 portal was found to be the most perilous. The radial sensory nerve exits from under the brachioradialis approximately 5 cm proximal to the radial styloid and bifurcates into a major volar and a major dorsal branch at a mean distance of 4.2 cm proximal to the radial styloid[15] (Figure 1.2). Branches of the superficial radial nerve (SRN) that were radial to the portal were within a mean of 3 mm (range 1 to 6 mm), whereas branches that were ulnar to the portal were at a mean of 5 mm (range 2 to 12 mm).

The radial artery was found at an average of 3 mm radial to the portal (range 1 to 5 mm). Either partial or complete overlap of the lateral antebrachial cutaneous nerve (LABCN) with the SRN occurs up to 75% of the time.[16] In an anatomical study by Steinberg et al., the LACBN was present within the anatomical snuffbox in 9 of 20 (45%) specimens. Based on these findings, they recommended a more palmar, proximal portal in the snuffbox that was no more than 4.5 mm dorsal to the first extensor compartment and within 4.5 mm of the radial styloid.[15]

Branches of the SRN that were radial to the 3-/,4 portal were located at a mean distance of 16 mm (range 5 to 22 mm). In one specimen, an ulnar branch of the SRN was found 6 mm ulnar to the portal. The distance to the radial artery was a mean of 26.3 mm (range 20 to 30 mm). Sensory nerves were remote to the 4-/,5 portal, except in one case (where an aberrant SRN branch was found 4 mm radial to the portal).

The dorsal cutaneous branch of the ulnar nerve (DCBUN) arises from the ulnar nerve an average of 6.4 cm (SD = 2.3 cm) proximal to the ulnar head and becomes subcutaneous 5 cm proximal to the pisiform. It crosses the ulnar snuffbox and gives off three to nine branches that supply the dorsoulnar aspect of the carpus, small finger, and ulnar ring

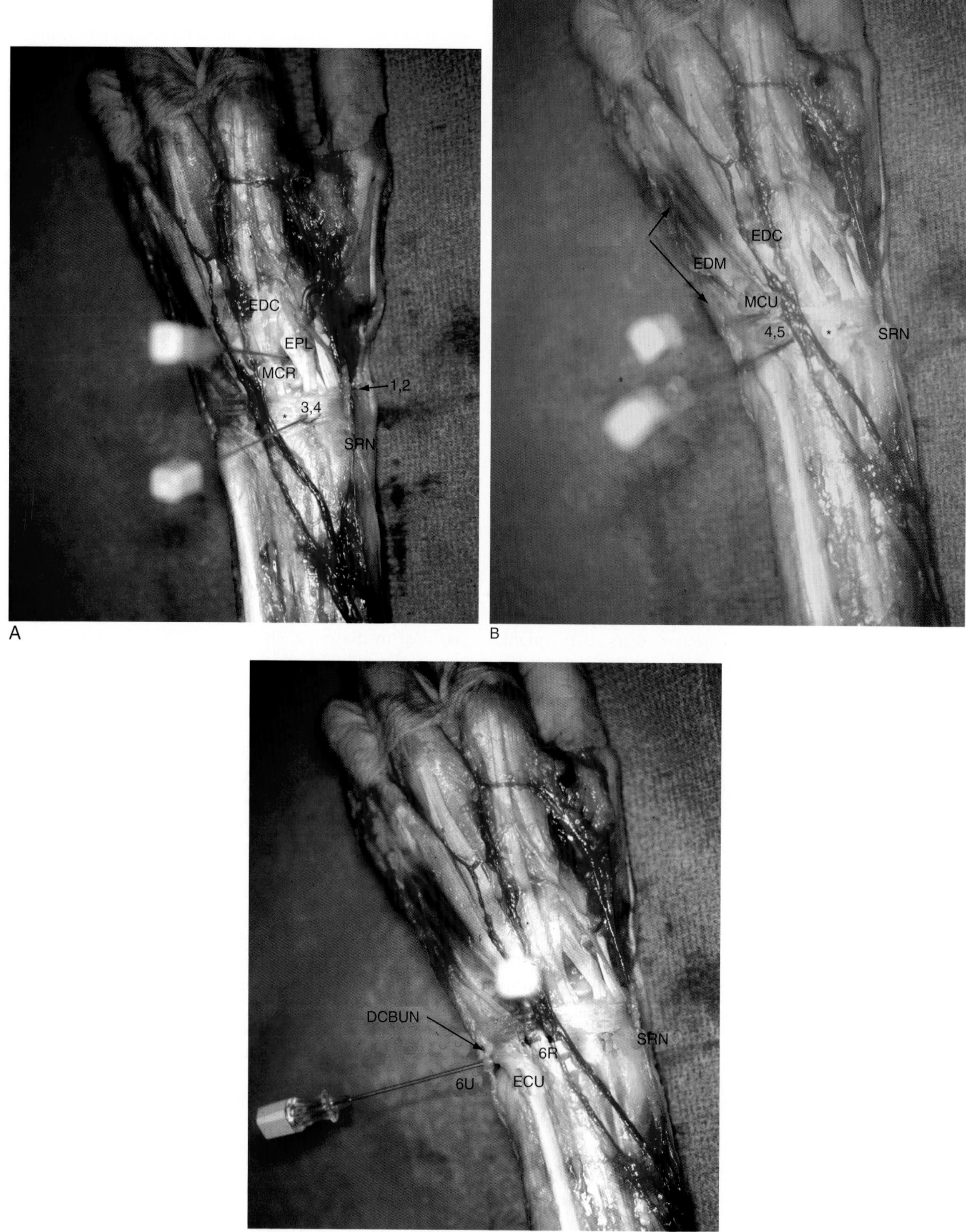

FIGURE 1.1. Dorsal portal anatomy. (A) Cadaver dissection of the dorsal aspect of a left wrist demonstrating the relative positions of the dorsoradial portals (EDC = extensor digitorum communis, EPL = extensor pollicus longus, SRN = superficial radial nerve, Lister's tubercle = *). (B) Relative positions of the dorsoulnar portals (EDM = extensor digiti minimi, DCBUN = dorsal cutaneous branch of the ulnar nerve). (C) Positions of the 6R and 6U portals.

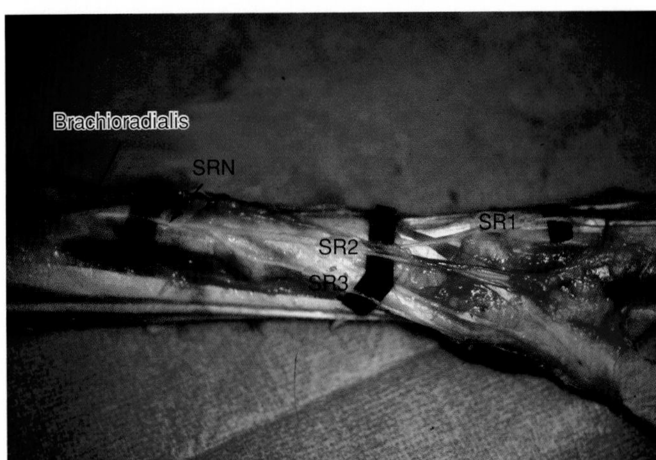

FIGURE 1.2. Branches of the superficial radial nerve (SRN; SR1 = minor dorsal branch, SR2 = major dorsal branch, SR3 = major palmar branch).

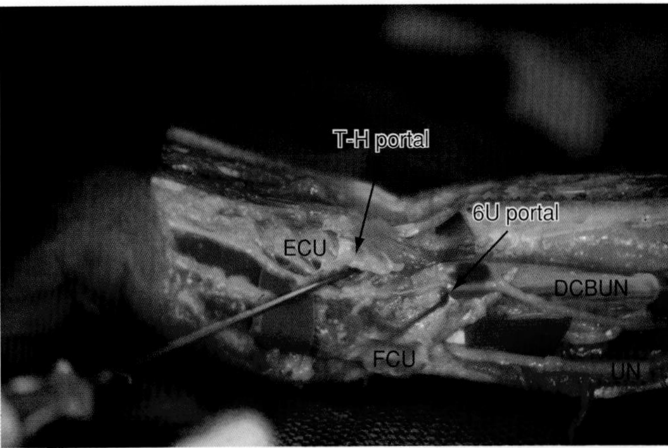

FIGURE 1.3. View of the ulnar aspect of a left wrist demonstrating the relative positions of the triquetro-hamate (T-H) portal and the 6U portal (DCBUN = dorsal cutaneous branch of the ulnar nerve, UN = ulnar nerve).

finger.[17] The mean distance of the dorsal cutaneous branch of the ulnar nerve (DCBUN) to the 6R portal was 8.2 mm (range 0 to 14 mm). Transverse branches of the DCBUN were found in 12 of 19 specimens and were noted to be within 2 mm of the portal (range 0 to 6 mm). The mean distance of branches of the dorsal cutaneous branch of the ulnar nerve (DCBUN) that were radial to the 6U portal was 4.5 mm (range 2 to 10 mm), whereas branches that were ulnar to the portal ranged from 1.9 to 4.8 mm on average. Any transverse branches of the DCBUN were generally proximal to the portal, at an average of 2.5 mm.

Dorsal Midcarpal Portals

Branches of the SRN were found radial to the MCR portal at a mean of 7.2 mm (range 2 to 12 mm; SD = 2.7) Two specimens contained SRN branches ulnar to the portal at 2 and 4 mm. Branches of the SRN were generally remote from the MCU portal except in one specimen (1 mm). Branches of the DCBUN were found at a mean distance of 15.1 mm (range 0 to 25 mm; SD = 4.6).

Triquetro-Hamate (TH) Portal

This portal enters the midcarpal joint at the level of the triquetro-hamate joint ulnar to the ECU tendon. The entry site is both ulnar and distal to the MCU. Branches of the DCBUN are most at risk (Figure 1.3).

Dorsal Radioulnar Portals

These portals lie between the ECU and the EDM tendons. Transverse branches of the DCBUN were the only sensory nerves in proximity to the dorsal radioulnar portal at a mean of 17.5 mm distally (range 10 to 20 mm) (Figure 1.4a and b).

Volar Portals

Volar Radial (VR) Portal

An anatomical study was performed on the arms of five fresh frozen cadavers to determine the safe landmarks for a volar radial (VR) portal after arterial injection studies to highlight the vascular anatomy.[6] The proximal and distal wrist creases were marked. The volar skin was then removed and the flexor carpi radialis tendon (FCR) sheath was divided. The tendon was retracted ulnarly and a trochar was inserted into the radiocarpal joint at the level of the proximal wrist crease. The trochar was noted to enter the radiocarpal joint between the radioscaphocapitate ligament (RSC) and the long radiolunate ligament (LRL) in four specimens and through the LRL ligament in one specimen (Figure 1.5). The median nerve was 8 mm (range 6 to 10 mm) ulnar to the VR portal, whereas the palmar cutaneous branch passed 4 mm (range 3 to 5 mm) ulnar to the portal.

The radial artery was 5.8 mm (range 4 to 6 mm) radial to the portal and its superficial palmar branch was located 10.6 mm (range 6 to 16 mm) distal to the portal. The superficial radial nerve lay 15.6 mm (range 12 to 19 mm) radial to the portal. The portal was 12.8 mm (range 12 to 14 mm) distal to the border of the pronator quadratus, which roughly corresponds to the palmar radiocarpal arch.[18] The palmar cutaneous branch was closest in proximity but always lies to the ulnar side of the FCR.[19,20] The superficial palmar branch of the radial artery passed through the subcutaneous tissue over the tuberosity of the scaphoid and was out of harms way with an incision at the proximal wrist crease.[21,22] When the trochar was placed through the floor of the FCR tendon sheath at the proximal palmar crease, the carpal canal was not violated. It was thus apparent that there was a safe zone comprising the width of the FCR tendon and at least 3 mm or more in all directions. This zone was free of any neurovascular structures.

Volar Radial Midcarpal (VRM) Portal

The volar aspect of the midcarpal joint was identified with a 22-gauge needle through the same skin incision and a blunt trochar was inserted. It was necessary to angle the trochar in a distal and ulnar direction (approximately 5 degrees) in

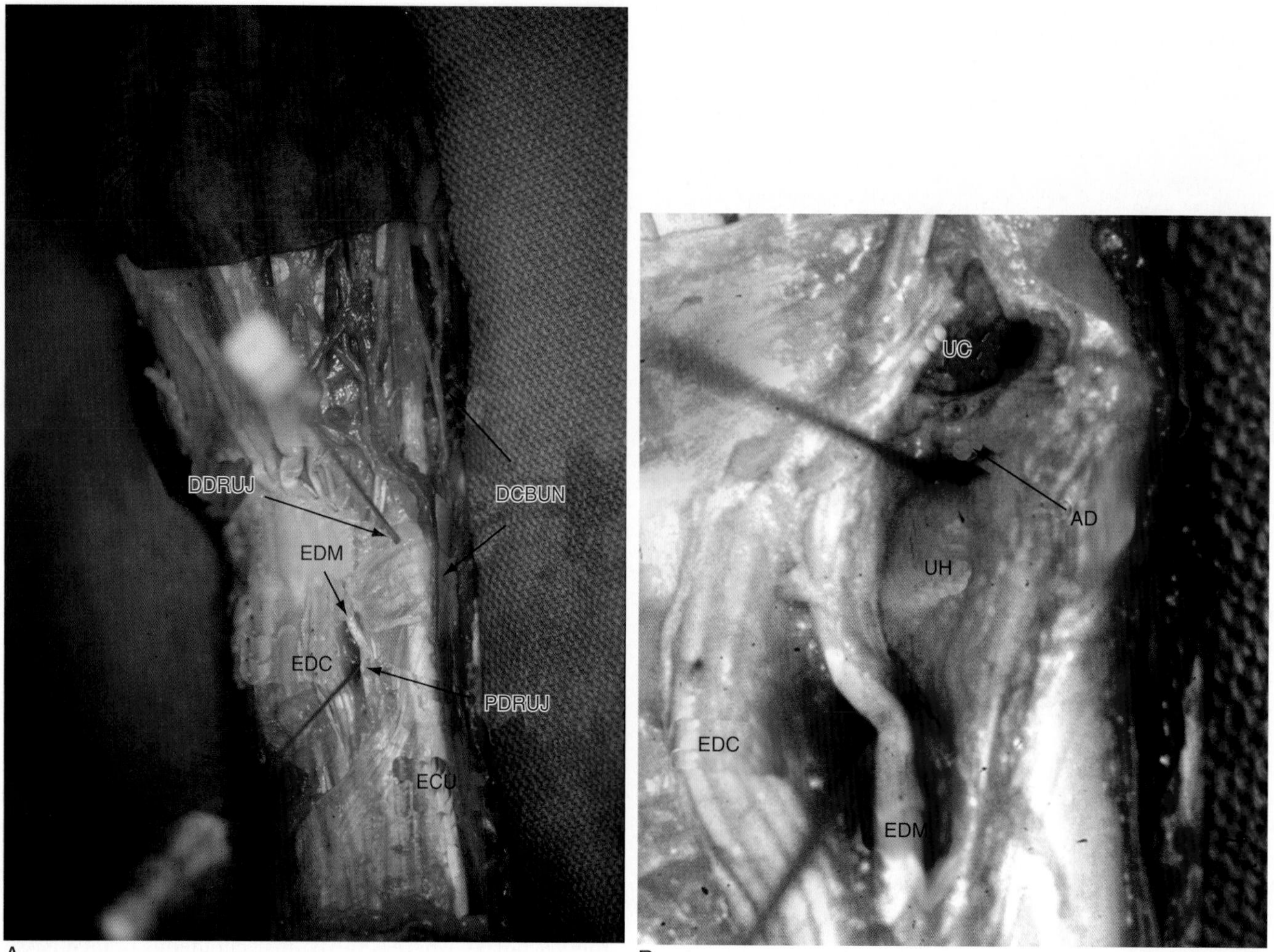

A B

FIGURE 1.4. Dorsal DRUJ portal anatomy. (A) Relative position of the proximal (PDRUJ) and distal (DRUJ) portals. (B) Close-up with the dorsal capsule removed, demonstrating the position of the needles in relation to the dorsal radioulnar ligament [(*); AD = articular disk, UC = ulnocarpal joint, UH = ulnar head].

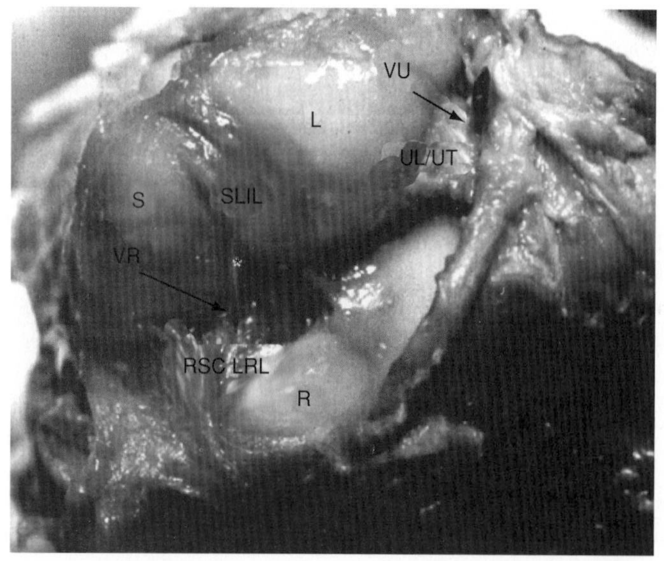

FIGURE 1.5. Ligamentous interval of VR and VU portals. Radiocarpal joint viewed from the dorsal aspect of a hyperflexed wrist. A needle in the VR portal (*) enters between the radioscaphocapitate (RSC) and long radiolunate (LRL) ligaments. A needle in the VU portal enters between the ulnolunate and ulnotriquetral ligaments (UL/UT). Abbreviations: S = scaphoid, L = lunate, R = radius, RSL = radioscapholunate ligament, SLIL = scapholunate interosseous ligament.

order to access the midcarpal joint through the same skin incision. The trochar passed closer to (but still deep to) the superficial palmar branch of the radial artery, which coursed more superficially over the scaphoid tuberosity at that level. The distance between the volar radiocarpal and volar midcarpal entry sites averaged 11 mm (range 7 to 12 mm).

Volar Ulnar (VU) Portal

In a companion study, a volar ulnar (VU) portal was established via a 2-cm longitudinal incision made along the ulnar edge of the finger flexor tendons at the proximal wrist crease.[13] The flexor tendons were retracted radially and a trochar was introduced into the radiocarpal joint. The ulnar styloid marked the proximal point of the VU portal, approximately 2 cm distal to the pronator quadratus. The portal was in the same sagittal plane as the ECU subsheath and penetrated the ulnolunate ligament (ULL) adjacent to the radial insertion of the triangular fibrocartilage. The ulnar nerve and artery were generally more than 5 mm from the trochar, provided the capsular entry point was deep to the ulnar edge of the profundus tendons.

The palmar cutaneous branch of the ulnar nerve (nerve of Henlé) was highly variable and not present in every specimen. This inconstant branch provides sensory fibers to the skin in the distal ulnar and volar part of the forearm to a level 3 cm distal to the wrist crease. Its territory may extend radially beyond the palmaris longus tendon.[23] This branch tends to lie just to the ulnar side of the axis of the fourth ray, but it was absent in 43% of specimens in one study.[24] Martin et al. demonstrated that there was no true internervous plane due to the presence of multiple ulnar-based cutaneous nerves to the palm, which puts them at risk with any ulnar incision.[19] Because there is no true safe zone, careful dissection and wound spread technique should be observed.

Volar Distal Radioulnar (VDR) Portal

The topographical landmarks and establishment of the portal are identical to those of the VU portal. The same risks also apply. The capsular entry point for the VDR lies 5 mm to 1 cm proximal to the ulnocarpal entry point (Figure 1.6a and b).

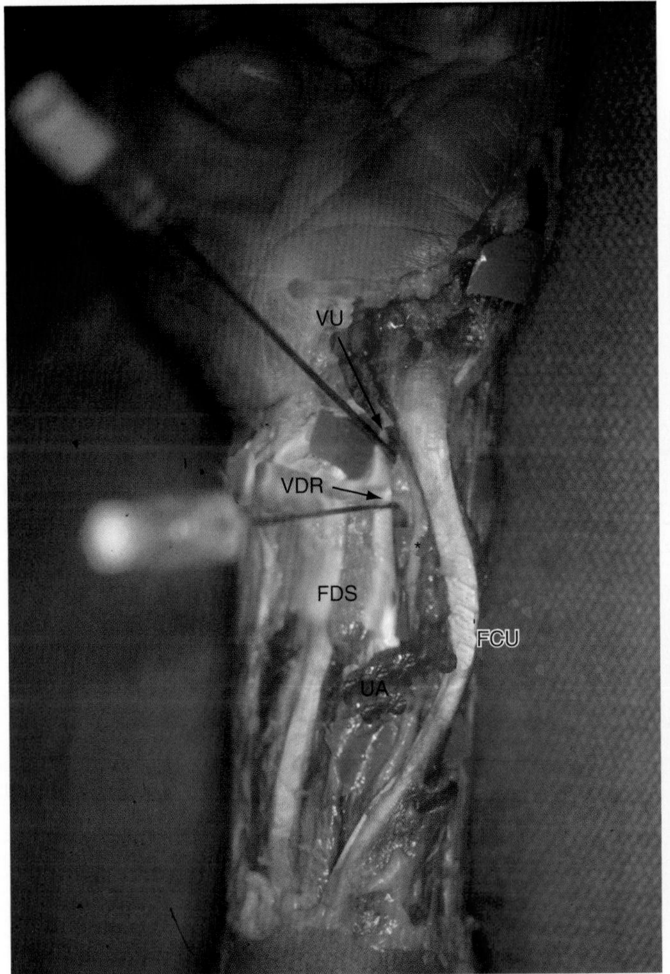

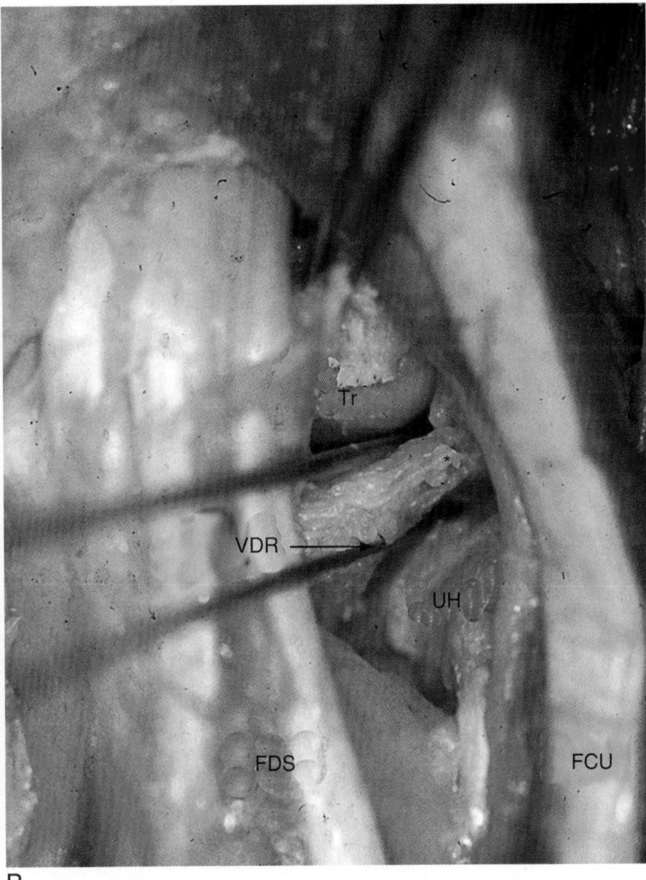

FIGURE 1.6. Volar DRUJ portals. (A) Volar aspect of a left wrist demonstrating the relative positions of the VU and volar DRUJ (VDR) portals in relation to the ulnar nerve (*) and ulnar artery (UA). Abbreviations: FDS = flexor digitorum sublimus, FCU = flexor carpi ulnaris. (B) Close-up view after the volar capsule is removed, showing position of needles in relation to the volar radioulnar ligament (*). Abbreviations: Tr = triquetrum, UH = ulnar head.

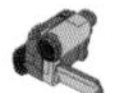

Field of View

The following sections describe the typical field of view as seen through a 2.7-mm arthroscope under ideal conditions.[25,26] Synovitis, fractures, ligament tears, and a tight wrist joint may limit the field of view (which necessitates the use of more portals to adequately assess the entire wrist).

1-/,2 Portal

Structures visualized are limited to the radial half of the wrist.

- *Radius:* Scaphoid and lunate fossa and dorsal rim of radius
- *Carpus:* Proximal and radial scaphoid, proximal lunate
- *Volar capsule:* Oblique views of the radioscaphocapitate (RSC) ligament, long radiolunate ligament (LRL), and short radiolunate ligament (SRL)
- *Dorsal capsule:* Oblique views of the dorsal radiocarpal ligament (DRCL)
- *TFC:* Poorly visualized

3-/,4 Portal

This is almost a complete panoramic view of the entire volar radiocarpal joint.

- *Radius:* Scaphoid and lunate fossa and volar rim of radius
- *Carpus:* Proximal scaphoid and lunate, dorsal and membranous SLIL
- *Volar capsule:* RSC, radioscapholunate ligament (RSL), LRL, and ulnolunate ligament (ULL)
- *Dorsal capsule:* Oblique views of the DRCL insertion onto the dorsal SLIL
- *TFC:* Radial insertion, central portion, ulnar attachment, palmar and dorsal radioulnar ligaments (PRUL, DRUL), and prestyloid recess ∀ piso-triquetral orifice

4-/,5 Portal

This portal gives improved views of the ulnar aspect of the radiocarpal joint, including TFCC, and is useful for instrumentation when combined with the 6R.

- *Radius:* Lunate fossa and volar rim of radius
- *Carpus:* Proximal lunate, triquetrum, and dorsal and membranous LTIL
- *Volar capsule:* RSL, LRL, and ULL
- *Dorsal capsule:* Poorly seen
- *TFC:* Radial insertion, central portion, ulnar attachment, PRUL, and prestyloid recess ∀ piso-triquetral orifice

6R Portal

This gives a more direct line of sight with the dorsal LTIL and is typically used for instrumentation or outflow.

- *Radius:* Poorly seen
- *Carpus:* Proximal lunate, triquetrum, dorsal, and membranous LTIL
- *Volar capsule:* ULL and ulno-triquetral ligament (ULT)
- *Dorsal capsule:* Poorly seen
- *TFC:* Radial insertion, central portion, ulnar attachment, PRUL, and prestyloid recess ∀ piso-triquetral orifice

6U Portal

This is also largely used for outflow, but is also useful for instrumentation for debridement of palmar LTIL tears in combination with the VU portal.

- *Radius:* Sigmoid notch
- *Carpus:* Proximal triquetrum and membranous LTIL
- *Volar capsule:* Oblique views of the ULL and ULT
- *Dorsal capsule:* Oblique views of the DRCL
- *TFC:* Dorsal rim and radial attachment

VR Portal

This portal is largely indicated to assess the palmar SLIL and the DRCL. It is also of use for arthroscopically assisted fixation of distal radius fractures due to the direct line of sight with the dorsal rim fragments.[10]

- *Radius:* Scaphoid and lunate fossa, and dorsal rim of radius
- *Carpus:* Proximal palmar scaphoid and lunate, and palmar and membranous SLIL
- *Volar capsule:* Oblique views of the radioscapholunate ligament (RSL), LRL, and ulnolunate ligament (ULL)
- *Dorsal capsule:* Direct in-line views of the DRCL
- *TFC:* Oblique views of the radial insertion, central portion, ulnar attachment, PRUL, and DRUL

VU Portal

This portal is largely indicated to assess the palmar LTIL and the dorsal ulnar capsule. It is also of use for debridement of palmar LTIL tears.

- *Radius:* Sigmoid notch region of lunate fossa
- *Carpus:* Proximal palmar lunate and triquetrum, and palmar and membranous LTIL
- *Volar capsule:* Poorly seen
- *Dorsal capsule:* Direct in-line views of the dorsoulnar capsule, including the ECUS
- *TFC:* Radial insertion, central portion, ulnar attachment, and DRUL

Radial Midcarpal Portal

- *Volar:* Continuation of the RSC ligament
- *Radial:* STT joint and distal scaphoid pole
- *Proximal:* SLIL joint, LTIL joint, distal scaphoid, and distal lunate
- *Distal:* Proximal capitate, capitohamate ligament, and oblique views of proximal hamate

Ulnar Midcarpal Portal

- *Volar:* Continuation of the volar ulnocarpal ligament (important in midcarpal instability)
- *Radial:* Distal articular surface of the lunate and triquetrum and partial scaphoid
- *Proximal:* LTIL joint and SLIL joint
- *Distal:* Proximal hamate, capitohamate ligament, and oblique views of proximal capitate

Dorsal DRUJ Proximal and Distal Portals

- *Volar:* Palmar radioulnar ligament
- *Radial:* Sigmoid notch and radial attachment of TFC
- *Ulnar:* Limited view of dorsal radioulnar ligament
- *Distal:* Proximal surface of articular disc

Volar DRUJ Portal

- *Volar:* Dorsal radioulnar ligament
- *Radial:* Sigmoid notch and radial attachment of TFC
- *Ulnar:* Foveal attachment of deep fibers of TFCC
- *Distal:* Proximal surface of articular disc

Relevant Clinical and Biomechanical Studies

The publications on the use of wrist arthroscopy through the standard dorsal portals are too numerous to list here. There are, however, a number of excellent reviews the reader is directed to.* A number of reports highlight the safety and clinical application of volar arthroscopy portals on the radial side of the wrist. Levy and Glickel[27] described the use of an accessory volar portal after volar plating of a Barton's fracture that was accessed through a standard carpal tunnel incision. Tham et al.[28] used a volar radial portal in 14 cases (for synovectomy, radial styloidectomy, and fracture reduction). Bain and co-workers published their early experience with a volar portal in the European literature.[29] They subsequently reported on the use of a volar portal for arthroscopic release of wrist contracture,[30] as an adjunct for arthroscopic-assisted fixation of distal radius fractures,[31] and for decompression of intraosseous ganglia of the lunate.[32]

Osterman described the use of a volar radial portal for arthroscopic release of dorsal wrist contractures.[33] Doi et al. used a volar radial portal in 34 cases of arthroscopically assisted reduction of distal radius fractures.[10] Abe et al. reported on the use of this portal for viewing the palmar aspects of the SLIL and LTIL ligaments in 230 cases.[34,35] Del Piñal and co-workers recently reported on the use of a volar radial portal for an inside-out osteotomy technique for correction of malunited intra-articular distal radius fractures.[36] Dr. Andrea Atzei and Riccardo Luchetti of Italy have used a palmar distal radioulnar joint portal that is ulnar to the TFCC. They presented their three year results at the FESSH meeting in 2005.[37]

*Atlas of the Hand Clinics 8(1) 2003; Atlas of the Hand Clinics 9(1) 2004; Hand Clinics 10(4) 994; Hand Clinics 2(1)1995; Hand Clinics 15(3)1999.

Author's Experience

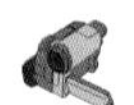

The volar radial portal has been used in 77 patients since 1998. Additional pathology was evident in 37 of the patients that was not visible from any standard dorsal portal. This included one case of hypertrophic synovitis of the dorsal capsule (Figure 1.7); one patient with an avulsion of the radioscapholunate ligament, which exposed the volar scapholunate cleft (Figure 1.8); two patients with tears restricted to the palmar region of the SLIL; and 35 patients with tears of the dorsal radiocarpal ligament. In five patients an isolated DRCL tear alone was responsible for chronic dorsal wrist pain (Figure 1.9a and b).

The midcarpal joint was accessed from the volar radial portal in three cases. In one patient with Preiser's disease the use of the volar radial midcarpal portal (VRM) allowed a more complete assessment of the distal articular surface of the scaphoid. Another patient had an unrecognized osteochondral fracture of the capitate head following a perilunate dislocation. The VRM portal admirably demonstrated the intact dorsal portion of the SLIL in the patient with the palmar tear (Figure 1.10). Using the dorsal midcarpal portals, one patient was found to have a chondral defect on the proximal hamate, along with a midcarpal loose body (Figure 1.11a and b).

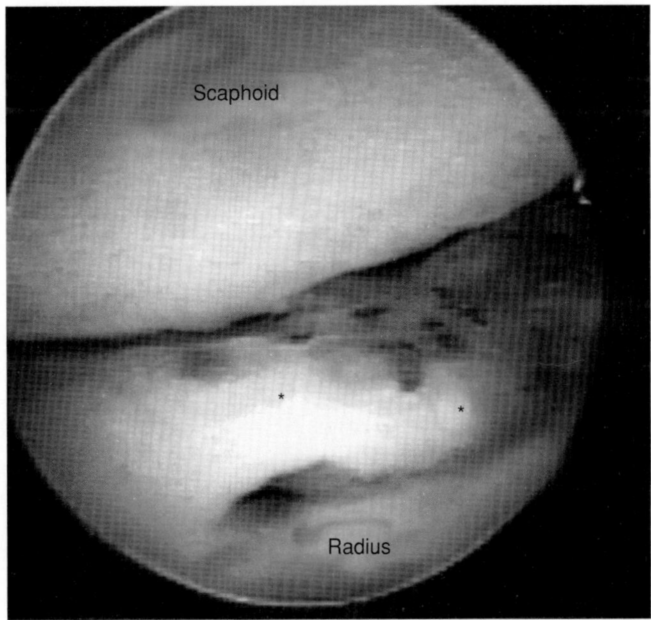

FIGURE 1.7. Hypertrophic synovitis (*) of the dorsal capsule in a case of Preiser's disease as seen through the VR portal. *(From Slutsky DJ. Wrist arthroscopy through a volar radial portal. Arthroscopy: The Journal of Arthroscopic and Related Surgery 2002;18(6):624–30. Used with permission.)*

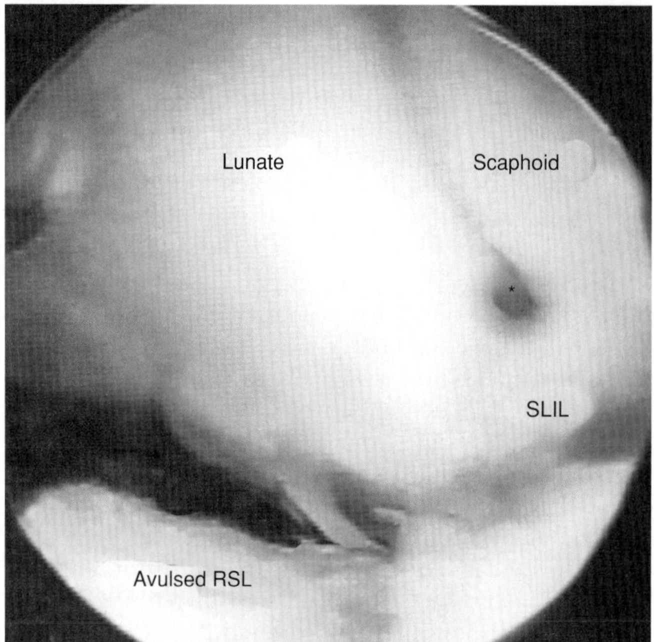

FIGURE 1.8. Radioscapholunate ligament avulsion. Note unmasking of the palmar cleft (*) between the scaphoid and lunate (SLIL= scapholunate interosseous ligament, RSL = radioscapholunate ligament). *(From Slutsky DJ. Wrist arthroscopy through a volar radial portal. Arthroscopy: The Journal of Arthroscopic and Related Surgery 2002;18(6):624–30. Used with permission.)*

The VU portal was used in 49 of these patients. The ulnar sided pathology included 13 tears of the LTIL ligament, 11 TFC tears, and 2 ulnolunate ligament tears. In one patient a TFC tear was found to extend into the dorsoulnar ligament (see Figure 1.12a and b). The VU portal facilitated debridement of the palmar region of the LTIL ligament through the 6R or 6U portals (Figure 1.13). In 2 of these patients unrecognized chondromalacia of the palmar aspect of the lunate was identified (see Figure 1.14). In 1 patient, the palmar aspect of the LTIL was found to be intact despite a large dorsal tear.

The volar aspect of the DRUJ portal was used in six of these patients to rule out a peripheral detachment of the TFC (2 with ulnar styloid fracture/nonunion). This would normally require a formal open arthrotomy and a high index of clinical suspicion.[41] The DRUJ was well visualized and the foveal attachment of the TFC was clearly identified (see Figure 1.15). In one patient with a TFC and LTIL tear, a wafer resection was performed by inserting the bur through the dorsal DRUJ portal while viewing through the VDRU. This allows for a more conservative TFC debridement since the ulnar head resection if performed underneath the TFC tear and not through it. The DRUJ wafer also facilitates preservation of the volar and dorsal radioulnar ligaments as well as the deep foveal attachment.

Complications

One patient in whom a dorsal capsulodesis was performed for dynamic scapholunate instability complained of numbness over the thenar eminence. Another patient who underwent debridement of a palmar LTIL tear complained of diminished sensation over the hypothenar eminence. There were otherwise no complications in the way of neurovascular or tendon injury in the previously cited series.

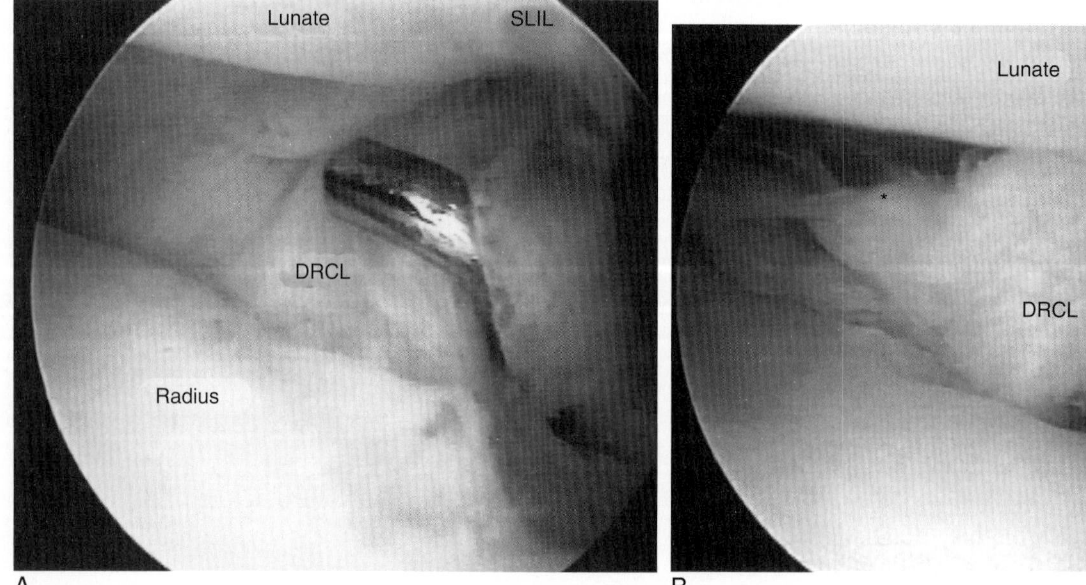

FIGURE 1.9. VR portal view. (A) Normal dorsal radiocarpal ligament. Hook probe is inserted through the 3/-,4 portal (SLIL = scapholunate interosseous ligament, DRCL = dorsal radiocarpal ligament). (B) DRCL tear (*). Hook probe inserted through the 3/-,4 portal. *(From Slutsky DJ. Wrist arthroscopy through a volar radial portal. Arthroscopy: The Journal of Arthroscopic and Related Surgery 2002;18(6):624–30. Used with permission.)*

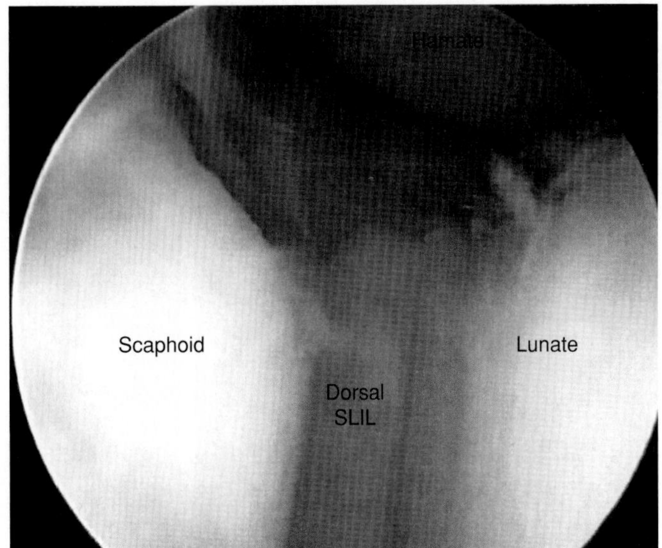

FIGURE 1.10. Volar midcarpal portal. Tear of the palmar region of the SLIL (scapholunate interosseous ligament) as viewed from the volar radial midcarpal portal. Note the intact dorsal fibers of the SLIL.

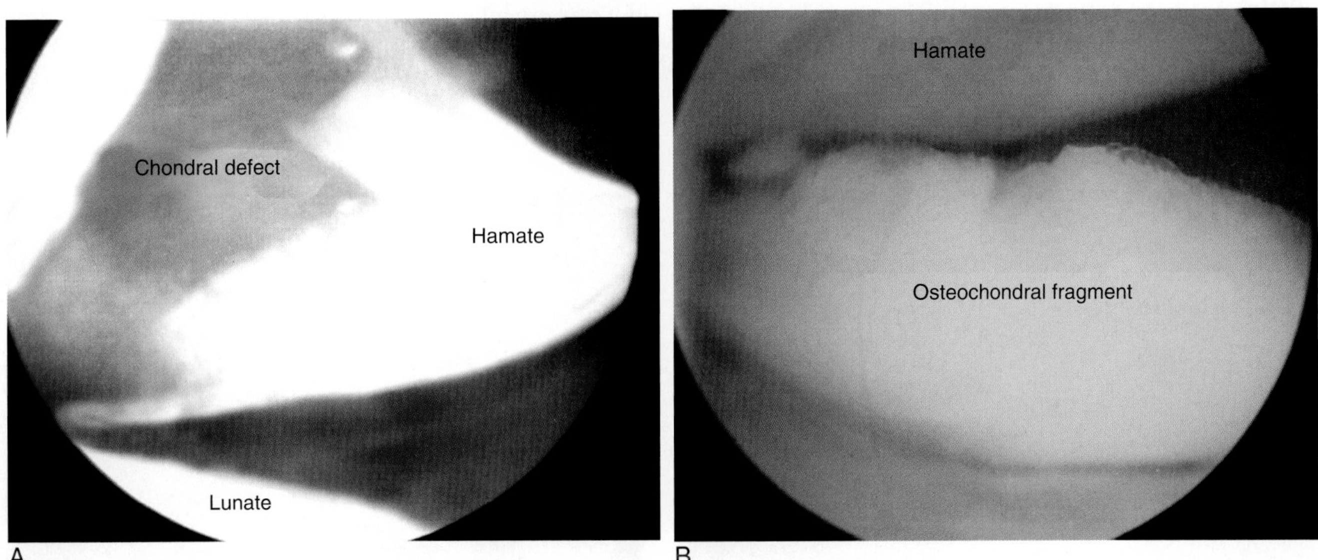

FIGURE 1.11. Dorsal midcarpal portal. (A) Chondral defect on proximal hamate. (B) Loose body in midcarpal joint.

Equipment and Implants

Required

In general, a 2.7-mm 30-degree angled scope along with a camera attachment is used. A fiberoptic light source, video monitor, and printer have become the standard of care. Digital systems allow direct writing to a CD and superior video quality compared to analog cameras. A 3-mm hook probe is needed for palpation of intracarpal structures. Some method of overhead traction is useful. This may include traction from the overhead lights or a shoulder holder along with 5- to 10-pound sandbags attached to an arm sling. A traction tower such as the Linvatec tower (Conmed - Linvatec Corporation, Largo, FL) or the ARC traction tower designed by Dr. William Geissler (Arc Surgical LLC, Hillsboro, OR) greatly facilitates instrumentation. The use of a motorized shaver or diathermy unit such as the Oratec probe (Smith and Nephew, NY) are useful for debridement. A motorized 2.9-mm bur is needed for bony resection.

Optional

There are a variety of commercially available suture repair kits, including the TFC repair kit by Arthrex or Linvatec (Conmed - Linvatec Corporation, Largo, FL). Ligament repairs can also be facilitated by use of a Tuohy needle, which is generally found in any anesthesia cart. Specially designed jigs have been made to facilitate repair of radial TFC tears,[38] although Trumble et al. have described a method with meniscal repair needles passed through a suction cannula in the 6U portal.[39]

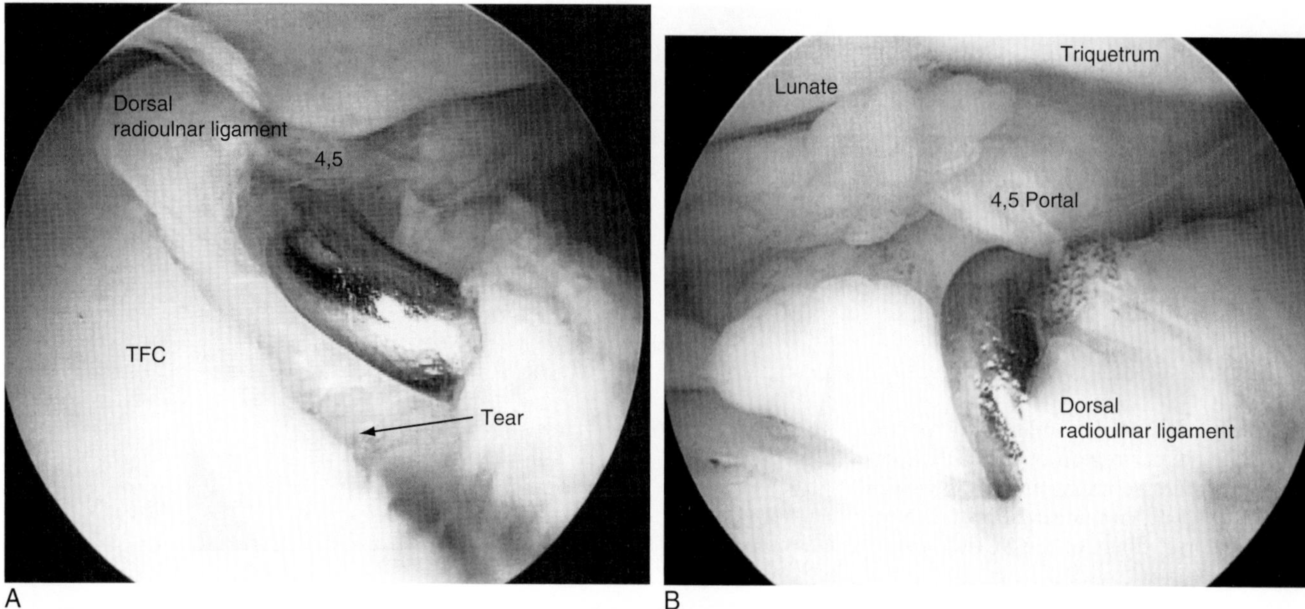

FIGURE 1.12. VU portal view. (A) Triangular fibrocartilage (TFC) tear extending into the dorsal radioulnar ligament. Probe inserted through the dorsal 4/-,5 portal. (B) Palpation of the dorsal radioulnar ligament tear with the hook probe. *(From Slutsky DJ. The use of a volar ulnar portal in wrist arthroscopy. The Journal of Arthroscopic and Related Surgery 2004;20(2):158–63. Used with permission.)*

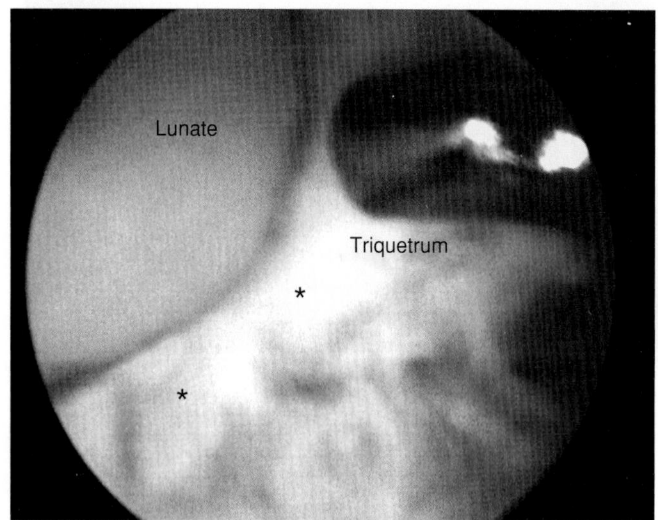

FIGURE 1.13. Palmar lunotriquetral ligament tear as viewed from the volar ulnar (VU) portal. Note the avulsed ligament (*) still attached to the triquetrum, with the exposed cleft between the lunate and triquetrum. *(From Slutsky DJ. Wrist arthroscopy through a volar radial portal. Arthroscopy: The Journal of Arthorscopic and Related Surgery 2002;18(6):624–30. Used with permission.)*

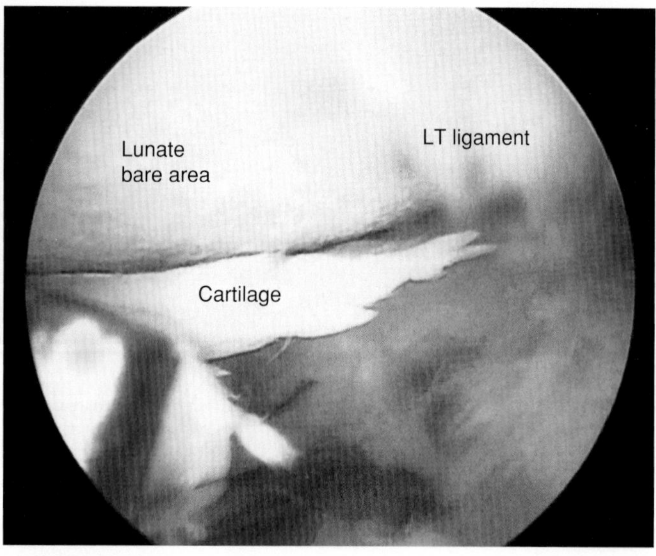

FIGURE 1.14. Unsuspected region of chondromalacia on the palmar surface of the lunate (LT = lunotriquetral). *(From Slutsky DJ. The use of a volar ulnar portal in wrist arthroscopy. The Journal of Arthroscopic and Related Surgery 2004;20(2): 158–63. Used with permission.)*

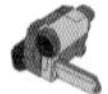

Methodology

It is useful to have a systematic approach to viewing the wrist. The structures that should be visualized as part of a standard exam include the radius articular surface, the proximal scaphoid and lunate, the SLIL and LTIL (palmar and dorsal for each), RSC, LRL, RSL, ULL, ULT, and the radial and peripheral TFCC attachments. It is my practice to establish the dorsal portals first but then to start the arthroscopic examination with the VR portal in order to visualize the palmar SLIL and the DRCL ligament to minimize any error from iatrogenic trauma to the dorsal capsular structures. This is followed by the VU portal to assess

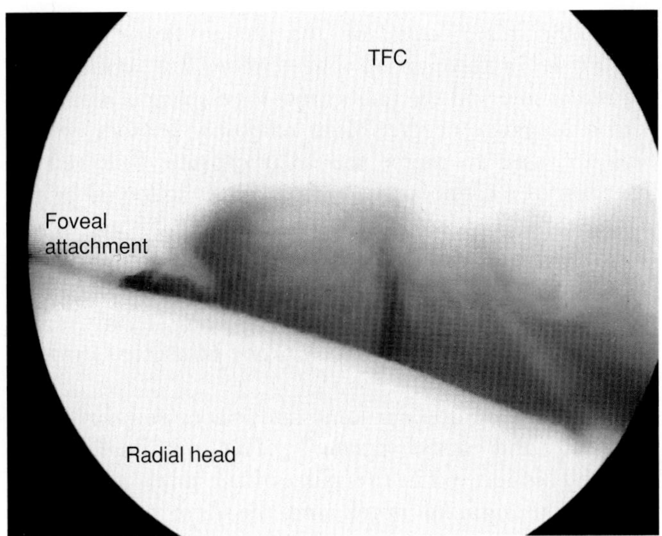

FIGURE 1.15. View from the palmar DRUJ portal. The undersurface of the TFC (triangular fibrocartilage) demonstrates no tears, with a solid attachment to the fovea of the ulnar styloid.

the palmar LTIL and dorsal radioulnar ligament, ECU subsheath, and radial TFC attachment.

The scope is then inserted in the 3-/,4 portal, followed by various combinations of the 4-/,5 portal and 6R portal. The 6U portal is mostly used for outflow but may be used for instrumentation when debriding palmar LTIL tears. Midcarpal arthroscopy is then performed to probe the SLIL and LTIL joint spaces for instability, to examine the capitohamate interosseous ligament (CHIL), and to look for chondral lesions on the proximal capitate and hamate and loose bodies. The special use portals such as the dorsal and volar DRUJ portals and the 1-/,2 portal are used as needed. The accompanying video illustrates the portal placement and technique.

3-/,4 Portal

Under general anesthesia, the patient's hand is suspended from either an overhead pulley or a traction tower with 10 to 15 pounds of counter-traction. The arm is exsanguinated and an upper arm tourniquet inflated to 250 mmHg. The surgeon is initially seated facing the dorsal surface of the wrist. The concavity overlying the lunate between the EPL and the EDC is located just distal to Lister's tubercle, in line with the second web space. The radiocarpal joint is identified with a 22-gauge needle that is sloped 10 degrees palmar to account for the volar inclination of the radius. The joint is injected with 5 cc of saline. A shallow incision is made to avoid injuring small branches of the SRN or superficial veins.

Tenotomy scissors or blunt forceps are then used to spread the soft tissue and pierce the dorsal capsule. The vascular tuft of the radioscapholunate ligament is directly in line with this portal. Superior to the RSL is the membranous portion of the SLIL. By rotating the scope while dorsally looking in an ulnar direction, the insertion of the DRCL onto the dorsal aspect of the SLIL can often be visualized. This is a common origin for the stalk of a dorsal ganglion. The RSL and LRL are radial to the portal and can be probed with a hook in the 4-/,5 portal. The LTIL, TFC, and ULL are ulnar to the portal.

4-/,5 Portal

The interval for the 4-/,5 portal is identified with the 22-gauge needle between the EDC and EDM, in line with the ring metacarpal. Due to the normal radial inclination of the distal radius, this portal lies slightly proximal and about 1 cm ulnar to the 3-/,4 portal. Care must be taken when inserting the scope because the LTIL lies directly ahead of this portal. One encounters the ulnar half of the lunate when moving the scope radially, and the oblique surface of the triquetrum in a superior and ulnar direction. The LTIL is seen obliquely from this portal, and unless a tear is present is often difficult to differentiate from the carpal bones without probing.

The ULL and ULT can be seen on the far end of the joint. Proximally, the radial insertion of the TFC blends imperceptibly with the sigmoid notch of the radius. However, it can be palpated with a hook probe in either the 3-/,4 or 6R portal. The peripheral insertion of the TFC slopes upward into the ulnar capsule. Peripheral TFC tears are often located ulnarly and dorsally. The volar radioulnar ligament can be probed and visualized (especially if torn), but the dorsal radioulnar ligament is poorly seen. The pisotriquetral recess can sometimes be identified by a small tuft of protruding synovium, and when probed may yield views of the articular facet of the pisiform.

6R and 6U Portals

The 6R portal is identified on the radial side of the ECU tendon, just distal to the ulnar head. The scope should be angled 10 degrees proximally to avoid hitting the triquetrum. The TFC is immediately below the entry site. The LTIL is located radially and superiorly, whereas the ulnar capsule is immediately adjacent to the scope. The 6U portal is found on the ulnar side of the ECU tendon. Angling the needle distally and ulnar deviation of the wrist help avoid running into the triquetrum. This portal can be used to view the dorsal rim of the TFC or for instrumentation when debriding the palmar LTIL.

Midcarpal Portals

The MCR portal is found 1 cm distal to the 3-/,4 portal. Flexing the wrist and firm thumb pressure help identify the soft spot between the distal pole of the scaphoid and the proximal capitate. The STT joint lies radially and can be seen by rotating the scope dorsally. The scapholunate articulation can be seen proximally and ulnarly, which can be probed for instability or step-off. Further ulnarly, the lunotriquetral articulation is visualized. Superiorly, oblique views of the proximal surface capitate and hamate as well as the CHIL are obtained. The continuation of the RSC ligament can occasionally be seen across the midcarpal space.

The MCU is found 1 cm distal to the 4-/,5 portal, and 1.5 cm ulnar and slightly proximal to the MCR portal (in line with the fourth metacarpal axis). This entry site is at the intersection of the lunate, triquetrum, hamate, and capitate with a type I lunate facet and directly over the lunotriquetral joint with a type II lunate facet[4] (which allows preferential views of this articulation). Directly volar, the continuation of the volar ulnocarpal ligament can be assessed (which is especially important in midcarpal instability).

Normally there is very little step-off between the distal articular surfaces of the scaphoid and lunate. Direct pressure from the scope combined with traction may force the carpal joints out of alignment. The traction should be released and the scapholunate joint should be viewed with the scope in the MCU, whereas the lunotriquetral joint should be viewed with the scope in the MCR.

Volar Portals

To establish the volar radial portal the surgeon is now seated, facing the volar aspect of the wrist. A 2-cm transverse or longitudinal incision is made in the proximal wrist crease overlying the flexor carpi radialis (FCR) tendon. It is not necessary to specifically identify the adjacent neurovascular structures, provided the anatomical landmarks are adhered to. The tendon sheath is divided and the FCR tendon is retracted ulnarly. The radiocarpal joint space is identified with a 22-gauge needle and distended with 5 cc of saline. Blunt tenotomy scissors or forceps are used to pierce the volar capsule. A blunt trochar is then introduced, followed by a 2.7-mm 30-degree angled arthroscope (Figure 1.16a through c). The midcarpal joint can be accessed through the same skin incision by angling the trochar 1 cm distally and approximately 5 degrees ulnarward. Outflow is established via an 18-gauge needle in the 6U portal or a cannula.

The standard dorsal portals (including the 3/-,4 and 4/-,5 portals as well as the radial and ulnar midcarpal portals) are established in a similar fashion. A hook probe is inserted through the 3/-,4 portal and used to assess the palmar aspect of the SLIL and the DRCL. A useful landmark when viewing from the VR portal is the intersulcal ridge between the scaphoid and lunate fossae. The radial origin of the DRCL is seen immediately ulnar to this, just proximal to the lunate.

The volar ulnar portal is established via a 2-cm longitudinal incision centered over the proximal wrist crease along the ulnar edge of the finger flexor tendons (Figure 1.17a through c). The tendons are retracted to the radial side and the radiocarpal joint space is identified with a 22-gauge needle. Blunt tenotomy scissors or forceps are used to pierce the volar capsule, followed by insertion of a cannula and blunt trochar, followed by the arthroscope. The ulnar nerve is protected by use of the cannula and a more radial entry site. The median nerve is protected by the adjacent flexor tendons. The palmar region of the LTIL can usually be seen slightly distal and radial to the portal. A hook probe is inserted through the 6R or 6U portal.

The dorsal radioulnar joint can be accessed through a proximal and distal portal.[40] The proximal portal (PDRUJ) is located in the axilla of the joint, just proximal to the sigmoid notch and the flare of the ulnar metaphysis. This portal is easier to penetrate and should be used initially to prevent chondral injury from insertion of the trochar. The forearm is held in supination to relax the dorsal capsule, to move the ulnar head volarly, and to lift the central disc distally from the head of the ulna. Reducing the traction to 1 to 2 pounds permits better views between the ulna and the sigmoid notch by reducing the compressive force caused by axial traction.

The joint space is identified by first inserting a 22-gauge needle horizontally at the neck of the distal ulna. Fluoroscopy facilitates the needle placement. The joint is infiltrated with saline and the capsule is spread with tenotomy scissors through a small incision. A small cannula and trochar for the 1.9-mm scope are introduced, followed by insertion of a 1.9-mm 30-degree angle scope. Entry into this portal provides views of the proximal sigmoid notch cartilage and the articular surface of the neck of the ulna. One should systematically look for loose bodies or synovial hypertrophy.

The distal portal (DDRUJ) is identified 6 to 8 mm distally with the 22-gauge needle, and just proximal to the 6R portal. This portal can be used for outflow drainage or for instrumentation. It lies on top of the ulnar head but underneath the TFC. Hence, it cannot be used in the presence of a positive ulnar variance. The TFC has the least tension in neutral rotation of the forearm, which is the optimal position for visualizing the articular dome of the ulnar head, the undersurface of the TFC, and the proximal radioulnar ligament from its attachment to the sigmoid notch to its insertion into the fovea of the ulna. Because of the dorsal entry of the arthroscope, the course of the dorsal radioulnar ligament is not visible until its attachment into the fovea is encountered.[25] Proximal surface tears of the TFC (which are usually caused by severe axial load) may be detected through this portal.

The volar DRUJ portal is accessed through the VU skin incision. A 1.9-mm small joint arthroscope is used since gaining access to the DRUJ can be difficult, especially in a small wrist. The joint is first identified by angling a 22-gauge needle 45° proximally, and then injecting the DRUJ

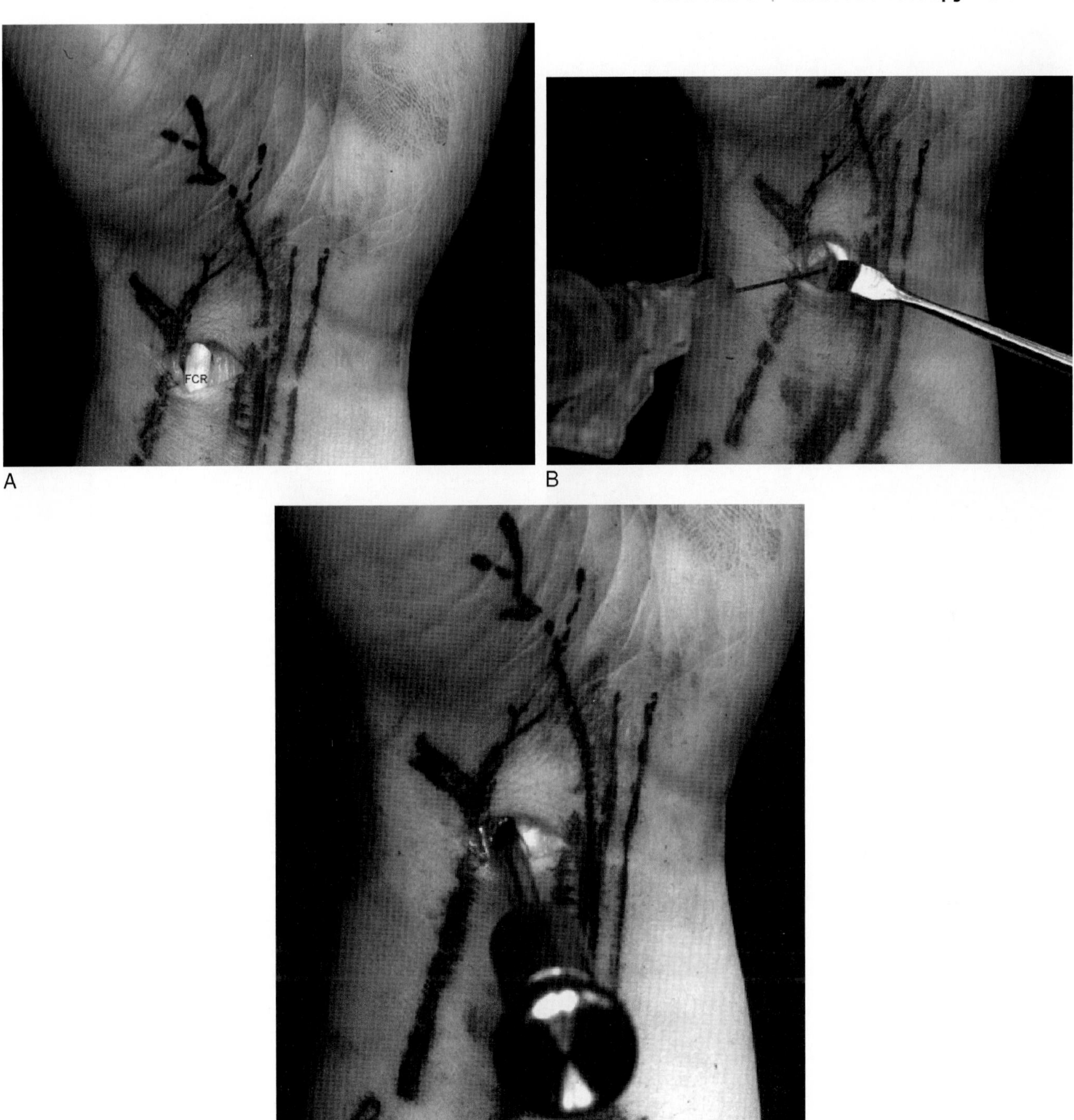

FIGURE 1.16. Technique for VR portal. (A) Skin incision for VR portal (FCR = flexor carpi radialis tendon). (B) Saline injection of radiocarpal joint. (C) Insertion of cannula through floor of the FCR sheath. *(From Slutsky DJ. Volar portals in wrist arthroscopy. JASSH 2002;2(4):225–32. Used with permission.)*

with saline. It is useful to leave a needle or cannula in the ulnocarpal joint for reference during this step. Alternatively, a probe can be placed in the distal dorsal radioulnar joint portal and advanced through the palmar incision to help locate the joint space. Care is taken to situate the portal underneath the ulnar edge of the flexor tendons and to apply retraction in a radial direction alone, in order to avoid injury to the ulnar nerve and artery. Once the correct plane is identified, the volar DRUJ capsule is pierced with tenotomy scissors followed by a cannula with a blunt trochar and then the arthroscope. The dorsal distal DRUJ portal can be used for instrumentation such as a thermal probe or bur while viewing through the VDRU portal (Figure 1.18a and b).[40]

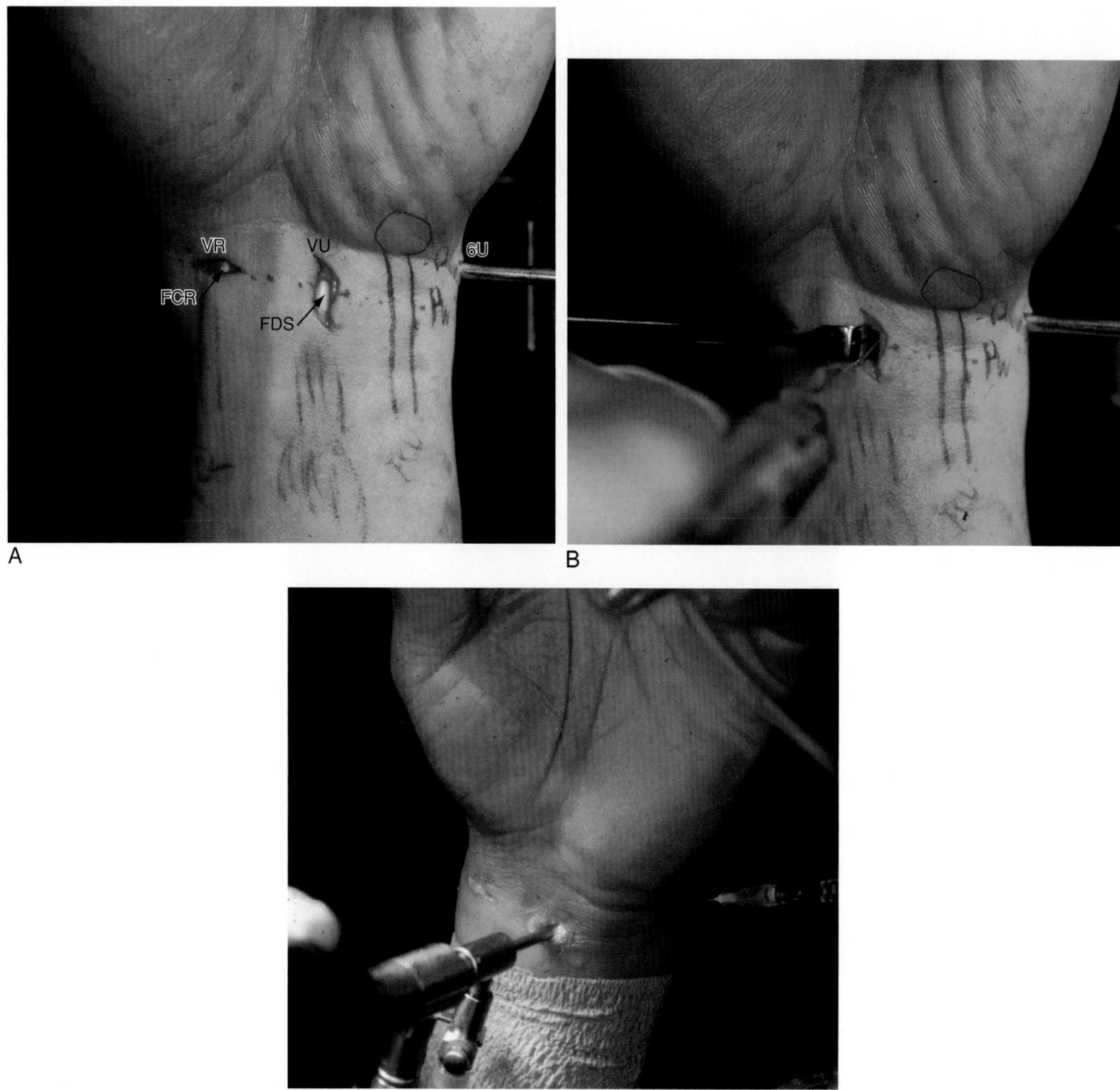

FIGURE 1.17. Technique for VU portal. (A) Skin incision for VU portal (FCR = flexor carpi radialis tendon, FDS = flexor digitorum sublimes). (B) FDS retracted, saline injection of radiocarpal joint. (C) Insertion of cannula through capsule deep to FDS tendons. *(From Slutsky DJ. The use of a volar ulnar portal in wrist arthroscopy. The Journal of Arthroscopic and Related Surgery 2004;20(2):158–63. Used with permission.)*

The Dry Technique of Wrist Arthroscopy

Dr. Francisco del Piñal of Santander, Spain, has pioneered a dry technique for diagnostic wrist arthroscopy.[41] In his experience, this technique is as effective as the standard procedure but without the disadvantages of fluid extravasation, which minimizes the risk of compartment syndrome during the arthroscopic treatment of distal radius fractures. The hand is suspended from a custom-made traction bow that allows one to easily change the hand from a horizontal to a vertical position while maintaining a sterile field. The arthroscopy portals are made and instruments inserted as in the usual fashion, except for the fact that no irrigation fluid is used to distend the joint. To periodically dry the joint out, he uses neurosurgical patties cut into small triangles.

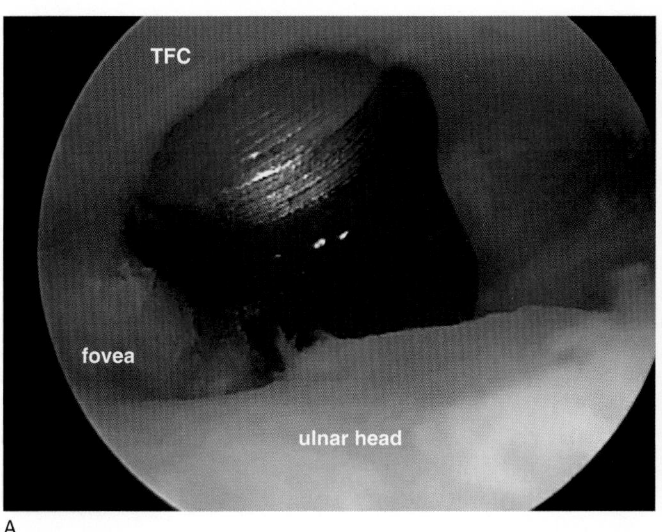

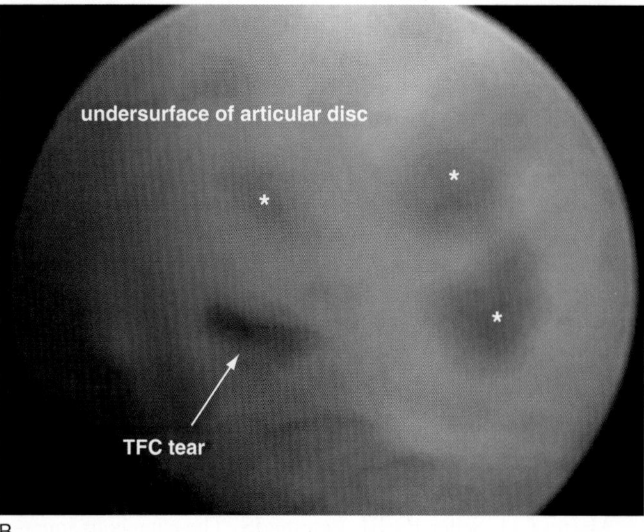

FIGURE 1.18 View from the volar DRUJ portal. (A) Thermal probe is in the dorsal DRUJ portal. (B) Tear of the TFC as seen from the VDRU portal.

One must avoid getting too close with the tip of the scope when working with burs or osteotomes, in order to avoid splashes that might impede vision. Blood clots or debris are first wetted with 10 or 20 cc of saline through the side valve of the scope and then aspirated with a synoviotome. He has thus far carried out the dry technique in more than 100 wrist arthroscopies without any complications (personal communication, del Piñal June 2006). In my experience, it is still necessary to use fluid to make the diagnosis of a DRC ligament tear. Copious joint irrigation is also necessary whenever a thermal probe is used, to minimize the risk of heat necrosis of the articular cartilage.

Rehabilitation

The postoperative rehabilitation is dictated by the treatment of the specific pathology. Finger motion and edema control are instituted immediately. TFC repairs and interosseous pinning may require up to six to eight weeks of immobilization. If an arthroscopic DRCL is repaired the patient is placed in a below-elbow cast or splint for six weeks, with the restriction of all wrist motion. Forearm pronation and supination is permitted. This is followed by wrist motion exercises and gradual strengthening. Following arthroscopic debridement alone, wrist range of motion exercises are instituted within three to five days postoperatively.

Summary

Advances in wrist arthroscopy continue to expand the indications and treatment options for myriad wrist disorders. A systematic approach and a thorough understanding of the topographical and internal anatomy of the wrist are integral to minimizing complications while maximizing the chances of a successful outcome.

References

1. Slutsky DJ. Wrist arthroscopy portals. In DJ Slutsky, DJ Nagel (eds.), *Techniques in Hand and Wrist Arthroscopy.* Philadelphia: Elsevier 2007 (in press).
2. Geissler WB, Freeland AE, Savoie FH, McIntyre LW, Whipple TL. Intracarpal soft-tissue lesions associated with an intra-articular fracture of the distal end of the radius. J Bone Joint Surg Am 1996;78:357–65.
3. Harley BJ, Werner FW, Boles SD, Palmer AK. Arthroscopic resection of arthrosis of the proximal hamate: A clinical and biomechanical study. J Hand Surg [Am] 2004;29:661–67.
4. Viegas SF. Midcarpal arthroscopy: Anatomy and portals. Hand Clin 1994;10:577–87.
5. Slutsky DJ. Volar portals in wrist arthroscopy. Journal of the American Society for Surgery of the Hand 2002; 2:225–32.
6. Slutsky DJ. Wrist arthroscopy through a volar radial portal. Arthroscopy 2002;18:624–30.
7. Slutsky DJ. Clinical applications of volar portals in wrist arthroscopy. Techniques in Hand and Upper Extremity Surgery 2004;8:229–38.
8. Slutsky DJ. Arthroscopic repair of dorsal radiocarpal ligament tears. Arthroscopy 2002;18:E49.
9. Slutsky DJ. Management of dorsoradiocarpal ligament repairs. Journal of the American Society for Surgery of the Hand 2005;5:167–74.
10. Doi K, Hattori Y, Otsuka K, Abe Y, Yamamoto H. Intra-articular fractures of the distal aspect of the radius: Arthroscopically assisted reduction compared with open reduction and internal fixation. J Bone Joint Surg Am 1999;81:1093–110.
11. Ritt MJ, Berger RA, Kauer JM. The gross and histologic anatomy of the ligaments of the capitohamate joint. J Hand Surg [Am] 1996;21:1022–28.
12. Garcia-Elias M, An KN, Cooney WPd, Linscheid RL, Chao EY. Stability of the transverse carpal arch: An experimental study. J Hand Surg [Am] 1989;14:277–82.

13. Slutsky DJ. The use of a volar ulnar portal in wrist arthroscopy. Arthroscopy 2004;20:158–63.
14. Abrams RA, Petersen M, Botte MJ. Arthroscopic portals of the wrist: An anatomic study. J Hand Surg [Am] 1994;19:940–44.
15. Steinberg BD, Plancher KD, Idler RS. Percutaneous Kirschner wire fixation through the snuff box: An anatomic study. J Hand Surg [Am] 1995;20:57–62.
16. Mackinnon SE, Dellon AL. The overlap pattern of the lateral antebrachial cutaneous nerve and the superficial branch of the radial nerve. J Hand Surg [Am] 1985;10:522–26.
17. Botte MJ, Cohen MS, Lavernia CJ, et al. The dorsal branch of the ulnar nerve: An anatomic study. J Hand Surg [Am] 1990;15:603–07.
18. Gelberman RH, Panagis JS, Taleisnik J, Baumgaertner M. The arterial anatomy of the human carpus. Part I: The extraosseous vascularity. J Hand Surg [Am] 1983; 8:367–75.
19. Martin CH, Seiler JG III, Lesesne JS. The cutaneous innervation of the palm: An anatomic study of the ulnar and median nerves. J Hand Surg [Am] 1996;21:634–38.
20. DaSilva MF, Moore DC, Weiss AP, Akelman E, Sikirica M. Anatomy of the palmar cutaneous branch of the median nerve: Clinical significance. J Hand Surg [Am] 1996; 21:639–43.
21. Kamei K, Ide Y, Kimura T. A new free thenar flap. Plast Reconstr Surg 1993;92:1380–84.
22. Omokawa S, Ryu J, Tang JB, Han J. Vascular and neural anatomy of the thenar area of the hand: Its surgical applications. Plast Reconstr Surg 1997;99:116–21.
23. Balogh B, Valencak J, Vesely M, et al. The nerve of Henle: An anatomic and immunohistochemical study. J Hand Surg [Am] 1999;24:1103–08.
24. McCabe SJ, Kleinert JM. The nerve of Henle. J Hand Surg [Am] 1990;15:784–88.
25. Berger RA. Arthroscopic anatomy of the wrist and distal radioulnar joint. Hand Clin 1999;15:393–413. vii.
26. Bowers WH. Arthroscopic anatomy of the wrist. In J McGinty (ed.), *Operative Arthroscopy.* New York: Raven Press 1991:613–23.
27. Levy HJ, Glickel SZ. Arthroscopic assisted internal fixation of volar intraarticular wrist fractures. Arthroscopy 1993; 9:122–24.
28. Tham S, Coleman S, Gilpin D. An anterior portal for wrist arthroscopy: Anatomical study and case reports. J Hand Surg [Br] 1999;24:445–47.
29. Bain GI, Pederini L. Procedure artroscopishe capsulari del polso. In L Pederini (ed.), *Ortpedia E Chirugia Mini-invasiva.* London: Springer-Verlag 1999.
30. Verhellen R, Bain GI. Arthroscopic capsular release for contracture of the wrist: A new technique. Arthroscopy 2000;16:106–10.
31. Mehta JA, Bain GI, Heptinstall RJ. Anatomical reduction of intra-articular fractures of the distal radius: An arthroscopically-assisted approach. J Bone Joint Surg [Br] 2000;82: 79–86.
32. Ashwood N, Bain GI. Arthroscopically assisted treatment of intraosseous ganglions of the lunate: A new technique. J Hand Surg [Am] 2003;28:62–68.
33. Osterman AL, Bednar JM. The Arthroscopic Release of Wrist Contracture. Presented at the American Society for Surgery of the Hand. 55th Annual Meeting. Seattle, WA 2000.
34. Abe Y, Doi K, Hattori Y, Ikeda K, Dhawan V. Arthroscopic assessment of the volar region of the scapholunate interosseous ligament through a volar portal. J Hand Surg [Am] 2003;28:69–73.
35. Abe Y, Doi K, Hattori Y, Ikeda K, Dhawan V. A benefit of the volar approach for wrist arthroscopy. Arthroscopy 2003;19:440–45.
36. del Piñal F, Delgado J, Sanmartín M, Regalado J. Correction of malunited intra-articular distal radius fractures with an inside-out osteotomy technique. J Hand Surg (Am) 2006 (in press).
37. Atzei A, Luchetti R, Carità E, Papin Zorli I, Cugola L. Arthroscopically assisted faveal reinsertion of peripheral avulsions of the TFCC. J Hand Surg B 2005;30:S1:40.
38. Trumble TE, Gilbert M, Vedder N. Isolated tears of the triangular fibrocartilage: Management by early arthroscopic repair. J Hand Surg [Am] 1997;22:57–65.
39. Whipple TL. Arthroscopy of the distal radioulnar joint: Indications, portals, and anatomy. Hand Clin 1994;10:589–92.
40. Slutsky DJ. Distal radioulnar joint arthroscopy and the volar ulnar portal. Techniques in Hand and Upper Extremity Surgery. 2007;11(1):1–7.
41. del Piñal F. Correction of malunited intra-articular distal radius fractures with an inside-out osteotomy technique. In DJ Slutsky, DJ Nagel (eds.), *Techniques in Hand and Wrist Arthroscopy.* Philadelphia: Elsevier 2007 (in press).

Further Reading

1. Jantea CL, Baltzer A, Ruther W. Arthroscopic repair of radial-sided lesions of the triangular fibrocartilage complex. Hand Clin 1995;11:31–36.

David J. Slutsky

CHAPTER 2

Trapeziometacarpal and Scaphotrapezial Arthroscopy Portals

Trapeziometacarpal Joint Portals

Standard Portals

Menon initially presented his work on arthroscopy of the trapeziometacarpal joint as a meeting exhibit in 1994.[1] He then published his experience with the arthroscopic management of trapeziometacarpal arthritis in 1996.[2] He described two working portals: a volar portal just radial to the abductor pollicus longus tendon (APL) and a dorsal portal that is just ulnar to the APL along the line of the joint. Berger independently developed his technique for arthroscopic evaluation of the first carpometacarpal joint, which he first presented as an instructional course in 1995. He then published his clinical work in 1997. He named the volar radial portal the 1-R portal and the dorsal ulnar portal the 1-U.[3] He defined the term *dorsal* as being in the plane of the thumb nail and volar in the plane of the distal pulp.

Radial and ulnar referred to the thumb when its nail is parallel to the fingernails, with the thumb supinated and radially abducted. He noted that the plane of the 1-R portal passes through the nonligamentous capsule just lateral to the anterior oblique ligament (AOL). This portal is preferred for viewing the dorsoradial ligament (DRL), the posterior oblique ligament (POL), and the ulnar collateral ligament (UCL). The plane of the 1-U portal, which is just posterior and ulnar to the extensor pollicus brevis (EPB), passes between the DRL and PRL. This portal provides views of the AOL and UCL. Both portals are along the radial border of the thumb, which makes it difficult to assess the lateral side of the joint.[4] There is no true internervous plane because branches of the superficial radial nerve surround the field and are at risk for injury with improper technique. The radial artery courses immediately posterior and ulnar to the arthroscopic field.

Modified Radial Portal

Orrellana and Chow described a modified radial portal (RP) for improving the radial view of the TMJ.[5] The RP is located just distal to the oblique ridge of the trapezium, following a line along the radial border of the flexor carpi radialis (FCR) tendon rather than the APL. In an anatomic study of six cadaver arms, the superficial radial nerve (SRN) was located a mean of 6.3 mm (range 4 to 8 mm) from the 1-U portal and 7.8 mm (range 4 to 12 mm) from the RP. The radial artery passed within 2.7 mm (range 2 to 3.5 mm) of the 1-U portal and 10 and 15 mm from the RP. To establish the RP, the scope is placed in the 1-U portal. The light source is pointed to the RP, which lies just radial to the AOL. A 22-gauge needle is inserted just distal to the ridge of the trapezium. The skin is incised, followed by blunt dissection through the capsule and insertion of the trocar and cannula, and then the arthroscope.

Thenar Portal

A thenar portal was subsequently described by Walsh et al.[6] This portal is placed by illuminating the thenar eminence with the arthroscope in the 1-U portal, and then inserting an 18-gauge needle through the bulk of the thenar muscles at the level of the TMJ (approximately 90 degrees from the 1-U portal). This portal did not appear to violate the important deep anterior oblique ligament, which is the major restraint against thumb metacarpal dorsal subluxation. They measured the distances of the surrounding neurovascular structures to three portals in a cadaver study of seven limbs. The superficial radial nerve typically has a major volar branch (SR1) and a major dorsal branch that subdivides into a volar (SR2) and dorsal (SR3) branch. SR1 generally parallels the first extensor compartment, whereas SR2 crosses the first web space.[7]

The mean distance from SR2 was 11.6 ∀ 1.0 mm for the 1-U, 25.7 ∀ 1.2 mm for the 1-R, and 33.7 ∀ 1.68 mm for the thenar portal. The mean distance from SR3 was 12.9 ∀ 1.1 mm for the 1-U, 7.4 ∀ 1.3 mm for the 1-R, and 19.07 ∀ 1.17 mm for the thenar portal. The mean distance from the radial artery was 13.3 ∀ 1.1 mm for the 1-U, 20.7 ∀ 0.9 mm for the 1-R, and 29.4 ∀ 1.15 mm for the thenar portal. The motor branch of the median nerve was an average of 23.0 ∀ 1.6 mm from the thenar portal. There are no published clinical series on the use of these two accessory portals as of yet.

Distal/Dorsal (D-2) Portal

Access to medial osteophytes may sometimes be difficult. Hence, I have found the use of a distal/dorsal (D-2) accessory portal to be of some value. Its main utility is that it allows one to look down on the trapezium rather than across it, which facilitates resection of medial osteophytes. This accessory portal allows views of the dorsal capsule with rotation of the scope and facilitates triangulation of the instrumentation. It is situated in the dorsal aspect of the first web space. An anatomical study of five cadaver hands revealed that the D-2 portal surface landmark is ulnar to the EPL tendon and 1 cm distal to the V-shaped cleft at the juncture of the index and thumb metacarpal bases. The portal lies just distal to the dorsal intermetacarpal ligament (DIML).[8]

The DIML is an extracapsular ligament that originates from the dorsoradial aspect of the index metacarpal radial to the extensor carpi radialis longus insertion. It inserts onto the palmar-ulnar tubercle of the base of the thumb metacarpal along with the POL and UCL.[4] A trocar placed through the D-2 portal was found to pass through the first dorsal interosseous muscle and penetrate the DIML, entering the joint either through or between the ulnar collateral ligament (UCL) and the posterior oblique ligament (POL) (Figure 2.1a through d). Branches of the superficial radial nerve passed within 3.2 mm (range 1 to 5 mm) of this portal. The radial artery was 3.8 mm away (range 3 to 5 mm) from this portal, the FDMA was within 2.8 mm (range 2 to 4 mm) of this portal, and the cephalic vein was within 2.8 mm (range 1 to 5 mm) of this portal. On average, the D-2 portal was 17.2 mm from the 1-U portal (range 12 to 20 mm).

There is no true safe zone for the D-2 portal, with branches of the SRN or the FDMA or one of its branches coming with 1 mm of the portal. The first dorsal metacarpal artery (FDMA) originates from the radial artery just distal to the extensor pollicus longus tendon (EPL), before the radial artery dives between the two heads of the first dorsal interosseous muscle (FDI). It is 1.2 to 1.5 mm near its origin, and is accompanied by at least one vein and by terminal branches of the radial nerve.

The FDMA runs within the deep fascia overlying the FDI, parallel to the radial side of the index metacarpal. It divides into an ulnodorsal branch to the thumb (FDM_R), a radiodorsal branch to the index (FDMA), and a muscular branch to the FDI. The radial artery dives between the two heads of the first dorsal interosseous and divides intramuscularly. Hugging the ulnar border of the thumb metacarpal and moving 1 cm distal to the thumb/index metacarpal juncture increases the space between the portal and the radial artery. Careful wound spread technique is of paramount importance when establishing this portal, especially in the presence of a dominant FDMAu.

Scaphotrapeziotrapezoidal Joint Portals

(Figure 2.2a through d.)

STT-U Portal

Bowers and Whipple have described a scaphotrapeziotrapezoidal joint (STT-U) portal they used to facilitate arthroscopic resections of the distal scaphoid with scaphotrapezial osteoarthritis. They used this portal in conjunction with the radial midcarpal portal (RMC) for evaluation and treatment of disorders of the STT joint. The STT-U portal is located in line with the midshaft axis of the index metacarpal, just ulnar to the EPL.[9] Entry into this portal requires traction on the index finger. Leaving the EPL to the radial side of the STT portal protects the radial artery in the snuffbox from injury.

STT-R Portal

A radial portal for STT arthroscopy (STT-R) has also been recently reported.[10] This portal is radial to the abductor pollicus longus (APL) tendon at the level of the STT joint. Access to the joint is facilitated by use of a 1.9-mm 30E angled arthroscope. Cadaver dissections demonstrated that maintaining a position palmar and radial to the APL tendon at the STT joint level avoids the radial artery by a mean of 8.8 mm (range 6 to 10 mm). The angle between the two portals is 130E, which facilitates triangulation of the instrumentation. As with the 1-/,2 portal, branches of the superficial radial nerve virtually surround the arthroscopic field.

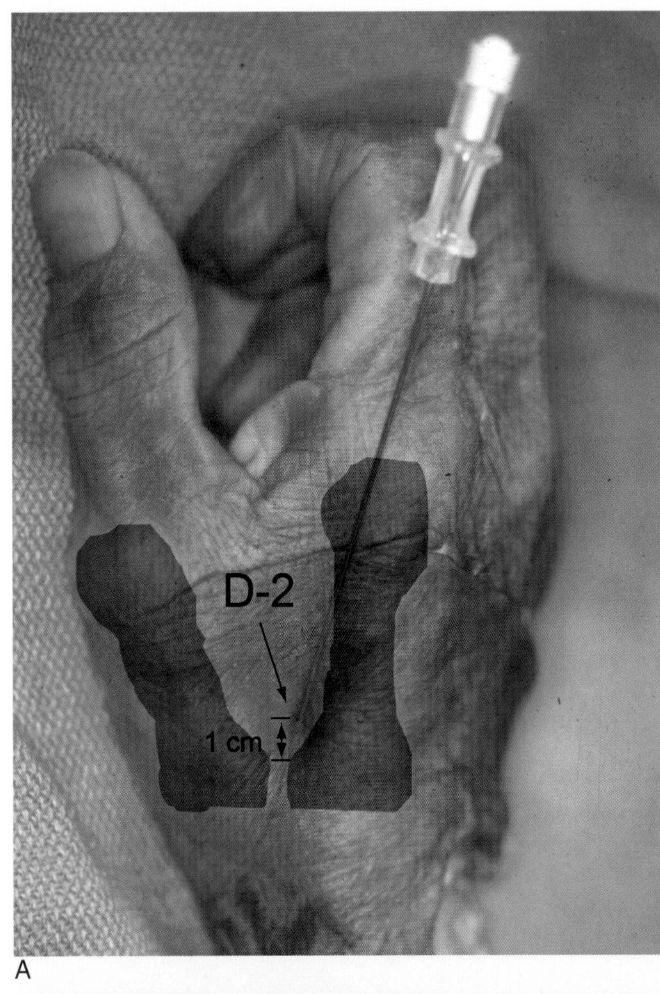

A

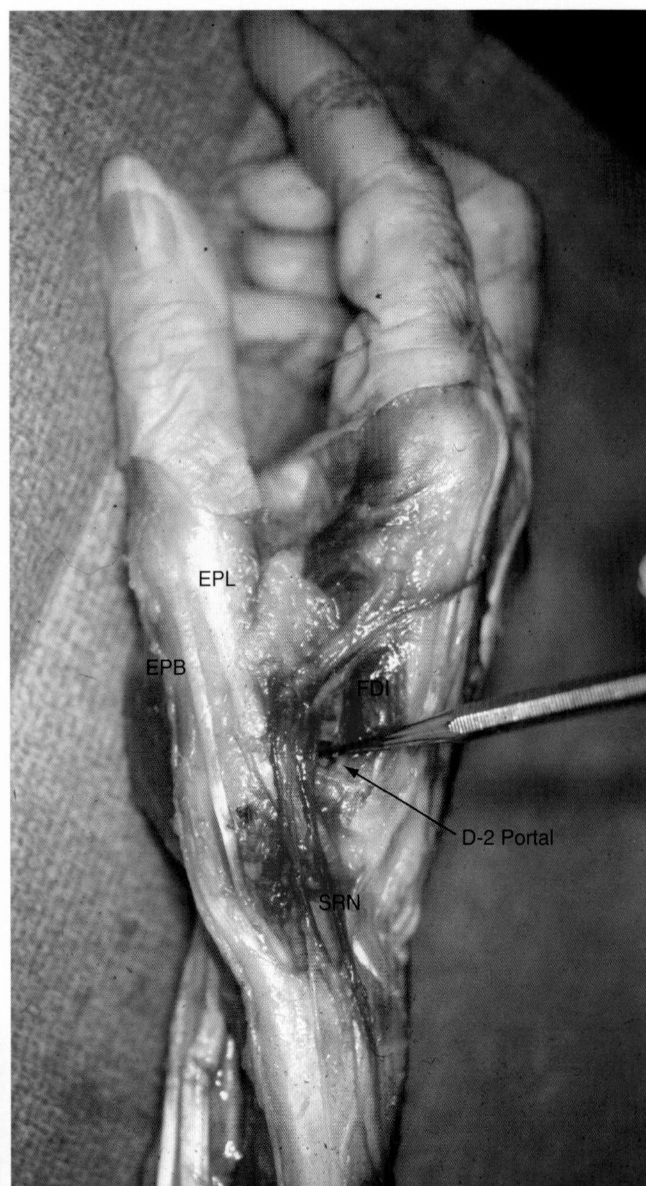

B

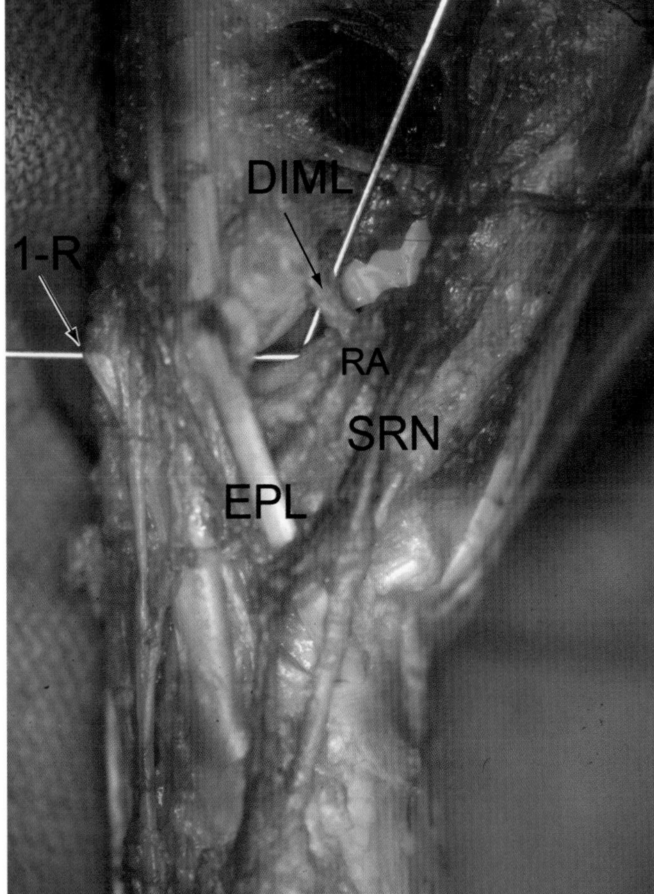

C

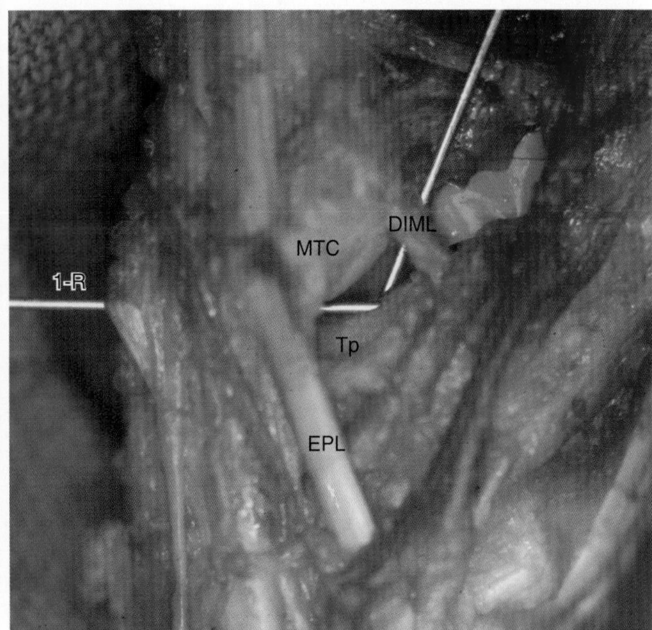

D

(Continued)

FIGURE 2.1. (A) Surface landmarks for D-2 portal. (B) Relative position of D-2 portal (EPB = extensor pollicus brevis, EPL = extensor pollicus longus, SRN = superficial radial nerve, FDI = first dorsal interosseous). (C) Deep anatomy of D-2 portal (RA = radial artery, DIML = deep intermetacarpal ligament). (D) Close-up view. Note that the D-2 portal needle points directly over the medial trapezium, whereas the 1-R portal needle moves parallel to the trapezium (MTC = metacarpal, Tp = trapezium).

Hence, blunt dissection of the capsule and knowledge of the regional anatomy are essential.

STT-P Portal

Baré and co-workers described another accessory palmar portal (STT-P) based on a dissection of 10 cadaver arms.[11] They identified a safe portal of entry that was midway between the radial styloid and the base of the first metacarpal, 3 mm ulnar to the APL tendon and 6 mm radial to the scaphoid tubercle. The trocar is inserted into the ST joint, aiming toward the base of the fifth metacarpal while holding the thumb in extension and adduction. This portal lay 7.6 mm (range 5 to 11 mm) from the radial artery, 6.5 mm (range 4 to 11 mm) from the superficial branch of the radial artery, and 11.6 mm (range 3 to 20 mm) from the closest radial sensory nerve branch.

Bain et al. used a portal that was radial to the EPL tendon (STT-R), along with the RMC, for arthroscopic debridement of isolated STT OA.[12] They recommended a 1.5-cm skin incision to enable safe blunt dissection.

Methodology

The patient is positioned supine on the operating table, with the arm extended on a hand table. The thumb is suspended by Chinese finger traps with 5 pounds of

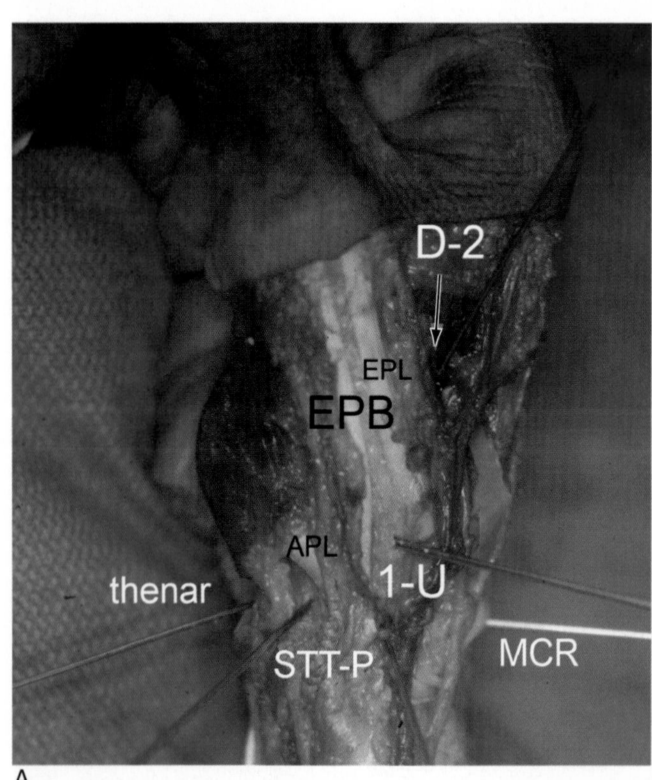

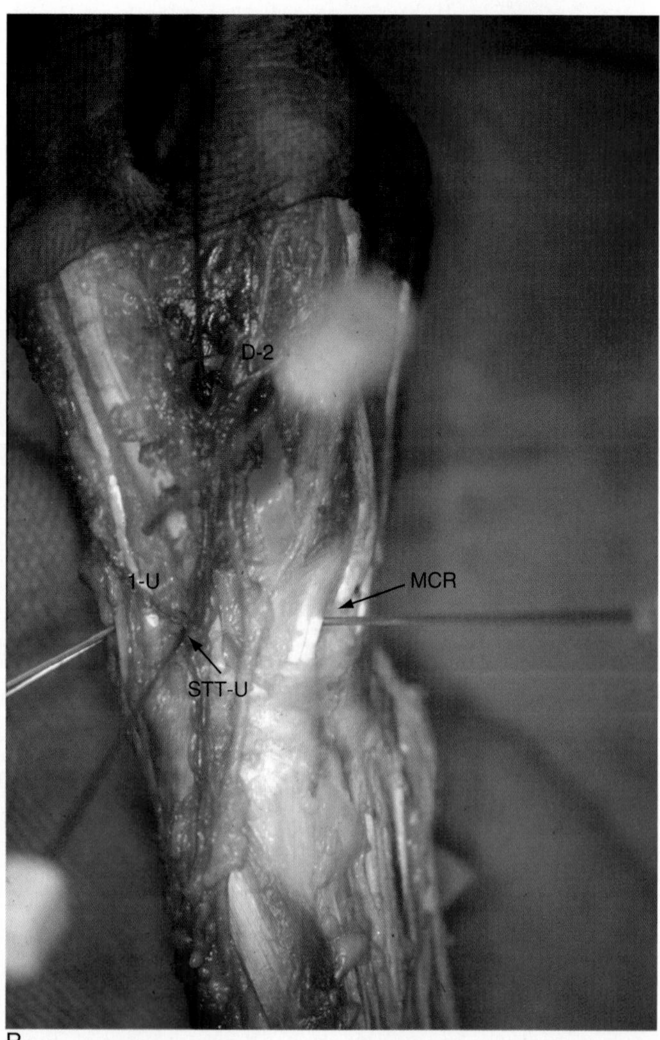

FIGURE 2.2. (A) Palmar oblique view of the wrist demonstrating the relative positions of the STT-P and MCR portals (MCR = midcarpal radial portal). (B) Lateral view of the wrist demonstrating the STT-U portal relative to TM portals.

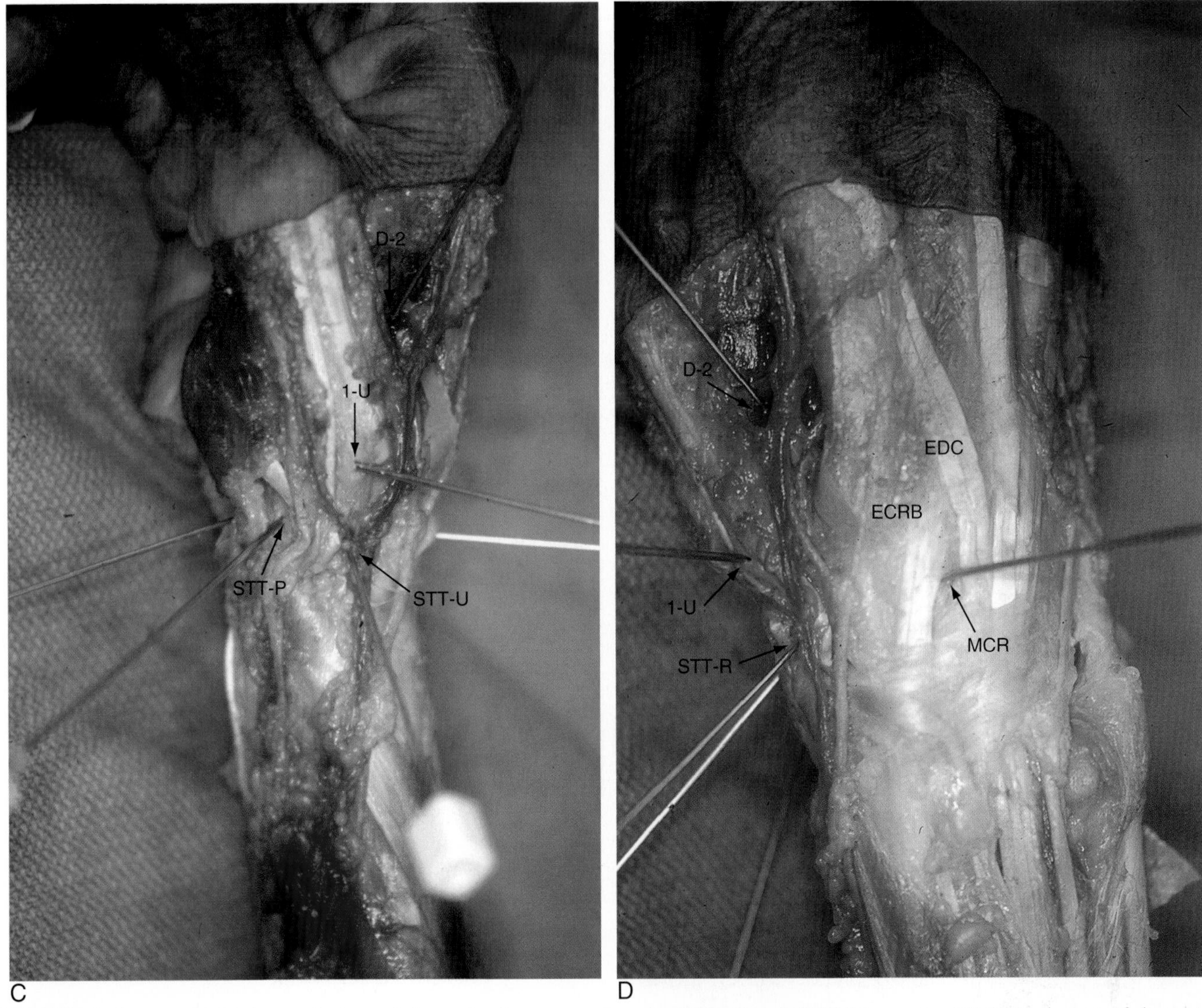

FIGURE 2.2. Cont'd (C) Lateral view of the wrist demonstrating the STT-P and STT-U portals. (D) Dorsal view of the wrist highlighting the MCR portal.

counter-traction, which forces the wrist into ulnar deviation. A traction tower facilitates this procedure, although any means of traction will suffice. The relevant landmarks are palpated and outlined, including the proximal and dorsal edge of the thumb metacarpal base, the APL and EPL tendons, and the radial artery in the snuffbox.

The procedure is performed under tourniquet control at 250 mmHg. Saline inflow irrigation is provided through the arthroscope and a small joint pump or pressure bag. To establish the 1-R portal, the thumb metacarpal base is palpated and the joint is identified with a 22-gauge needle just radial to the APL, followed by injection of 2 cc of saline. This step may be facilitated by fluoroscopy. A small skin incision is made, followed by wound spread technique with tenotomy scissors. The capsule is pierced and a cannula and blunt trocar are inserted, followed by the arthroscope. An identical procedure is used to establish the 1-U portal, just ulnar to the EPB tendon, followed by insertion of a 3-mm hook probe. The portals are used interchangeably to systematically inspect the joint, which is facilitated by judicious use of a 2.0-mm synovial resector.

To establish the D-2 portal, the junction of the base of the index and thumb metacarpal is palpated just distal and ulnar to the extensor pollicus longus (EPL) tendon. The entry site is marked, with the tourniquet down to allow palpation or Doppler of the radial artery. A 22-gauge needle is inserted at this juncture, angling proximally radial and palmar to penetrate the joint space (which is viewed from the 1-R or 1-U portal). A small skin incision is made and tenotomy scissors are used to spread the soft tissue and pierce the joint capsule. This is followed by use of a blunt trocar and cannula and then the arthroscope (or hook probe, motorized shaver, or 2.9-mm bur) (Figure 2.3a through e).

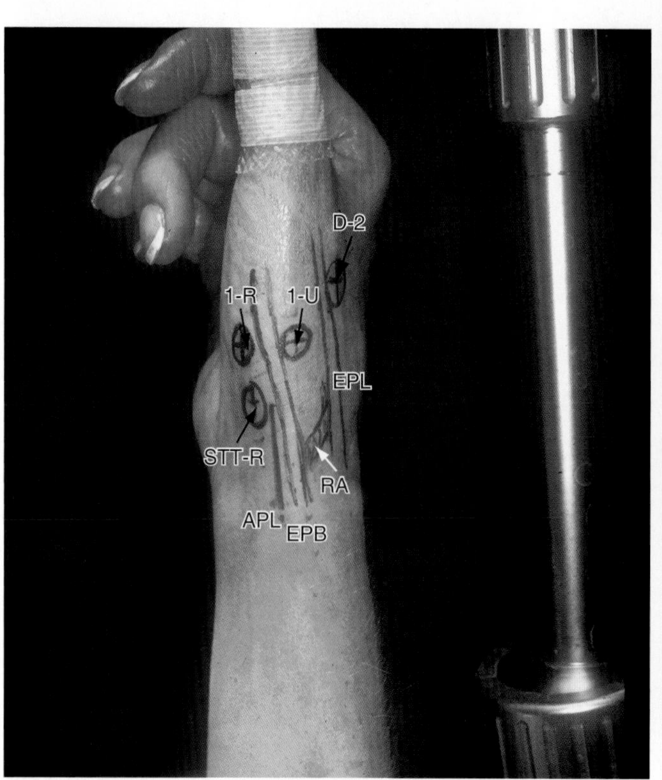

A

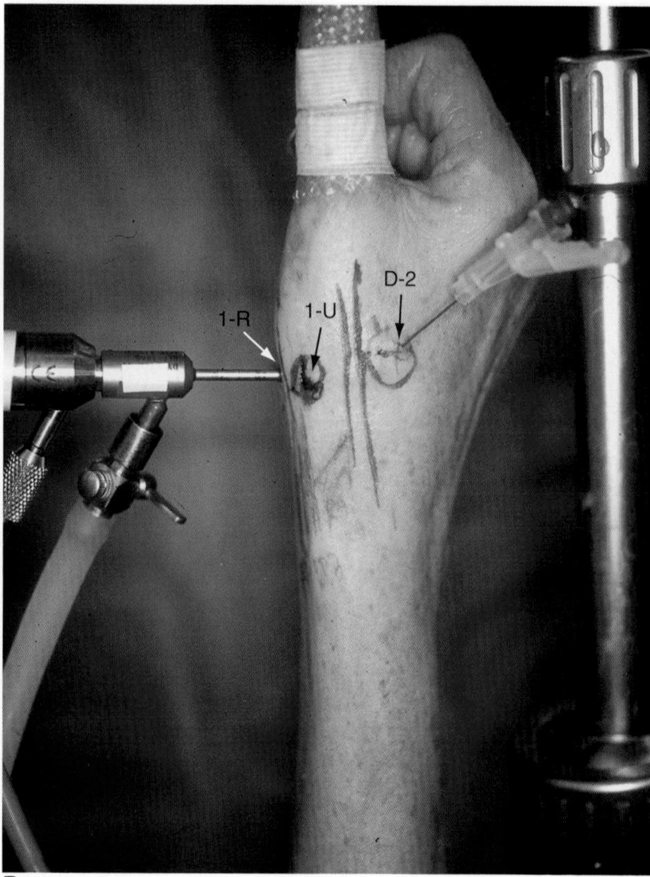

B

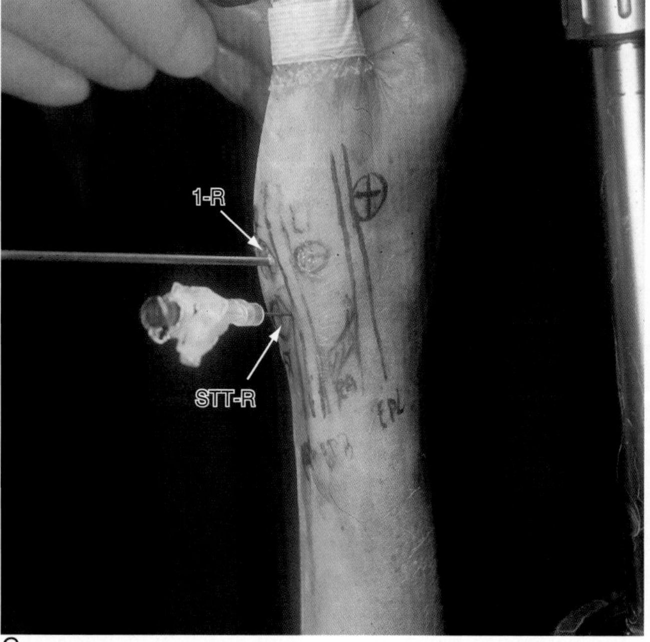

C

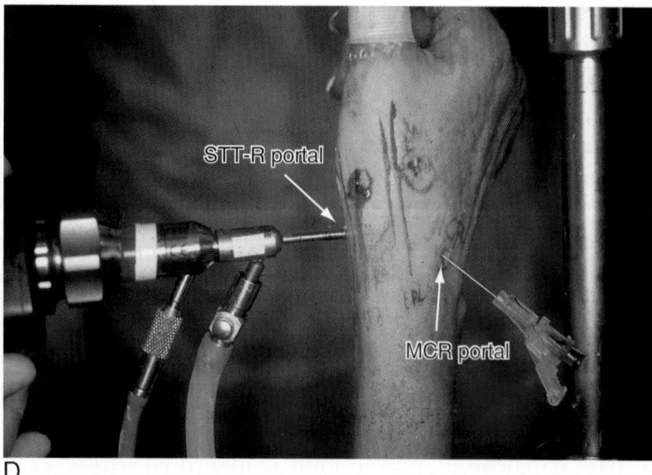

D

FIGURE 2.3. Clinical applications. (A) Surface landmarks for TM and STT portals. (B) Needle inserted in D-2 portal. Note the relative position to the 1-U portal. (C) Needle localization of the STT-R portal relative to the 1-R portal. (D) Needle localization of the MCR portal while viewing from the STT-R portal.

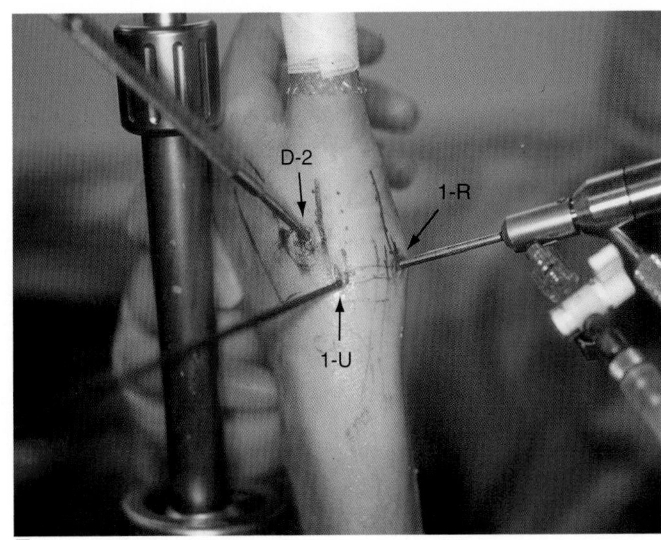

FIGURE 2.3. Cont'd (E) Percutaneous reduction of a Bennet's fracture. Freer elevator introduced through D-2 portal and probe in 1-U portal while viewing through 1-R portal.

References

1. Menon J. Arthroscopic evaluation of the first carpometacarpal joint. J Hand Surg [Am] 1998;23:57.
2. Menon J. Arthroscopic management of trapeziometacarpal joint arthritis of the thumb. Arthroscopy 1996;12:581–87.
3. Berger RA. A technique for arthroscopic evaluation of the first carpometacarpal joint. J Hand Surg [Am] 1997;22:1077–80.
4. Bettinger PC, Berger RA. Functional ligamentous anatomy of the trapezium and trapeziometacarpal joint (gross and arthroscopic). Hand Clin 2001;17:151–68, vii.
5. Orellana MA, Chow JC. Arthroscopic visualization of the thumb carpometacarpal joint: Introduction and evaluation of a new radial portal. Arthroscopy 2003;19:583–91.
6. Walsh EF, Akelman E, Fleming BC, DaSilva MF. Thumb carpometacarpal arthroscopy: A topographic, anatomic study of the thenar portal. J Hand Surg [Am] 2005;30: 373–79.
7. Steinberg BD, Plancher KD, Idler RS. Percutaneous Kirschner wire fixation through the snuff box: An anatomic study. J Hand Surg [Am] 1995;20:57–62.
8. Slutsky DJ. The use of a dorsal distal portal in trapeziometacarpal arthroscopy. Arthroscopy: The Journal of Arthroscopic and Related Surgery. In press 2007.
9. Bowers WH. Arthroscopic anatomy of the wrist. In J McGinty (ed.), *Operative Arthroscopy*. New York: Raven Press 1991:613–23.
10. Carro LP, Golano P, Farinas O, Cerezal L, Hidalgo C. The radial portal for scaphotrapeziotrapezoid arthroscopy. Arthroscopy 2003;19:547–53.
11. Bare J, Graham AJ, Tham SK. Scaphotrapezial joint arthroscopy: A palmar portal. J Hand Surg [Am] 2003;28:605–09.
12. Ashwood N, Bain GI, Fogg Q. Results of arthroscopic debridement for isolated scaphotrapeziotrapezoid arthritis. J Hand Surg [Am] 2003;28:729–32.

SECTION 2

The Ulnocarpal Joint

Daniel J. Nagle

CHAPTER 3

To my son, Peter

Arthroscopically Assisted Ulnar Shortening

Basic Science and Anatomy

Ulnocarpal Joint Anatomy

The base of the triangular fibrocartilage attaches to the distal radius at the distal edge of the sigmoid notch. Its distal surface blends imperceptibly with the hyalin cartilage of the lunate fossa of the distal radius. The triangular fibrocartilage narrows as it passes from radial to ulnar to insert in the fovea at the base of the ulnar styloid. Dorsally and palmarly, the TFCC thickens to form the distal radioulnar ligaments. The integrity of these two ligaments is critical to the stability of the distal radioulnar joint. The triangular fibrocartilage meniscal homologue passes distally to attach at the ulnar aspect of the triquetrum. The interval between the ulnotriquetral ligament and the meniscal homologue and ulnar collateral ligament is known as the pre-styloid recess (or the pisotriquetral recess).[1]

Biomechanics

Palmer and others have demonstrated an inverse relationship between the thickness of the triangular fibrocartilage and ulnar variance.[2] That is, the more positive the ulnar variance the thinner the triangular fibrocartilage. This relationship explains the observed coincidence of ulnar plus variance and TFCC tears (ulnar abutment syndrome). The ulnar abutment syndrome is characterized by an ulnar plus variance, central tears of the triangular fibrocartilage, and chondromalacia of the adjacent articular surfaces of the lunate, triquetrum, and ulnar head.

Werner et al.[3] have studied the effect of ulnar length on load transmission across the triangular fibrocartilage. They demonstrated a direct relationship between the length of the ulna and the amount of force transmitted across the TFCC. As the ulna gets longer, the force transmitted across the TFCC increases. The opposite occurs with ulnar shortening.

The vascular supply of the triangular fibrocartilage is characterized by a peripheral vascular zone and a central avascular zone.[4] The lack of central blood supply precludes any healing of central TFCC tears and dictates the choice of debridement as the treatment for such tears.

Indications

Patients presenting with a symptomatic triangular fibrocartilage complex (TFCC) tear, either acute or chronic, in combination with an ulnar zero or ulnar plus variance are unlikely to respond to a simple debridement of the TFCC. These patients are suffering from an ulnar abutment syndrome in which the TFCC is "pinched" between the ulnar head and the proximal surface of the lunate. Such patients are candidates for arthroscopic debridement of the TFCC combined with an arthroscopic ulnar shortening.

Contraindications

Arthroscopic ulnar shortening is unlikely to help those patients who present with an ulnar abutment syndrome combined with additional ulnocarpal and/or lunatotriquetral pathology. A lunatotriquetral ligament instability or ulnocarpal ligament laxity in the presence of an ulnar abutment syndrome will not respond to an arthroscopic ulnar shortening because the arthroscopic ulnar shortening does not address the LT or ulnocarpal instability. An ulnar shortening osteotomy combined with an arthroscopic TFCC debridement would be a reasonable approach in this case. The LT and ulnocarpal instability cannot be treated with ulnocarpal capsular shrinkage because the capsular shrinkage demands immobilization for six to eight weeks. The postoperative regimen for an arthroscopically assisted ulnar shortening consists of early range of motion of the wrist and distal radioulnar joint.

Technique

The initial approach to the TFCC and distal ulna is through the 3-4 and 4-5 portals or through the 6-R portal. The arthroscope is placed in the 3-4 portal, whereas the 4-5 or 6-R portals are used as instrument portals. The arthroscopic treatment of the ulnar abutment syndrome is facilitated by using the Holmium:YAG laser.[5] Hyaline cartilage is very efficiently removed with the laser at higher energy settings (2.0 joules at 20 pulses per second). Not only is the ulnar head hyalin cartilage and subchondral bone rapidly removed but in contrast to burring is removed without producing much debris.

Once the cancellous bone of the ulnar head is exposed, however, the bur becomes the most effective tool for completing the ulnar shortening. This is because it becomes very time consuming to focus the laser beam on each trabecula. During the ulnar head resection, care must be taken to not injure the sigmoid notch with either the laser or the bur. Care must also be taken to not detach the insertion of the triangular fibrocartilage from the fovea at the base of the ulnar styloid. The successful arthroscopic ulnar shortening relies on teamwork. The assistant brings the surfaces of the ulnar head to be resected to the laser being held by the operating surgeon. By progressively supinating and pronating the forearm, an appropriate amount of ulnar head is excised.

The resection should be carried out in a systematic fashion. For example, start the cartilage ablation with the wrist fully pronated and gradually rotate the radius around the ulna, bringing the forearm into full supination. Next, ablate the subchondral plate rotating from pronation to supination. Finally, the ablation of the cancellous bone is accomplished while rotating the radius from supination into pronation. The depth of the first pass with the bur is easily kept uniform by burying the bur head in the bone to the level of its guard and using that depth as a guide for the rest of the burring.

The goal is to resect sufficient ulna to produce a 2-mm negative ulnar variance. The amount of ulna resected must be verified with intraoperative fluoroscopy. Occasionally, complete visualization of the ulnar head requires the scope to be placed in the 4-5 portal (with the laser and bur entering the distal radioulnar joint through the distal radioulnar joint portal). This portal is established just proximal to the 4-5 portal and TFCC.

An effort is made to leave a smooth surface on the remaining distal ulna. The trabeculae of the distal ulna always produce a somewhat rough distal ulnar surface at the completion of the procedure. However, these irregularities disappear during the months following the surgery (Figures 3.1 and 3.2). Large irregularities must be avoided because they can catch on the proximal surface of the residual TFCC during supination and pronation. Once the ulnar shortening is complete, the traction should be removed from the wrist and the wrist should be ulnarly deviated, axially loaded, and taken through a full range of supination and pronation. If this maneuver produces no popping and clicking or catching, the ulnar head surface is probably smooth.

The postoperative regimen after ulnar shortening includes providing the patient with a wrist splint to be worn as needed, as well as a home therapy program consisting of active and passive range-of-motion exercises. Early range-of-motion exercises are essential. Immobilization of the wrist leads to a loss of motion due to postoperative scar contracture. The sutures (wounds are closed using subcuticular sutures of 4–0 Prolene) are removed at two weeks. Strengthening exercises can be started at six weeks if needed. Premature resumption of heavy lifting or repetitive activities will lead to radiocarpal synovitis. The recovery after an ulnar shortening can be as long as six months (as suggested by Feldon).[6] However, the majority of patients will be improved long before six months.

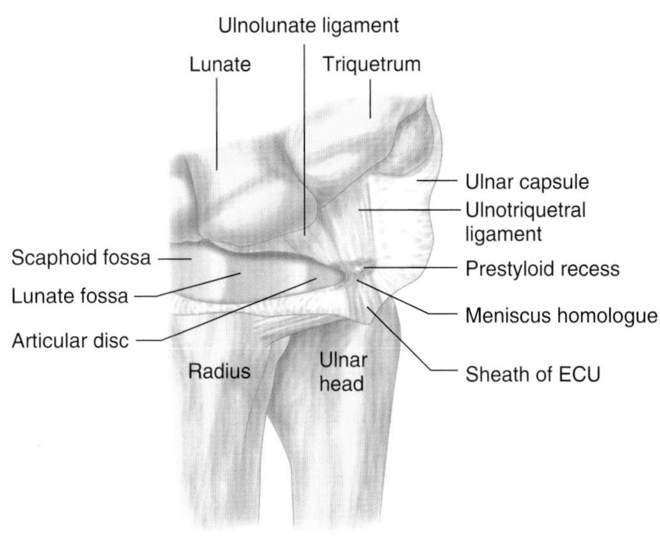

FIGURE 3.1. Anatomy of the triangular fibrocartilage. *(Redrawn from Ishii S, Palmer AK, Werner FW, Short WH, Fortino MD. An anatomic study of the ligamentous structure of the triangular fibrocartilage complex. J Hand Surg [Am] 1998; 23:977–85.)*

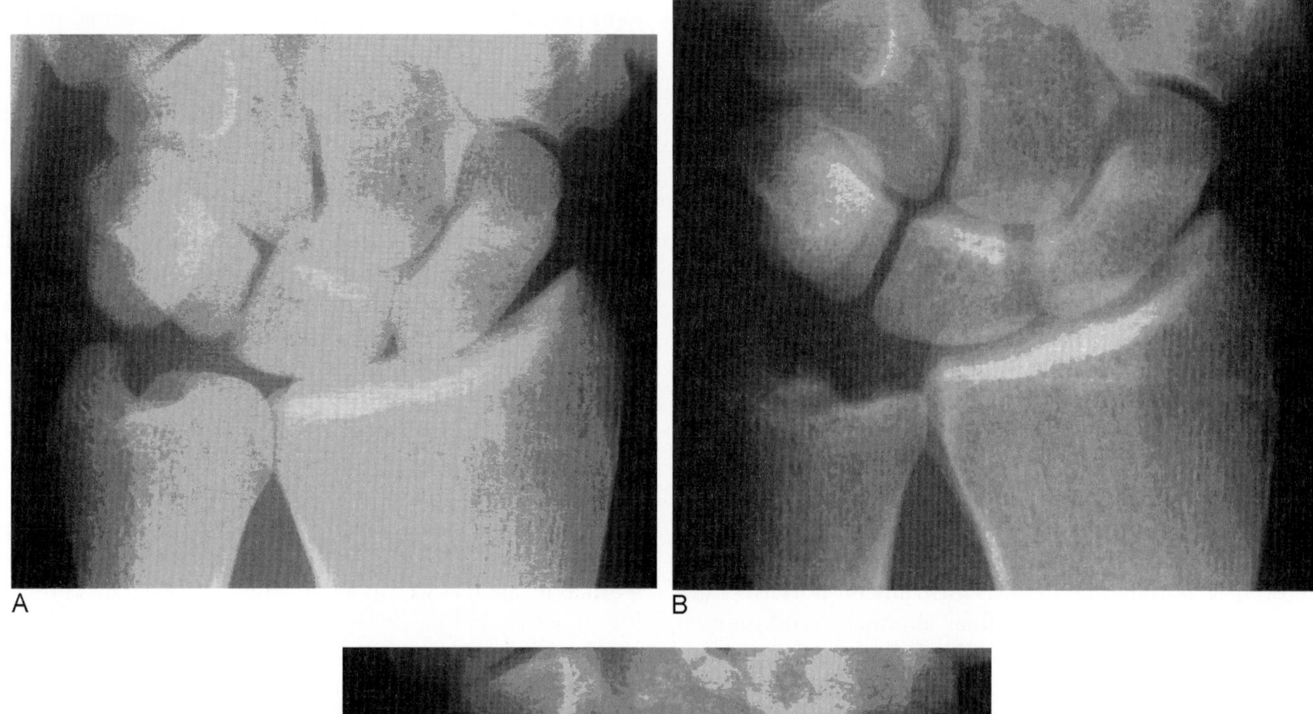

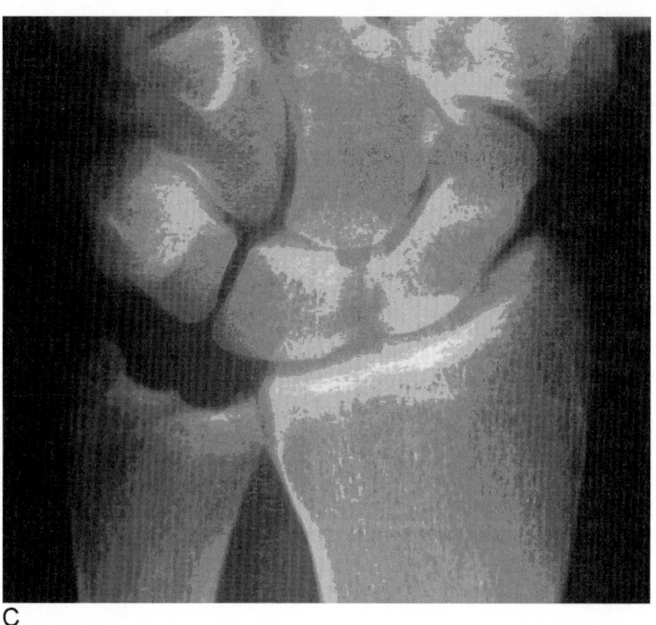

FIGURE 3.2. Early and late post laser-assisted arthroscopic ulnar shortening demonstrating smoothing of resection site with time: (A) ulnar abutment, (B) six weeks postoperatively, and (C) six months postoperatively.

Results

Arthroscopically assisted ulnar shortening has proven to be an effective method of treating patients with an ulnar abutment syndrome.[7,8] Eighty-one percent of our patients had an excellent or good outcome. Eight of Tomaino's 12 patients were pain free, and 4 had minimal symptoms.

This technique has been shown to be as effective as formal ulnar shortening osteotomy for the treatment of ulnar abutment syndrome.[9] Arthroscopically assisted ulnar shortening has the advantage of being less invasive and is not associated with complications associated with plate fixation of an osteotomy, such as nonunion and the need for subsequent plate removal (56%).

References

1. Ishii S, Palmer AK, Werner FW, Short WH, Fortino MD. An anatomic study of the ligamentous structure of the triangular fibrocartilage complex. J Hand Surg [Am] 1998;23:977–85.
2. Palmer AK, Glisson RR, Werner FW. Relationship between ulnar variance and triangular fibrocartilage complex thickness. J Hand Surg [Am] 1984;9:681–82.
3. Werner FW, Glisson RR, Murphy DJ, Palmer AK. Force transmission through the distal radioulnar carpal joint: Effect of ulnar lengthening and shortening. Handchir Mikrochir Plast Chir 1986;18:304–08.
4. Bednar MS, Arnoczky SP, Weiland AJ. The microvasculature of the triangular fibrocartilage complex: Its clinical significance. J Hand Surg [Am] 1991;16(6):1101–05.

5. Nagle DJ, Bernstein MA. Laser-assisted arthroscopic ulnar shortening. Arthroscopy 2002;18(9):1046–51.
6. Feldon P, Terrono AL, Belsky MR. The "wafer" procedure: Partial distal ulnar resection. Clin Orthop 1992;275:124–29.
7. Nagle DJ, Bernstein MA. Laser assisted arthroscopic ulnar shortening. Arthroscopy 2002;18(9):1046–51.
8. Tomaino MM, Weiser RW. Combined arthroscopic TFCC debridement and wafer resection of the distal ulna in wrists with triangular fibrocartilage complex tears and positive ulnar variance. J Hand Surg [Am] 2001;26 (6):1047–52.
9. Bernstein MA, Nagle DJ, Martinez A, Stogin JM Jr., Wiedrich TA. A comparison of combined arthroscopic triangular fibrocartilage complex debridement and arthroscopic wafer distal ulna resection versus arthroscopic triangular fibrocartilage complex debridement and ulnar shortening osteotomy for ulnocarpal abutment syndrome. Arthroscopy 2004;20(4):392–401.

Jennifer Weintraub, A. Lee Osterman, and Jeffrey Yao

CHAPTER 4

From A. Lee Osterman: This chapter is dedicated to all those hand fellows who have taught me to see more with less.

Arthroscopic Treatment of Radial-Sided TFCC Lesions

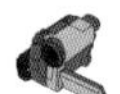

Functional Anatomy of TFCC

The triangular fibrocartilage complex (TFCC) is a ligamentous structure composed of fibrocartilage located between the distal ulna and the ulnar carpus.[1,2] The TFCC has several functions, the most important of which is to stabilize the ulnar carpus.[3] The TFCC also provides a continuous gliding surface across the distal face of the radius and ulna for flexion-extension and translational movements. It provides a flexible mechanism for stable rotational movements of the radiocarpal unit around the ulnar axis, and cushions the forces transmitted through the ulnocarpal axis.[4] The TFCC improves functional stability of the wrist while allowing 6 degrees of motion: flexion, extension, supination, pronation, and radial and ulnar deviation. The TFCC functionally enhances the surface area of joint contact between the radius and ulna to the carpus.

The TFCC consists of several discrete anatomical structures that when combined form a functional unit.[2] The dorsal and volar radioulnar ligaments encase the articular disc and create the distal radioulnar joint. The ulnar collateral ligament, the meniscal homologue, the tendon sheath of the extensor carpi ulnaris, and the ulnocarpal ligaments intimately attach to the articular disc. This broadly based disc adheres to the radial sigmoid notch and extends to the ulnar styloid.

The TFCC transmits axial load from the wrist to the forearm in a longitudinal direction across the ulnar column of the wrist.[3] Force is transmitted across the ulnar aspect of the lunate, the triquetrum, and the TFCC on the distal radioulnar joint. The bony morphology of these structures reflects an adaptation to the unique demands on this part of the wrist. Densitometric studies have demonstrated patterns of enhanced subcortical mineralization in the bones of the ulnar wrist. The patterns of increased mineralization correspond to the distribution of force in a longitudinal direction across the ulnar column of the wrist.[5]

The vascular anatomy of the TFCC is variable, and is in part responsible for the differences in outcomes resulting from different patterns of injuries. Perfusion to the TFCC arises from dorsal and palmar branches of the anterior interosseus artery. Dorsal and palmar branches of the ulnar artery supply the ulnar styloid and the ulnar aspect of the volar periphery (Figure 4.1).[6,7] Studies of the vascular anatomy of the TFCC have demonstrated that vessels supply the TFCC from the palmar, ulnar, and dorsal attachments of the joint capsule in a radial fashion—and that the blood flow penetrates less than 20% of the periphery (Figure 4.2).[6,8,9] The central portion of the TFCC is therefore relatively avascular. Although the radial aspect of the disc is hypovascular compared to the ulnar side, some radial-sided vascularity has been documented in cadaveric studies—suggesting that healing is possible in this region.[9]

The radial insertion of the TFCC is vulnerable to injury when axial load is combined with pronation and ulnar deviation or extension of the wrist. This motion exposes the TFCC to shear stress, which if substantial enough causes distortion of the TFCC. Extreme stress loads can result in a TFCC tear and subsequent degeneration of the TFCC from its radial insertion (Figures 4.3 and 4.4).[10]

Patterns of TFCC Injury

The TFCC transmits force from the wrist to the forearm, and injuries to the TFCC are a common cause of ulnar-sided wrist pain. When evaluating TFCC injuries, it is important to distinguish between age-related (degenerative) and traumatic

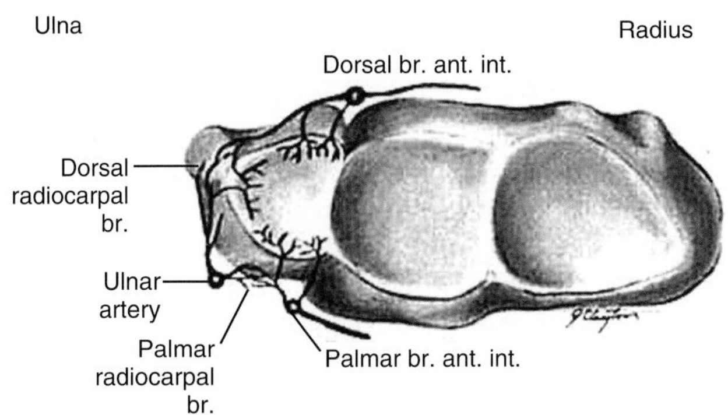

FIGURE 4.1. Blood supply to the TFCC arises from the dorsal and palmar branches of the anterior interosseus artery, as well as from the dorsal and palmar branches of the ulnar artery. *(Reproduced with permission from Thiru-Pathi RG, Ferlic DC, Clayton ML, McClure DC. Arterial anatomy of the triangular fibrocartilage of the wrist and its surgical significance. J Hand Surg [Am] 1986;11:258–63.)*

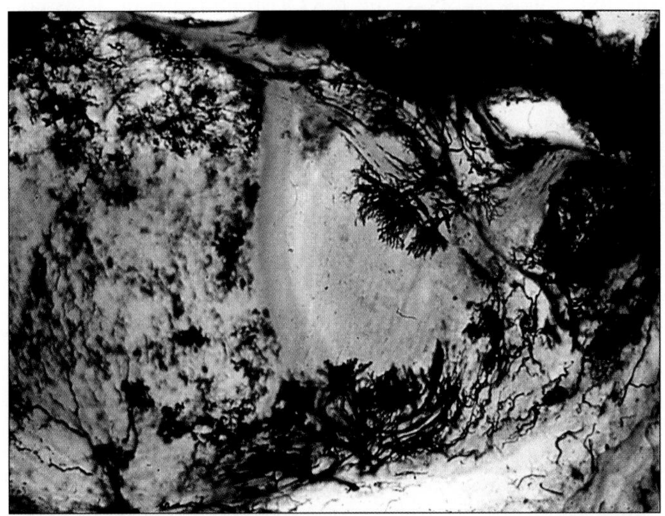

FIGURE 4.2. Anatomic studies of the vascular supply to the TFCC demonstrate that blood vessels penetrate less than 20% of the periphery of the disc, leaving the central portion relatively avascular. *(Reproduced with permission from Bednar MS, Arnoczky SP, Weiland AJ. The microvasculature of the triangular fibrocartilage complex: Its clinical significance. J Hand Surg [Am] 1991;16(6):1101–05.)*

etiologies. A useful classification system for TFCC injuries was established by Palmer (Figure 4.5 and Table 4.1).[11]

Age-related nontraumatic lesions to the TFCC are typically characterized by central perforations.[8,12] In a study of 180 wrist joints in 100 cadavers ranging in age from fetuses to 94 years, Mikic demonstrated that degeneration of the TFCC begins in the third decade of life. He showed that this degeneration increases in frequency and severity as people age. After the fifth decade of life, he noted 100% of TFCCs to be abnormal appearing. It is important to note, however, that these age-related TFCC lesions are often asymptomatic.[13]

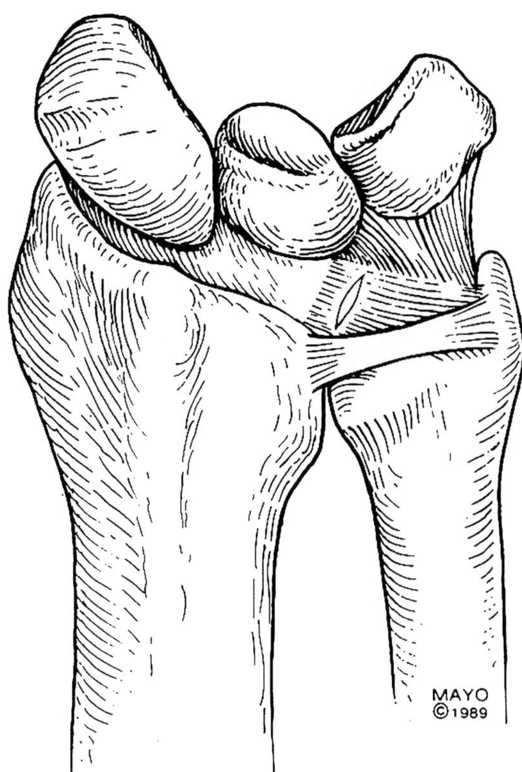

FIGURE 4.3. The TFCC is located between the distal ulna and the ulnar carpus. The radial insertion of the TFCC is particularly vulnerable to injury when axial load and pronation are combined with ulnar deviation and wrist extension. *(Reproduced with permission from the Mayo Foundation.)*

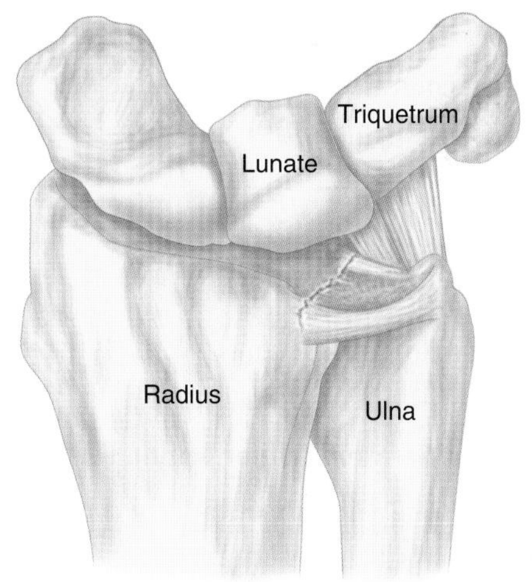

Class 1D

FIGURE 4.4. Extreme stress loads can cause tears of the TFCC from its radial insertion. *(Adapted from Palmer AK. Triangular fibrocartilage complex lesions: A classification. J Hand Surg [Am] 1989;14:594–606.)*

In contrast to degenerative age-related lesions, traumatic injuries to the TFCC are characterized by peripheral, radial, or dorsal ruptures or avulsions. In cases of underlying degenerative changes, such lesions can exist in combination with one another.

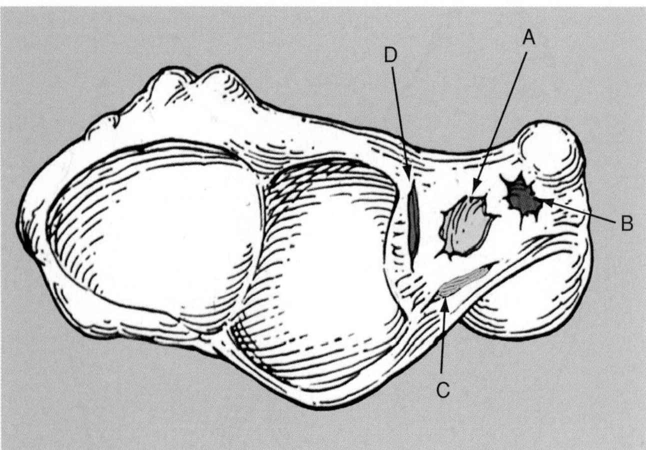

FIGURE 4.5. Traumatic lesions are further classified by location within the disc. Class A lesions are located in the center of the disc, class B tears occur along the ulnar aspect, class C lesions are located distally, and class D lesions are along the radial attachment to the sigmoid notch. *(Reproduced with permission from the Mayo Foundation.)*

Table 4.1.

Palmer's Classification of TFCC Lesions (Acute and Degenerative)

Class 1: Traumatic
• Central perforation of the TFCC disc
• Ulnar avulsion
• With styloid fracture
• Without styloid fracture
• Distal avulsion from carpus
• Radial avulsion
• With sigmoid notch fracture
• Without sigmoid notch fracture
Class 2: Degenerative (Ulnar Impaction Syndrome)
• TFCC wear
• TFCC wear + lunate and/or head chondromalacia
• TFCC perforation + lunate and/or head chondromalacia + lunotriquetral ligament perforation
• TFCC perforation + lunate and/or head chondromalacia + lunotriquetral ligament perforation
• + ulnocarpal arthritis

Classification from Palmer AK. Triangular fibrocartilage complex lesions: A classification. J Hand Surg [Am] 1989;14:594–606.

Evaluation of Radial-Sided TFCC Injuries

Patients with radial-sided TFCC injuries typically present with ulnar-sided wrist pain and clicking.[14–16] Frequently, a history of a fall onto a pronated and hyperextended wrist can be elicited. Class 1D injuries are frequently associated with distal radius fractures.[17] Upon clinical examination, the examiner may note crepitus of the DRUJ during active supination and ulnar deviation. The patient may experience pain in the region of the DRUJ, with dorsopalmar translation of the distal ulna. As a provocative test, the examiner can fix the patient's wrist in ulnar deviation while rotating the forearm between pronation and supination. A click may indicate a tear of the TFCC, which is interposed between the carpus and the ulnar head. If the injury is advanced, and osteoarthritis has caused deterioration of the sigmoid notch, the patient may experience pain when lateral force is applied to the ulna (compressing it into the radius). The stability of the DRUJ should also be assessed.

Numerous modalities are useful in evaluating the location of injury within the TFCC. Triple-injection wrist arthrography is particularly valuable in detecting Palmer class 1D lesions.[18,19] With this procedure, 5 to 10 ml of contrast agent is injected into the ulnar aspect of the wrist, tangent to the triquetrum, under continuous radiographic visualization. This allows examination of the distribution and flow of contrast through the wrist (Figure 4.6).

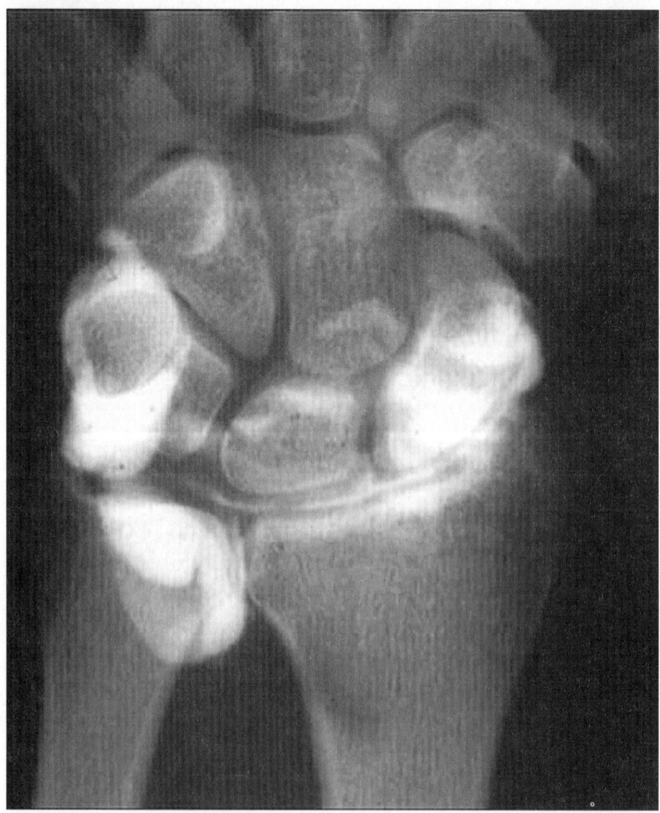

FIGURE 4.6. An arthrogram of the wrist. Injection of contrast tangent to the triquetrum under continuous radiography allows visualization of contrast flow through a tear in the TFCC.

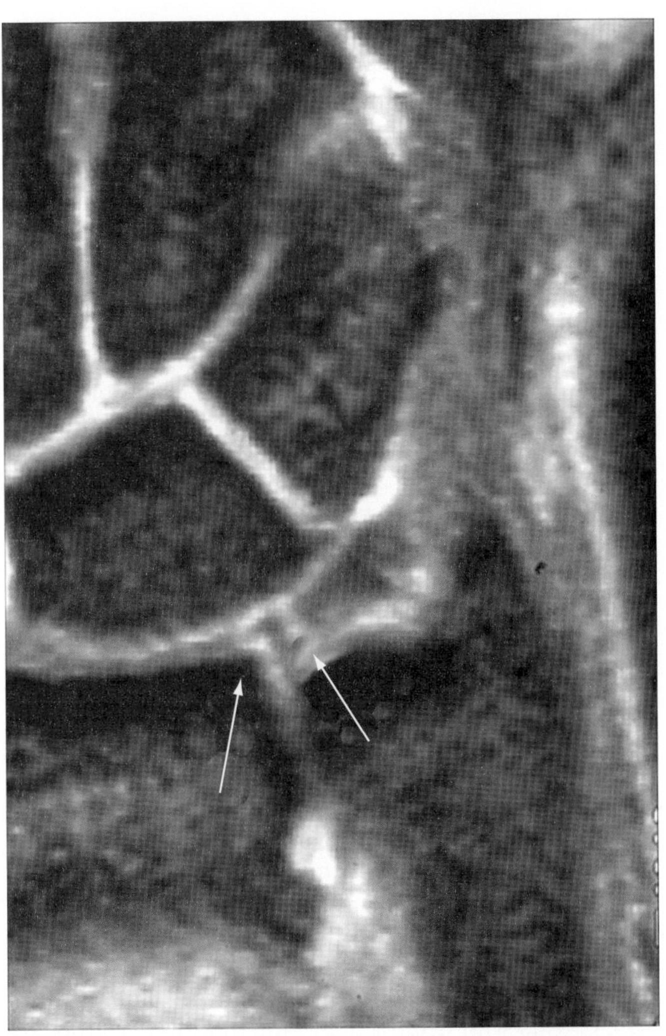

FIGURE 4.7. MRI of the wrist. A T2-weighted coronal image shows a tear at the radial attachment of the TFCC.

MRI has become the most widely utilized imaging modality for the evaluation of TFCC injuries.[20,21] Using dedicated small-joint wrist coils, MRI predicts lesions of the TFCC with approximately 80% sensitivity and 70% specificity.[22] Fat suppression T2-weighted images in the coronal plane can best elucidate the precise anatomical details of the TFCC. MRI has the capacity to localize lesions to the central part of the disc, the periphery, and the radial insertion (Figure 4.7). This specificity can aid in the surgical planning for the treatment of such lesions.

Wrist arthroscopy has recently become the criterion standard for both diagnosing and treating lesions of the TFCC. When compared to MRI and arthrography, arthroscopy most accurately determines the location of lesions and the size of tears. It also allows determination of whether a flap is unstable.[23,24] Scar and vascular invasion along the periphery of the TFCC, as well as tears within the lunotriquetral interosseous ligament or ECU subsheath, indicates injury. Specifically, a trampoline test is positive when the surgeon's probe fails to bounce off the TFCC, indicating laxity of the disc and the presence of a tear (Figure 4.8).[25] It is important to note, however, that laxity of the TFCC does not necessarily translate into instability of the DRUJ.[26]

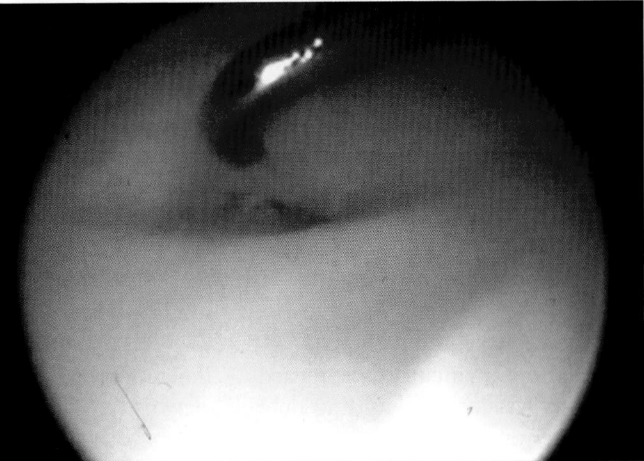

FIGURE 4.8. Arthroscopy of the wrist. A trampoline test is positive when the surgeon's probe fails to bounce off the TFCC, indicating laxity of the disc and the presence of a tear.

Surgical Treatment of Radial-Sided TFCC Lesions

The anatomy and patterns of injury to the TFCC are well elucidated. Efforts now focus on the optimal treatment of different types of lesions. With recent advances in small-joint arthroscopy, arthroscopic debridement and repair of TFCC lesions are now possible. Historically, treatment of most tears of the TFCC (particularly those involving the avascular horizontal disc) emphasized debridement or excision.[14,27,28] This practice stemmed from two important principles. First, the variable vascular perfusion to the different regions of the TFCC was thought to create a suboptimal biologic environment for the healing of repairs. This is known to be especially true in the central portion of the disc, where vascular penetration is negligible.[6,8,9]

Several investigators also questioned whether there was significant penetration of vessels in the radial aspect of the TFCC, and proposed that class 1D lesions be treated in a similar fashion to central lesions (with debridement).[6] Second, biomechanical studies of the stability of the horizontal disc showed that no significant kinematic or structural changes result if debridement involves less than two-thirds of the disc and spares the peripheral 2 mm of the disc.[5]

Currently, the optimal treatment for radial-sided avulsions of the TFCC is a subject of considerable controversy. When compared to arthroscopic repair, the advantages of arthroscopic debridement include decreased operative time, decreased recovery time (with a shorter period of immobilization), fewer complications, and better range of motion.[14]

We have previously shown that in 52 patients arthroscopic debridement of TFCC tears provided complete relief of pain in 73%. Of these lesions, 34% were radial-sided tears. Our technique consisted of using small pituitary rongeurs or punches, as well motorized shavers to debride the defect edges. We noted no clinical ulnar wrist instability in follow-up. Similar outcomes were recently reported by Husby and Haugstvedt, who demonstrated excellent clinical outcomes after arthroscopic debridement of central and radial TFCC tears (with high patient satisfaction and no complications).[29]

Despite convincing data regarding the functional outcomes in patients undergoing debridement of radial-sided TFCC lesions, further research has emphasized the importance of the peripheral attachments of the TFCC in stabilizing the distal radioulnar joint. These attachments also provide support for the ulnocarpal joint.[4,11] This observation has led several investigators to advocate repair of certain peripheral TFCC tears in order to increase stability.[25,30,31] A number of techniques for reattachment of class 1B and 1C TFCC tears have been described with positive clinical results, confirming the ability of lesions in these regions to heal. The optimal treatment of radial-sided class 1D lesions remains controversial.

It is uncommon for a class 1D tear to cause instability of the DRUJ in the absence of a distal radius fracture, which is the most common cause of DRUJ instability.[26] The examiner should examine the volar and dorsal aspects of the wrist and forearm for swelling and symmetry with the other wrist. Increased anteroposterior translation of the ulna on the radius during passive movement of the DRUJ when compared to the contralateral side provides evidence for instability.[32] A provocative maneuver for DRUJ instability can be performed by depressing the patient's distal ulna from dorsal to volar with the wrist in pronation. A positive piano-key sign is characterized by volar laxity of the ulnar head in the affected wrist when compared with the contralateral wrist.

In the setting of a distal radius fracture with concomitant DRUJ instability, accurate fracture reduction and maintenance of the reduction are imperative for healing of the disrupted joint.[33] After reduction of a distal radius fracture, it is important to test the stability of the DRUJ. The secondary stabilizers of the DRUJ (namely, the ulnocarpal ligaments, ECU subsheath, interosseous membrane, and lunotriquetral interosseous ligament) typically maintain sufficient stability of the joint to allow healing after fracture reduction.[34] If, however, a radial TFCC tear is identified during the arthroscopic treatment of a distal radius fracture securing the radial side of the disc to the sigmoid notch using a 0.035-inch Kirschner wire will typically promote healing of the radial attachment. Severe or bidirectional DRUJ instability that persists after fracture reduction and fixation indicates that the secondary stabilizers of the DRUJ, including the TFCC, have been progressively injured and may be contributing to joint instability. In this situation, open repair of the TFCC may be indicated.

Repairing the torn TFCC to the sigmoid notch of the radius has been described using both open and arthroscopic approaches. Cooney described a technique for an open suture repair of peripheral lesions through a dorsal approach (Figure 4.9).[35] Thirty-three patients with peripheral rim tears *not* associated with instability of DRUJ joint underwent open repair, combined with debridement of the ulnar border of the radius to promote vascular ingrowth. He reported good to excellent results in 80% of the patients. At two-year follow-up, MRI showed continuity of the repair in a small subgroup of patients within the series.

Miniami coupled open reattachment of peripheral TFCC tears with hemiresection-interposition arthroplasty of the DRUJ to avoid impingement of the ulnar head against the reconstructed disc. He reported complete relief of pain in 63% of patients.[31]

Numerous arthroscopic techniques have subsequently been described for radial-sided TFCC lesions. Jantea reported a series of 12 patients with radial-sided TFCC

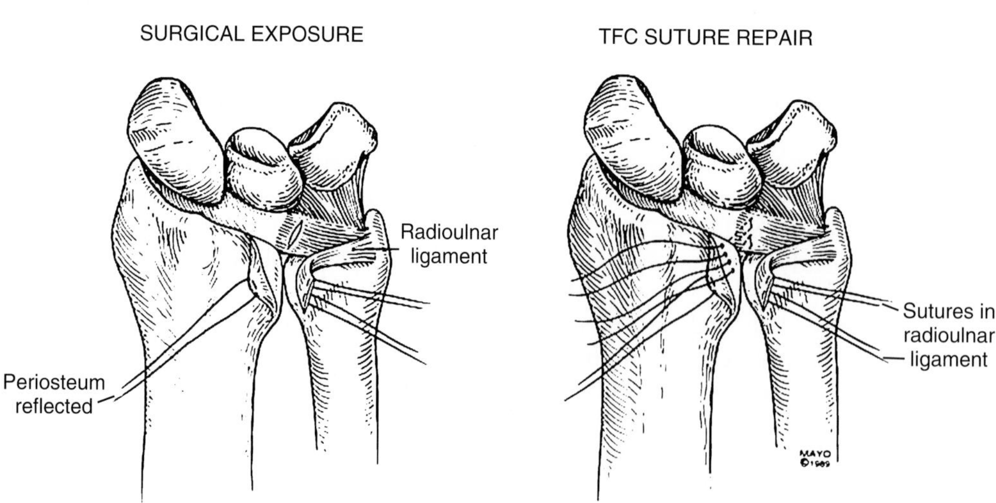

FIGURE 4.9. Repair of a class 1D injury using an open, dorsal approach and placement of transosseus sutures. *(Reproduced with permission by Cooney WP, Linscheid RL, et al. Triangular fibrocartilage tears. J Hand Surg [Am] 1994;19:143–54.)*

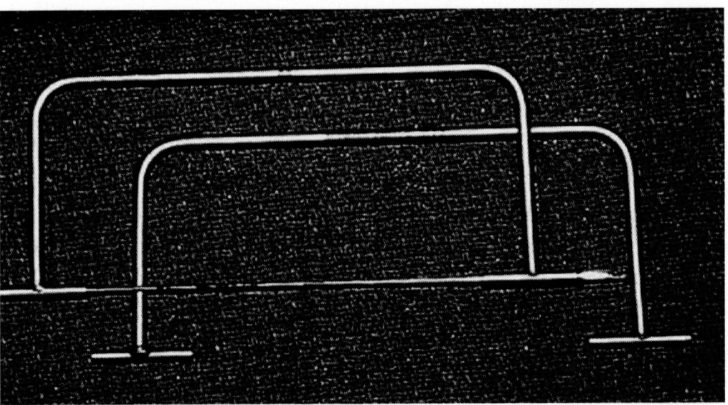

FIGURE 4.10. Jantea's arthroscopic technique utilizes rectangular wire guides mounted on the dorsal wrist to allow accurate underpinning of the TFCC tear.

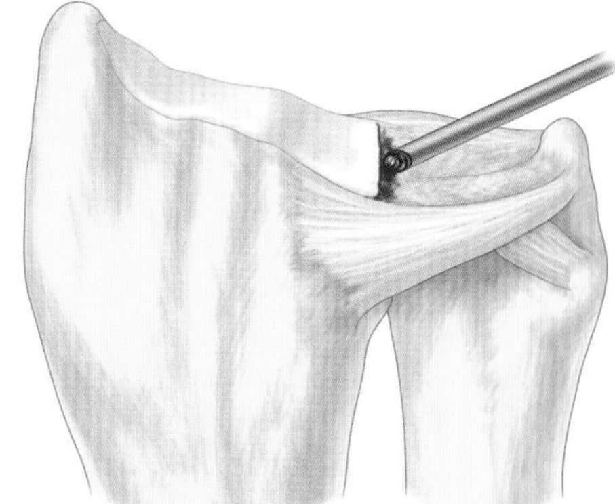

FIGURE 4.11. Burring of the attachment site along the sigmoid notch of the radius to bleeding bone introduces additional vascularity and promotes wound healing. *(Adapted from Sagerman SD, Short W. Arthroscopic repair of radial-sided triangular fibrocartilage complex tears. Arthroscopy 1996;12(3):339–42.)*

tears who underwent arthroscopic repair by means of transosseus sutures.[36] His technique involves using a rectangular guiding device mounted on the dorsal wrist, which allows accurate underpinning of the TFCC tear (Figure 4.10). A 0.045-inch Kirschner wire is first inserted through the ulnar wrist in the interval between the ECU and FCU tendons. The wire exits at the point on the sigmoid notch where the TFCC inserts. A small skin incision is made on the radial side of the wrist between the first and second compartment, carefully avoiding injury to the superficial branch of the radial nerve, the radial artery, and the extensor tendons.

The dorsally placed jig fits over the K-wire and guides the placement of a second K-wire through the radius, exiting at the TFCC insertion point on the sigmoid notch. This process is repeated so that two parallel drill holes are made through the radius, with exit points at the TFCC insertion. Eighteen-gauge spinal needles are introduced through the parallel drill holes through the radius and the trocars are removed. Absorbable monofilament suture is inserted through one needle and retrieved with a wire loop suture retriever through the second needle. The suture is tied on the radial aspect of the distal radius. The repair is inspected arthroscopically and additional sutures are placed if reinforcement of the repair is required. Among Jantea's 12 patients, one required another operation with an open procedure due to persistent pain, and three experienced temporary neuropraxia of the sensory branches of the ulnar nerve. Short-term follow-up showed 11 patients to be pain free after their arthroscopic repair.

Trumble described an alternative technique that employs a cannula and preloaded meniscal repair needle instead of a wire guide.[37] In his series, which emphasized repair of class 1D lesions, postoperative range of motion and grip strength averaged greater than 80% compared to the contralateral side. Follow-up studies showed that repairs were intact in 12 out of 15 patients.

Sagerman and Short treated 14 patients with class 1D TFCC tears with arthroscopic reattachment in a similar fashion using a direct suture technique.[38] In accordance with Chidgey's theory that introducing additional vascularity to the radial attachment of the TFCC improves healing, the authors emphasized the use of a motorized bur to abrade the edge of the sigmoid notch (Figure 4.11) before reconnecting the radial attachment (Figure 4.12).[1] Follow-up yielded 67% of patients with good or excellent clinical results.

Fellinger described repair of the torn disc to the radial sigmoid notch using a T-Fix device (Acufex).[39] With this procedure, a K-wire is passed from distal to proximal through an ulnar skin incision and into the sigmoid notch under arthroscopic guidance. The wire is advanced until it reaches the opposite radial cortex, which is then over-reamed using a cannulated 2.5-mm drill. Through a separate radial-sided skin incision, the T-Fix device is inserted into the canal until the tip reaches the sigmoid notch.

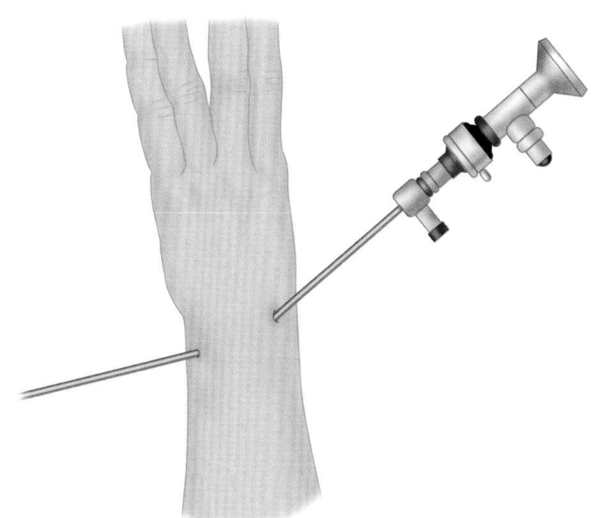

FIGURE 4.12. Arthroscopic repair of a 1D radial TFCC tear using cannulated suture needles.

Using arthroscopic guidance and assistance, the base of the disc is perforated with the tip of the application device.

The mandrel then pushes out to deploy a T-shaped anchor into the sigmoid notch, which reattaches the disc into its insertion point. The mandrel and application device are then retracted. The anchor is sutured to the periosteum through a small radial-sided skin incision and the repair is inspected arthroscopically. Among the 26 patients in this series, three were found to have class 1D lesions These were treated with the T-Fix anchor. An arthrogram performed at six weeks showed no contrast leakage, which suggested that these tears have the potential to heal.

Personal Series

We performed a retrospective study of 19 patients with Palmer class 1D TFCC lesions between 1999 and 2001 to compare the clinical outcomes after reattachment of the disc versus debridement. Patients were excluded from the study if their TFCC injuries were acute, or if they had concomitant intra-articular distal radius fractures. In addition, patients were excluded from the study if they were found to have other wrist pathology requiring surgical repair (with the exception of ulnar-sided TFCC tears). Of the 19 patients who were treated surgically, 10 underwent debridement and 9 underwent repair.

In the debridement group, the average age was 30 years (age ranged between 16 and 44 years). Of these, 60% were male and 40% were female. Eighty percent reported a history of trauma to the affected wrist. The average duration of symptoms was 11 months. Twenty percent had associated non-articular distal radius fractures, 80% reported ulnar-sided wrist pain, and 60% of the patients had involvement of their dominant hand. Upon physical examination, 60% had a notable click but none had instability of the DRUJ. Imaging studies revealed an ulnar positive variance in one patient, ulnar neutral variance in six patients, and ulnar negative variance in three patients. MRI was positive for a class 1D lesion in 90%. Intraoperatively, 100% of patients in the group were found to have a class 1D tear, 30% had a concomitant ulnar-sided tear, 10% had a perforation of the scapholunate ligament, and 40% were noted to have chondromalacia.

In the repair group, the average age was 28 years (age ranged between 17 and 38 years). Of these, 55% were male and 45% were female. Eighty-eight percent reported a history of trauma to the involved wrist, and 77% complained of ulnar-sided wrist pain and were symptomatic for an average of 9 months. Twenty-two percent had associated distal radius fractures and 66% had injured their dominant hand. Upon physical examination, a click was observed in 66% and no patients had instability of the DRUJ. Imaging studies showed an ulnar positive variance in two patients, ulnar neutral variance in five patients, and ulnar negative variance in two patients. MRI was positive for a class 1D lesion in 100% of patients in this group. Intraoperatively, a radial-sided tear was confirmed in 100% of patients. A concomitant ulnar-sided tear was noted in 22%, 11% had perforation of the lunotriquetral ligament, and 33% were found to have chondromalacia.

Five patients underwent an in-out suture repair similar to that described by Short and Sagerman. Three patients were treated with a repair similar to that described by Jantea, utilizing a jig type of pin-guiding device (Figure 4.10). Three patients underwent repair with the T-Fix bone anchor device, as described by Fellinger. Regardless of the technique employed, all repairs utilized 2–0 PDS suture on meniscal needles. The suture limbs were tied over a bone bridge on the radial aspect of the distal radius (Figure 4.13). In addition, in order to promote vascular in-growth to the radial portion of the disc the sigmoid notch was abraded with a bur before the ligament was reattached in each of the repairs (Figure 4.11).

In both the debridement and the repair group, all ulnar-sided lesions were repaired. The average total operative time was 92 minutes for the repair group, compared to 43 minutes for the debridement group. The postoperative protocol for the debridement group included splinting for one week, followed by free wrist range of motion thereafter.

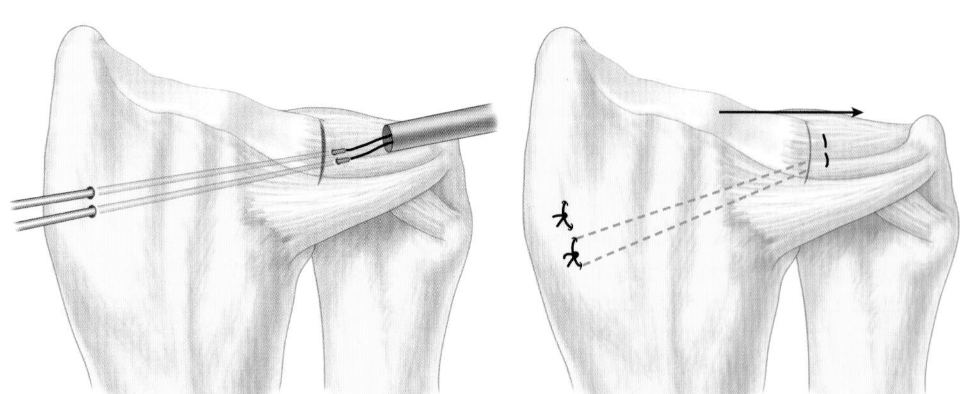

FIGURE 4.13. Class 1D TFCC tears are repaired with suture on meniscal needles, tied over a bone bridge on the radial aspect of the distal radius.

Sixty percent of patients participated in formal hand therapy, and the average time to return to work was seven weeks. In contrast, the patients who underwent repair were kept immobilized for three weeks. One hundred percent of patients in this group participated in formal hand therapy, and the average time to return to work was 16 weeks.

The average follow-up for the debridement group was 4.2 years, with 100% of patients expressing satisfaction with the procedure. Grip strength measured 87% compared to the contralateral hand, and wrist range of motion reached 95% of pre-injury levels. No complications were reported in the debridement group. Based on the Mayo wrist scores, 80% of patients in the debridement group had good to excellent results (with an average score of 85.5%). In the repair group, the average follow-up time was 3.9 years.

Sixty-seven percent of patients in the repair group had good to excellent results. Postoperatively, three patients (33%) complained of transient nerve irritation—two in the region of the radial sensory nerve and one in the region of the ulnar sensory nerve. One patient (11%) also suffered from prolonged wrist stiffness despite physical therapy. Seven patients (78%) expressed satisfaction with the procedure. Grip strength measured 91% compared to the uninjured hand, and range of motion averaged 87% of pre-injury levels.

This study, which focuses specifically on the treatment of class 1D TFCC lesions, provides data that suggests that debridement is equally effective as repair in alleviating wrist pain—improving grip strength and restoring range of motion. Debridement is simple, with a short operative time. Functional return is more rapid with debridement of the disc, with less complication compared to reattachment. We therefore now advocate debridement rather than repair of isolated radial-sided lesions of the TFCC.

Author's Preferred Technique

For radial-sided tears of the TFCC, the first issue to address is whether the DRUJ is stable or unstable. If the DRUJ is stable, the next factor in determining the appropriate treatment of a class 1D TFCC lesion is the acuity of the injury. The treatment of most acute TFCC injuries is nonsurgical, and involves immobilization for four weeks. However, if wrist pain persists after a trial of conservative measures (including a period of immobilization, rest, and anti-inflammatory medication) further studies (such as MRI, arthrography, or arthroscopic surgery) are indicated for proven or suspected TFCC injury.

When an isolated radial-sided TFCC tear exists with a stable DRUJ, debridement of the lesion is a simple procedure that removes the reactive tissue and allows early return of wrist motion and function. Under regional anesthesia, the patent's wrist is reexamined to confirm stability of the DRUJ and to identify abnormal clicking or ECU subluxation. A well-padded pneumatic tourniquet is applied to the upper arm, and the wrist is placed in traction using a standard traction tower set to 12 pounds (Figure 4.14). After gravity exsanguination of the limb, the tourniquet is inflated to 250 mmHg. A standard 3-/,4 portal is made using a #11 scalpel. The subcutaneous tissues are dissected down to the level of the joint capsule using a small curved clamp in order to protect the branches of the radial sensory nerve. A small capsulotomy is performed, and a 30-degree 2.3-mm-diameter arthroscope is inserted into the portal.

Initially, the radial side of the wrist is systematically examined. The arthroscope is then directed ulnarly to evaluate the entire TFCC. Once a class 1D lesion is confirmed, the ulnar portal is placed (typically in the 6-R location)—being mindful to avoid injury to the sensory branch of the ulnar nerve (Figure 4.12). Through this portal a small arthroscopic probe is inserted to assess the stability of the torn flap and the TFCC tension. A 3.5 motorized suction shaver is then inserted and used to debride any synovitis and to smooth the edges of the defect. Unstable flaps are resected using small-joint suction punches. Once the lesion is debrided, the midcarpal joint is inspected.

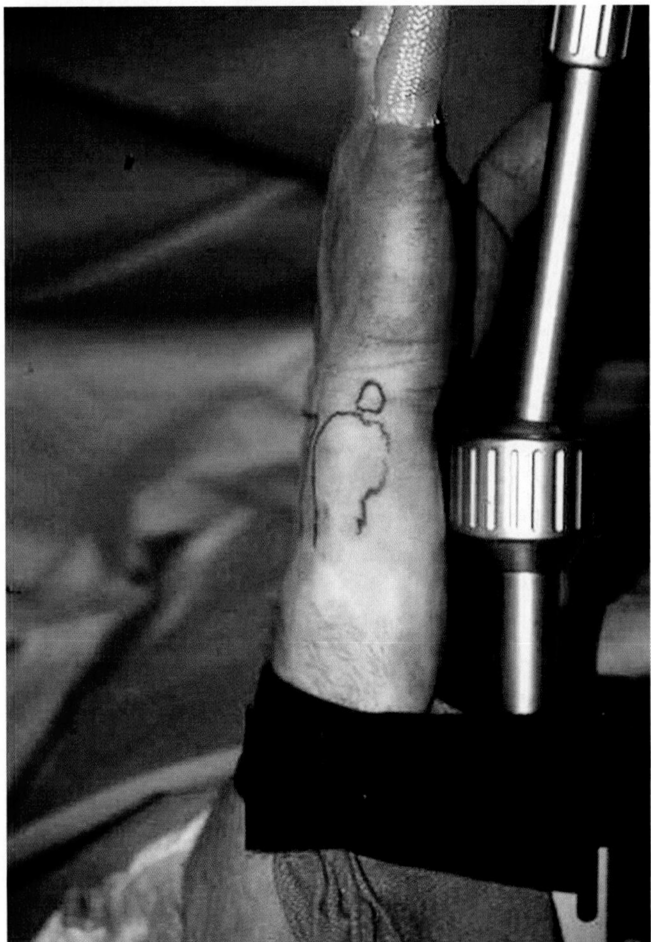

FIGURE 4.14. A standard arthroscopy set-up: Index and long fingers are placed in finger traps and the wrist is placed in a traction tower set to 12 pounds.

Once the arthroscopic procedure is complete, the wrist is reexamined under anesthesia. The clicks that were noted previously have typically resolved. The portal sites are then closed with a single suture using 4–0 nylon, and a splint is applied. The splint is worn continuously for the first week to support the wrist, and then worn intermittently for an additional three weeks while the patient avoids repetitive rotatory wrist activity or forceful grasping. The critical points are summarized in Table 4.2.

Table 4.2.

Critical Points: Arthroscopic Debridement of Isolated Class 1D TFCC Tears

Indications

- Class 1D radial-sided TFCC tears in patient of any age with negative, neutral, or positive ulnar variance
- Class 1D TFCC tears associated with distal radius fractures
- Failure of ulnar-sided wrist pain to resolve after a trial of nonoperative treatment, including immobilization, splinting, and anti-inflammatory medication

Contraindications

- Concomitant DRUJ instability
- Acute injury, less than 2 months old
- Sigmoid notch fracture

Preoperative Evaluation

- History of fall onto outstretched, pronated wrist
- Ulnar-sided wrist pain with clicking, positive TFCC compression test
- Documented stability of the DRUJ upon exam, with a negative piano key sign
- Arthrography or MRI evidence of class 1D tear (not necessary for procedure)

Technical Pearls

- Debride edges and unstable flaps with full-radius shaver
- Probe to confirm debridement to a stable rim of TFCC
- Reexamine DRUJ stability and wrist range of motion at end of procedure

Pitfalls

- Failure to recognize concomitant DRUJ instability

Postoperative Care

- One week of continuous splinting
- Three additional weeks of intermittent splinting
- Avoidance of repetitive rotatory wrist motion or forceful grasping for four weeks

Controversies

The results of arthroscopic reattachment of isolated radial-sided TFCC lesions have been promising. Despite studies suggesting hypovascularity of the radial aspect of the TFCC, vascular in-growth and/or synovial fluid diffusion presumably provide adequate nutritional support to allow 1D lesions of the TFCC to heal. Clearly, arthroscopic repair of TFCC tears has the potential to offer advantages—including increased stability of the DRUJ. This is especially true for class 1B and 1C lesions. Many techniques have been described for arthroscopic repair of class 1D lesions, with promising short-term results.[20,36–38,40] Few long-term results, however, are available from these studies. In addition, further studies are necessary to clarify the optimal suture technique and the size, number, and placement of sutures.

Whether the outcomes after arthroscopic reattachment of class 1D lesions are superior to those following simple debridement has yet to be proven. A retrospective study by Miwa of 62 wrists treated with either arthroscopic debridement or repair of TFCC lesions showed no statistically significant difference in clinical outcomes between the debridement group and the repair group in any class, including class 1D lesions.[41] These results are similar to those from our own series, suggesting that debridement remains a simple and effective means of treating radial-sided TFCC tears.

Arthroscopic debridement of class 1D lesions offers the advantages of being technically simple and safe, with a low potential for complications and short operative time. Long-term data suggests that DRUJ stability is not compromised after disc debridement, which calls into question the theoretical advantage of repair.[29] Furthermore, if arthroscopic debridement is unsuccessful in relieving pain or providing stability it does not preclude a future repair.

References

1. Chidgey LK, Dell PC, Bittar ES, Spanier SS. Histologic anatomy of the triangular fibrocartilage. J Hand Surg [Am] 1991;16(6):1084–100.
2. Kauer JMG. The articular disc of the hand. Acta Anat 1975;93:590–605.
3. Palmer AK, Glisson RR, Werner FW. Relationship between ulnar variance and TFCC thickness. J Hand Surg [Am] 1984;9:681–83.
4. Palmer AK, Werner FW. The triangular fibrocartilage complex of the wrist: Anatomy and function. J Hand Surg [Am] 1981;6:153–62.
5. Adams BD. Partial excision of the triangular fibrocartilage complex articular disk: A biomechanical study. J Hand Surg [Am] 1993;18:334–40.
6. Bednar MS, Arnoczky SP, Weiland AJ. The microvasculature of the triangular fibrocartilage complex: Its clinical significance. J Hand Surg [Am] 1991;16(6):1101–05.
7. Osterman AL, Hunt TR, Bednar JM, Bozentka DJ. Vascularity of the triangular fibrocartilage as measured in vivo.

Presented at the 49th annual meeting of the American Society for Surgery of the Hand, Cincinnati, OH, 1994.
8. Mikic ZD. Age changes in the triangular fibrocartilage of the wrist joint. J Anat 1978;126(2):367–84.
9. Thiru-Pathi RG, Ferlic DC, Clayton ML, McClure DC. Arterial anatomy of the triangular fibrocartilage of the wrist and its surgical significance. J Hand Surgery [Am] 1986; 11:258–63.
10. Melone CP, Nathan R. Traumatic disruption of the triangular fibrocartilage complex. Clin Orthop 1992;275:65–73.
11. Palmer AK. Triangular fibrocartilage complex lesions: A classification. J Hand Surg [Am] 1989;14:594–606.
12. Viegas SF, Ballantyne G. Attritional lesions of the wrist joint. J Hand Surg [Am] 1987;12:1025–29.
13. Culp R, Osterman L, Kaufmann R. Wrist arthroscopy: Operative procedures. In D Green, R Hotchkis, W. Pederson, S. Wolfe (eds.), *Green's Operative Hand Surgery, Fifth Edition*. Philadelphia: Elsevier 2005;786.
14. Osterman AL. Arthroscopic debridement of triangular fibrocartilage complex tears. Arthoscopy 1990;6:120–24.
15. Osterman AL, Terrill RG. Arthroscopic treatment of TFCC lesions. Hand Clinics 1991;7:277–81.
16. Terrill RQ. Use of arthroscopy in the evaluation and treatment of chronic wrist pain. Hand Clinics 1994;10:593–604.
17. Lindau T, Arner M, Hagberg L. Intraarticular lesions in distal fractures of the radius in young adults: A descriptive arthroscopic study in 50 patients. J Hand Surg [Br] 1997; 22B:638–43.
18. Levinsohn EM, Rosen ID, Palmer AK. Wrist arthrography: Value of the three compartment injection method. Radiology 1991;179:231–39.
19. Zinberg EM, Palmer AK, Coren AB, Levinsohn EM. The triple injection wrist arthrogram. J Hand Surg [Am] 1988; 13:803–09.
20. Giovagnoni A, Misericordia M, Terrilli F, et al. Magnetic resonance in the diagnosis of lesions of the carpal triangular fibrocartilage: The experience with 49 patients with chronic pain at the wrist. Radiol Med (Torino) 1993;85:12–16.
21. Oneson SR, Timins ME, Scales LM, et al. MR imaging diagnosis of triangular fibrocartilage pathology with arthroscopic correlation. Am J Roentgenol 1997;168:1513–18.
22. Nakamura T, Yabe Y, Horiuchi Y. Fat suppression magnetic resonance imaging of the triangular fibrocartilage complex: Comparison with spin echo, gradient echo pulse sequences and histology. J Hand Surg [Br] 1999;24(1):22–26.
23. Pederzini L, Luchetti R, Soragni O, et al. Evaluation of the triangular fibrocartilage complex tears by arthroscopy, arthrography, and magnetic resonance imaging. Arthroscopy 1992;8:191–97.
24. Weiss APC, Akelman E, Lambiase R. Comparison of the findings of triple injection cine-arthrography of the wrist with those of arthroscopy. J Bone Joint Surg Am 1996; 78:348–56.
25. Hermansdorfer JD, Kleinman WB. Management of chronic peripheral tears of the triangular fibrocartilage complex. J Hand Surg [Am] 1991;16:340–46.
26. Adams BD. Distal radioulnar instability. In D Green, R Hotchkis, W. Pederson, S. Wolfe (eds.), *Green's Operative Hand Surgery, Fifth Edition*. Philadelphia: Elsevier 2005;612–16.
27. Imbriglia JE, Boland DS. Tears of the articular disc of the triangular fibrocartilage complex: Results of excision of the articular disc. J Hand Surg [Am] 1984;9:527–30.
28. Menon J, Wood VE, Schoene HR, Frykman GK, Hohl JC, Bestard EA. Isolated tears of the triangular fibrocartilage of the wrist: Results of partial excision. J Hand Surg [Am] 1984;9(4):527–30.
29. Husby T, Haugstvedt JR. Long-term results after arthroscopic resection of lesions of the triangular fibrocartilage complex. Scand J Plast Reconstr Hand Surg 2001;35:79–83.
30. Nagle DJ, Benson LS. Wrist arthroscopy: Indications and results. Arthroscopy 1992;8(2):198–203.
31. Minami A, Kaneda K, Itoga H. Hemiresection-interposition arthroplasty of the distal radioulnar joint associated with repair of triangular fibrocartilage complex lesions. J Hand Surg [Am] 1991;16(6):1120–25.
32. Morrissy RT, Nalebuff EA. Dislocation of the distal radioulnar joint: Anatomy and clues to prompt diagnosis. Clin Orthop 1979;144:154–58.
33. Ekenstam F, Jakobsson OP, et al. Repair of the triangular ligament in Colles' fracture: No effect in a prospective randomized study. Acta Orthop Scand 1989;60:393–96.
34. Pardubsky P, Adams BD. The distal radioulnar joint in fracture of the wrist. Tech Orthop 2000;15:353–58.
35. Cooney WP, Linscheid RL, et al. Triangular fibrocartilage tears. J Hand Surg [Am] 1994;19:143–54.
36. Jantea CJ, Baltazar A, Ruther W. Arthroscopic repair of radial-sided lesions of the fibrocartilage complex. Hand Clinics 1995;11(1):31–36.
37. Trumble TE, Gilbert M, Vedder N. Arthroscopic repair of the triangular fibrocartilage complex. Arthroscopy 1996; 12(5):588–97.
38. Sagerman SD, Short W. Arthroscopic repair of radial-sided triangular fibrocartilage complex tears. Arthroscopy 1996; 12(3):339–42.
39. Fellinger M, Peicha G, Seibert FJ, Grechenig W. Radial avulsion of the triangular fibrocartilage complex in acute wrist trauma: A new technique for arthroscopic repair. Arthroscopy 1997;13(3):370–74.
40. Trumble TE, Gilbert M, et al. Ulnar shortening combined with arthroscopic repairs in the delayed management of triangular fibrocartilage complex tears. J Hand Surg [Am] 1997;22:807–13.
41. Miwa H, Hashizume H, Fujiwara K, Nishida K, Inoue H. Arthroscopic surgery for traumatic triangular fibrocartilage complex injury. J Orthop Sci 2004;9(4):354–59.

Thomas E. Trumble and
Seth D. Dodds

CHAPTER 5

We hope that this text emphasizes the value of being prepared. The experienced surgeon checks that all the necessary equipment and implants are available and functioning.

Peripheral Tears of the TFCC: Arthroscopic Diagnosis and Management

Introduction

Ulnar-sided wrist pain is a common disorder that encompasses a broad range of diagnoses. One cause of ulnar-sided wrist pain can be triangular fibrocartilage complex (TFCC) trauma. The TFCC and its supporting ligaments suspend the ulnar carpus, bear carpal load through the wrist to the ulna, and permit the carpus and radius to rotate as a unit around the axis of the ulna.

Because the TFCC plays a vital role in normal wrist function, any injury that does not heal on its own can lead to pain, stiffness, loss of strength, and significant patient dissatisfaction. The TFCC is frequently compared to the menisci of the knee because they have similar biomechanical roles, biochemical composition, diminished blood supply, and poor intrinsic healing capacity. As in the meniscus, peripheral tears of the TFCC are more amenable to healing after repair than central lesions due to a greater peripheral blood supply. Arthroscopic repair techniques for peripheral tears of the TFCC have been shown to provide a successful and minimally invasive approach to a difficult problem.

Anatomy and Biomechanics

The anatomy of the triangular fibrocartilage complex (TFCC) is primarily composed of the articular disc (or triangular fibrocartilage), a meniscus homologue, dorsal and volar radioulnar ligaments, the extensor carpi ulnaris (ECU) tendon subsheath, and the ulnocarpal ligaments (ulnolunate, ulnotriquetral, and ulnocapitate)—as depicted in Figures 5.1 and 5.2. The triangular fibrocartilage is a meniscus-like structure composed predominantly of type I collagen. Surrounding the periphery of the triangular fibrocartilage is the meniscal homologue, a fibrocartilaginous rim of dense irregular connective tissue that confluences with the dorsal and volar radioulnar ligaments.[1]

The ligaments and the triangular fibrocartilage form a three-walled structure that supports the distal radioulnar joint and ulnar portion of the carpus. The TFC, with its bordering volar and dorsal radioulnar ligaments, acts as the base of this structure. These ligaments originate as a unit from the fovea of the ulnar head and the very base of the ulnar styloid (Figure 5.3) and diverge distally into dorsal and volar stabilizers for the distal radius as it rotates around the distal ulna to achieve forearm rotation.[2] The ulnotriquetral, ulnolunate, and ulnocapitate ligaments form the volar wall of this box, and the dorsal radial triquetral ligament (along with the dorsal fibers of the ECU subsheath) forms the dorsal wall.

The dorsal ECU subsheath has Sharpey fiber connections to the ulnar head at the fovea.[2] The ulnar fibers of the ECU subsheath make up the ulnar-sided wall. The ulnotriquetral and ulnolunate ligaments along the volar wall of the TFCC have been shown to extend distally from the volar margin of the triangular fibrocartilage and the volar radioulnar ligament, rather than from the ulna itself.[2,3] This confluence of many ligaments on the ulnar aspect of the wrist stabilizes the ulnar carpus to the triangular fibrocartilage as the radius rotates around the ulna.

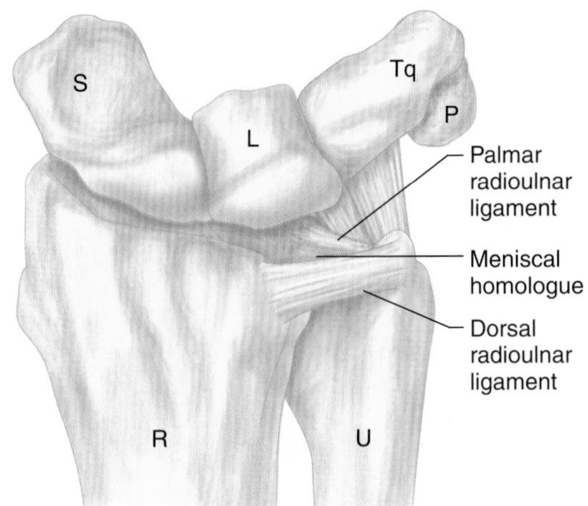

FIGURE 5.1. The distal radioulnar ligaments extend from the sigmoid notch of the distal radius to the base of the ulnar styloid. The triangular fibrocartilage is suspended between these ligaments.

The blood supply and innervation of the triangular fibrocartilage enters from the periphery.[4,5] Thiru et al. evaluated the vascular perforators to the TFCC in a cadaveric study.[6] The ulnar artery provides the blood supply to the ulnar portion of the TFCC through dorsal and palmar radiocarpal branches. This ulnar periphery of TFCC has the richest blood supply and the best potential for healing after repair. The dorsal and palmar branches of the anterior

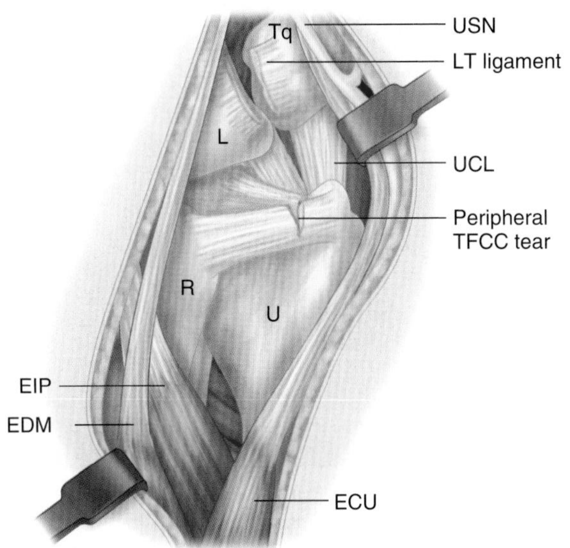

FIGURE 5.2. An open approach to the TFCC typically occurs between the fifth (extensor digiti minimi or EDM) and sixth (extensor carpi ulnaris or ECU) compartments. After flap exposure of the dorsal joint capsule overlying the DRUJ, the TFCC as well as the ulnar carpus can be visualized (USN = dorsal sensory branch of the ulnar nerve, UCL = ulnocarpal ligaments, Tq = triquetrum, L = lunate, LT = lunotriquetral, R = radius, U = ulna, EIP = extensor indicis proprius, TFCC = triangular fibrocartilage complex).

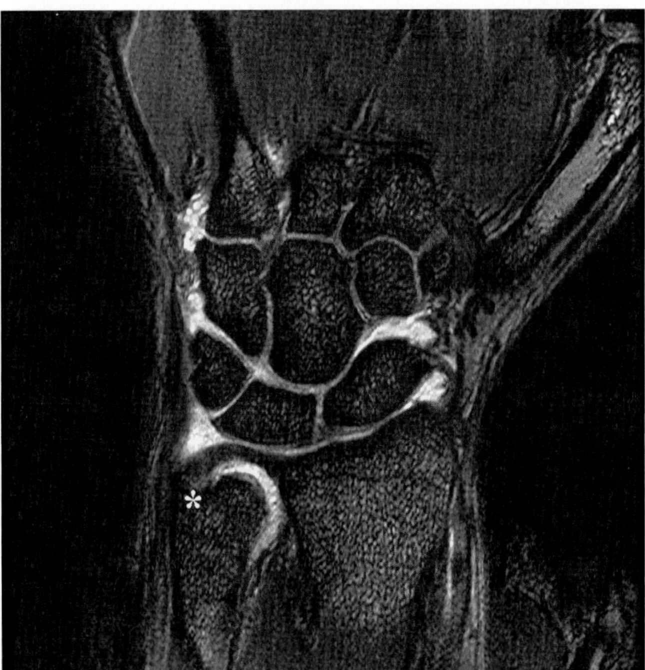

FIGURE 5.3. A normal MRI demonstrates the insertion of the distal radioulnar ligaments of the TFCC at the ulnar fovea and base of ulnar styloid (marked by the asterisk).

interosseous artery supply the more radial periphery and the attachment to the distal radius. The central portion of the TFCC is essentially avascular and is not amenable for repair. Similarly, the radial/central portion has been shown to have essentially no innervation.[7] The majority of nerve supply to the TFCC is also peripheral, with contributions from the posterior interosseous nerve, the ulnar nerve, and the dorsal sensory branch of the ulnar nerve (DSBUN).

The volar and dorsal radioulnar ligaments are the primary stabilizers of the distal radioulnar joint (DRUJ) during rotation and translation at the DRUJ. As the forearm supinates from a position of full pronation, the volar radioulnar ligament is under stress and lengthens in a viscoelastic manner to accommodate.[8,9] Pronation, from a position of full supination, causes the dorsal radioulnar ligament to be stressed and subsequently lengthen.[8,9] A majority of the load from the carpus are directed to the radius (80%), whereas the remainder (20%) is directed to the ulna through the TFCC.[10]

There continues to be dispute among authors as to the advantages of either arthroscopic or open surgery for tears of the TFCC. Significant DRUJ instability has been demonstrated with complete release of the foveal attachments of the TFCC.[11,12] In one study, the DRUJ instability was corrected with an open suture repair of the volar and dorsal radioulnar ligaments through bone tunnels to the fovea or an open version of the arthroscopic repair of the ulnar TFCC to the ECU subsheath.[12] Biomechanical testing demonstrated significant improvements in the stability of the DRUJ for both groups. However, it was noted that the weakest aspect of each repair was not the type of repair but the bioabsorbable polydioxanone suture used.

Patient Presentation

Isolated injuries to the TFCC commonly occur with extension and pronation of the axially loaded carpus, as with falling on an outstretched hand. Activities involving rapid twisting of the hand in relationship to the forearm with ulnar-sided loading (as in racquet sports or golf) may cause subluxation, dislocation, or fracture of the structures of the distal radioulnar joint and the TFCC. Patients often delay treatment or are misdiagnosed as having a "wrist sprain" that fails to get better. Symptoms of TFCC injury include ulnar-sided wrist pain characterized by a diffuse and sometimes burning deep ache that can radiate dorsally or volarly. A clicking sensation in the wrist may be experienced by the patient as the forearm is rotated and the wrist is held in ulnar deviation, as when using a key to unlock a door.

Upon physical examination, acute TFCC injuries present with ulnar-sided wrist swelling. Point tenderness occurs when palpating the ulnar side of the wrist in the ballotable region between the ulnar styloid and the triquetrum. Forearm rotation with the wrist maintained in ulnar deviation may also elicit pain or a wrist click. The TFCC compression test is positive if axial loading of the ulnar side of the hand with ulnar deviation of the wrist results in significant pain. Similarly, de Araujo et al.[13] described an ulnar impaction test that elicits pain by wrist hyperextension and ulnar deviation with axial compression. Although radiographs may not directly diagnose soft-tissue pathology in cases of suspected TFCC tears without carpal or distal radioulnar joint instability, indirect information can be obtained from the ulnar variance, the distal radioulnar joint congruency, and the presence or absence of a prior ulnar styloid or distal radius fracture.

Magnetic resonance imaging (MRI) with intra-articular gadolinium has become the imaging modality of choice for the diagnosis of soft-tissue injuries, and TFCC injuries are no exception (Figures 5.4 and 5.5). Although an MRI arthrogram may be both sensitive and specific in diagnosing a tear,[14] at this point it has not been shown to be accurate in assessing tear size. In one study, Fulcher and Poehling felt that MRI understaged some TFCC pathology and overstaged others.[15] Pederzini et al. performed arthrography, MRI, and arthroscopy on 11 patients with TFCC injuries.[16] Although these authors found 100% specificities with sensitivities of 80 and 82% for arthrography and MRI (respectively), arthroscopic visualization of a TFCC tear continues to be the gold standard for definitive diagnosis.

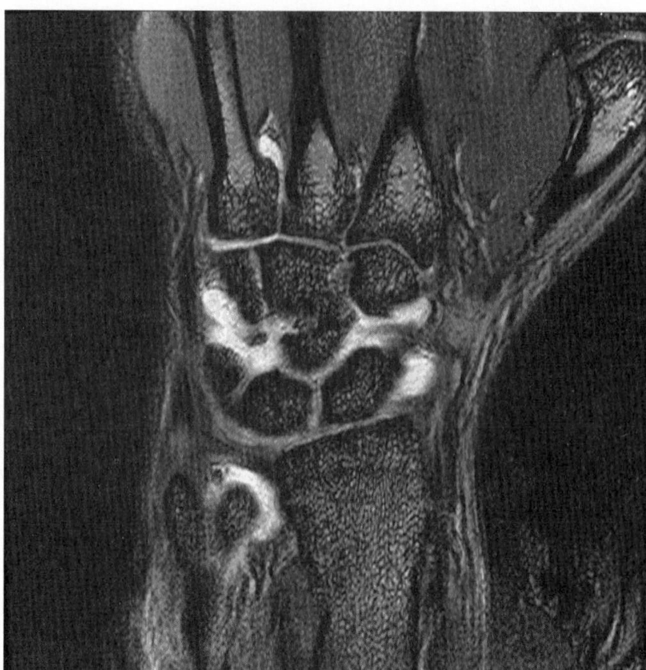

FIGURE 5.4. This coronal MRI demonstrates a normal peripheral attachment of the TFCC.

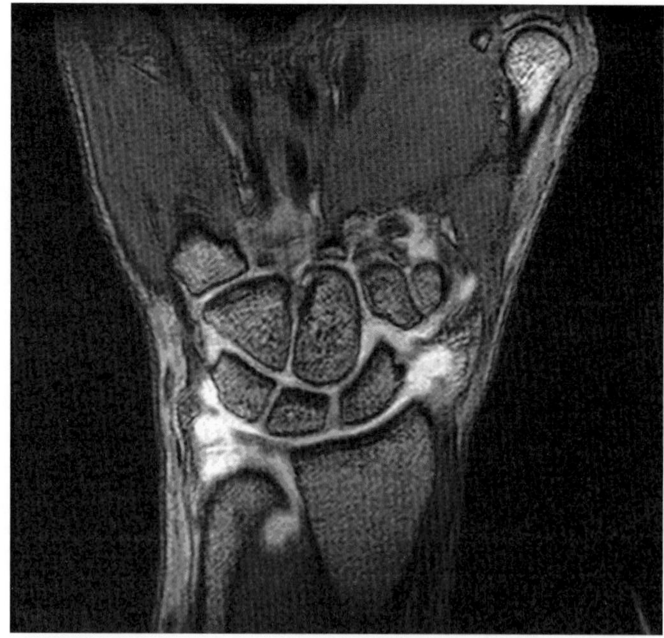

FIGURE 5.5. Here, the coronal MRI shows a tear or disruption of the peripheral TFCC at its ulnar and distal attachment, just proximal to the articular base of the triquetrum.

Classification of TFCC Injuries

Anatomic, clinical, and biomechanical investigations have led to a classification of the triangular fibrocartilage complex injuries. Originally proposed by Palmer,[17] this classification helps differentiate between traumatic and degenerative lesions. Repairable peripheral tears are generally classified as either type 1B or type 1C tears. Type 1B lesions are peripheral tears that occur as the ulnar side of the TFCC complex is avulsed from its capsule ulnar ligamentous attachments. These injuries are amenable to arthroscopic repair of the TFCC if there is no associated ulnar styloid fracture and no associated DRUJ instability. The type 1C injury involves rupture along the volar attachment of the TFCC or tears of the ulnocarpal ligaments. Type 1C tears may be amenable to repair if the ligamentous injury is vertically oriented. Arthroscopic repair of transverse or horizontally oriented tears of the ulnocarpal ligaments has not yet been described to our knowledge.

TFCC tears can be subdivided further by their time course from injury to treatment (Table 5.1).[18] Tears are classified as acute when treated within three months from the time of injury. Arthroscopic repairs of acute tears can result in the recovery of up to 85% of the contralateral grip strength and range of motion.[18] Acute injuries have a better prognosis than subacute injuries and chronic injuries.[19] Subacute tears are treated from three months to one year after injury. Although subacute tears are still amenable to direct repair, in general they tend to regain less strength and range of motion than patients with repair of acute injuries.[19] Chronic tears (more than one year) are repairable, but the results are inconsistent—presumably due to contraction of TFCC ligaments and degeneration of the torn fibrocartilage margins. Chronic injuries frequently require ulnar shortening osteotomy with or without TFCC debridement to decrease the load distributed to the ulna via the TFCC.

Indications

Whereas repair of the peripheral triangular fibrocartilage attempts to recreate the original anatomy with direct suture of a rent in the fibrocartilage or its peripheral attachment, arthroscopic repairs involve imbrication of the peripheral-most aspect of the TFCC to the neighboring wrist capsule. This imbrication restores the tautness and trampoline effect of the TFCC and thus improves the stability of the TFCC as well as the patient's symptoms, but does not precisely replicate the pre-injury anatomy. If DRUJ instability exists, only an open and direct reattachment of the foveal origin of the volar and dorsal radioulnar ligaments can reliably and completely restore stability.[20] However, patients frequently present with acute or subacute peripheral TFCC tears in the setting of a stable DRUJ. These patients are amenable to arthroscopic repair.

The specific indications for arthroscopic repair of periphery tears of the TFCC continue to evolve. If clinical assessment and diagnostic studies suggest a TFCC tear, a wrist arthroscopy is warranted for adolescent or adult patients assuming a few key prerequisites (presented in Table 5.2). The type of peripheral tear also plays a role in the indications for repair. Horizontal, oblique, and vertical tears of the periphery of the TFCC can be addressed. However, distal transverse tears involving the volar ulnocarpal ligaments (within the type 1C category) are not amenable to arthroscopic repair at this point. More proximal split tears can be repaired and these ligaments can be imbricated to augment lunotriquetral instability, as has been demonstrated by Moskal et al.[21]

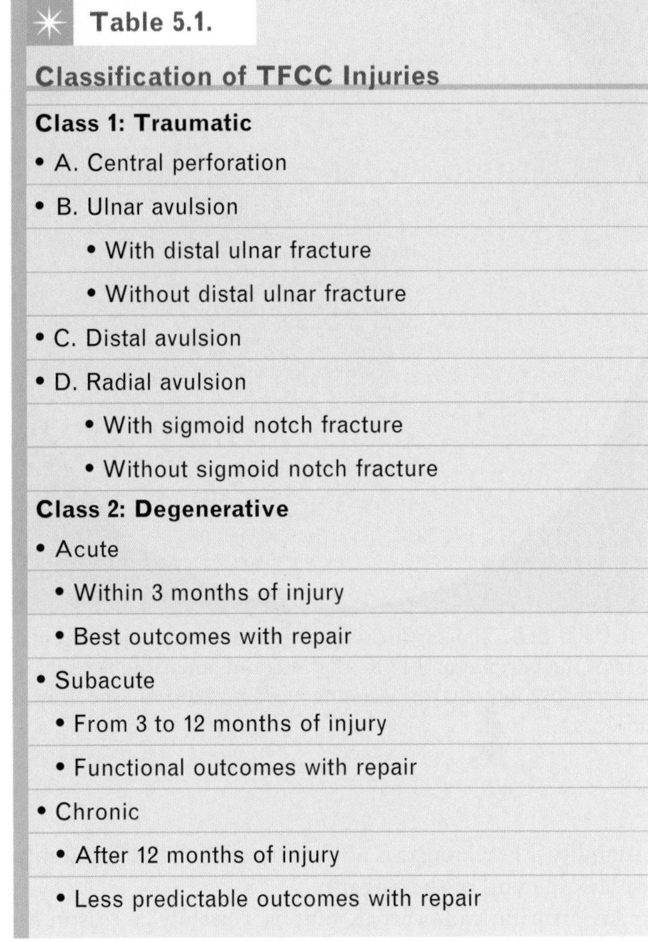

Table 5.1.

Classification of TFCC Injuries

Class 1: Traumatic
• A. Central perforation
• B. Ulnar avulsion
• With distal ulnar fracture
• Without distal ulnar fracture
• C. Distal avulsion
• D. Radial avulsion
• With sigmoid notch fracture
• Without sigmoid notch fracture
Class 2: Degenerative
• Acute
• Within 3 months of injury
• Best outcomes with repair
• Subacute
• From 3 to 12 months of injury
• Functional outcomes with repair
• Chronic
• After 12 months of injury
• Less predictable outcomes with repair

Table 5.2.

Prerequisites for Arthroscopic Repair of Peripheral TFCC Tears

• Clinical stability of the distal radioulnar joint
• Peripheral tears of the TFCC, excluding avulsions from the ulnar fovea
• No untreated fractures or malalignment of the distal radius, ulna, or carpus
• No significant symptomatic arthrosis of the radiocarpal joint

Contraindications

Contraindications to arthroscopic repair begin with DRUJ instability. If the DRUJ is unstable due to fracture or complete disruption of the distal radioulnar ligaments, fracture repair and open repair of the origin of the distal radioulnar ligaments should be considered. In chronic cases of symptomatic DRUJ instability, reconstruction of the ligamentous stabilizers of this joint is warranted. Similarly, in chronic Essex-Lopresti injuries and cases of interosseous

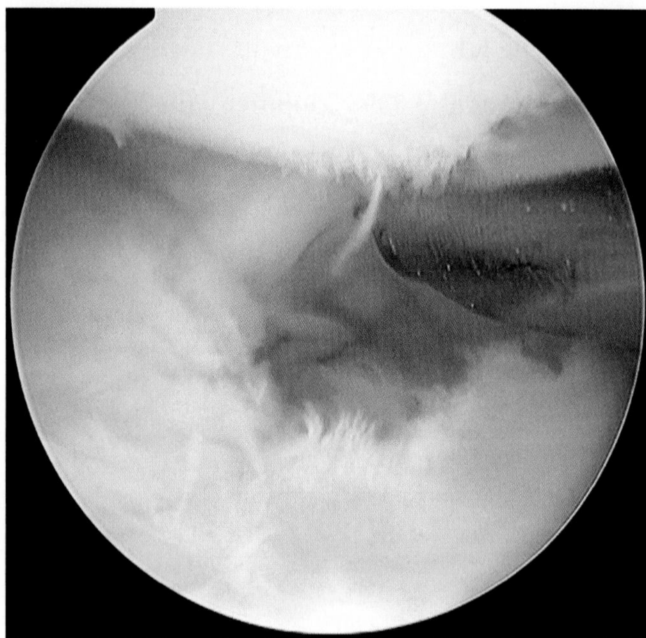

FIGURE 5.6. This arthroscopic view depicts a wide circular tear of the peripheral TFCC that was not amenable for repair. An arthroscopic shaver is being used to smooth the frayed surfaces.

instability TFCC repair is unlikely to alter the axial stability (or lack thereof) of the forearm.

An arthritic radiocarpal joint is certainly a reason to reconsider the outcome of an isolated arthroscopic TFCC repair. If the arthritis remains untreated, the return of the trampoline effect of the TFCC will unlikely change a patient's entire wrist pathology. Last, cases of ulnar positive variance—where the ulna abuts the ulnar carpus with the TFCC sandwiched between—demand ulnar shortening osteotomy (either alone or in concert with arthroscopic TFCC repair).[19] A final relative contraindication exists for cases in which the TFCC tear is irreducible, either due to its large size or contracture (Figure 5.6). TFCC tears that cannot be adequately reapproximated or reduced should undergo debridement to a smooth rim.

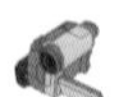

Surgical Technique

Preparation

Preoperative preparation begins with a thorough review of the patient's history and physical exam. Diagnostic studies should be reviewed and should be available intraoperatively. If there are questions or concerns with MRI or arthrogram findings, communication with a bone and joint radiologist about the case and pertinent clinical findings may be helpful.

In our practice, which involves a consistent surgical staff and a team approach, a diagnostic wrist arthroscopy with peripheral TFCC repair is scheduled for 75 minutes of total operative time. The surgery should be scheduled to allow sufficient time for anesthesia as well as operative preparation and positioning. Certainly, scheduling also depends on the institution's preparedness for wrist arthroscopic procedures and the surgical staff's (circulating nurse, scrub technician, and surgical assistants) familiarity with the arthroscopic equipment, the wrist traction tower, and the steps of the surgical technique. All of these factors should be considered when arranging the operative time schedule.

For any surgical procedure it is imperative to have the equipment required to perform the operation available to the surgeon. This is primarily the surgeon's responsibility. It is important to engage the staff responsible for operating room equipment prior to the day of surgery to ensure all of the necessary equipment will be available. This section details some of the surgical equipment specific to arthroscopic TFCC repairs that we use at our institution. We use a Concept wrist traction tower (Linvatec, Largo, FL), which allows the wrist to be deviated into any position with up to 15 pounds of traction applied via sterile finger traps (separate item). Most wrist traction towers have this capability, but they are set up and work differently with various strapping options to secure the arm and forearm to the tower and the hand table. Becoming comfortable with the traction tower set-up and function preoperatively will decrease the operative time and intraoperative frustration.

For arthroscopic equipment, there is great variety. We use a short 30-degree 2.7-mm arthroscope for a majority of wrist arthroscopy. For particularly small or tight joints, a 1.9-mm arthroscope should also be available. We use a 2.5-mm full-radius arthroscopic shaver and have a radiofrequency probe available for cautery or ablation. A set of small-joint arthroscopy instruments (including an arthroscopic probe, biters, and graspers) should also be available for intra-articular debridement. Although a meniscal repair needle set (such as by Smith and Nephew, Memphis, TN) or a TFCC-specific repair kit (such as by Linvatec, Largo, FL) can facilitate the operation and minimize trauma to the wrist capsule, such sets are not a prerequisite of performing a peripheral TFCC repair. Last, it is necessary to have a standard hand surgery instrument set open at the beginning of the operation.

Some consideration should also be given preoperatively to the suture material used for the TFCC repair. Although nearly any nonabsorbable or long-lasting absorbable suture that can be threaded through an 18-gauge needle will suffice for the TFCC repair, some sutures have unique characteristics that facilitate the procedure. For example, a suture that is dark in color substantially improves suture visualization, grasping, and retrieval during the arthroscopy. A particularly stiff suture will frequently facilitate intra-articular retrieval as well. At our institution, either a nonabsorbable 2-0 Prolene (Ethicon, Somerville, NJ) or an absorbable 2-0 PDS suture (Ethicon, Somerville, NJ) is utilized. The PDS suture will typically begin to be reabsorbed at six weeks and is used in patients with excellent healing potential.

Arthroscopic Repair: Step-by-step Technique

In regard to this section, see Table 5.3. After a general anesthetic, the affected extremity is positioned on a hand table to allow full access to the hand, wrist, and elbow. Diagnosis commences with a physical exam of the radiocarpal joint and the distal radioulnar joint under anesthesia. In isolated peripheral tears of the TFCC, the examination under anesthesia may have no dramatic positive findings other than catching or grind with ulnar-sided compression and simultaneous forearm rotation. However, previously undiagnosed scapholunate or lunotriquetral instability can often be elicited in an anesthetized patient. A nonsterile upper arm tourniquet is placed with plenty of clearance for free elbow flexion after surgical prep and application of the impervious sterile drapes. The traction tower is assembled at this time, with 10 to 15 pounds of traction applied through finger traps on the index through small fingers. It is also possible to apply the finger traps to just the ulnar three digits for more pronounced traction on the ulnar side of the wrist, although this arrangement does make diagnostic arthroscopy of the radial side of the wrist more difficult.

 **Table 5.3.**

Preoperative Planning for Arthroscopic Repair of Peripheral TFCC Tears

Anesthesia
• General with or without axillary block for post-op pain (intra-articular pain pump postoperatively)
Patient Position
• Supine
• Affected hand on hand table
• Upper arm tourniquet
Instrument List
• Hand surgery set
• Wrist arthroscopy traction tower
• Sterile finger traps
• Arthroscope (2.7-mm, 30-degree) and cannula
• 1.9-mm arthroscope as a backup for smaller wrists
• Arthroscopy instruments—all small scale for wrist
• Soft-tissue shaver (2.5 mm)
• Arthroscopic probe
• Arthroscopic biters (straight, left, and right bend)
• Arthroscopic grasper (a Jacobson hemostat can be used as an alternative)
• Radiofrequency or ablation probe
• 18-gauge needles
• 2-0 Prolene (nonabsorbable) or PDS (absorbable) suture

Next, the placement of the arthroscopic portals should be planned (Figure 5.7). Landmarks such as Lister's tubercle, the DRUJ, the ulnar styloid, and the potential path of the dorsal sensory branch of the ulnar nerve are outlined. The 3-/,4 portal is placed between the extensor pollicis longus (EPL) tendon and the extensor digitorum communis (EDC) tendons, one centimeter distal to Lister's tubercle between the scaphoid and the lunate. The 4-/,5 portal is positioned also 1 cm distal to Lister's tubercle, but between the EDC and the EDQ tendons. If desired, a 6-R portal can be marked at the same axial level but just radial to the ECU. The point of outflow can also be designated at the 6-U position just ulnar or volar to the ECU tendon. Midcarpal portals should also be outlined, but will not be used specifically for the TFCC repair.

At this point, the arm can be exsanguinated with an esmarch bandage and the tourniquet inflated to a pressure of 250 mmHg of mercury. Not all surgeons perform wrist arthroscopy under tourniquet control, but it is our preference—especially in cases of TFCC repair, in that a bloodless field facilitates identification of the dorsal branch of the ulnar sensory nerve. Lidocaine or marcaine with epinephrine is injected to distend the radiocarpal joint, through the area of the planned 3-/,4 portal.

A #15 blade is used to create a 5- to 7-mm vertical skin incision at the planned location for the 3-/,4 portal. Blunt dissection with a fine hemostat (Jacobson) or a tenotomy scissors is carried down to the wrist capsule. The wrist capsule should be palpated and balloted with this instrument to ensure accurate placement of this radiocarpal portal in the proximal to distal axis. Once a soft spot in the

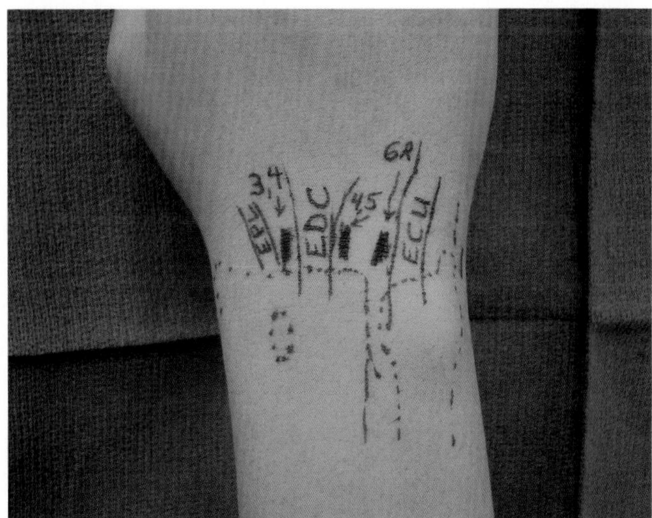

FIGURE 5.7. The 3,4 arthroscopic portal is typically located distal to Lister's tubercle between the third and fourth extensor compartments. The 4,5 portal is created just ulnar to the fourth extensor compartment, also at the level of the radiocarpal joint.

capsule is confirmed, the tips of the fine hemostat or tenotomy scissors are gently driven into the radiocarpal joint, with the utmost care taken to avoid iatrogenic chondral injury. It is reasonable to check the traction across the wrist prior to entering the joint, as the initial level of traction often changes as the wrist is manipulated throughout the case. Once the joint has been entered, the tips of the instrument are spread to expand the size of the aperture to allow placement of the blunt arthroscopic trocar followed by the arthroscope itself. Most hand surgeons are comfortable with this technique, which relies on a knowledge of the anatomy, palpation of anatomic landmarks, and a tactile sense of the joint capsule.

Alternatively, a fluoroscopic-guided technique has been advocated and utilized by some wrist arthroscopists.[22,23] Although this technique may seem burdensome at first, it can prevent iatrogenic chondral injury in a reliable fashion. A small or mini fluoroscopy unit is required, such as a XiScan (XiTec, East Windsor, CT). The fluoroscopy unit is positioned with the arm parallel rather than perpendicular to the floor. It is brought in directly from the end of the hand table at the height of the wrist joint. With a minimal adjustment, the fluoroscopy unit can be directed at the wrist joint in such a way that it avoids the vertical steel rod of the wrist arthroscopy tower. Under direct fluoroscopic control, 18-gauge needles can then be placed easily and atraumatically into the radiocarpal joint (marking the 3-/,4, 4-/,5 or 6-R, and 6-U portals). The small fluoroscopy unit is simply pulled from the field and the formal portals are made using the 18-gauge needles as guides to portal placement and direction.

Once the 3-/,4 portal has been established, a 2.7-mm arthroscope inserted, and flow of the arthroscopic fluid has begun (either by pump or gravity feed—our preference), it is critical to initiate and maintain an outflow portal. The outflow portal will allow controlled clearance of the arthroscopic lavage and improved intra-articular visualization. We prefer to use a single 1.5-inch 18-gauge needle at the 6-U location for radiocarpal outflow. In placing this needle under direct arthroscopic visualization (so as to not inadvertently injure the triangular fibrocartilage), we direct the sharp bevel of the needle longitudinally or vertically to avoid injury to the dorsal sensory branch of the ulnar nerve. A transverse or horizontally directed bevel of a sharp 18-gauge neeedle could conceivably transect nerve fibers rather than separating them along a vertical axis, as in the case of a vertically directed bevel.

For the initial diagnostic examination, the arthroscope is placed into the 3-/,4 portal and a small probe is placed into either a 4-/,5 or 6-R portal. The 3-/,4 portal is the workhorse visualization portal for radiocarpal arthroscopy. A majority of the TFCC repairs performed at our institution are completed with the arthroscope in the 3-/,4 portal throughout the repair. The 4-/,5 or 6-R portal provides an aperture for instrumentation, specifically a probe or nerve hook, the arthroscopic shaver, a grasper, or a radiofrequency probe. Typically, we will use a 4-/,5 portal as our working portal for instrumentation. The radioscaphoid articulation, scapholunate interval, volar ligaments, radiolunate articulation, lunotriquetral interval, and TFCC should all be assessed with direct arthroscopic visualization and probe examination. Next, it is important to examine the midcarpal joint for intercarpal instability through separate portals typically 1 cm distal to the 3-/,4 and 4-/,5 radiocarpal portals.

After complete arthroscopic examination of the wrist, attention can be directed to the TFCC repair. First, it is important to have undisturbed visualization of the TFCC tear itself. If synovitis impedes direct visualization, a partial synovectomy may be performed using a 2.5-mm small-joint shaver/debrider (e.g., Stryker, Sunnyvale, CA) with a full-radius blade. If visualization of the TFCC is not satisfactory after debridement of synovitis or redundant dorsal capsule, consideration can be made to placing the arthroscope into the 4-/,5 portal.

This portal is slightly more ulnar and will provide a great view of the volar and ulnar aspects of the TFCC, but may limit the view of the dorsal-most aspect of the TFCC's periphery. In cases of poor visualization from the 3-/,4 portal, we prefer to bring the arthroscope back to the scapholunate interval and then advance the arthroscope directly volar under the scapholunate ligament until it is just past the convexity of the lunate. At this point, the arthroscope can frequently be swept ulnarly in an atraumatic fashion from its current position toward the TFCC. This maneuver with the arthroscope slid under the lunate provides a more direct view of the TFCC from the 3-/,4 portal. Now, the camera is looking directly ulnar and in a right wrist its view can be rotated toward the 9 o'clock position to look volarly or toward the 3 o'clock position to look dorsally.

Using a small arthroscopic probe, the diagnosis of peripheral detachment is made by the trampoline test of the TFCC as described by Hermansdorfer and Kleinman.[24] A normal TFCC is taut when indented with the probe, as shown in Figure 5.8. With release of indentation pressure the probe will be felt to "bounce" off the robust intact TFCC, similar to rebounding off a trampoline. If the TFCC is redundant or easily deformed when pressed by the arthroscopic probe, the diagnosis of a TFCC injury can be made. Careful arthroscopic inspection is required to differentiate radial-sided (type 1D), central (type 1A), and peripheral (ulnar type 1B or distal type 1C) lesions. One easy intra-articular landmark for TFCC tears is the ulnar head.

If the ulnar head is visible from the 3-/,4 or 4-/,5 portal, the TFCC is incompetent either centrally (type 1A or 2C) or radially (type 1D). A TFCC with a typical ulnar-sided lesion will usually still cover the ulnar head. To improve visualization of the more common dorsal ulnar-sided lesion, the camera on the arthroscope needs to be angled toward the ulnar and dorsal aspect of the wrist (looking toward the 3 o'clock position in a right wrist and the 9 o'clock position in a left wrist). Volar ulnar-sided lesions may require slight radial deviation of the wrist (accomplished by angling the pull of the traction tower radially) to better visualize the volar attachment of the TFCC and its ulnolunate and ulnotriquetral ligaments.

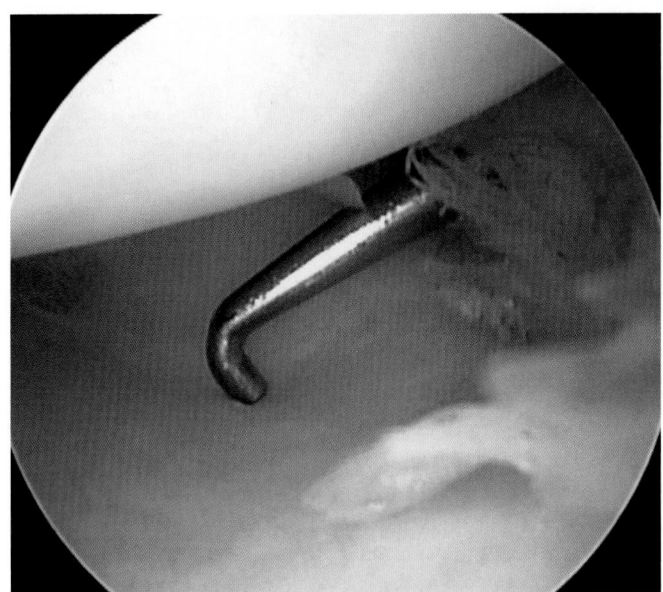

FIGURE 5.8. The trampoline sign can be visualized by downward pressure on the TFCC with an arthroscopic probe. An intact TFCC (as depicted here) will be taut against the pressure of the probe.

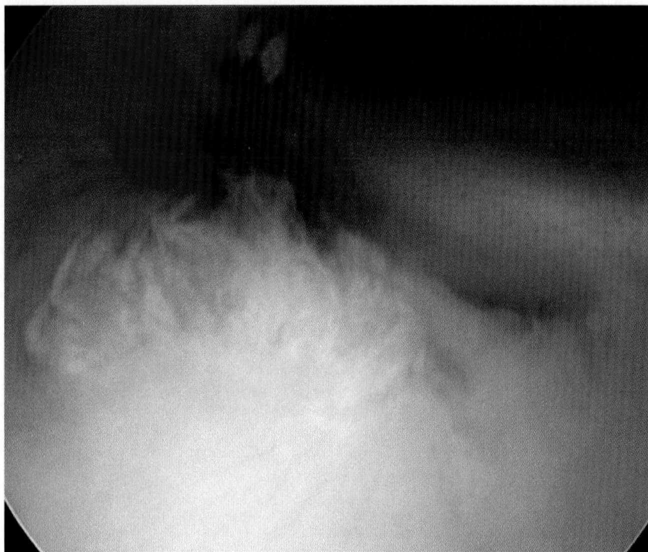

FIGURE 5.9. Debridement of the edges of the TFCC tear can be performed with an arthroscopic shaver and should help stimulate the formation of a fibrin clot.

Once a peripheral lesion is identified, it must be debrided to clean edges. A full-radius 2.5-mm shaver is the ideal tool for this debridement, but occasionally a small biter may be necessary to debride larger flaps of torn or redundant tissue (Figures 5.9 and 5.10). An adequate debridement allows for complete assessment of the tear and provides a stimulus for a fibrin clot to form at the repair site. This fibrin clot will incite an appropriate repair response at the biological level. At this point, the size of the tear can be assessed with an arthroscopic probe (by knowing the length of the probe hook, one can measure the intra-articular extent of the TFCC tear). Tears greater than 5 mm in length will typically require at least two sutures to appropriately maintain the TFCC in a reduced position.

After the tear is identified, a 25- or 27-gauge 1.5-inch needle (with the bevel vertically aligned) is placed into the wrist joint at the level of the tear. The small-diameter needle is used to localize a 1- to 1.5-cm longitudinal incision over the ulnar aspect of the wrist. This ulnar incision is a prerequisite to avoiding injury to the DSBUN, which is the most common complication following these repairs. Using a blunt spreading technique with tenotomy scissors or a fine hemostat, the DSBUN is localized as it travels obliquely from proximal-volar to distal-dorsal at the level of the ulnar head distally. Dissection should be carried down to wrist capsule if possible. If visualization is not sufficient to comfortably document protection of the DSBUN and neighboring tendons, this limited incision should be extended until adequate visualization is obtained.

Our preferred repair method of ulnar-sided TFCC injuries is an outside-in technique. Prior to beginning the repair, the surgeon should decide if the repair suture will be horizontally or vertically oriented. A horizontal mattress-type suture is very effective in drawing a peripherally

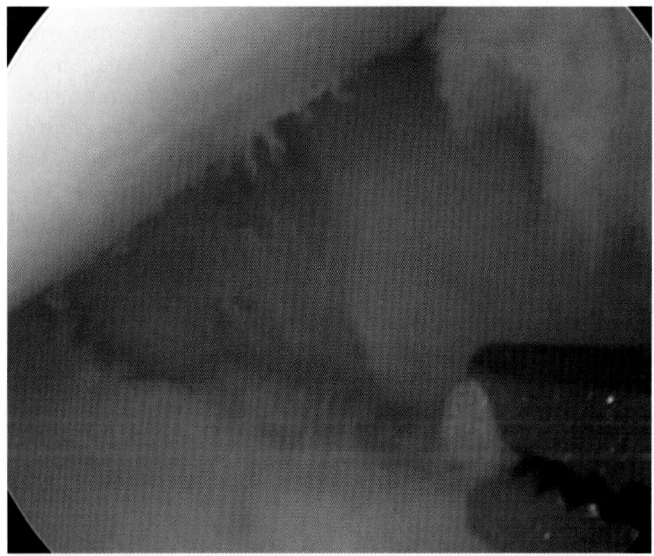

FIGURE 5.10. After debridement, the torn peripheral edge of this TFCC can then be approximated to the overlying wrist capsule just dorsal and ulnar to it.

torn edge of the triangular fibrocartilage out toward the ulnar wrist capsule to reestablish the trampoline effect. Similarly, multiple vertically oriented sutures can be effective in coapting the edges of a peripheral tear. Either technique begins with puncturing the ulnar wrist capsule and TFCC using an 18-gauge needle after localization of the stitch with the finer 25-gauge needle to avoid iatrogenic trauma caused by multiple passes with the larger-bore needle. The needle should pass just inferior (for horizontal tears) or radial (for vertical tears) to the torn edge of the TFCC. The repair suture is then threaded into an 18-gauge needle and inserted into the wrist joint via the ulnar-sided 6-U incision under arthroscopic control (Figure 5.11).

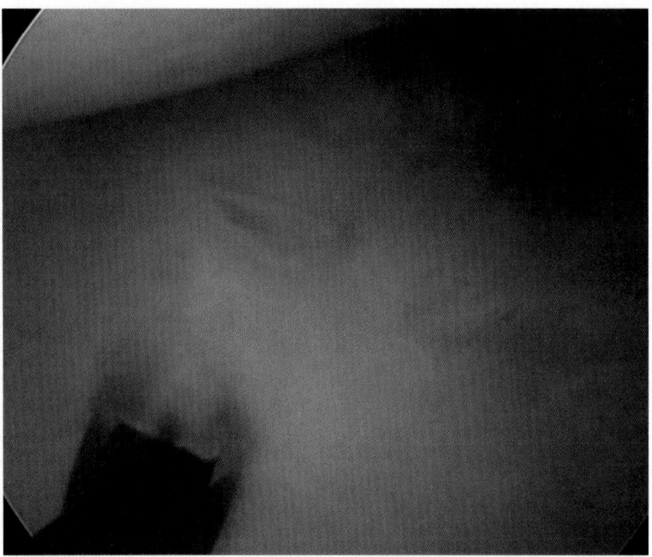

FIGURE 5.11. In this case, a nonabsorbable 2–0 suture was passed through the intact portion of the TFCC via an 18-gauge needle.

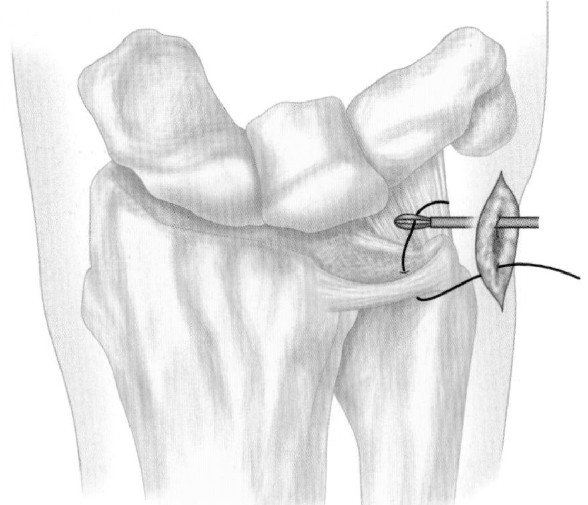

FIGURE 5.13. This line drawing demonstrates the incision utilized for ulnar-sided arthroscopic repairs. In a majority of cases, a single small incision can be used to pass all of the sutures required for repair. By creating a small incision and protecting the dorsal sensory branch of the ulnar nerve, sutures can be retrieved and tied safely.

There are different suture retrieval techniques that work well. The intra-articular suture can be grasped using a small arthroscopic grasping forceps or wire suture grasper. With either instrument, a separate intra-articular puncture is required to retrieve the suture (Figures 5.12 and 5.13). The tissue bridge between the just-inserted suture grasper and the 18-gauge needle is the area over which the repair will be tied down. Although all of this work can be done through the small ulnar-sided incision, it is not necessary. The needles and suture must be passed such that the best possible repair is obtained.

Frequently, one limb of the suture may need to be passed more dorsal (at the 6-R position, for example). In these circumstances, the overlying subcutaneous tissues can be undermined off the dorsal capsule—and with the DSBUN safely retracted, the sutures can still be retrieved into the ulnar-sided 6-U portal incision and tied under direct visualization. Certainly, when tying the repair sutures it is imperative that the DSBUN or an extensor tendon is not trapped under the tie. Tension is then placed on the sutures to ensure that there is reestablishment of TFCC tension and obliteration of any gapping between the articular disc and peripheral capsular tissue (Figure 5.14). In some cases, to establish a tension-free reduction of the torn edges the hand may be taken out of the traction device and the sutures tied with the wrist in slight ulnar deviation and forearm in

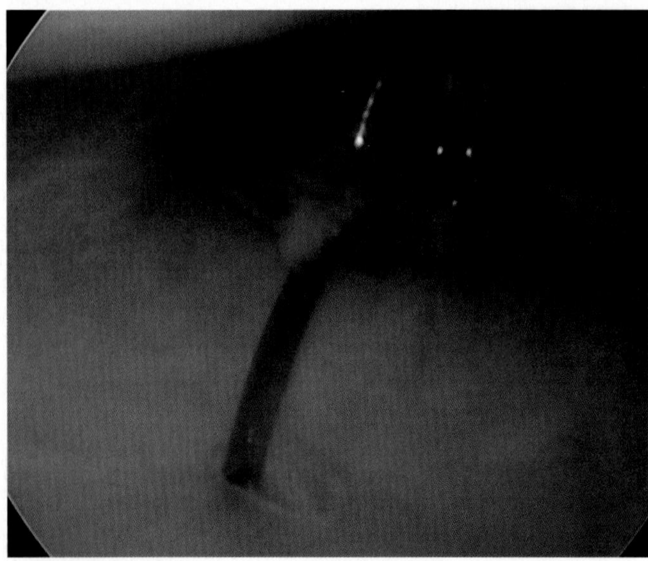

FIGURE 5.12. Next, the suture can be retrieved from the joint using a suture grasper.

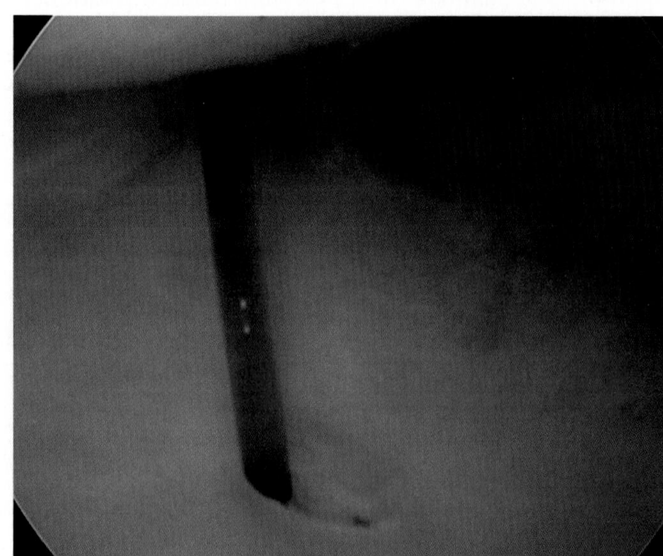

FIGURE 5.14. Prior to tying the suture, the reduction of the tear can be assessed. Here, the avulsed edge of the TFCC has been reapproximated to the overlying wrist capsule.

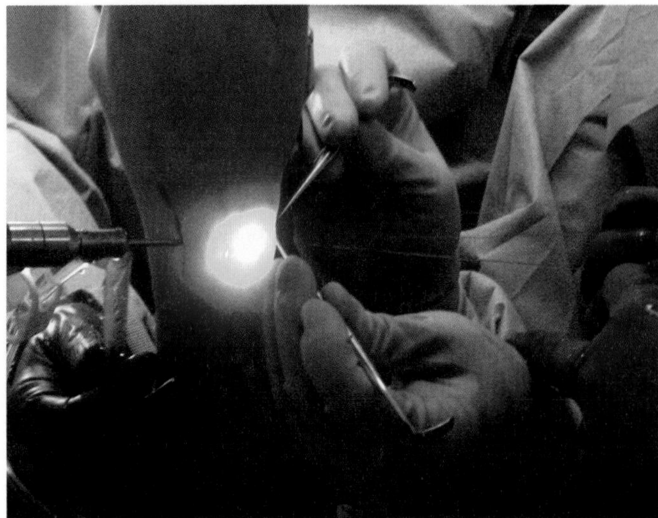

FIGURE 5.15. This outside view of the wrist demonstrates retraction of the ulnar-sided soft tissues and safe protection of the sensory nerve branches while tying the suture with simultaneous direct and arthroscopic visualization.

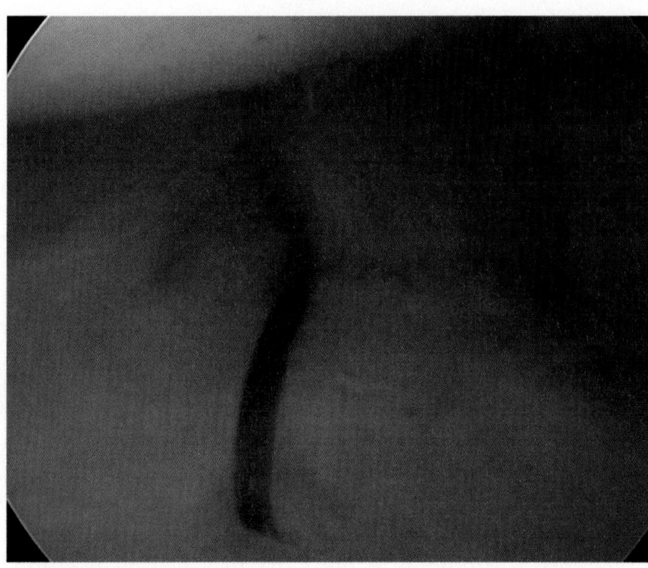

FIGURE 5.16. After the suture is tied, the repaired edge of the TFCC is now held firmly against the ulnar wrist capsule to allow for peripheral healing.

neutral rotation. However, in a majority of cases the torn edges have not contracted and the suture can be tied with the wrist remaining in the traction tower (Figures 5.15 and 5.16). Two or three sutures are passed and tied using these techniques.

In cases of coincidental lunotriquetral ligament injury or longitudinal injury to the ulnolunate and lunotriquetral ligaments, the repair of these structures follows. Two 0.045-inch Kirschner wires can then be driven across the lunotriquetral articulation to stabilize the joint after reduction of the lunate using a percutaneously placed Kirschner wire (0.045 inch). The palmar ulnolunate and ulnotriquetral ligaments are then lassoed by sutures passed through the 6-U portal to augment the pinning of the lunotriquetral interval (Figure 5.17). Great care is to be taken to avoid inadvertent injury to the ulnar neurovascular bundle lying just volar to the ulnar wrist capsule and ulnocarpal ligaments. If necessary, the ulnar nerve and artery can be identified through the ulnar-sided 6-U incision and safely retracted. The sutures are tied over the capsule after the 6-U portal is enlarged, to bring all sutures out through this portal so that they can be tied under direct vision while protecting the dorsal sensory branch of the ulnar nerve. The pins are left in place for six weeks while the wrist is immobilized following the combined repair of the TFCC and the lunotriquetral ligament.

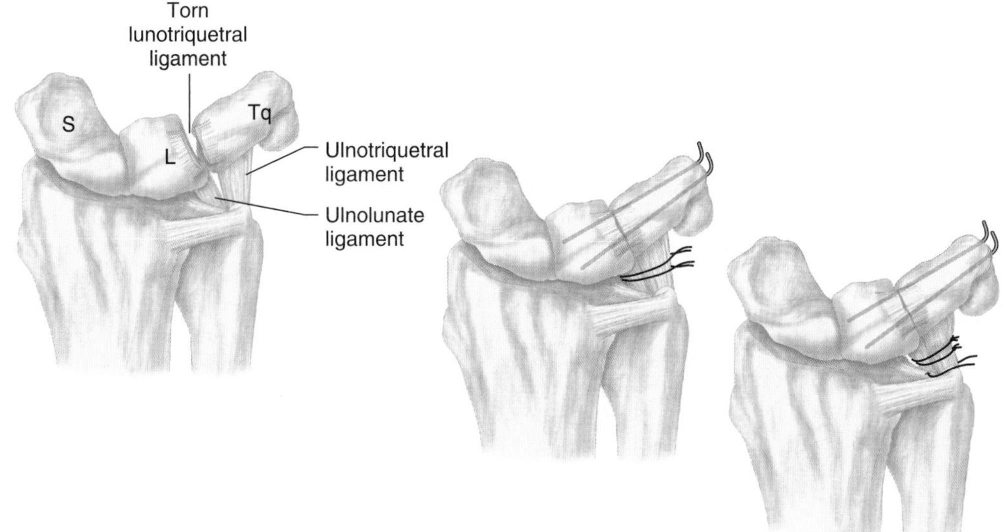

FIGURE 5.17. Tears of the ulnocarpal ligaments often occur in concert with lunotriquetral ligament tears. After pinning of the reduced lunotriquetral interval under arthroscopic and fluoroscopic control, vertical tears between the ulnolunate and lunotriquetral ligaments can be reapproximated arthroscopically with one or two sutures passed using outside-in techniques.

If there has been prior surgery involving the ulnar radiocarpal joint or DRUJ, scar tissue formation can make arthroscopy extremely difficult. With an open exposure of the TFCC using an approach between the fifth and sixth compartments (Figure 5.2), the same technique can be applied to repair peripheral tears of the TFCC. As previously mentioned, when clinically significant instability of the DRUJ exists open reattachment of the distal radioulnar ligaments to the ulnar fovea or open reconstruction should be considered.

Rehabilitation

Postoperatively, forearm rotation and wrist motion should be restricted with an above-elbow splint that accommodates swelling and egress of arthroscopic fluid. It is our preference to immobilize the wrist in a neutral position, which theoretically minimizes stress at the repair site. Typically, the splint is maintained until the initial postoperative visit after two weeks. During this time, patients are encouraged to maintain supple finger joints with range-of-motion exercises. Sutures are removed at 10 to 14 days and then the patient is placed in a custom-molded long-arm cast or Munster-type brace to control wrist rotation.

At the fourth postoperative week, the cast or brace is changed to a removable short-arm wrist brace for an additional two weeks. Gentle active wrist and forearm motion can be started at this time, but radial and ulnar deviation should be avoided to protect the repair. After the sixth postoperative week, passive range-of-motion exercises and gentle strengthening may be added to the regimen as the patient is gradually weaned from the brace. Typically, patients return to full activities after approximately 10 to 12 weeks.

Results

To evaluate the efficacy of arthroscopic repair of the TFCC, functional outcome was determined after arthroscopic repair of 22 wrists.[25] Average follow-up was 36 months, with a range from 26 to 48 months. There was a significant relief of pain and increase in work and sports activities ($p < 0.01$). Postoperative range of motion averaged 86% +/− 9% of the contralateral side and grip strength averaged 82% +/− 20% of the contralateral side. There were significant correlations between the delay from injury to surgical repair and the final total range of motion and grip strength, with repairs of acute tears having better outcomes. Arthroscopic repair of peripheral TFCC tears results in significant relief of pain and increased function during work or sports.

References

1. Benjamin M, Evans EJ, Pemberton DJ. Histological studies on the triangular fibrocartilage complex of the wrist. J Anat 1990;172:59–67.
2. Nakamura T, Takayama S, Horiuchi Y, Yabe Y. Origins and insertions of the triangular fibrocartilage complex: A histological study. J Hand Surg [Br] 2001;26(5):446–54.
3. Nakamura T, Yabe Y. Histological anatomy of the triangular fibrocartilage complex of the human wrist. Ann Anat 2000;182(6):567–72.
4. Chidgey LK, Dell PC, Bittar ES, Spanier SS. Histologic anatomy of the triangular fibrocartilage. J Hand Surg [Am] 1991;16(6):1084–100.
5. Bednar MS, Arnoczky SP, Weiland AJ. The microvasculature of the triangular fibrocartilage complex: Its clinical significance. J Hand Surg [Am] 1991;16(6):1101–05.
6. Thiru RG, Ferlic DC, Clayton ML, McClure DC. Arterial anatomy of the triangular fibrocartilage of the wrist and its surgical significance. J Hand Surg [Am] 1986;11 (2):258–63.
7. Gupta R, Nelson SD, Baker J, Jones NF, Meals RA. The innervation of the triangular fibrocartilage complex: Nitric acid maceration rediscovered. Plast Reconstr Surg 2001; 107(1):135–39.
8. DiTano O, Trumble TE, Tencer AF. Biomechanical function of the distal radioulnar and ulnocarpal wrist ligaments. J Hand Surg [Am] 2003;28(4):622–27.
9. Nakamura T, Makita A. The proximal ligamentous component of the triangular fibrocartilage complex. J Hand Surg [Br] 2000;25(5):479–86.
10. Trumble T, Glisson RR, Seaber AV, Urbaniak JR. Forearm force transmission after surgical treatment of distal radioulnar joint disorders. J Hand Surg [Am] 1987;12(2):196–202.
11. Haugstvedt JR, Berger RA, Nakamura T, Neale P, Berglund L, An KN. Relative contributions of the ulnar attachments of the triangular fibrocartilage complex to the dynamic stability of the distal radioulnar joint. J Hand Surg [Am] 2006;31(3):445–51.
12. Ruch DS, Anderson SR, Ritter MR. Biomechanical comparison of transosseous and capsular repair of peripheral triangular fibrocartilage tears. Arthroscopy 2003;19(4):391–96.
13. de Araujo W, Poehling GG, Kuzma GR. New Tuohy needle technique for triangular fibrocartilage complex repair: Preliminary studies. Arthroscopy 1996;12(6):699–703.
14. Zanetti M, Bram J, Hodler J. Triangular fibrocartilage and intercarpal ligaments of the wrist: Does MR arthrography improve standard MRI? J Magn Reson Imaging 1997; 7(3):590–94.
15. Fulcher SM, Poehling GG. The role of operative arthroscopy for the diagnosis and treatment of lesions about the distal ulna. Hand Clin 1998;14(2):285–96.
16. Pederzini L, Luchetti R, Soragni O, Alfarano M, Montagna G, Cerofolini E, et al. Evaluation of the triangular fibrocartilage complex tears by arthroscopy, arthrography, and magnetic resonance imaging. Arthroscopy 1992;8(2):191–97.
17. Palmer AK. Triangular fibrocartilage complex lesions: A classification. J Hand Surg [Am] 1989;14(4):594–606.
18. Trumble TE, Gilbert M, Vedder N. Isolated tears of the triangular fibrocartilage: Management by early arthroscopic repairs. J Hand Surg 1997;22A:57–65.
19. Trumble TE, Gilbert M, Vedder N. Ulnar shortening combined with arthroscopic repairs in the delayed management of triangular fibrocartilage complex tears. J Hand Surg [Am] 1997;22(5):807–13.
20. Nakamura T, Nakao Y, Ikegami H, Sato K, Takayama S. Open repair of the ulnar disruption of the triangular fibrocartilage complex with double three-dimensional mattress

suturing technique. Tech Hand Up Extrem Surg 2004;8(2): 116–23.

21. Moskal MJ, Savoie FH III, Field LD. Arthroscopic capsulodesis of the lunotriquetral joint. Clin Sports Med 2001; 20(1):141–53. ix, x.
22. Slade JF III, Geissler WB, Gutow AP, Merrell GA. Percutaneous internal fixation of selected scaphoid nonunions with an arthroscopically assisted dorsal approach. J Bone Joint Surg Am 2003;85(4):20–32.
23. Slade JF III, Dodds SD. Minimally invasive management of scaphoid nonunions. Clin Orthop Relat Res 2006;445: 108–19.
24. Hermansdorfer JD, Kleinman WB. Management of chronic peripheral tears of the triangular fibrocartilage complex. J Hand Surg Am 1991;16(2):340–46.
25. Trumble TE, Gilbert M, Vedder N. Arthroscopic repair of the triangular fibrocartilage complex. Arthroscopy 1996;12(5): 588–97.

Ericka A. Lawler and
Brian D. Adams

CHAPTER 6

Arthroscopy of the Distal Radioulnar Joint

Introduction

Arthroscopy of the distal radioulnar joint (DRUJ) is a natural extension of radiocarpal and midcarpal arthroscopy. It provides a minimally invasive means of evaluating the DRUJ, including visualization of the articular cartilage, synovium, and triangular fibrocartilage complex (TFCC). This chapter discusses the relevant anatomy and biomechanics of the DRUJ, indications for DRUJ arthroscopy, and the surgical technique. In addition, open distal radioulnar ligament reconstruction is described for patients with DRUJ instability found to have an irreparable TFCC.

Anatomy and Biomechanics

The DRUJ is a trochoid diarthrodial articulation that allows both rotation and translation during normal forearm motion. The overall dimensions of the sigmoid notch average 15 mm in the transverse plane and 10 mm in the coronal plane. Its dorsal bony rim is typically acutely angled, whereas the volar rim is more rounded and is frequently augmented by a cartilaginous lip. The shape of the notch varies considerably in both planes, which plays a role in both joint stability and ease of arthroscopic access.[1] Due to its relatively shallow and incongruent articulation, the DRUJ relies strongly on the soft tissues for stability. The structures that contribute to DRUJ stability are the pronator quadratus, extensor carpi ulnaris (ECU), interosseous membrane (IOM), DRUJ capsule, and components of the triangular fibrocartilage complex (TFCC).[2]

The TFCC is generally accepted as the major static soft-tissue stabilizer. The palmar and dorsal radioulnar ligaments are the prime components of the TFCC that stabilize the DRUJ. These ligaments appear as thickenings at the junctures of the triangular fibrocartilage, DRUJ capsule, and ulnocarpal capsule. As each ligament extends from its respective distal margins of the sigmoid notch, it divides in the coronal plane into two limbs. The deep (proximal) limb attaches at the fovea, and the superficial (distal) limb attaches to the base and midportion of the ulnar styloid. The palmar ligament provides origins for the ulnolunate and ulnotriquetral ligaments, whereas the dorsal ligament is confluent with the ECU sheath.

During forearm rotation, DRUJ translation occurs because the sigmoid notch is shallow (with a radius of curvature 50% greater than that of the ulnar head). At the extremes of pronation and supination, the ulnar head slides palmarly and dorsally in the sigmoid notch (respectively)—resulting in only 2 to 3 mm of articular contact area at the rims.[3] Although DRUJ motion has a substantial translational component (with a changing axis of rotation), its instant axis generally passes near the center of the ulnar head—moving dorsally with pronation and palmarly with supination. The ulnar head serves as the seat for the sigmoid notch, around which the radius rotates.[3] The amount of articular cartilage that covers the head varies from a 50-degree to a 130-degree arc.

The ulnar styloid is a continuation of the subcutaneous ridge of the ulna, providing increased area for soft-tissue attachments. At the base of the styloid lies a shallow concavity termed the fovea, which is replete with vascular foramina and is an attachment site for ligaments. Identification of this site is essential for anatomical repair and reconstructive procedures because the axis of forearm motion passes through it.

Indications

The DRUJ is susceptible to trauma, post-traumatic degenerative changes, and inflammatory conditions. Arthroscopy allows for inspection of the articular surfaces of both the sigmoid notch and the ulnar head. Chondromalacia, cartilage defects, and articular shear injuries may be visualized. Systemic inflammatory conditions (including gout and rheumatoid arthritis) are sources of DRUJ synovitis that can be evaluated and treated arthroscopically. PVNS leading to synovial hypertrophy, loose bodies from fracture, or osteophytes can be removed. Undersurface partial- or full-thickness tears of the TFCC can be seen and debrided. Occasionally, the competency of the volar ulnocarpal ligaments may be evaluated.

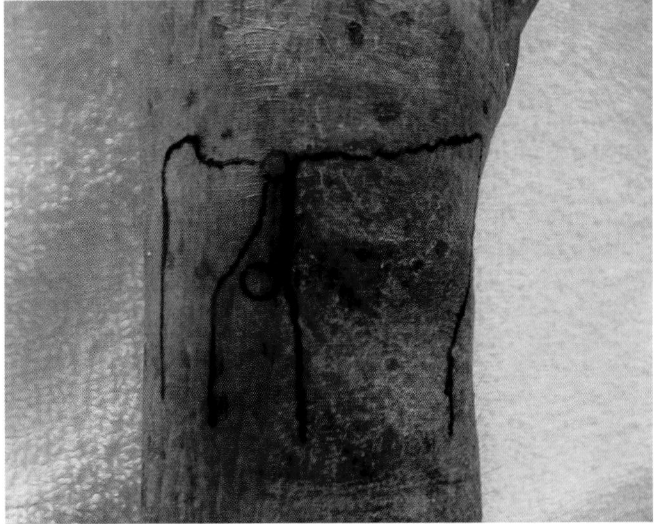

FIGURE 6.1. Sites of the proximal and distal DRUJ portals are marked on the skin. The proximal portal is located just proximal to the confluence of the radius and ulna, and the distal portal enters between the TFCC and the ulnar head.

Contraindications

There are no absolute contraindications to DRUJ arthroscopy. However, the joint is very small and access is limited. Thus, relative contraindications include surgical proficiency and a tight joint that does not allow passage of the scope or instruments without undo joint damage. Radiographic evidence of degenerative changes is a sign that navigating the joint arthroscopically could be very difficult, especially if the joint is stiff.

Surgical Technique

A regional or general anesthetic is administered. The patient is positioned supine on the operating table. An upper-arm tourniquet is applied over cotton padding. The elbow is flexed to 90 degrees and the upper extremity is mounted in a traction tower using finger traps applied to the long and ring fingers. Placing the wrist in full supination facilitates access to the DRUJ, unless the joint becomes excessively tight in this position. In neutral rotation the opposing surfaces of the sigmoid notch and the ulnar head are congruent, whereas in full supination the opposing surfaces have only a marginal contact area of 2 to 3 mm.[4]

The joint is insufflated with 3 to 5 cc of sterile saline using a 20-gauge needle. The needle is punctured through the skin just proximal to the confluence of the radius and ulna and angled 45 degrees distally to enter the proximal aspect (axilla) of the DRUJ, which will serve as the proximal DRUJ portal. After distension of the joint, a small longitudinal incision is made at the injection site using a number 11 or 15 blade. Care is taken to avoid the EDQ tendon. A hemostat can be used to spread the subcutaneous tissue and penetrate the capsule.

A cannula with bullet-tipped trocar is inserted into the joint. The trocar is then removed and the arthroscope is inserted. A 2.0- or 2.7-mm arthroscope is preferred, depending on the size and tightness of the joint. Inflow is directed through the cannula, and outflow (if needed) is provided with a needle inserted just distal to the ulnar head and proximal to the TFCC. To maintain appropriate pressure, a three-way stopcock with an attached syringe filled with saline can be used to pump fluid into the joint when needed. Some surgeons prefer an arthroscopy pump system.

A distal DRUJ portal can be established for instrumentation and improved visualization of the ulnar dome and TFCC. This portal enters between the TFCC central disc and the head of the ulna (Figure 6.1). It should first be localized with a needle while viewing with the arthroscope in the proximal portal.[5] The portal is typically used for instruments such as shavers, graspers, and radiofrequency devices.

Arthroscopic Evaluation of the DRUJ

Beginning proximally, the axilla of the joint is inspected for loose bodies, synovial hypertrophy, and marginal osteophytes. Continuing distally, the cartilaginous surfaces of the sigmoid notch and ulnar head are evaluated. Chondromalacia, articular fractures, and full-thickness cartilage defects can be visualized and debrided. Relaxing traction on the fingers may increase space and visualization. Pronation and supination allow a more complete evaluation of the articular surfaces. Directing the arthroscope distally, the undersurface of the TFCC is evaluated for full- or partial-thickness tears.

By passing the arthroscope between the TFCC and the dome of the ulnar head, the distal radioulnar ligaments may be visualized from their attachments on the sigmoid notch to their insertion at the fovea of the ulna head. With the arm in neutral rotation, the TFCC is under the least amount of tension—allowing for easier evaluation of the distal articular surface of the ulna. At the fovea, the ulnocapitate ligament may be seen inserting into the ulnar head—just slightly ulnar to the attachments of the radioulnar ligaments.[5,6]

Pitfalls

Entry into the joint is the most difficult aspect of DRUJ arthroscopy. Keeping the forearm positioned in supination during entry into the DRUJ is important to maximize the dorsal space of the DRUJ. At times, a 1.9-mm scope may be necessary if the joint is tight. Absorption of fluid by the distal radioulnar joint synovium can easily obscure one's view of the small DRUJ. In the presence of a TFCC tear, fluid inflow from the radiocarpal joint may have already affected the DRUJ.[6,7]

Postoperative Management

The portals are closed with 5-0 nylon sutures or Steri-Strips (some surgeons prefer to leave the sites open). The wrist is dressed in a compressive bandage with an ulnar gutter plaster splint to immobilize the wrist in a position of comfort. The splint is removed at 10 to 14 days when the patient returns for the initial postoperative visit. At this time, the sutures are removed and gentle wrist range of motion is initiated. A second postoperative visit two to three weeks later allows for a clinical assessment of function. Patient activities are typically advanced as tolerated, but unrestricted use is not usually achieved for several weeks.

DRUJ Instability

Arthroscopically assisted TFCC repair, especially for peripheral tears, is common practice (see Chapter 5). In the presence of DRUJ instability, an open TFCC repair directly to the fovea with transosseous sutures is more effective at restoring joint stability. If an arthroscopic or open TFCC repair is not possible due to chronicity and attenuation of the tissues, a secondary reconstruction is indicated. The author's preferred technique for chronic instability reconstructs both radioulnar ligaments to restore normal joint stability and mechanics.[8–11]

A 5-cm incision is made between the fifth and sixth extensor compartments over the DRUJ. The fifth compartment is opened over the radioulnar joint, and the extensor digiti minimi tendon is retracted. An L-shaped DRUJ capsulotomy is made with one limb along the dorsal rim of the sigmoid notch and the other just proximal to the dorsal radioulnar ligament (Figure 6.2). The ECU sheath is not opened or dissected from the ulnar groove during the procedure. Scar is debrided from the fovea. Functioning remnants of the TFCC are retained.

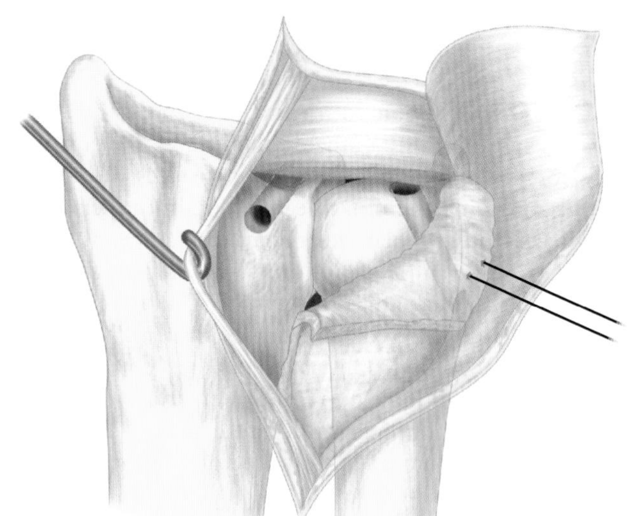

FIGURE 6.2. Dorsal exposure of the DRUJ for ligament reconstruction is obtained by incising the fifth compartment and raising a triangular capsular flap.

The periosteum beneath the fourth dorsal extensor compartment is elevated from the dorsal margin of the sigmoid notch. A guide wire for a 3.5-mm cannulated drill bit is driven through the radius several millimeters proximal to the lunate fossa and approximately 5 mm radial to the articular surface of the sigmoid notch. The site is chosen so that a tunnel can be enlarged if necessary to accommodate the graft without disrupting the subchondral bone of the lunate fossa or sigmoid notch. Fluoroscopic views confirm proper guide-wire position, and the tunnel is made with a cannulated drill.

A tunnel is created in the distal ulna between the fovea and ulnar neck. A 4- to 5-mm drill hole is made in the ulnar neck at its subcutaneous border. A guide wire is inserted in the hole and driven through the fovea. Alternatively, the wrist is flexed and the guide wire may be driven through the fovea and out the ulnar neck. A 3.5-mm cannulated drill bit is used to create the tunnel. If necessary, the tunnel may be further enlarged with larger drill bits or gouges to accommodate both limbs of the graft.

A palmaris longus or plantaris tendon graft is harvested. The palmar opening of the radius tunnel is exposed through a 3- to 4-cm longitudinal incision extending proximally from the proximal wrist crease between the ulnar neurovascular bundle and finger flexor tendons. A suture retriever is passed through the radius tunnel from dorsal to palmar, and one end of the graft is pulled back through the tunnel. A hemostat is passed over the ulnar head but proximal to the remaining TFCC and pushed through the volar DRUJ capsule.

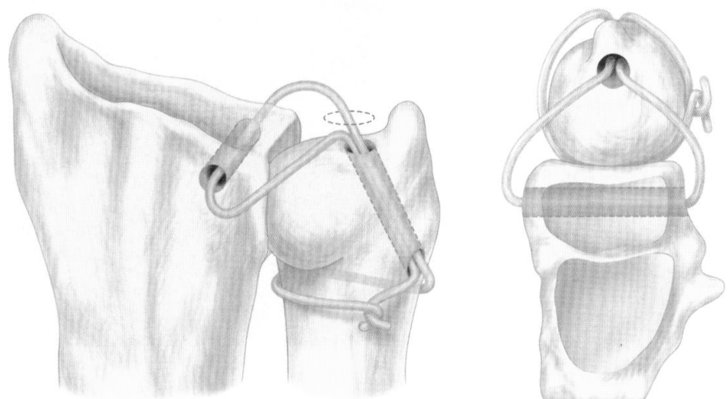

FIGURE 6.3. Tendon graft reconstruction of the DRUJ through bone tunnels.

The other end of the graft is grasped with the hemostat and pulled back along this tract. Both graft limbs are then passed through the ulnar tunnel to exit the ulnar neck. The limbs are passed in opposite directions around the ulnar neck, one passing deep to the ECU sheath. With the forearm in neutral rotation and the DRUJ manually compressed, the limbs are pulled taut, tied together, and secured with sutures (Figure 6.3). The dorsal DRUJ capsule and extensor retinaculum are closed in layers with 3-0 sutures, leaving the EDQ subcutaneous.

Postoperative Management

The patient is placed in a long arm splint with the forearm in neutral to slight supination or pronation, depending on the most stable position. At the first postoperative visit at about 10 days, the patient is converted to a long arm cast extending just above the elbow to control forearm rotation. At three weeks, the cast is changed to a short arm well-molded cast that partially limits forearm rotation for an additional two to three weeks.

The patient is then converted to a removable commercial or custom wrist brace to be used for at least two more months as motion and strength are recovered. Therapy begins with active and gentle passive wrist flexion, extension, pronation, and supination. No limitations are placed on active motion, but only gentle passive motion should be used during the first month of therapy. Strengthening is started early, but high forces with the arm in full pronation and supination are avoided. At four months postoperatively, more aggressive passive ROM and strengthening are added (with the goal to recover 85% of "normal" forearm rotation by six months). No use of the hand for sports or lifting greater than ten pounds is allowed until at least four months postoperatively.

References

1. Tolat AR, Stanley JK, Trail IA. A cadaveric study of the anatomy and stability of the distal radioulnar joint in the coronal and transverse planes. J Hand Surg 1996;21B(5):587–94.
2. Kihara H, Short WH, Werner FW, Fortino MD, Palmer AK. The stabilizing mechanism of the distal radioulnar joint during pronation and supination. J Hand Surg 1995;20A: 930–36.
3. Ekenstam FA, Hagert CG. Anatomical studies on the geometry and stability of the distal radio ulnar joint. Scand J Plast Reconstr Surg 1985;19:17–25.
4. Ekenstam FA. Anatomy of the distal radioulnar joint. Clin Orthop 1992;275:14–18.
5. Whipple TL. Arthroscopy of the distal radioulnar joint. Hand Clinics 1994;10(4):589–92.
6. Leibovic SJ, Bowers WH. Arthroscopy of the distal radioulnar joint. Ortho Clinics of North America 1995;26(4): 755–57.
7. Zelouf DS, Bowers WH. Arthroscopy of the distal radioulnar joint. Hand Clinics 1999;15(3):475–77.
8. Adams BD, Berger RA. An anatomic reconstruction of the distal radioulnar ligaments for posttraumatic distal radioulnar joint instability. J Hand Surg 2002;27A:243–51.
9. Petersen MS, Adams BD. Biomechanical evaluation of distal radioulnar reconstructions. J Hand Surg 1993;18A:328–34.
10. Adams BD. Anatomic reconstruction of the distal radioulnar ligaments for DRUJ instability. Techniques in Upper Extremity Surgery 2000;4:154–60.
11. Adams BD. Distal radioulnar joint instability. In DP Green (ed.), *Operative Hand Surgery, Fifth Edition*. Philadelphia: Elsevier Churchill Livingstone 2005;621–24.

Matthew M. Tomaino

CHAPTER 7

To Jim Herndon for launching my career and to my patients—past, present, and future—for sustaining it. And to ML for his tireless support and friendship.

Class IIA and B Ulnar Impaction: Treatment with Arthroscopic TFCC Disc Excision and Wafer Distal Ulna Resection

Introduction

The ulnar impaction syndrome refers to a painful overload of the ulnocarpal joint[1,2] and has been classified by Palmar based on pathoanatomy (Table 7.1).[3] Palmer and Werner have shown that positive ulnar variance results in an increase in ulnocarpal load,[4] and this has been implicated in the etiology of degenerative triangular fibrocartilage complex (TFCC) tears.[4,25] Ulnar impaction also develops in the wrists with neutral or negative ulnar variance, however.[5,6]

Dynamic increases in ulnar variance may occur with forearm pronation and grip,[7,8,9] and an inverse relationship may exist between TFCC thickness and ulnar variance.[10] Further, it is known that TFCC wear and undersurface fibrillation occur clinically prior to perforation[11] and that innervation of the TFCC may in part explain pain early in the pathologic spectrum of this condition.[12] Palmer's classification of ulnar impaction accounts for the existence of TFCC wear without central disc perforation class IIA and B lesions.[3] This chapter addresses the feasibility of arthroscopic TFCC disc excision and wafer distal ulna resection as treatment of ulnar impaction when TFCC perforation has not yet occurred. This procedure is a viable alternative to ulnar shortening osteotomy.

Biomechanics

Palmer and Werner have shown that in the ulnar neutral wrist 80% of the load is transferred across the radiocarpal joint compared to 20% across the ulnocarpal joint.[4] When variance increases from neutral to 2.5 cm positive, however, ulnocarpal load increases by approximately 20%. Decreasing variance by 2.5 cm lowers force transmission from 20 to 5% in the neutral variant.

This data provides a basis for treating ulnar impaction syndrome with a shortening osteotomy of the ulna.[1,2] Feldon advocated a wafer resection as an alternative in 1992,[13] and in that same year Wnorowski et al. showed that an arthroscopic wafer procedure successfully diminished load across the ulnocarpal joint.[14] Most recently, Markolf et al. have shown that wafer resection decreases distal ulna forces under all conditions of ulnar variance—although less effectively when variance exceeds 4 mm positive.[15]

Although Palmer and Werner have shown that increasing ulnar length results in an increase in force transmission across the distal ulna, and it is known that forearm pronation and forceful grip increase ulnar variance,[5,16,17] few studies have investigated loads across the distal ulna when the forearm is pronated.[10,18] In nine cadaver specimens in different wrist and forearm positions, Glisson et al. showed

Table 7.1.

Classification of Traumatic and Degenerative Conditions of the TFCC

Class I: Traumatic
• Central perforation
• Medial avulsion (ulnar attachment)
• With distal ulnar fracture
• Without distal ulnar fracture
• Distal avulsion (carpal attachment)
• Lateral avulsion (radial attachment)
• With sigmoid notch fracture
• Without sigmoid notch fracture
Class II: Degenerative (Ulnocarpal Impaction Syndrome)
• A. TFCC wear
• B. TFCC wear + lunate and/or ulnar chondromalacia
• C. TFCC perforation + lunate and/or ulnar chondromalacia
• D. TFCC perforation + lunate and/or ulnar chondromalacia + LT ligament perforation
• E. TFCC perforation + lunate and/or ulnar chondromalacia + LT ligament perforation + ulnocarpal arthritis

that loads across the distal ulna increased in pronation, wrist flexion, and ulnar deviation.[18]

Pfaeffle et al. evaluated the effect of axial load and forearm pronation on ulnar variance and distal ulna load in seven cadaver forearms.[10] They found that ulnar variance increased an average of 2 mm in four ulnar positive and three ulnar neutral specimens. Distal ulna load increased in the ulnar neutral wrists and decreased in the ulnar positive wrists, in which greater dorsal subluxation of the distal radioulnar joint occurred. Accurate measurement of variance is important, therefore, when addressing ulnar wrist pain because the radioulnar length relationship has profound impact on load transfer across the wrist.[19]

Diagnosis

Our current diagnostic work-up for ulnar impaction syndrome revolves around the physical examination and plain radiographs. Patients typically complain of ulnar wrist pain. Thus, an evaluation of the ulnocarpal and distal radioulnar joint is required. One must evaluate the TFCC, LT ligament, extensor carpi ulnaris (ECU), flexor carpi ulnaris (FCU) tendons, and pisotriquetral joint and assess for the presence of a midcarpal clunk.

Nakamura's ulnar stress test is routinely performed by ulnarly deviating the pronated wrist while axially loading, flexing, and extending.[20] The "fovea test" is performed by asking the patient to flex the wrist. This allows palpation of the FCU, which facilitates locating the fovea of the TFCC between the FCU and ulnar styloid process. Positive ulnar stress and fovea tests, in combination, are roughly 98% sensitive in terms of correlation with an objective problem with the TFCC and/or LT ligament. Exclusion of other sources of discomfort—such as pisotriquetral arthritis, distal radioulnar joint (DRUJ) instability or arthritis, and ECU tendonitis or hypermobility—increases the suspicion for pathology. An X-ray series is then obtained to evaluate ulnar variance and to assess for the presence of cystic changes in the ulnar corner of the lunate.

Imaging

Various methods of measuring ulnar variance have been described, but each uses neutral rotation posteroanterior (PA) radiographs of the wrist[5,19,21] because pronation will slightly increase the length of the ulna. We routinely check a zero-rotation PA and a lateral view. In addition, a "pronated grip" radiograph is typically taken with the patient making a fist of maximum intensity while the forearm is in pronation.[16] This X-ray may reveal positive ulnar variance not present on a neutral rotation X-ray because of dynamic changes in length when radial shortening occurs during forceful grip.[16,17]

Minami et al. were the first to report using a pronated-grip X-ray, and showed that positive ulnar variance was associated with poorer outcome following TFCC debridement alone.[22] Their suggestion that persistent pain was related to positive ulnar variance is consistent with the message of two other reports that have shown the efficacy of ulnar shortening osteotomy in two situations: with TFCC repair to improve pain relief[23] and to provide successful treatment of persistent ulnar wrist pain following TFCC debridement.[7] Most recently, Minami and Kato have reported successful treatment of TFCC tears associated with positive ulnar variance using ulnar shortening osteotomy alone.[24]

The use of the pronated-grip X-ray attempts, therefore, to image the dynamic increase in ulnar variance—which may accompany forceful grip and pronation. Friedman et al. have reported that a maximum grip-effort grip resulted in an average increase in ulnar variance of 1.95 mm in asymptomatic volunteers.[5] Tomaino showed an identical average increase in the measurement of ulnar variance in light of the fact that measurements in both reports were to the nearest 0.5 mm.[17] Although these two studies do not prove that ulnar recession is required when variance becomes positive on the pronated-grip X-ray, pathomechanical and pathoanatomical data suggests that such positive variance may cause a problem.[1,2,11]

Indeed, high-resolution MR imaging has shown that the TFCC disc is thinner during forearm pronation.[25] It is also known that the undersurface of the TFCC is innervated[12] and undergoes degeneration prior to perforation.[11] Although MR imaging may reveal marrow edema in the ulnar corner of the lunate, TFCC perforation, ulnar chondrosis, and a tear of the LT ligament,[26,27] we no longer routinely order an MRI if the clinical suspicion is high for ulnar impaction and variance is positive on a pronated-grip X-ray.

Treatment

When the history lacks a discrete traumatic precipitant for pain, in the presence of a suggestive examination (as described previously) and when ulnar variance is positive on a neutral rotation X-ray we hypothesize that a class II lesion is present. When a neutral rotation X-ray demonstrates neutral or negative ulnar variance but the pronated-grip view demonstrates positive ulnar variance, we have found that a positive ulnar stress test in combination with a tender fovea correlates highly with a positive finding at the time of wrist arthroscopy. We routinely perform a corticosteroid injection into the ulnocarpal joint at presentation. This frequently provides transient relief at least of symptoms, but not always.

For degenerative TFCC tears, ulnar recession with either ulnar-shortening osteotomy or open wafer resection commonly provides satisfactory pain relief *without* the need for concomitant debridement of associated TFCC or LT tears. Indeed, even post-traumatic perforations of the TFCC have been treated with ulnar recession[28] or by partial excision.[29] For class IIA and B ulnar impaction pre-TFCC perforation lesions, ulnar shortening osteotomy[1,2,30,31] is an option. However, our current preference is arthroscopic TFCC disc excision and wafer distal ulna resection.

Arthroscopic Wafer Procedure

Because TFCC debridement alone may not provide complete pain relief in wrists with positive ulnar variance—and in light of the efficacy of wafer distal ulna resection as a treatment for ulnar impaction syndrome,[6,13,32,33] as well as the biomechanical effect of an arthroscopic wafer procedure in unloading the ulnocarpal joint[14]—Tomaino and Weiser evaluated the efficacy of an arthroscopic wafer procedure and TFCC debridement as a treatment for both post-traumatic and degenerative TFCC tears associated with positive ulnar variance.[9]

At final review, nine patients were very satisfied and three were satisfied. Among the former group, complete resolution of pain occurred in eight and one rated pain as minimal. Among the three patients who were only satisfied with the procedure, one had no pain but complained of portal sensitivity ulnarly, one complained of minimal pain referable to the SL joint, and one had minimal ulnar wrist pain during gripping activities.[9] The ulnocarpal stress test failed to elicit pain in any patient, and the postoperative pronated-grip X-ray revealed that ulnar variance was neutral in all wrists.

Our appreciation of class IIA and B lesions (TFCC wear and lunate chondrosis) at the time of the arthroscopic evaluation has allowed confirmation of the diagnosis of early stages of ulnar impaction (Figure 7.1). TFCC thinning and "pitting" are rather easily noted. Because of favorable results of arthroscopic wafer resection in the setting of TFCC perforation[9]—and the knowledge that isolated TFCC disc excision decreases ulnocarpal load and may address painful undersurface fibrillation[11,12]—we have been prospectively evaluating the results of arthroscopic TFCC disc excision and wafer resection for class IIA and B ulnar impaction for more than two years.

Inclusion criteria have included TFCC wear without perforation and positive ulnar variance on either the zero-rotation or pronated-grip X-ray. The volar and dorsal radioulnar ligaments and the attachment of the TFCC to the ulnar styloid are preserved. A wafer resection is then performed as described by Tomaino and Weiser (Figure 7.2).[9] Our initial prospective evaluation has shown that 16 of 18 patients have experienced satisfactory pain relief at a minimum follow-up of one year. Having performed disc excision and wafer resection in more that 50 patients between 2002 and 2005, we have observed favorable results in 95% of cases.

Surgical Technique

Wafer resection is performed using the 3–4 and 6-R portals with the wrist in 10 pounds of traction via finger traps placed on the index and long fingers. A radiofrequency probe is used to excise the central disc of the TFCC. It is imperative that the dorsal and volar radioulnar ligaments be preserved. Thus, it is safest to use the probe centrally on the disc first, proceeding radially to the sigmoid notch cartilage. After the ulna is visualized, it is easier to complete the disc excision moving ulnarly but not so far that the foveal attachment of the TFCC is disrupted. A shaver or the radiofrequency probe is then used to remove the cartilage on the ulnar head.

A 2.9-mm bur is then brought in through the 6-R portal and a groove is made in the central portion of the ulnar head, proceeding volarly and dorsally as the wrist is pronated and supinated by an assistant. Initially a round bur is used, which is seated its full width to a depth of approximately 2.9 mm. Thereafter, subsequent planing may be achieved more easily—particularly when the bone is hard—using a conical 2.9-mm bur. After debris is removed with a shaver, it is critical to visualize the resected ulnar

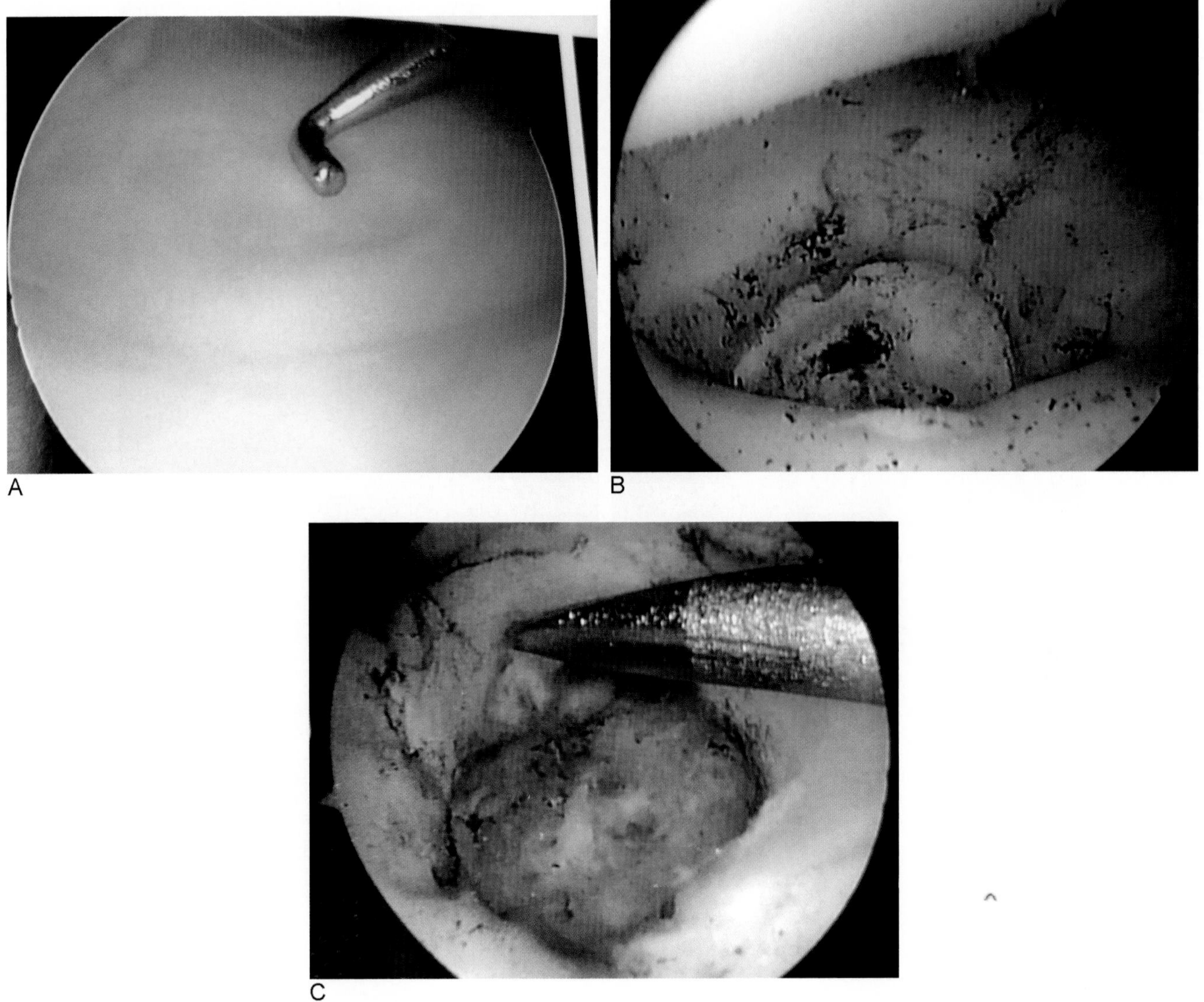

FIGURE 7.1. (A) Intraoperative picture shows TFCC wear. (B) After TFCC disc excision. (C) After wafer resection.

head completely to ensure that a full resection has been performed.

This is performed as the forearm is pronated and supinated. A probe placed through the 6-R portal can be used to lift up the volar and dorsal radioulnar ligaments to facilitate visualization. In addition, when the arthroscope is advanced a bit more ulnarly via the 3–4 portal and the light is rotated to look back toward the sigmoid notch it is possible to verify that a smooth and complete resection has been performed at the sigmoid notch articulation (more radially).

Summary

Although Palmer's classification of TFCC lesions differentiates post-traumatic central perforations (1A tears) from degenerative tears secondary to ulnocarpal impaction (2C),[3] the distinction is not always clear clinically. In the final analysis, the literature suggests that as many as 25% of wrists with TFCC tears have residual symptoms following arthroscopic debridement alone.[22] It is also likely that either static or dynamic ulnar positive variance plays a role.[2,5,17,24]

Our observations suggest that combined arthroscopic TFCC debridement and wafer resection is feasible and provides efficacious treatment for all stages of ulnar impaction syndrome. When class IIA and B changes are observed (that is, when a TFCC perforation has not yet developed), we have observed favorable results in the majority of patients at one-year follow-up following arthroscopic TFCC central disc excision and wafer resection as an alternative to either ulnar shortening osteotomy[31] or open wafer excision.[6]

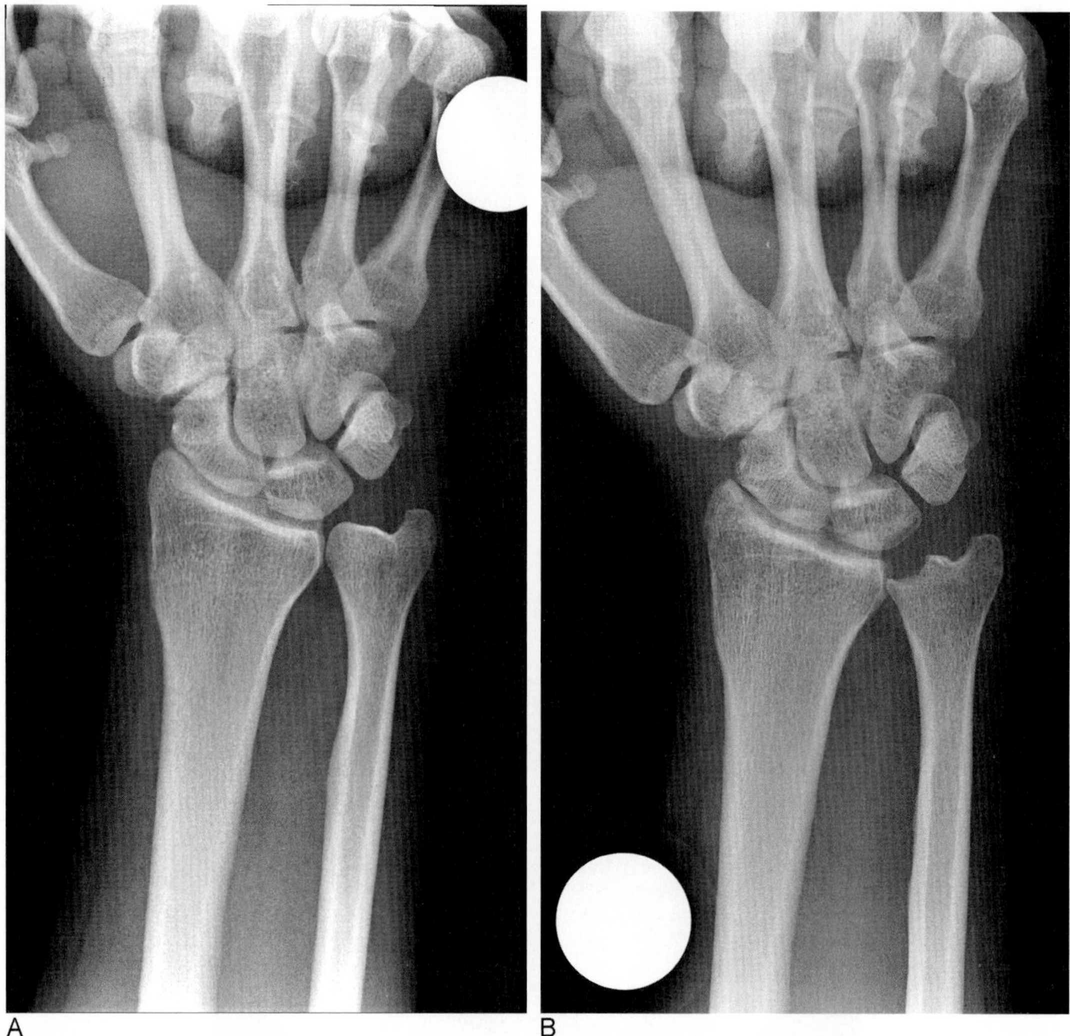

FIGURE 7.2. (A) Preoperative pronated-grip X-ray. (B) Postoperative grip X-ray.

References

1. Chun S, Palmer AK. The ulnar impaction syndrome: Follow-up of ulnar shortening osteotomy. J Hand Surg 1993; 18A:46–53.
2. Friedman SL, Palmer AK. The ulnar impaction syndrome. Hand Clinics 1991;7(2):295–320.
3. Palmer AK. Triangular fibrocartilage complex lesions: A classification. J Hand Surg 1989;14A:594–606.
4. Palmer AK, Werner FW. Biomechanics of the distal radioulnar joint. Clin Orthop 1984;187:26–35.
5. Friedman SL, Palmer AK, Short WH, Levinsohn EM, Halperin LS. The change in ulnar variance with grip 1993; 18A:713–16.
6. Tomaino MM. Results of the wafer procedure in ulnar impaction syndrome in the ulnar negative and neutral wrist. J Hand Surg [Br] 1999;24B:671–75.
7. Hulsizer D, Weiss AC, Akelman E. Ulna-shortening osteotomy after failed arthroscopic debridement of the triangular fibrocartilage complex. J Hand Surg 1997; 22A:694–98.
8. Tomaino MM, Towers JD, Gainer M. Carpal impaction with the ulnar styloid process: Treatment with partial resection. J Hand Surg 2001;26B:252–55.
9. Tomaino MM, Weiser RW. Combined arthroscopic TFCC debridement and wafer resection of the distal ulna in wrists with triangular fibrocartilage complex tears and positive ulnar variance. J Hand Surg 2001;26A:1047–52.
10. Pfaeffle HJ, Manson T, Fischer KJ, Herndon JH, Woo S L-.Y., Tomaino MM. Axial loading alters ulnar variance and distal ulna load with forearm pronation. Pittsburgh Orthopaedic Journal 1999;10:101–02.
11. Tomaino MM. Ulnar impaction syndrome in the ulnar negative and neutral wrist: Diagnosis and pathoanatomy. J Hand Surg 1998;23B:754–57.
12. Ohmori M, Azuma H. Morphology and distribution of nerve endings in the human triangular fibrocartilage complex. J Hand Surg 1998;23B:522–25.
13. Feldon P, Terrono AL, Belsky MR. Wafer distal ulna resection for triangular fibrocartilage tears and/or ulna impaction syndrome. J Hand Surg 1992;17A:731–37.
14. Wnorowski DC, Palmer AK, Werner FW, Fortino MD. Anatomic and biomechanical analysis of the arthroscopic wafer procedure. Arthroscopy 1992;8:204–12.
15. Markolf KL, Tejwani SG, Benhaim P. Effects of wafer resection and hemiresection from the distal ulna on load-sharing at the wrist: A cadaveric study. J Hand Surg 2005;30A: 351–58.

16. Tomaino MM, Rubin DA. The value of the pronated grip view radiograph in assessing dynamic ulnar positive variance: A case report. Am J of Ortho 1999;3:180–81.
17. Tomaino MM. The importance of the pronated grip X-ray. J Hand Surg 2000;25A:352–57.
18. Ekenstam FW, Palmer AK, Glisson RR. The load on the radius and ulna in different positions of the wrist and forearm: A cadaver study. Acta Orthop Scand 1984;55(3):363–65.
19. Palmer AK, Glisson RR, Werner FW. Ulnar variance determination. J Hand Surg 1982;7:376–79.
20. Nakamura R, Horii E, Imaeda T, Nakao E, Kato H, Watanabe K. The ulnocarpal stress test in the diagnosis of ulnar-sided wrist pain. J Hand Surg 1997;22B:719–23.
21. Steyers CM, Blair WF. Measuring ulnar variance: A comparison of techniques. J Hand Surg 1989;14A:607–12.
22. Minami A, Ishikawa J, Suenage N, Kasashima T. Clinical results of treatment of triangular fibrocartilage complex tears by arthroscopic debridement. J Hand Surg 1996;21A: 406–11.
23. Trumble TE, Gilbert M, Vedder N. Ulnar shortening combined with arthroscopic repairs in the delayed management of triangular fibrocartilage complex tears. J Hand Surg 1997;22A:807–13.
24. Minami K, Kato H. Ulnar shortening for triangular fibrocartilage complex tears associated with ulnar positive variance. J Hand Surg 1998;23A:904–08.
25. Nakamura T, Yabe Y, Horiuchi Y. Dynamic changes in the shape of the triangular fibrocartilage complex during rotation demonstrated with high resolution magnetic resonance imaging. J Hand Surg 1999;24B:338–41.
26. Escobedo EM, Bergman G, Hunter JC. MR imaging of ulnar impaction. Skeletal Radiology 1993;24:85–90.
27. Imaeda T, Nakamura R, Shionoya K, Makino N. Ulnar impaction syndrome: MR imaging findings. Radiology 1996; 201:495–500.
28. Boulas JH, Milek MA. Ulnar shortening for tears of the triangular fibrocartilagenous complex. J Hand Surg 1990; 15A:415–20.
29. Menon J, Wood VE, Schoene HR. Isolated tears of the triangular fibrocartilage of the wrist: Results of partial excision. J Hand Surg 1984;9A:527–30.
30. Loh YC, Van Den Abbeele K, Stanley JK, Trail IA. The results of ulnar shortening for ulnar impaction syndrome. J Hand Surg 1999;24B:316–20.
31. Tatebe M, Nakamura R, Horii E, Nakao E. Results of ulnar shortening osteotomy for ulnocarpal impaction syndrome in wrists with neutral or negative ulnar variance. J Hand Surg 2005;30B:129–32.
32. Schuurman AH, Bos KE. The ulno-carpal abutment syndrome. J Hand Surg 1995;20B:171–77.
33. Tomaino MM, Shah M. Treatment of ulnar impaction syndrome with the wafer procedure. Am J Ortho 2001; 30:129–33.

SECTION 3

Carpal Ligament Injury

Steven H. Goldberg, Robert E. Carroll, Kongkhet Riansuwan, and Melvin P. Rosenwasser

CHAPTER 8

To Robert E. Carroll, MD for his past and continued enthusiasm and generosity as a mentor, surgeon, and researcher.

Arthroscopic Treatment of Scapholunate Ligament Tears

Introduction

Scapholunate interosseous ligament (SLIL) injuries are one of the most common causes of mechanical wrist pain. Despite an increased knowledge of carpal injuries and improvements in radiologic evaluation, the diagnosis of an SLIL tear can be difficult or missed unless the evaluating physician has a high index of suspicion and an appropriate level of understanding of wrist anatomy and injury patterns. Usually a detailed history, physical examination, and a series of plain radiographs are sufficient to make a diagnosis of SLIL injury (Figure 8.1). Occasionally, advanced imaging (such as MRI with or without intra-articular contrast) can be helpful in establishing a diagnosis and evaluating the wrist for associated injuries.[1–3] However, MRI usually detects large complete tears better than partial smaller tears, particularly if the tear configuration is oblique to the imaging plane or the tear is smaller than the distance between contiguous image slices.

After successful introduction in the knee and shoulder, arthroscopy gained popularity as one of the most useful modalities for diagnosing and treating a wide spectrum of wrist pathology.[4,5] This procedure has become the gold standard for diagnosis of SLIL injuries.[6–8] Arthroscopy is a minimally invasive procedure allowing direct observation of intrinsic and extrinsic carpal ligaments as well as articular cartilage integrity under static and dynamic conditions. Therefore, comprehensive and accurate diagnosis and treatment of all carpal injuries can be performed concurrently.

Because a delayed or missed diagnosis of an SLIL tear can lead to progressive carpal instability and predispose the patient to a predictable pattern of carpal arthritis called scapholunate advanced collapse (SLAC),[9–11] we believe that wrist arthroscopy should be considered early during the evaluation and management of a patient with a suspected SLIL injury. However, it should be used selectively for patients with significant symptoms (a mechanism of injury consistent with SLIL injury) and in whom conservative treatment has failed or for whom acute operative management is indicated.

Anatomy of the Scapholunate Complex

The wrist is a complex structure comprised of multiple small-joint articulations with stability resulting from a complex linkage of intrinsic intercarpal ligaments and extrinsic capsular ligaments. The wrist can be thought of as 2 separate rows—with hand motion being the composite effect of motion among the radius, ulna, proximal carpal row (scaphoid, lunate, and triquetrum) and distal carpal row (scaphoid, trapezium, trapezoid, capitate, and hamate). Thus, the scaphoid is uniquely situated in both rows on an oblique axis to stabilize the carpus while still permitting coordinated relative motion between the two rows and the radius and ulna. The scaphoid is stabilized by many ligaments, including the SLIL, radioscaphocapitate, scaphotrapeziotrapezoid, scaphocapitate, and dorsal intercarpal ligament.[12]

The SLIL is a C-shaped structure connecting the dorsal, proximal, and palmar surfaces between the scaphoid and the lunate—leaving the distal aspect of the joint bare of soft tissue and allowing the evaluation of scapholunate articular congruity, preservation, and instability. This midcarpal visualization is essential in assessing the degree of instability between the two bones and in grading the spectrum of partial to complete injury.[13] The dorsal and palmar portions of

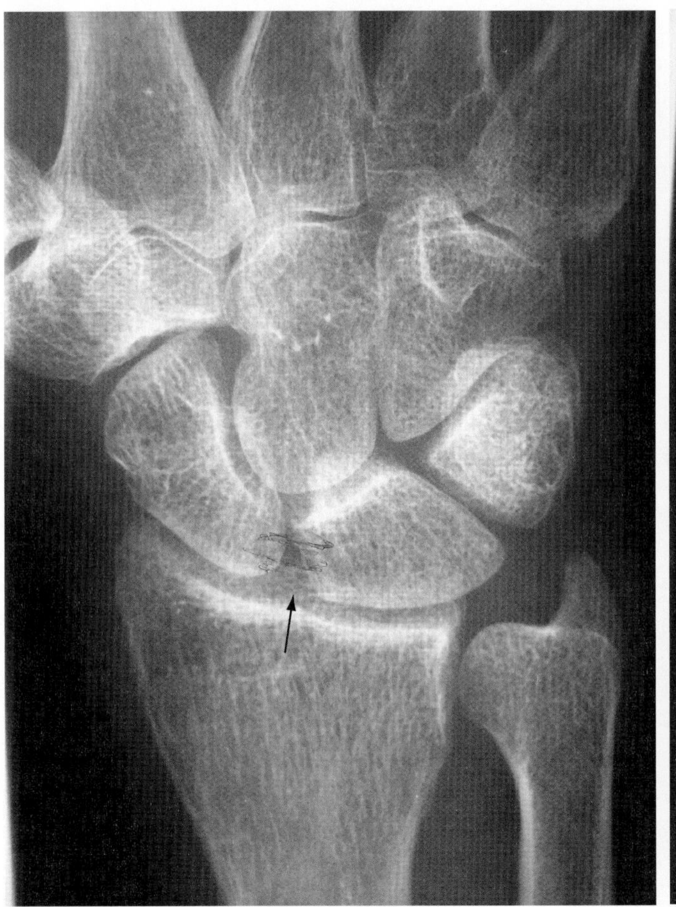

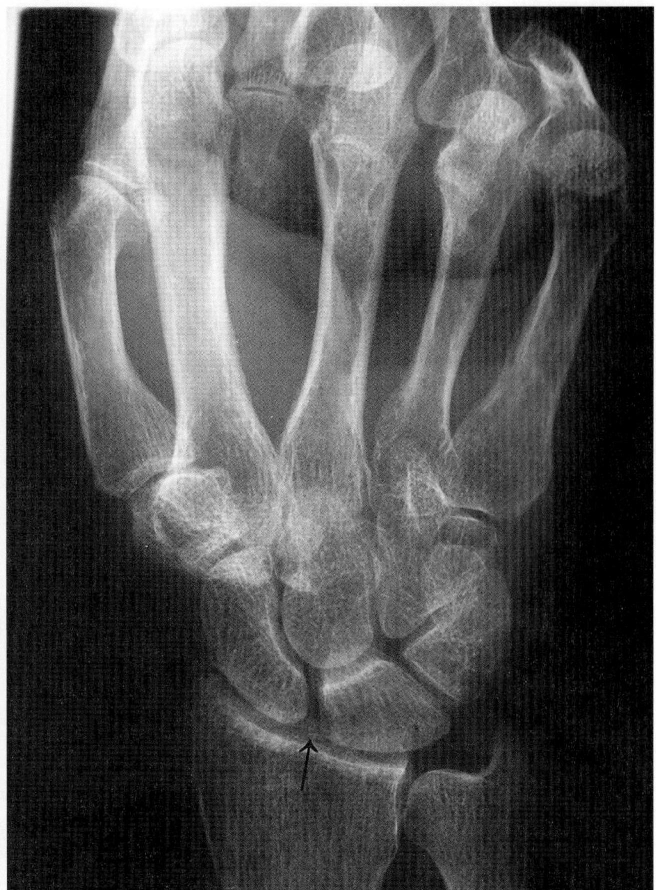

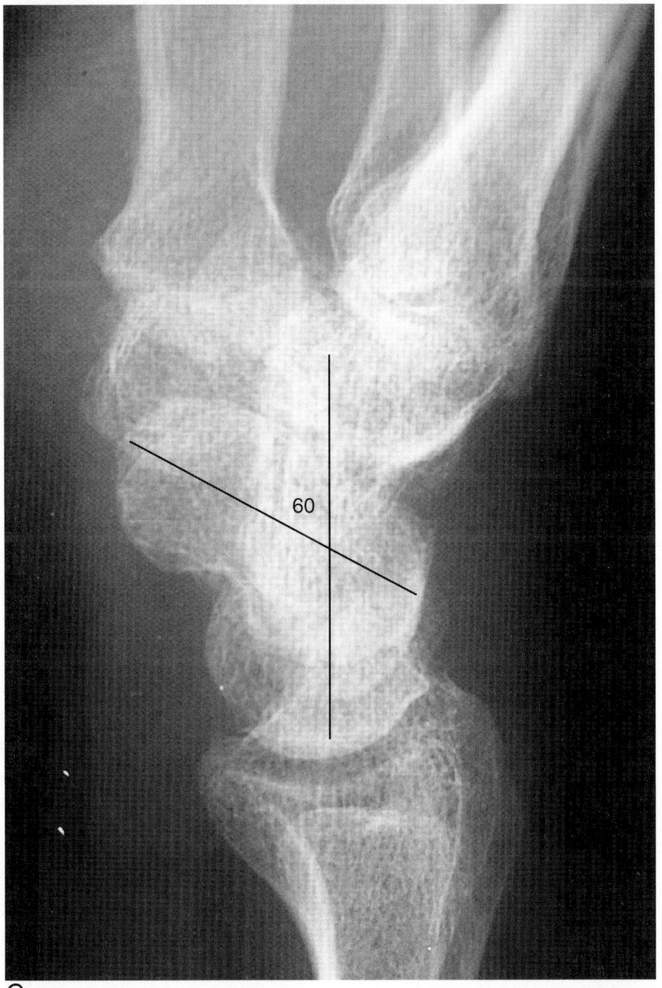

FIGURE 8.1. A 54-year-old patient has 8 years of dorsal radial wrist pain after a snowboarding injury treated with nonoperative management. New radiographs were obtained. (A) Posteroranterior (PA) image, unstressed with possible very early radial styloid-scaphoid joint space narrowing and styloid pointing (SLAC 1). (B) Clenched fist PA image showing no change in width of scapholunate interval or scapholunate step-off. (C) Lateral radiograph.

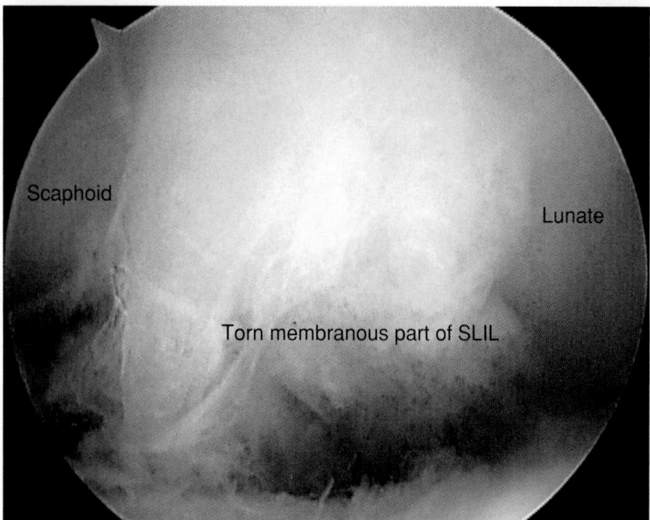

FIGURE 8.2. Intraoperative radiocarpal view of patient in Figure 8.1 showing patulous lax membranous portion of the scapholunate ligament with a complex fibrillated palmar tear.

the SLIL are true ligamentous structures.[14] The proximal portion is a membranous structure composed mainly of fibrocartilaginous tissue.

In the absence of a tear, the transition between the dorsal and proximal portions is not readily visualized during arthroscopy. However, palpation of the SLIL with a probe permits differentiation between the thick taut dorsal ligament and the softer thin proximal portion. A partial SLIL tear may appear as a patulous convex outpouching rather than as a confluent (barely discernible) structure (Figure 8.2). Furthermore, the probe may uncover a complete disruption of the insertion of the SLIL—often from the lunate, which could not be perceived with observation alone. Partial tears may require palpation in the radiocarpal joint with a probe (to appreciate the laxity) and a thorough evaluation of the distal scapholunate joint articular surface congruity in the midcarpal joint to observe subtle incongruity or diastasis. A significant complete intrasubstance SLIL tear will be readily visualized in both the radiocarpal and midcarpal joints.

Biomechanical and Kinematics Considerations

The three different portions of the SLIL have different biomechanical properties. The dorsal portion of the SLIL has highest load at ultimate failure, followed by the palmar portion, and then the proximal portion.[15] Serial sequential ligament sectioning studies in cadavers have found that the SLIL is the primary ligament scapholunate stabilizer.[16–21] However, no significant dissociation between the scaphoid and the lunate is shown on static radiographs with an isolated complete SLIL disruption.[16,22] This is explained by the presence of secondary stabilizers of the SL joint, which must be injured either acutely or chronically to demonstrate radiographic instability. Injury to the volar extrinsic (radiolunate, radioscaphocapitate),[16,23] distal intrinsic (scaphotrapezial),[16,24] or dorsal intercarpal ligament and the SLIL is needed to radiographically visualize pathologic carpal bone rotation.[25]

An isolated tear of the SLIL changes carpal loading and kinematics even without demonstrable radiographic abnormalities. Isolated loss of this major stabilizer of the carpus may lead to attenuation of the secondary supporting structures and progressive dissociation and rotation of the scaphoid and the lunate. With axial loading over time and without proximal restraint by the intact scapholunate joint, the capitate can descend proximally—further driving the scaphoid and lunate apart like a wedge. This results in midcarpal instability, loss of carpal height, and increased clinical symptoms as the bones increase their abnormal rotation.

Changes in the radiocarpal, intercarpal, and midcarpal joint contact areas and loads in conjunction with the altered kinematics result in predictable SLAC arthritis. This begins with radial styloid beaking and radial styloid-scaphoid joint narrowing (stage 1), which then progresses proximally to alter the radial scaphoid facet proximal pole scaphoid articulation (stage 2) and then the midcarpal capitolunate joint (stage 3).[9]

Treatment Options

Several factors need to be considered to aid the clinical judgment indicating an arthroscopic procedure, not only to diagnose but to treat symptomatic scapholunate injuries (Figure 8.3). Acute repairable lesions have heretofore been treated with open suture repair or reattachment with bone anchors. Previous reports have sought to separate acute injuries from chronic by using an arbitrary and unproven 6 weeks as a cutoff, with the implied understanding that only acute injuries could be repaired. However, because the patient history is often unreliable as to the first subtle injury versus the most recent and now symptomatic injury dates alone should not indicate irreparable ligaments.

We believe all such presumed SLIL injuries should be evaluated arthroscopically to properly stage and treat all injured structures. If possible, repair is of course preferred. Arthroscopy has the added advantages that it is performed in real time, can include direct palpation of structures, and can assess the dynamic nature of the instability and its reducibility (neither of which can be known from even the best MRI).

Stable wrists with symptomatic tears (pre-dynamic radiographic instability) are assumed after obtaining normal static and stress radiographs. Unstable wrists with tears demonstrable on grip films or cineradiography only (dynamic radiographic instability) have abnormal carpal alignment on stress radiographs (for example, pronated posterior-anterior grip) but normal alignment on unloaded routine radiographs. Unstable wrists with static instability

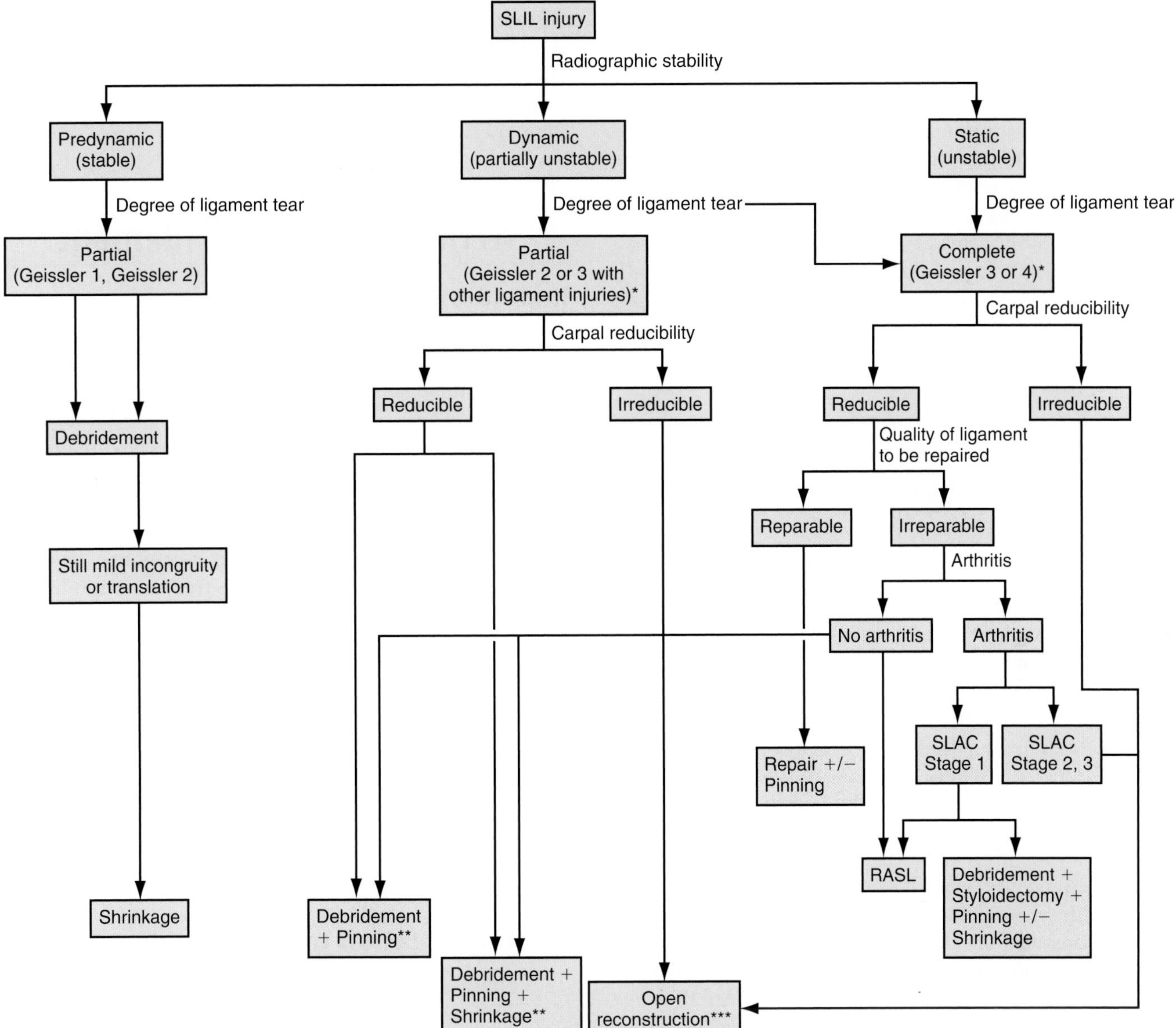

FIGURE 8.3. Algorithm of management of scapholunate ligament tears. (A) Depending on degree of associated ligament injuries, Geissler 2 or 3 can result in dynamic or static instability. (B) Transarticular Kirschner wire fixation of the scapholunate joint is necessary when carpal malrotation is present so that normal alignment can be maintained after carpal bone reduction. (C) Depending on injury pattern, degree of arthritis, and surgeon preference, open reconstruction options include ligament reconstruction by tendon weaves, bone-retinaculum-bone contructs, limited intercarpal fusion, proximal row carpectomy, scaphoidectomy, and 4-corner fusion. Abbreviations: SLAC = scapholunate advanced collapse, RASL = reduction and association of scapoid and lunate procedure.

on routine plain films (static radiographic instability) are the injuries that are obvious and thus not missed. However, these wrists may have advancing cartilage degeneration that is often underappreciated (especially at the capitolunate joint). The presence of significant polyarticular arthritis changes treatment options and often precludes reconstruction and indicates salvage procedures that usually fall outside the purview of arthroscopy (save for the master arthroscopist).

Arthroscopic assessment guides and rationalizes the potential for repair by confirming the degree of injury and the severity of instability.[13] Arthroscopic treatment options include the following, either in isolation or in combination: ligament debridement, ligament thermal shrinkage, transarticular Kirschner wire fixation, and radial styloidectomy (Figure 8.3).

Complete repairable tears in the senior author's (MPR) experience are best managed with open techniques. If the dorsal ligament has been avulsed from its attachment, it can and should be primarily repaired either with transosseous suture or suture anchor. Depending on the amount of associated soft-tissue injuries, this can be augmented with any of the numerous variations on dorsal capsulodesis.[26–28]

SLAC wrist evolution beyond the radial styloid and scaphoid wrist articulation often requires more extensive open surgical procedures. Complete irreparable tears in a young and active patient with a wide scapholunate diastasis and significant carpal mal-rotation should be considered for any procedure that can realign the carpus and preserve carpal kinematics so that the natural history of end-stage SLAC wrist can be forestalled. One such procedure used by the senior author since 1989 is the reduction and association of the scaphoid and lunate (RASL), creating an SLIL neoligament and protecting the repair with a transosseous SL headless bone screw.

Standard Arthroscopic Technique

Similar patient positioning and technique are used in each of the arthroscopic surgical techniques. The patient is placed supine, with the symptomatic arm abducted on a hand table. Regional anesthesia is preferred, and prophylactic intravenous antibiotics are administered. The arm is elevated, prepped, and draped in the usual manner and then a sterile tourniquet is applied to the upper arm. The index and middle fingers are placed in finger traps and suspended from a traction tower, with the elbow flexed 90 degrees. The upper arm is strapped to the hand table and traction tower for counter-traction. Care is taken to ensure all of the ulnar nerve and all bony prominences are well padded and protected. Ten pounds of traction is applied.

All arthroscopic portals are outlined with a skin marker before exsanguination so that the superficial veins are noted and avoided during portal creation. The arm is exsanguinated and the tourniquet is inflated to 250 mmHg. An 18-gauge needle is used to confirm the location of each arthroscopic portal, ensuring that the entry angle corresponds to the volar tilt and radial inclination of the distal radius. The radiocarpal joint is then distended with 3 to 5 cc of normal saline to increase the working space of the joint and to reduce the risk of iatrogenic chondral injury. A #11 blade is used to make a push incision through the skin only, which minimizes the chance for an injury to any adjacent cutaneous nerve branches.

Then a fine curved hemostat is used to bluntly penetrate the capsule. The hemostat is then spread to establish a viewing portal and a blunt-tipped trocar within a cannula is inserted in a controlled manner with a gentle pressure. If there is any resistance to instrument advancement, the needle should again be used to confirm portal location. Iatrogenic damage to the articular cartilage or intercarpal ligaments usually occurs during forced introduction of the trocar at the wrong angle or starting point. After successful cannula placement, the trocar is removed and a 30-degree-angled 2.7-mm arthroscope is inserted.

Distention of the radiocarpal space is maintained by a pressurized irrigation system through the cannula, with outflow through a separately placed 18-gauge needle into the radiocarpal joint in the 1-2 portal or into the ulnocarpal joint through the 6-R or 6-U portals. The 3-4, 4-5, 6-U, 6-R, midcarpal radial, and midcarpal ulnar portals are necessary to complete a thorough diagnostic evaluation and to allow therapeutic procedures.

Arthroscopic Debridement

Indications

Arthroscopic debridement alone is indicated for acute or chronic partial but stable tears of the volar or membranous portion of the ligament in a patient with mechanical symptoms (Figure 8.4). These patients usually have focal reproducible mechanical wrist pain over the dorsal scapholunate joint worsened by activity and normal X-rays. It is common to treat these patients conservatively for several months with splints and activity modification. Persistent symptoms often lead to an MRI, which rarely provides a definitive diagnosis and certainly does not illuminate the treatment options.

Arthroscopy in these patients typically reveals a stable Geissler grade 1 or 2 injury pattern with slight midcarpal incongruity and joint widening. Patients' symptoms are due to tears in the substance of the ligament that while not destabilizing create mechanical impingement during wrist motion, causing focal dorsal wrist pain and occasionally leading to a synovitis and dorsal capsular thickening. Debridement of these SLIL flap tears in either the dorsal or membranous portions and partial synovectomy often ameliorate symptoms.

Contraindication to Debridement Alone

An absolute contraindication is a complete reparable tear or a more advanced Geissler instability pattern that was underappreciated in the preoperative evaluation. Static

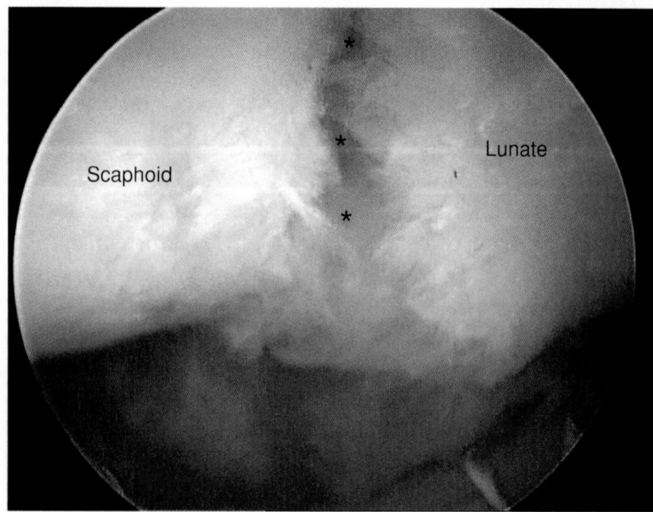

FIGURE 8.4. In the patient from Figures 8.1 and 8.2 the scapholunate joint (*) is visible after debridement of the membranous portion of the scapholunate ligament.

instability patterns with preexistent arthritis will not be helped save in a few selected cases of elderly patients with relatively low demand. A staged debridement and synovectomy can be offered with the full understanding that it may fail and necessitate a more comprehensive salvage procedure.

Technique

Evaluation of the instability is central in indicating the appropriate procedure and requires both radiocarpal and midcarpal arthroscopy to determine the Geissler grade. If the wrist is stable (Geissler grade 1 or 2 injuries), the tear can be debrided by alternating the arthroscope and working instruments between the 3-4 and 4-5 radiocarpal portals. The torn portion of the SLIL is debrided to stable margins, with care taken to preserve healthy intact fibers. This is facilitated by using the least aggressive shaver (such as a full-radius resector), which will not injure healthy intact tissue. After debridement, it is important to reprobe the midcarpal SL articulation to ensure that stability has not been affected.

Results

Isolated arthroscopic debridement has been reported in several small case series (Table 8.1).[5,7,29] Most patients have predynamic or dynamic radiographic instability and Geissler grade 1 or 2 tears. Good pain relief, grip strength improvement, and maintenance of range of motion have been reported. The need for postoperative immobilization is unclear because some studies treated patients in a soft dressing with immediate motion and some studies reported wrist immobilization for 6 to 8 weeks.

Radiofrequency Thermal Collagen Shrinkage

Indications

The indications for thermal collagen shrinkage are similar to those described in the debridement section. In particular, it may be most useful in partial membranous tears or ligament redundancy. If the surgeon appreciates increased motion between the scaphoid and lunate, particularly after debridement, without significant rotation radiofrequency thermal collagen shrinkage can be performed in an attempt to tighten the intact portions of the SLIL and improve carpal kinematics. If there is a redundancy or laxity in the SLIL, usually corresponding to Geissler grade 1, radiofrequency thermal shrinkage can be performed with or without debridement based on surgeon judgment.

Contraindications

Thermal collagen shrinkage alone is contraindicated in the presence of significant unstable flaps of ligamentous tissue because debridement of this tissue is necessary to decrease mechanical symptoms. It is also contraindicated as an isolated procedure in the presence of carpal bone rotation, in repairable ligament tears, and in patients with significant arthritis.

Technique

One study describes thermal stabilization using monopolar cautery (Oratec, Mountain View, CA) placed through the 4-5 portal.[30] The probe is applied to the SLIL, starting volarly and working dorsally until all lax and redundant SLIL has been made taut. The authors recommend continuous irrigation with a safety limit on the probe set to 75° C to prevent chondral thermal injury. When midcarpal examination reveals the scapholunate joint congruency without gapping, the thermal shrinkage is complete. The authors believe postoperative immobilization for 4 to 6 weeks is critical to allow ligament healing and to prevent recurrent laxity.

Another study uses a 2.3-mm bipolar probe (Vapr; Mitek, Westwood, MA) placed through the 4-5 portal.[31] The probe is carefully applied to the torn rim of the volar portion of the ligament, the proximal membranous, and a small part of the dorsal ligament using multiple strokes (like a paintbrush) until visual color changes occur. The probe is used intermittently, delivering energy for only a few seconds at a time to allow adequate outflow of warmed fluid. The tissue quality is palpated with a probe to confirm decreased laxity.

The senior author (MPR) often applies the radiofrequency probe (Microblator 30 1.4-mm, Arthrocare, Sunnyvale, CA) to the proximal membranous portion of the SLIL and to the palmar midcarpal ligaments. In the midcarpal joint, the palmar ligamentous tissue at the junction of the scaphoid and lunate corresponds to the distal edge of the palmar SLIL and the radioscaphocapitate ligament (Figure 8.5).

Careful, limited, short bursts of thermal energy applied to this palmar midcarpal ligamentous and capsular tissue tighten the scapholunate and scapholunocapitate articulations. Thus, this midcarpal application of thermal collagen shrinkage can address both proximal row intercarpal and midcarpal instability. Decreased gapping between the scaphoid and lunate is readily observable. Manual reciprocal palmar-dorsal translation between the scaphoid and lunate before and after thermal shrinkage should be performed without traction to determine if there are any changes in stability after shrinkage. Without reduction of traction, a false increased sense of stability may be appreciated. In addition, it should be more difficult to insert a probe in the midcarpal scapholunate interval.

Results

There are two published series of 10 and 16 patients treated with monopolar and bipolar electrothermal collagen shrinkage and postoperative immobilization ranging from

Table 8.1.

Summary of Literature Regarding Arthroscopic Treatment of SLIL Injuries

	West-Kaempfer[7]	Weiss[29]	Ruch[5]	Hirsh[30]	Darlis[31]	Rosenwasser (Unpublished)	Whipple[33]	Peicha[34]
No. of patients	23 cases	28 cases	7 cases	10 cases	16 cases	8 cases	40 cases	11 cases
Average age	30 years	32 years	41 years	37 years	34 years	38 years	Not mentioned	40 years
Average length of preoperative symptom	6 months	8 months	>6 months	2 (<6 months) 6 (>6 months) 2 unknown	5 months	25 months	Variable	Acute
No. of clinical instability	6 cases	30 cases	Not mentioned	10 cases	13 cases	4 cases	Not mentioned	7 cases
Radiographic instability							Not mentioned	Not mentioned
predynamic	23 cases	not mentioned	7 cases	8 cases	16 cases	5 cases		
dynamic		8 cases		2 cases		3 cases		
static		2 cases						
Geissler grade (number of cases)	1 or 2(21), 3(2)	Complete (15)	Not mentioned	2(10)	1(2), 2(14)	1(1), 2(7)	Not mentioned	3 or 4(7)
Procedure	Debridement	Debridement	Debridement	Monopolar thermal	Debridement + bipolar thermal	4 debridement + shrinkage (none)	Temporary pinning	Temporary pinning
Postoperative immobilization	6–8 weeks	2 weeks	None	Shrinkage (4–6 weeks)	Shrinkage (2 weeks)	4 debridement + shrinkage + pinning	Unknown	8 weeks
Average FU	15 months	27 months	34 months	28 months	19 months	3–8 months	24–96 months	36 months
Outcome	11 excellent 9 good 1 fair 2 poor	67% completed 85% partial Resolved	Good pain relief, minimal loss of motion	9/10 pain resolved, average DASH = 20	8 pain free, VAS 8 to 4 mm, grip 80%, flex/ext. 142 degrees	7 good pain relief, minimal loss of motion, 1 finally wrist fusion	85% pain relief if <3 months and <3 mm of scapholunate diastasis	4 pain relief, 3 mild pain; residual pain may be related to distal radial fractures

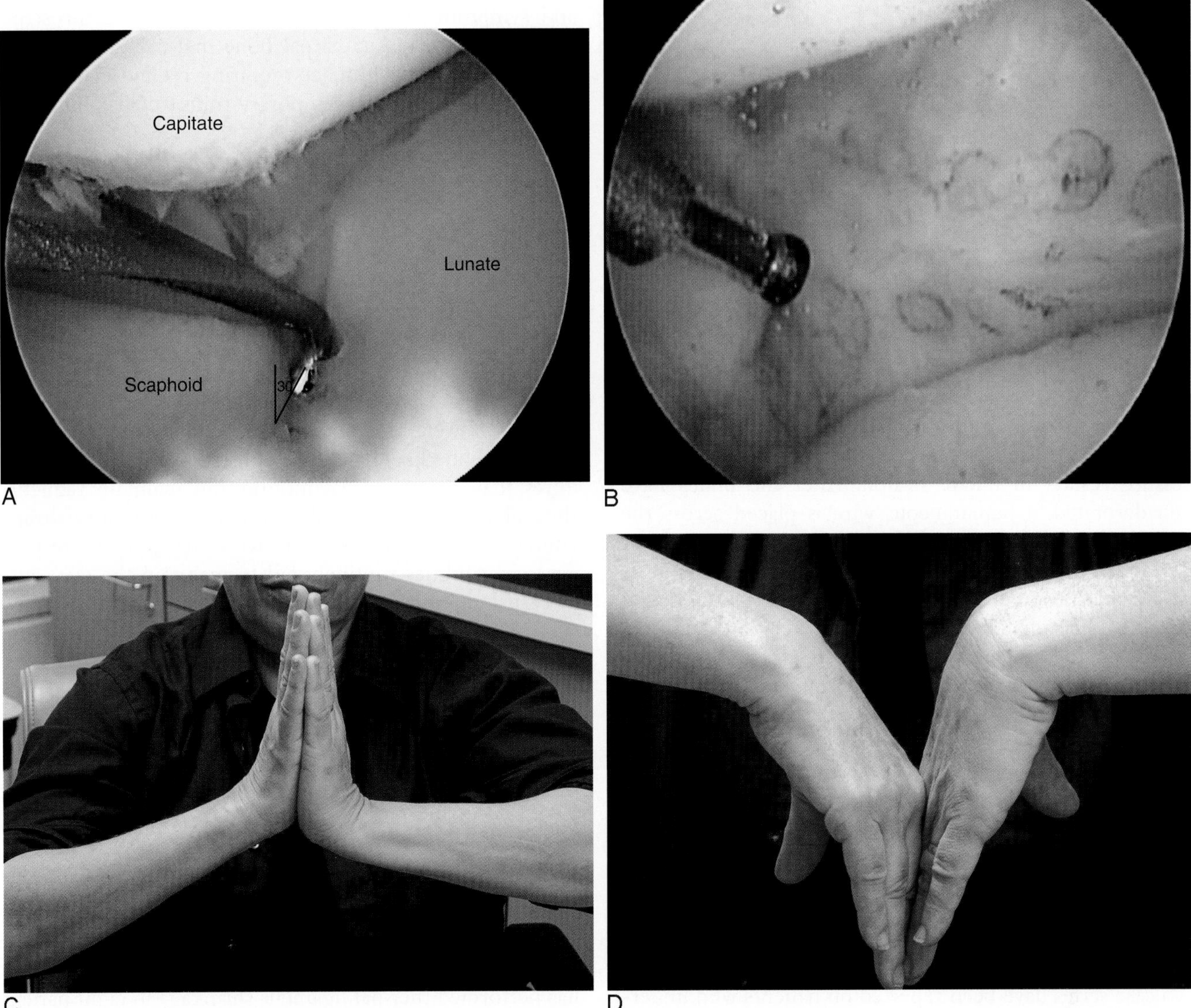

FIGURE 8.5. (A) Midcarpal joint picture of patient from prior figures with a probe inserted into scapholunate joint and able to rotate greater than 30 degrees, indicating at least a Geissler 2 tear. (B) After thermal capsular shrinkage of the palmar midcarpal ligaments, note the brown color change from A. (C) Clinical follow-up of patient four months after debridement, thermal shrinkage, and temporary Kirschner wire fixation. Wrist extension of 52 degrees (right) and 80 degrees (left). (D) Wrist flexion of 40 degrees (right) and 55 degrees (left).

two to six weeks (Table 8.1).[30,31] Complete pain relief ranged from 50 to 90%, with preservation of wrist motion and no postoperative radiographic instability.

Arthroscopic-Assisted Temporary Transarticular Wire Placement

Indications

Transarticular pinning has been hypothesized to result in ligament stiffening and the formation of fibrosis along the pin tract, which can lead to joint stability and alleviate symptoms in patients with mild scapholunate instability. This technique may be useful in patients with mild carpal bone malrotation and diastasis from partial SLIL injuries. When carpal bone anatomic position needs to be restored, transarticular pin placement is necessary to hold the bones in the reduced position until soft-tissue healing occurs. In patients with partial tears without carpal malrotation (in whom the surgeon would like to try to increase stability but does not want to perform radiofrequency thermal collagen shrinkage or in whom there is minimal remaining ligament to debride), the placement of temporary wires may result in increased scapholunate stability.

Contraindications

There are no absolute contraindications to transarticular wire placement. However, wire placement across the intercarpal joints may not be necessary in the absence of carpal malrotation.

Technique

Using manual pressure applied on the distal scaphoid tubercle, palmar to dorsal, the scaphoid can be rotated out of palmarflexion. Radial to ulnar pressure between the scaphoid and triquetrum can close the scapholunate gap. Fluoroscopy and arthroscopy should be used to confirm anatomic reduction. If the lunate is dorsiflexed on the lateral view, it is not possible to be reduced by closed manipulation. Therefore, separate wires can be placed into individual bones and then used as joysticks to derotate the scaphoid and lunate. The scaphoid joystick wire is placed obliquely into the scaphoid, aiming from distal-dorsal to proximal-palmar so that pressure applied to the wire from distal to proximal causes scaphoid extension.

The lunate joystick wire is placed obliquely from proximal-dorsal to distal-palmar so that proximal to distal pressure results in lunate flexion. After the bones have been derotated, a percutaneous wire is placed across the scapholunate joint from radial to ulnar. Either 0.045- or 0.062-inch wires can be used. Pin insertion technique is critical because the anatomic snuffbox contains the dorsal branch of the radial artery, the cephalic vein, and multiple sensory nerve branches with a narrow safe zone.[32] Thus, wires should be pushed through the skin and down to the scaphoid-free hand. Then the wire driver is placed over the wire and turned on. By having the wire tip fixed to the bone prior to wire rotation by the driver, soft-tissue injury is minimized. Several divergent pins can be placed across the scapholunate and scaphocapitate joint in this manner. This is the best way to maintain the reduction of the scapholunate diastasis achieved through derotation.

Results

Two case series have been reported on patients who underwent arthroscopic reduction of the scapholunate joint and temporary transarticular scapholunate joint fixation for isolated SLIL injury or associated with a distal radius fracture (Table 8.1).[33,34] It should be noted that these types of injuries are very different and do not act the same way clinically over long-term follow-up. Acute injuries recognized and treated following trauma have more predictable outcomes in contradistinction to chronic injuries with a vague history of significant antecedent trauma. This correlates with the quality of the tissue at the ligamentocapsular injury site and its capacity to heal.

Arthroscopic Debridement, Thermal Shrinkage, and Temporary Transarticular Pinning

Indications

SLIL debridement combined with thermal capsular shrinkage is indicated in the context of clinical localizing signs and symptoms, radiographic instability, and arthroscopic grading of injury. Any carpal bone mal-rotation (dynamic instability) or incongruence requiring reduction should be further supported with temporary transarticular pinning.

Contraindications

This procedure is contraindicated and inadequate for patients with static carpal malalignment. This corresponds to chronicity, which translates to a lack of adequate residual ligament as scaffolding that could foster repair and provide stability and improved carpal kinematics. These patients require supplemental tissue grafting utilizing open or closed techniques (such as capsulodeses in their many variations, as well as ligament reconstruction with tendon grafts or bone ligament bone constructs or salvage procedures that restrict carpal motion and maintain reduction through limited intercarpal fusions as scaphotrapezialtrapezoid). Simple debridement and Kirschner pinning for these static instabilities routinely fail to maintain the correction of carpal alignment achieved at surgery.[26,35,36]

Technique

Ligament debridement, thermal shrinkage, and temporary transarticular pinning are performed together in a similar fashion (as described in the previous sections).

Results

To date there are no published reports detailing the outcomes of patients treated with this protocol. Thus, this communication is the opinion of the senior author (who has performed thermal ligament shrinkage in eight patients with follow-up to an early clinical result). The patients averaged 38.3 years (range 21 to 54) (Table 8.1), and all met the clinical and radiographic inclusion criteria discussed previously. Procedures included eight ligament debridement—four scaphocapitate and four scapholunate transarticular pinning (0.045-inch K-wire)—one dorsal ganglionectomy, two debridement of the triangular fibrocartilage complex, and one posterior interosseous neurectomy. Predynamic and dynamic radiographic instability were observed in five and three patients, respectively.

The proximal scapholunate ligament was thermally shrunk in all patients, and the midcarpal palmar ligaments were shrunk in four patients. Postoperative immobilization was used in the four patients with reducible instability who underwent pinning. Seven out of eight patients had pain and symptom resolution. One patient with a worker's compensation claim and a prior wrist arthroscopy complained of persistent pain after thermal capsulorrhaphy by the senior author. He was revised to total wrist arthrodesis, which allowed him to return to work. During intraoperative assessment 12 months after thermal shrinkage, there was no visible evidence of cartilage or ligament injury from the thermal shrinkage.

Arthroscopic Styloidectomy

Indications

Arthroscopic radial styloidectomy eliminates the painful impingement between the distal scaphoid and the radial styloid in stage I SLAC. It is typically performed in combination with arthroscopic SLIL debridement. The presence of arthritis indicates long-standing carpal instability with secondary ligament attenuation. Thus, arthroscopic styloidectomy and SLIL debridement alone are usually recommended in older patients with low demand who present with localizing radial wrist pain during activities of daily living. They must be counseled that styloidectomy and debridement may only provide temporary relief of symptoms.

Contraindications

It is contraindicated when arthritis extends beyond the radial styloid-scaphoid waist articulation, as in stage II or III SLAC wrist. It is not recommended as the definitive intervention in a younger and more active person with higher demands because it will not treat the underlying chronic instability.

Technique

After diagnostic arthroscopy confirms advanced midcarpal and/or proximal radioscaphoid arthritis, the working instrumentation portal is the 1-2 portal (which is established between the extensor pollicis brevis and extensor carpi radialis longus tendons). A shielded bur is inserted in the 1-2 portal. Alternatively, the arthroscope may be placed in the 4-5 portal (with the bur placed through the 3-4 portal).

Radiocarpal synovectomy improves visualization of the radial styloid and volar extrinsic ligaments. Less than 4 mm of styloid should be removed to avoid detachment of the radioscaphocapitate (RSC) ligament. The RSC ligament prevents ulnar translation of the carpus. The diameter of the bur helps guide the resection depth, but the degree of resection and decompression should also be assessed with the mini-fluoroscope and in the provocative positions of wrist flexion and radial deviation.

Results

There are no published reports on the outcome of arthroscopic radial styloidectomy in the treatment of SLIL injury and its sequelae. Arthroscopic and open radial styloidectomy were discussed in relation to SLAC wrist in a study by Yao and Osterman,[37] without clinical results.

Reduction and Association of the Scaphoid and Lunate (RASL)

The RASL procedure was developed as an open reconstructive procedure to reassociate the scapholunate joint and foster a fibrous neoligament by dechondrification of the interface and maintaining the reduction through healing with a headless bone screw placed transarticularly by the senior author (MPR). The procedure can be (and is being) done arthroscopically, and although the follow-up is shorter the results are similar.[38–40]

Indications

The RASL procedure is a technique developed for treatment of a chronic static SL instability in which the ligament is irreparable and the resultant arthritis is focal. It is also indicated in salvage after a failed primary surgical reconstruction such as scapholunate ligament repair, scapholunate pinning, or a dorsal capsulodesis.

The RASL technique's premise is that it is important to maintain the obligatory intercarpal SL rotation while still controlling the aberrant scaphoid flexion and lunate extension by relinking the joints without fusing them. The crucial elements of a successful RASL procedure are the dechondrification of the opposing surfaces of the scaphoid and lunate; the anatomic reduction of the scaphoid, lunate, and capitate; and the maintenance of this normal carpal alignment during the reparative phase (in which the formation of a fibrous neoligament between the scaphoid and the lunate occurs).

The planned retention of a headless bone screw (Figure 8.6) augments and protects the fibrous neoligament while undergoing an expected lucency around the lunate screw threads because it permits near physiologic motion between the scaphoid and lunate. This concept has been confirmed by a cadaveric biomechanical study in which scapholunate motion after the RASL procedure was found to be preserved within 5 degrees of the preinjury state for all positions of wrist motion.[41]

Contraindications

The RASL procedure is contraindicated in partial tears without instability or in repairable unstable SLIL tears. In addition, this procedure will not relieve pain in the presence of advanced radiocarpal or midcarpal arthritis. Limited radial styloid-scaphoid arthritis is not a contraindication because a radial styloidectomy is an integral part of the procedure to gain access for the placement of the screw in the central axis of rotation of the lunate.

Technique: Open RASL

A longitudinal dorsal skin incision is made just ulnar to the Lister's tubercle. The third compartment is opened longitudinally and the extensor pollicis longus is retracted radially. The fourth compartment is elevated subperiosteally in an ulnar direction. Wrist arthrotomy is then performed in a ligament-sparing fashion through a transverse incision parallel and proximal to the dorsal intercarpal ligament. The dorsal radiotriquetral ligament is also preserved.

The radial styloid is approached through a separate, short, longitudinal radially based incision. Identification

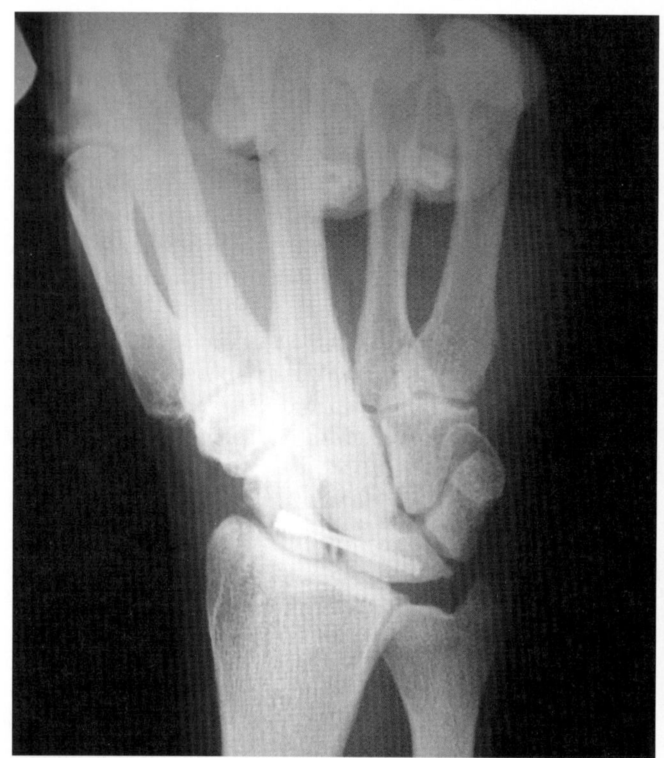

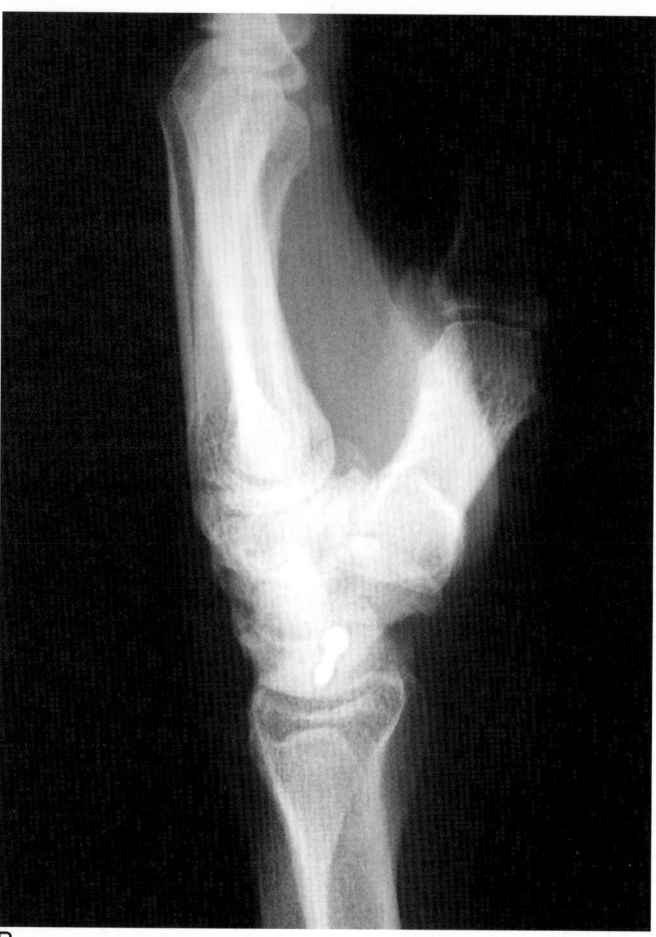

A B

FIGURE 8.6. Two years after RASL procedure, patient has 50 degrees of extension and 60 degrees of flexion, with no pain or activity restrictions. (A) PA grip view. Note central placement of screw into lunate vertex ulnarly. Expected radiolucent lines are seen around the screw ends within the scaphoid and lunate, indicating rotation of the bones around the screw. (B) Lateral radiograph showing slightly palmar position of screw with maintenance of neutral alignment among the radius, lunate, and capitate. Radiolucent lines are also visualized.

and protection of the superficial radial sensory nerve branches and the radial artery are mandatory. Next, the first dorsal compartment retinaculum is incised and reflected and is later used to imbricate the radial collateral ligament and capsule at closure. The thumb tendons are retracted and the capsule is opened longitudinally. A limited styloidectomy is performed, preserving the scaphoid fossa and most of the radioscaphocapitate ligament origin. This provides access to the radial proximal scaphoid for later screw placement and treats the concomitant radio-stylo-scaphoid arthritis. The dorsal capsulotomy is performed through two transverse windows that respect the dorsal intercarpal ligament, an important secondary stabilizer of the wrist.

To manipulate the scaphoid and the lunate during reduction, a 0.062-inch Kirschner wire (K-wire) is placed into each bone and used as a joystick. Each K-wire should be placed at an orientation that will not block the guide-wire placement in the center axis of rotation of the lunate and the subsequent headless screw fixation. If this is noted in subsequent passes of the guide wire, the joystick K-wire can be repositioned after reduction is obtained. One K-wire is placed distally near the scaphotrapezial joint and directed proximally into the palmarflexed scaphoid, and another is placed proximally and directed distally in the dorsiflexed lunate.

The cartilage of the scaphoid and the lunate at the articulation is then burred to induce punctate subchondral bleeding. This will facilitate the ingrowth of vascularity, leading to the development of fibrous tissue and a neoligament. The scapholunate joint is then anatomically reduced by derotation reciprocally by performing flexion of the lunate and extension of the scaphoid using the wire joysticks. This also results in reduction of the capitolunate joint, which is anatomic when the cartilage of capitate proximal pole is no longer visualized. A Kocher clamp is placed on the reduced K-wires to maintain the reduction, which is confirmed fluoroscopically and visually.

Then the wire for the cannulated Headless Bone Screw (Orthosurgical Implants, Inc., Miami, FL) is inserted through the radial incision just proximal to the scaphoid waist toward the lunate vertex. The wire should pass through the center of the scaphoid and lunate in both the coronal and sagittal planes to establish an isometric rotation point that will nearly restore carpal kinematics. The depth should be measured so that the screw can be countersunk slightly within the scaphoid. The screw is advanced, and fluoroscopy is used to confirm appropriate screw position and length. The K-wires are all removed. Interrupted absorbable sutures are used to close the radial capsule. The first dorsal retinaculum is closed over the relocated tendons. The dorsal wrist capsule is carefully repaired without imbrication, and no capsulodesis is performed to limit motion. The extensor pollicis longus remains transposed from its sheath.

A volar splint is used for comfort for two to three weeks. Then, early and active motion in a supervised occupational therapy program is initiated. Gradual resistance exercises are begun several weeks later, with unrestricted activity at four to six months.

The arthroscopic RASL procedure follows the same principles, but the wires and screw are placed percutaneously (often aided by stab wound incisions with a #11 blade). The radial styloidectomy and decortication of the opposing scaphoid and lunate articular surfaces are performed arthroscopically with mechanical burs. Rather than direct observation, scapholunate and lunocapitate reductions are observed fluoroscopically. Thus, time should be taken at the beginning of the procedure to ensure adequate fluoroscopic visualization. We teach that several open RASL procedures should be done before the arthroscopic RASL is attempted.

Results

A good outcome was achieved in 20 of 24 (83%) patients who have undergone an open RASL procedure for chronic scapholunate injury (22 static and 2 dynamic tears an average of 16 months post-injury), with mean follow-up time of 62 months. The postoperative average Visual Analog Score for pain was 1, and the average DASH score was 23. Mean grip strength of the affected hand was 79% compared to the unaffected hand. Mean range of motion in both flexion/extension was 103 degrees.

Postoperative radiographs showed significant improvement of scapholunate diastasis (5.1 to 1.6 mm) and of the scapholunate angle (81 degrees to 53 degrees), and no significant change in carpal height ratio. Three patients needed re-operation due to chronic instability and pain and required intercarpal fusion or proximal row carpectomy. Two patients required screw removal at an average 49 months after surgery due to screw head prominence. One patient is asymptomatic after screw removal and the second patient has persistent instability and progressive arthritis.

Summary

Scapholunate ligament injuries are common, but they are often difficult to diagnose (with many overlapping and confounding conditions). Inadequate treatment can lead to progressive instability due to changes in associated intrinsic and extrinsic ligaments. Arthroscopy plays a major role in staging the degree of chondral and ligamentous injuries and indicating treatment. Various arthroscopic procedures can be performed alone or in combination based on radiographic instability, location, and extent of the ligament injuries. These arthroscopic techniques include debridement, thermal capsuloligamentous shrinkage, transarticular wire placement, styloidectomy, and the RASL procedure. Increasingly severe static deformity resistant to reduction via the arthroscope should be opened. Advanced arthritis should proceed to accepted salvage procedures.

References

1. Morley J, Bidwell J, Bransby-Zachary M. A comparison of the findings of wrist arthroscopy and magnetic resonance imaging in the investigation of wrist pain. J Hand Surg [Br] 2001;26:544–46.
2. Haims AH, Schweitzer ME, Morrison WB, Deely D, Lange RC, Osterman AL, et al. Internal derangement of the wrist: Indirect MR arthrography versus unenhanced MR imaging. Radiology 2003;227:701–07.
3. Schmitt R, Christopoulos G, Meier R, Coblenz G, Frohner S, Lanz U, et al. Direct MR arthrography of the wrist in comparison with arthroscopy: A prospective study on 125 patients. Rofo 2003;175:911–19.
4. Rettig ME, Amadio PC. Wrist arthroscopy: Indications and clinical applications. J Hand Surg [Br] 1994;19:774–77.
5. Ruch DS, Poehling GG. Arthroscopic management of partial scapholunate and lunotriquetral injuries of the wrist. J Hand Surg [Am] 1996;21:412–17.
6. Dautel G, Goudot B, Merle M. Arthroscopic diagnosis of scapho-lunate instability in the absence of X-ray abnormalities. J Hand Surg [Br] 1993;18:213–18.
7. Westkaemper JG, Mitsionis G, Giannakopoulos PN, Sotereanos DG. Wrist arthroscopy for the treatment of ligament and triangular fibrocartilage complex injuries. Arthroscopy 1998;14:479–83.
8. Sennwald G. Diagnostic arthroscopy: Indications and interpretation of findings. J Hand Surg [Br] 2001;26:241–46.
9. Watson HK, Ballet FL. The SLAC wrist: Scapholunate advanced collapse pattern of degenerative arthritis. J Hand Surg [Am] 1984;9:358–65.
10. Watson HK, Weinzweig J, Zeppieri J. The natural progression of scaphoid instability. Hand Clin 1997;13:39–49.
11. Taleisnik J. Current concepts review: Carpal instability. J Bone Joint Surg Am 1988;70:1262–68.
12. Berger RA. The anatomy of the ligaments of the wrist and distal radioulnar joints. Clin Orthop Relat Res 2001;383:32–40.
13. Geissler WB, Freeland AE, Savoie FH, McIntyre LW, Whipple TL. Intracarpal soft-tissue lesions associated with an intra-articular fracture of the distal end of the radius. J Bone Joint Surg Am 1996;78:357–65.
14. Berger RA. The gross and histologic anatomy of the scapholunate interosseous ligament. J Hand Surg [Am] 1996; 21:170–78.
15. Berger RA, Imeada T, Berglund L, An KN. Constraint and material properties of the subregions of the scapholunate interosseous ligament. J Hand Surg [Am] 1999;24:953–62.
16. Short WH, Werner FW, Green JK, Masaoka S. Biomechanical evaluation of ligamentous stabilizers of the scaphoid and lunate. J Hand Surg [Am] 2002;27:991–1002.

17. Burgess RC. The effect of rotatory subluxation of the scaphoid on radio-scaphoid contact. J Hand Surg [Am] 1987;12:771–74.
18. Ruch DS, Smith BP. Arthroscopic and open management of dynamic scaphoid instability. Orthop Clin North Am 2001;32:233–40, vii.
19. Short WH, Werner FW, Green JK, Weiner MM, Masaoka S. The effect of sectioning the dorsal radiocarpal ligament and insertion of a pressure sensor into the radiocarpal joint on scaphoid and lunate kinematics. J Hand Surg [Am] 2002;27:68–76.
20. Meade TD, Schneider LH, Cherry K. Radiographic analysis of selective ligament sectioning at the carpal scaphoid: A cadaver study. J Hand Surg [Am] 1990;15:855–62.
21. Blevens AD, Light TR, Jablonsky WS, Smith DG, Patwardhan AG, Guay ME, et al. Radiocarpal articular contact characteristics with scaphoid instability. J Hand Surg [Am] 1989;14:781–90.
22. Berger RA, Blair WF, Crowninshield RD, Flatt AE. The scapholunate ligament. J Hand Surg [Am] 1982;7:87–91.
23. Ruby LK, An KN, Linscheid RL, Cooney WP III, Chao EY. The effect of scapholunate ligament section on scapholunate motion. J Hand Surg [Am] 1987;12:767–71.
24. Boabighi A, Kuhlmann JN, Kenesi C. The distal ligamentous complex of the scaphoid and the scapho-lunate ligament: An anatomic, histological and biomechanical study. J Hand Surg [Br] 1993;18:65–69.
25. Mitsuyasu H, Patterson RM, Shah MA, Buford WL, Iwamoto Y, Viegas SF. The role of the dorsal intercarpal ligament in dynamic and static scapholunate instability. J Hand Surg [Am] 2004;29:279–88.
26. Szabo RM, Slater RR Jr., Palumbo CF, Gerlach T. Dorsal intercarpal ligament capsulodesis for chronic, static scapholunate dissociation: Clinical results. J Hand Surg [Am] 2002;27:978–84.
27. Wintman BI, Gelberman RH, Katz JN. Dynamic scapholunate instability: Results of operative treatment with dorsal capsulodesis. J Hand Surg [Am] 1995;20:971–79.
28. Lavernia CJ, Cohen MS, Taleisnik J. Treatment of scapholunate dissociation by ligamentous repair and capsulodesis. J Hand Surg [Am] 1992;17:354–59.
29. Weiss AP, Sachar K, Glowacki KA. Arthroscopic debridement alone for intercarpal ligament tears. J Hand Surg [Am] 1997;22:344–49.
30. Hirsh L, Sodha S, Bozentka D, Monaghan B, Steinberg D, Beredjiklian PK. Arthroscopic electrothermal collagen shrinkage for symptomatic laxity of the scapholunate interosseous ligament. J Hand Surg [Br] 2005;31(4):458–59.
31. Darlis NA, Weiser RW, Sotereanos DG. Partial scapholunate ligament injuries treated with arthroscopic debridement and thermal shrinkage. J Hand Surg [Am] 2005;30:908–14.
32. Steinberg BD, Plancher KD, Idler RS. Percutaneous Kirschner wire fixation through the snuff box: An anatomic study. J Hand Surg [Am] 1995;20:57–62.
33. Whipple TL. The role of arthroscopy in the treatment of scapholunate instability. Hand Clin 1995;11:37–40.
34. Peicha G, Seibert F, Fellinger M, Grechenig W. Midterm results of arthroscopic treatment of scapholunate ligament lesions associated with intra-articular distal radius fractures. Knee Surg Sports Traumatol Arthrosc 1999;7:327–33.
35. Wyrick JD, Youse BD, Kiefhaber TR. Scapholunate ligament repair and capsulodesis for the treatment of static scapholunate dissociation. J Hand Surg [Br] 1998;23:776–80.
36. Muermans S, De Smet L, Van Ransbeeck H. Blatt dorsal capsulodesis for scapholunate instability. Acta Orthop Belg 1999;65:434–39.
37. Yao J, Osterman AL. Arthroscopic techniques for wrist arthritis (radial styloidectomy and proximal pole hamate excisions). Hand Clin 2005;21:519–26.
38. Lipton CB, Ugwonali OF, Sarwahi V, Chao JD, Rosenwasser MP. Reduction and association of the scaphoid and lunate for scapholunate ligament injuries (RASL). Atlas of the Hand Clinics 2003;8:249–60.
39. Rosenwasser MP, Miyasaka KC, Strauch RJ. The RASL procedure: Reduction and association of the scaphoid and lunate using the Herbert screw. Techniques in Hand and Upper Extremity Surgery 1997;1:263–72.
40. Lipton C, Ugwonali O, Sarwahi V, Chao JD, Rosenwasser MP. The treatment of chronic scapholunate dissociation with reduction and association of the scaphoid and lunate (RASL). Atlas of the Hand Clinics 2003;8:95–105.
41. Amin, F, Gardner, TR, Ko, BH, Grafe, MW, Raizman, NM, Rosenwasser MP. The RASL procedure (reduction and association of the scaphoid and lunate using the Herbert screw): An evaluation of inter-carpal kinematics in cadaveric wrists. Presented as a paper at the American Association for Hand Surgery Meeting, Tucson, Arizona, January 2006.

Michael R. Hausman

CHAPTER 9

"It is a very sad thing that nowadays there is so little useless information."
—Oscar Wilde

This chapter is dedicated to Esther and Sydney Hausman.

Arthroscopic RASL

Introduction

Treatment of scapholunate instability due to rupture of the scapholunate interosseous ligament remains a challenge, with no predictable or reproducible procedure. The natural progression of SL instability has been documented, and in the last 30 years several treatments have been described to halt the ensuing pathomechanics.[1] Soft-tissue reconstructions include capsulodesis procedures such as the Blatt procedure or the Szabo modification, which uses the dorsal intercarpal ligament. These techniques do not reduce the scapholunate (SL) interval, but are nonetheless thought to provide symptomatic relief.[2,3] Brunelli has described a tenodesis of the scaphotrapezial joint using a strip of the FCR tendon, but long-term follow-up is lacking.[4]

Bone procedures include arthrodesis of the scaphoid and lunate (which has a high complication and nonunion rate) and the scaphotrapezialtrapezoid arthrodesis advocated by Watson.[5,6] Results of this procedure have not been reproducible, and there is the suggestion of progressive arthrosis and limitation of motion over time. Unfortunately, both soft and bony techniques will ultimately impair grip strength and total arc of motion at the expense of scaphoid stabilization.[2]

Herbert initially described a surgical technique involving open reduction and reattachment of the ligament to the bone, combined with Herbert screw fixation across the scapholunate joint. The screw is normally left in situ for 12 to 18 months, allowing sufficient time for ligament healing and restoration of carpal stability.[7]

Rosenwasser and colleagues recently popularized this technique and endeavored to create a stable fibrous pseudarthrosis between the scaphoid and lunate by reducing and stabilizing the SL joint (or reduction association of the scaphoid-lunate RASL) with a Herbert bone screw (HBS). Long-term data is not available on this procedure, but early results are encouraging.[8] The procedure they describe uses both dorsal and radial incisions for joint preparation and reduction (as well as screw placement). Further experience with the procedure led us to develop an arthroscopic (ARASL) technique, which minimizes the tissue trauma and facilitates precise reduction of the joint and placement of the screw.

At the fifty-fifth annual meeting of the American Association of Hand Surgery (January 1996, Palm Springs, CA), a group of hand surgeons were presented with the scenario of a 34-year-old laborer who had suffered a scapholunate interosseous ligament (SLIL) tear. Nearly all believed surgical intervention was necessary. However, half of the group opted for a soft-tissue reconstruction and the other half recommended a bony procedure. The mixed consensus suggests that no clear mode of treatment or solution is suitable to this day, leaving the door open for new techniques to control the scaphoid.

History and Literature Review

As early as 1978, Palmar and colleagues tried to treat scapholunate instability with a tenodesis technique using the ERCL or ERCB. The reports led to modifications of the procedure by Glickel[7] and Almquist. However, the intervention often demonstrated a loss of grip strength and wrist motion of 20 to 25% (while many still complained of pain). By 1985, Watson described fusion of the scaphoid, trapezium, and trapezoid bones (triscaphe arthrodesis) to control scaphoid rotation (with improved results in grip strength).

Other authors were not able to duplicate his clinical results, and Watson modified the procedure by including a generous radial styloidectomy to prevent radioscaphoid arthrosis.[6] However, by spanning the proximal and distal carpal rows mobility was decreased 40% and complications often included nonunion. Although a fusion procedure was generally considered if the SL gap was >4mm, or if the scaphoid was nonreducible, many believed that post-traumatic arthritis was inevitable with limited arthrodeses due to the abnormal wrist kinetics.

Blatt subsequently used the dorsal capsule to tether the distal pole of the scaphoid in extension, whereas Szabo and colleagues demonstrated success utilizing the dorsal intercarpal ligament.[9] Although motion appears to improve at the expense of grip strength, these reconstructions tend to fail over time (as evidenced by radiographic carpal collapse and SL widening). Long-term outcomes are not well documented, but there is cause for concern that late degeneration may occur (because the abnormal carpal alignment is not corrected). Overall, the results are variable (with soft-tissue reconstructions wherein mobility decreases 10 to 44% and strength decreases to 13 to 35% of the contralateral limb).[2] Despite symptomatic improvement, Moran et al. recorded a 15% loss of motion and 20% decrease in grip strength with dorsal capsulodesis (with radiographic alignment lost at two-year follow-up).[3]

In 1991, Hom and Ruby attempted limited arthrodesis of the scaphoid and lunate with high rates of nonunion. However, the pseudoarthrosis rendered many patients symptom free.[5] This led to Rosenwasser to decribe the RASL procedure with encouraging clinical results in early 2000 (American Society for Surgery of the Hand meeting, October 2000, Seattle, WA). The RASL has been reported to minimize the loss of grip strength and mobility 10 to 15%. The technique uses a cannulated Herbert screw to stabilize the scaphoid and lunate.

The dumbbell-shaped screw allows for some rotation, while restoring the scapholunate interval and preventing AP translation at the joint. The RASL requires two incisions: one to perform the reduction and a second for a radial styloidectomy.[8] Shortly thereafter, the ARASL technique was developed using three portals to achieve similar results. Performing this procedure arthroscopically facilitates both establishing the initial diagnosis of a scapholunate injury as well as visualizing the adequacy of reduction of the scapholunate subluxation during HBS screw placement.

Anatomy and Biomechanics

The SLIL is an important intrinsic restraint that allows the scaphoid and lunate to seamlessly rotate in unison during wrist motion. As the wrist palmar or dorsiflexes, the scaphoid moves in concert with the lunate. As the wrist deviates ulnarly or radially, the scaphoid and lunate extend and flex (respectively).[10] If there is an isolated SLIL rupture, the extrinsic ligamentous complex maintains the position of the scaphoid and lunate, albeit with added stress, because the two bones are no longer internally coupled. Attrition of the extrinsic restraints occurs over time, and ultimately the SL interval widens and a dorsal intercalated segment instability (DISI) pattern appears. It is important to understand that both the intrinsic SLIL and extrinsic restraints have to be compromised in order to observe radiographic abnormalities. However, symptoms can still be present despite the lack of radiographic findings. One of the advantages of using the arthroscope is the ability to assess the integrity of the SLIL.

The SLIL consists of three segments, with the ligament being the strongest and thickest dorsally. The volar portion is less robust, and the mid-substance is the weakest (being comprised of fibrocartilagenous material).[2] The volar extrinsic ligaments include the radioscaphocapitate (RSC), long and short radiolunate ligaments (LRL, SRL), and the ulnotriquetral and ulnolunate ligaments. The RSC acts as a fulcrum for the scaphoid to flex and extend. Dorsally, the radiocarpal (DRC) and dorsal intercarpal (DIC) ligaments are stout restraints that prevent dorsal translation of the carpal bones.[10] When the SLIL, along with any of the external ligaments, is injured the scaphoid is free to flex over the RSC and pronate. During the ARASL, adequate reduction of the rotary subluxation is achieved by dorsiflexion and supination of the scaphoid at the same time the lunate is palmar flexed. If the SL instability is allowed to go untreated, the abnormal kinematics that ensue will lead to a scapholunate advanced collapse (SLAC) deformity.[1]

Indications

The ARASL is indicated in cases where there is clinical and radiographic evidence of SL instability. Upon physical examination, tenderness over the dorsum of the scapholunate joint as well as a positive scaphoid shift test (Watson test) is suggestive of SL instability. The Mayfield classification for radial-sided injuries (stage 1) is a useful method to stratify which patients require surgical intervention. Stage 1 injuries are subdivided into four classes with respect to the severity of injury to both the intrinsic and extrinsic restraints.

Class A injuries are the least severe (in which no radiographic signs are present). However, there is clinical suspicion of SL injury. Generally, this represents a partial simple tear of the intrinsic SL ligament and can often be treated conservatively. Class B is considered a "dynamic" state in which stress radiographic views reveal SL widening consistent with an injury to both the intrinsic and extrinsic restraints. Class C demonstrates a static SL gap on radiographs. Such injuries can be further classified into flexible and fixed deformities (Figure 9.1a and b).

Patients with a class A or "predynamic" state can be treated with splinting, pain medication, or cortisone injection until symptoms improve. However, attrition of the extrinsics may develop in which the patient will progress to class B. Patients who present with classes B and C injuries require surgical intervention to control the scaphoid instability and are candidates for the ARASL procedure. Some of the alternative methods of treatment may be contraindicated in the presence of radiocarpal arthritis. However, an

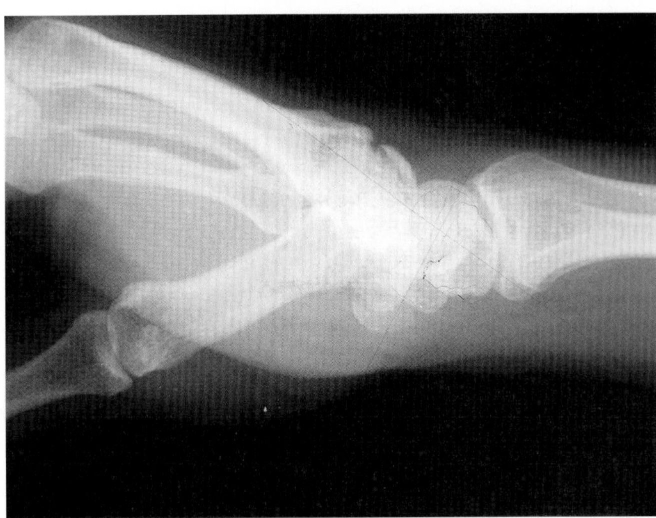

FIGURE 9.1. AP and lateral radiographs show a diastasis (Terri-Thomas) sign at the scapholunate interval, characteristic of a scapholunate ligament rupture. The lesion would be classified as CID (carpal instability dissociative) because of the disruption within the proximal carpal row. The diastasis suggests a Geissler grade IV ligament injury. DISI (dorsal intercalated segment instability) is seen on the lateral view, with the scapholunate angle of 90 degrees.

early SLAC wrist does not preclude one from undergoing the ARASL coupled with a radial styloidectomy. Patients with stage II SLAC wrist have demonstrated symptomatic improvement in our small series, and the ARASL can be performed prior to considering a salvage procedure. Absolute contraindications include SLAC wrists beyond stage II.

Technique

Preparation

The procedure is usually performed under regional anesthesia, with the patient in the supine position. An arthroscopy traction tower is used. Important landmarks include Lister's tubercle, the radial styloid, the abductor pollicis longus (APL) and extensor pollicis brevis (EPB) tendons, and the extensor carpi ulnaris tendon. Low-pressure inflow is used to prevent extravasation into the subcutaneous tissues.

The arthroscopic RASL procedure begins by creating a 3-/,4 portal between the third and fourth extensor compartments and a radial midcarpal portal. The arthroscope is initially inserted into the 3-/,4 portal for inspection of the scapholunate interval and radiocarpal joint. The midcarpal portal, which is located one centimeter distal to the 3-/,4 portal, is then used to evaluate the distal aspect of the scapholunate joint and to confirm the presence of instability. This is more easily seen from the midcarpal portal, in that the torn ligament remnants may obscure the view from the 3-/,4 portal.

Once the diagnosis is confirmed and a "drive-through" sign is seen (Figure 9.2), the arthroscope is placed in the radial midcarpal portal. A 2.9-mm shaver is placed in the 3-/,4 portal. The adjacent articular surfaces of the scaphoid and lunate are denuded of cartilage and excoriated until punctate bleeding is seen. The surfaces are not, however, completely decorticated.

Reduction Procedure

Step 1

Once the surfaces are prepared, a trial reduction is performed. A .062 Swanson pin is placed in the distal pole of the scaphoid. The wire should be placed in the distal pole so that it will not interfere with placement of the screw. The wrist is then flexed and a second .062 wire is inserted into the lunate so that when the wrist is then extended impingement of the K-wire on the dorsal lip of the radius holds the lunate in flexion. In chronic cases, mobilization of the distal pole of the scaphoid may be necessary. This can be accomplished by placing the arthroscope in the radial midcarpal portal and creating an additional palmar portal at the scaphotrapezial joint to permit localized soft-tissue debridement and mobilization.

Step 2

Next, a 1-/,2 portal is created just dorsal to the APL tendon. This will allow for insertion of the cannulated HBS

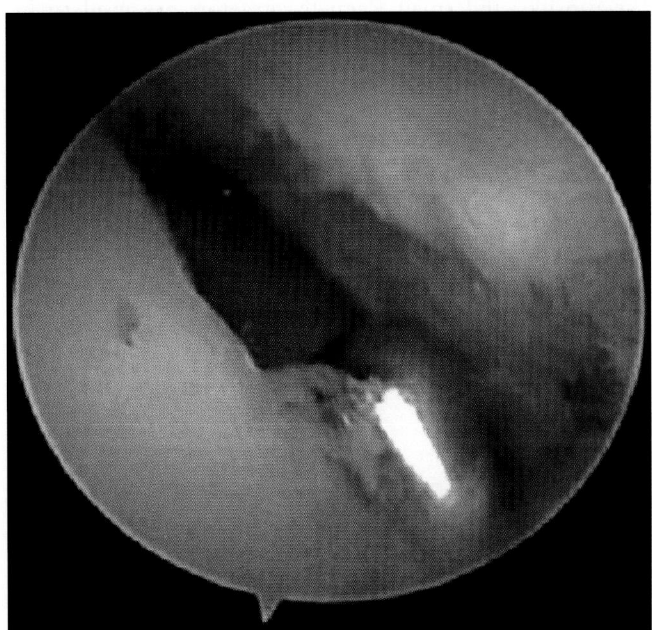

FIGURE 9.2. Radial midcarpal and 3-4 radiocarpal portals are established. With the arthroscope in the radial midcarpal portal, the ligament rupture is confirmed and a 2.9-mm shaver is placed in the 3-4 portal and used to excoriate the opposing surfaces of the scaphoid and lunate. Ideally, punctate bleeding should be seen, but the bones should not be decorticated because this will adverse affect the purchase of the screw.

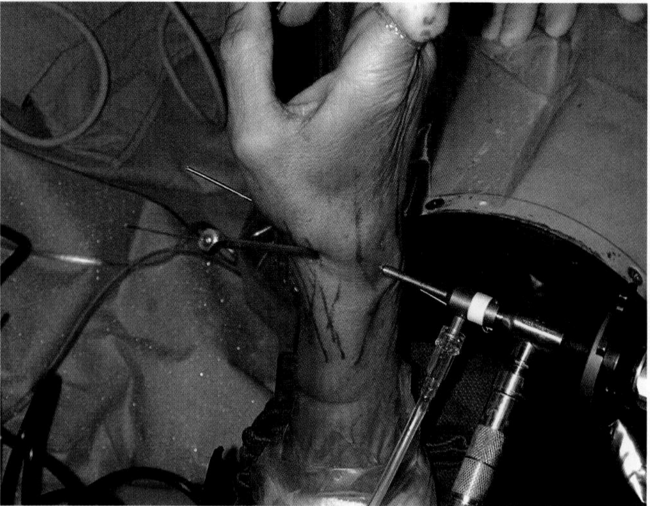

FIGURE 9.3. In chronic injuries, mobilization of the distal pole of the scaphoid may be necessary to anatomically reduce the joint. The shaver may be placed in a 1-2 portal or a palmar scaphotrapezial portal can be made for the shaver. Once mobilized, a .062 K-wire is placed in the distal pole of the scaphoid. The wrist is flexed and a second .062 K-wire is placed in the lunate. When the wrist is dorsiflexed, this pin impinges on the dorsal lip of the radius, stabilizing the lunate in flexion. The joint is then reduced by dorsiflexing and supinating the scaphoid (the supination is critical to an anatomic reduction). The scaphoid is then pinned to the capitate and the radius and the lunate is also pinned to the radius to help stabilize the reduction as the guide wire is passed into the lunate.

screw guide wire. The subcutaneous tissues are spread to the capsule, and small Ragnell retractors are used to introduce a protective cannula. The entrance position of the 0.35-mm guide wire may be observed from either the 3-/,4 portal or under fluoroscopic control (Figure 9.3).

The .035 Kirschner (K)-wire should enter near the waist of the scaphoid, in the mid portion of the bone on the lateral projection. The guide wire should exit just beneath the subchondral surface at the medial edge of the scaphoid. The exit of the pin can be observed from the 3-4 or radial midcarpal portal. The position of the guide wire is absolutely critical to the success of the operation. This may be the most time-consuming part of the operation, but malpositioning is the most common cause of failure.

Step 3

Once the correct position is confirmed, the pin is withdrawn slightly so as not to interfere with the reduction (Figure 9.4a). The scapholunate joint is anatomically reduced by levering the K-wire in the distal pole dorsally and rotating the pin to supinate the scaphoid. The scaphoid and lunate are then firmly fixed by pinning them to the radius and capitate (Figure 9.4b). Confirming again that an anatomic reduction has been achieved, the guide pin is advanced across the scapholunate joint and advanced to the proximomedial corner of the lunate.

The reduction is checked with the arthroscope, and the position of the wire and the carpal alignment are checked with the image intensifier. If correct, the length of the screw is determined by placing a second K-wire against the scaphoid from the 1-2 portal immediately adjacent to the guide wire. The pin is advanced to the surface of the scaphoid, and the difference between the two wires is the length inside the bones. The screw length is 4 to 5 mm *less* than this distance. A second wire may now be inserted parallel to the guide wire to further stabilize the joint. The guide wire is advanced out of the lunate to prevent inadvertent withdrawal during drilling.

Step 4

Next, a new cannulated drill is used. The two scaphoid cortices are perforated. Power may be desirable to penetrate the lunate cortex to avoid pressure that could distract the joint. Once in the lunate, the drill should be advanced by hand up to the medial corner of the lunate. The position is confirmed with the image intensifier and the scapholunate joint is checked to ensure there has been no distraction (Figure 9.4c). It is helpful to compress the joint with the .062 pins during drilling to prevent distraction.

Step 5

Once the drilling is completed, the screw is inserted. If the joint is well reduced, the standard compression screw is used. However, if there is any distraction the high-compression HBS screw can be used to compensate. The screw is advanced until it is barely beneath the subchondral surface of the scaphoid (Figure 9.5a through c). Motion is checked with the image intensifier while the position of the screw and reduction of the joint are confirmed. The instruments are then withdrawn and the portals closed. A short arm cast is applied.

Postoperative Care

Exercises are initiated for the fingers immediately after surgery. Use for light activities (such as typing, writing, and eating) is encouraged. Postoperatively, cast removal occurs at three weeks and gentle range-of-motion exercises are begun. Use, as tolerated, is permitted—except for heavy gripping, lifting, and contact sports, which are prohibited until week six.

Results

A total of seven patients (five males and two females, ages 28 to 77) were included in our study. Four patients had static deformities, whereas three had progressed to an SLAC pattern. Two patients had stage II, and one patient had a stage III SLAC pattern. Total arc of wrist motion was reduced 22.5% at a mean follow-up of 19 months. One patient, who had the SLAC III wrist, experienced

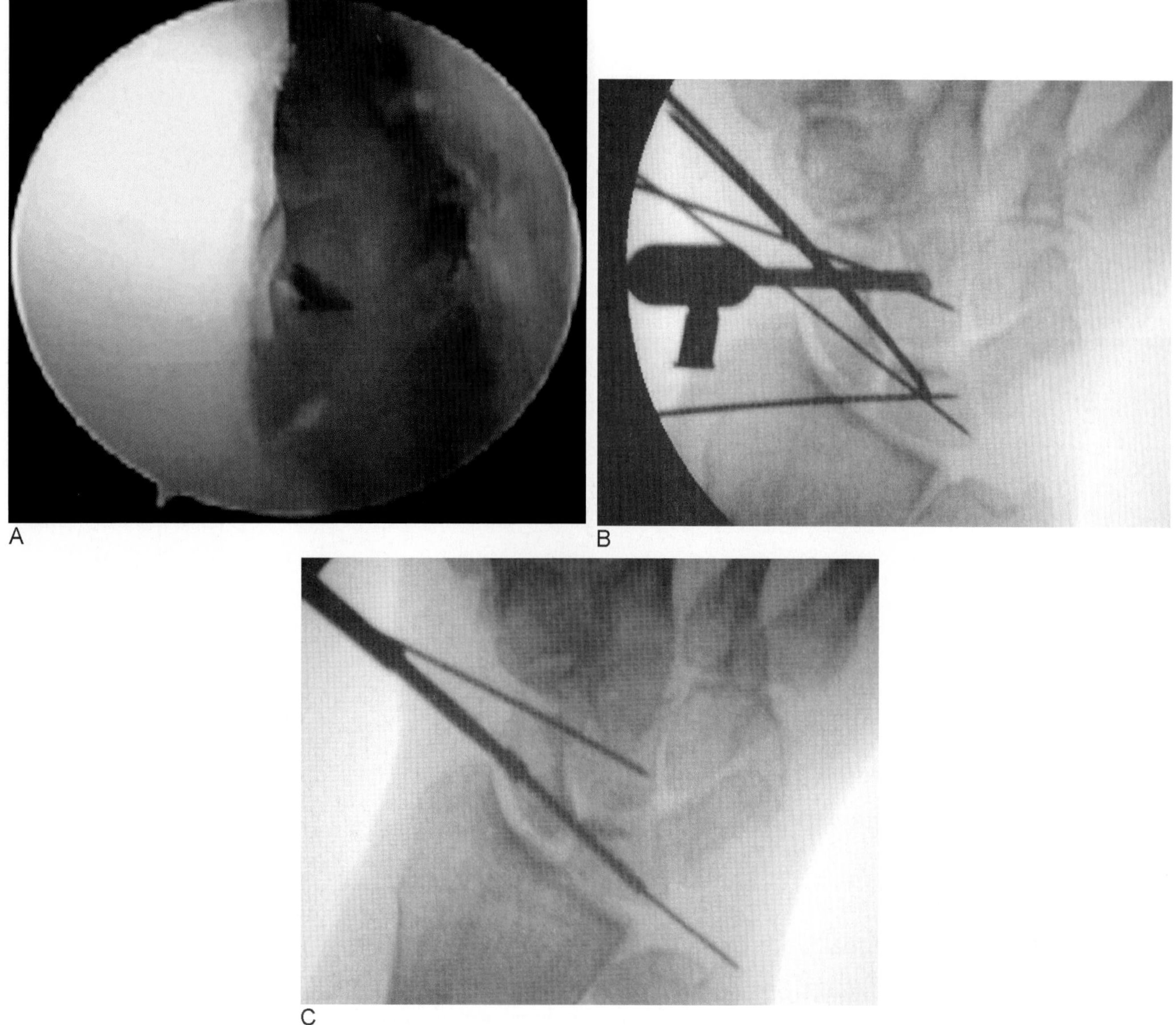

FIGURE 9.4. (A) The position of the guide wire is observed from the radial midcarpal portal. (B) It should pass just beneath the subchondral bone of the scaphoid and lunate and reach the proximomedial pole of the lunate. (C) The drill is then used, taking care not to force the bones apart when drilling the lunate cortex, and the screw is advanced.

a poor result (with a 47% reduction in wrist range of motion and persistent pain). This patient opted for the ARASL prior to having a salvage procedure to minimize her worsening mobility. Without this poor result, the mean reduction in wrist range of motion for the remaining six patients was 17.6%. Radiographically, the mean SL distance was reduced from 4.2 to 1.75 mm and the mean SL angle was reduced from 81.6 to 61.8 degrees.

The ARASL allows for wrist movement to begin more rapidly than the open procedure postoperatively and overall morbidity is minimized. Arthroscopic screw insertion is as precise as its counterpart open procedure, with the advantage of decreased soft-tissue damage. The key to a successful result, regardless of technique, lies within proper screw placement. We have seen fantastic results when the hardware is positioned perfectly. Unfortunately, with the slightest malpositioning the results have been less than favorable.

References

1. Watson HK, Ballet FL. The SLAC wrist: Scapholunate advanced collapse pattern of degenerative arthritis. J Hand Surg [Am] 1984;9:358–65.
2. Bloom HT, Freeland AE, Bowen V, Makonjic L. The treatment of chronic scapholunate dissociation: An evidence-based assessment of the literature. Orthopedics 2003;26: 195–203.
3. Moran SL, Cooney, Berger RA, Strickland J. Capsulodesis for the treatment of chronic scapholunate instability. J Hand Surg [Am] 2005;30:16–23.

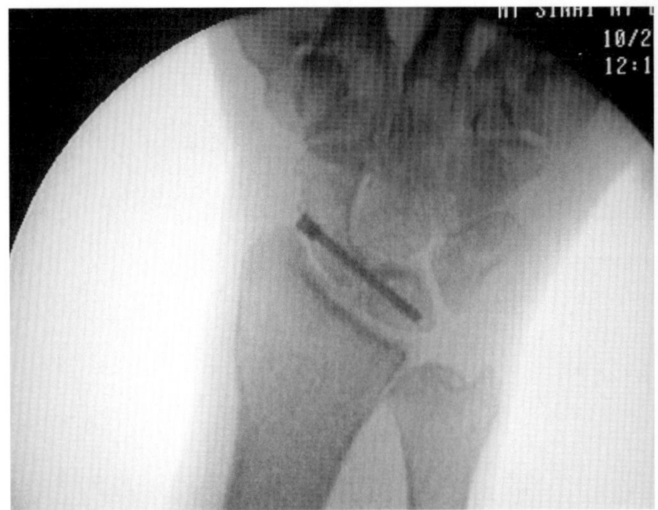

A

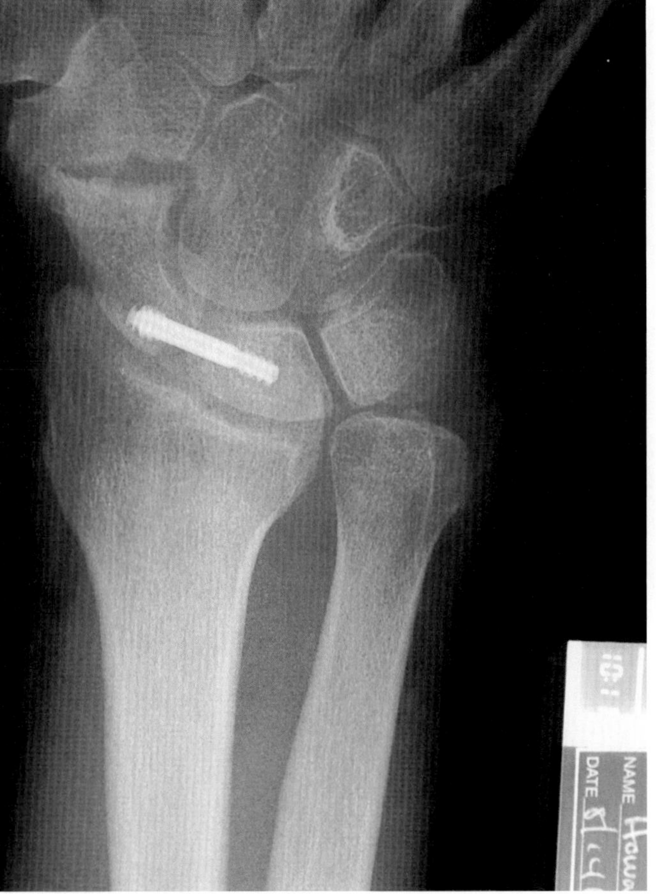

B

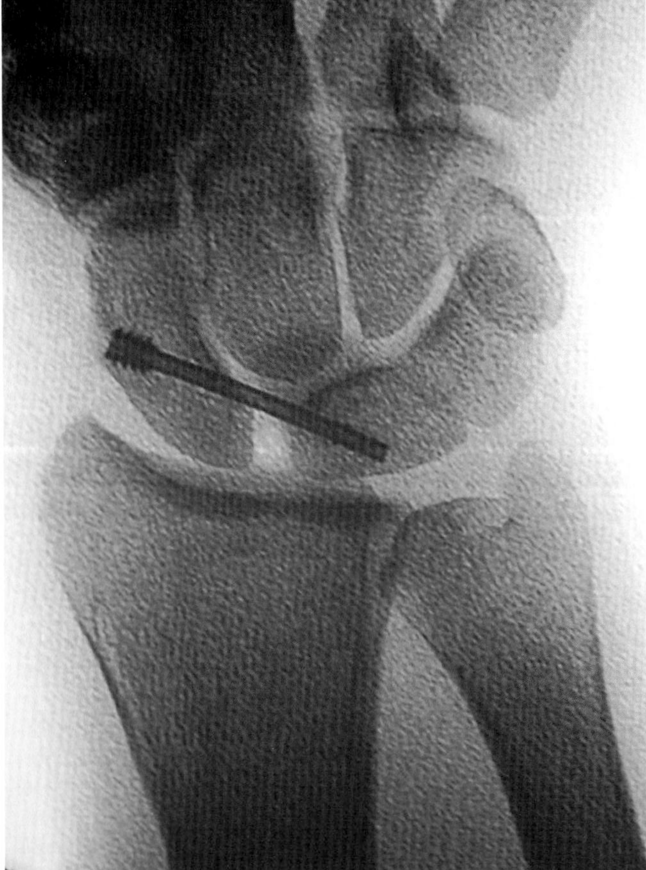

C

FIGURE 9.5. Improper positioning of the screw. Incomplete reduction and incorrect choice of hardware are the most common causes of failure. (A) The correct position of the screw. (B) The screw is placed too proximally in the scaphoid. In addition, the screw does not have enough step-off between the threaded and central diameters, increasing the chance of "pull-out." (C) The scapholunate joint is inadequately reduced, making it impossible for the screw to reach the proximal-medial corner of the lunate without entering the midcarpal joint. If the guide wire cannot be advanced from the waist of the scaphoid to the proximal-medial corner of the lunate without transgressing the midcarpal joint, either the SL joint is mal-reduced or the guide wire is being directed too distally.

4. Brunelli GA, Brunelli GR. A new technique to correct carpal instability with scaphoid rotary subluxation: A preliminary report. J Hand Surg [Am] 1995;20:S82–S85.
5. Hom S, Ruby LK. Attempted scapholunate arthrodesis for chronic scapholunate dissociation. J Hand Surg [Am] 1991; 16:334–39.
6. Watson HK, Ryu J, Akelman E. Limited triscaphoid intercarpal arthrodesis for rotatory subluxation of the scaphoid. J Bone Joint Surg [Am] 1986;68:345–49.
7. Glickel SZ, Millender LH. Ligamentous reconstruction for chronic intercarpal instability. J Hand Surg [Am] 1984;9: 514–27.
8. Lipton CB, Ugwonali OF, Sarwahi V, Chao JD, Rosenwasser MP. Reduction and association of the scaphoid and lunate for scapholunate ligament injuries (RASL). Atlas Hand Clin 2003;8:249–60.
9. Szabo RM, Slater PR Jr., Palumbo CF, Gerlach T. Dorsal intercarpal ligament capsulodesis for chronic, static scapholunate dissociation: Clinical results. J Hand Surg [Am] 2002;27:978–84.
10. Wolfe SW, Neu C, Crisco JJ. In vivo scaphoid, lunate and capitate kinematics flexion and extension. J Hand Surg [Am] 2000;5:860–69.

Ferdinando Battistella, Pau Golano, and Ettore Taverna

CHAPTER 10

The power of the mind is to never stop searching.

Arthroscopic Thermal Shrinkage for Scapholunate Ligament Injuries

Introduction

The use of arthroscopic thermal shrinkage with radiofrequency (RF) for the treatment of scapholunate (SL) ligament injuries is a recent technique, but the real effectiveness is undetermined.[1–3] The ability of RF probes to both debride and shrink tissues makes them an attractive alternative to the use of a mechanized resector for debridement of SL ligament tears, and provides a means of stabilizing the SL joint.

There is still uncertainty about the effectiveness of this technique in the wrist, which is also true with the use of thermal shrinkage in the shoulder or for ACL shrinkage. This may be because technology, rather than scientific clinical evidence, is often the driving force in orthopedic surgery today.

What Is Shrinkage?

Shrinkage is a physical phenomenon that occurs with heat modification of type I collagen in ligamentous tissue. When the collagen is heated to a critical temperature, the heat-labile intramolecular hydrogen bonds break.[4] The protein undergoes a phase transition from a highly ordered crystalline structure to a random-coil state (similar to a melted state) and the tissue tensile properties change.[5] Typically, this thermal denaturation of collagen type I occurs at approximately 60 to 65° C.

The heat in ligamentous tissues is generated by an RF pulse that results in the oscillation of molecules as their polarity changes (i.e., ohmic resistance occurs). The RF probe imparts a high-frequency (350 kHz to 1 MHz) alternating current from an electrical generator to the tissue. This creates an ionic agitation in the tissue as the ions attempt to follow the changes in direction of the alternating current. This ionic agitation results in frictional heating within the tissue. The current passes either between the probe tip and a grounding pad (monopolar) or between two points on the probe tip (bipolar).

Molecular Effects of Thermal Shrinkage

Transmission electron microscopy shows significant alterations in the collagen architecture. These changes are characterized by the loss of the classic 67-nm periodicity of the type I collagen fibril that is evidenced by the loss of the periodical cross-striations in the collagen fibril. There is also an increase in the cross-sectional area of the collagen fibril. The margins of the fibrils begin to lose their distinct edge, while maintaining their circular shape. These ultrastructural effects are caused by unwinding of the collagen triple-helix as a result of the temperature rise in the tissue.[6,7]

Biologic Response to Thermal Shrinkage

At time 0, after thermal shrinkage there is evidence under light microscopy of diffuse hyalinization and fusion of the collagen fiber. By day 7, there is fibroblast proliferation around and within the hyalinized regions. By day 30, large fibroblasts have migrated into the region and have produced a new matrix. These newly arrived fibroblasts use the acellular "hyalinized" collagen as a scaffold for migration and matrix synthesis. At three months, active reparative changes are evident (with an increase in vascularity). The fibroblasts have now regained a more normal appearance under transmission electron microscopy. At seven months, cell morphology and vascularity have returned to normal—without evidence of permanent tissue injury or severe inflammation.[8,9]

Biomechanical Effects of Thermal Shrinkage

The aim of thermal shrinkage is to improve joint stability when the ligaments or capsular tissue are lax or incompetent. There is, however, some conflicting data with regard to the biomechanical properties of thermally treated soft tissue. Some of these inconsistencies may be accounted for by differences in experimental protocols, which do not allow for direct comparison between studies. Only a few (but important) basic concepts may be extrapolated from these studies as they pertain to shrinkage of the scapholunate ligament.

Experimental studies have shown that (1) ligaments and joint capsular tissue can be modified significantly (shortened) by thermal energy at the temperature range of 70 to 80° C, (2) thermal energy causes immediate deleterious effects such as loss of the mechanical properties, collagen denaturation, and cell necrosis, (3) thermally treated tissue is repaired actively by a residual population of fibroblasts and vascular cells, with concomitant improvement of mechanical properties, (4) the shrunken tissue stretches with time if the tissue is subjected to physiologic loading immediately after surgery, and (5) leaving viable tissue between treated regions significantly improves the healing process.[10,11]

Near- and long-term biomechanical effects of thermal energy treatment are different, and the result will depend on the final tissue composition of the scapholunate complex (ligament SL and dorsal capsular ligament). Thus, the postoperative program should maintain the surgically achieved stability for enough time for cellular invasion matrix formation and healing.

Rationale for Shrinkage of Scapholunate Ligament Injuries

Our concept for the use of thermal shrinkage for the treatment of instability of the carpus with scapholunate ligament injuries arose from previous published work on the use of thermal shrinkage on other articulations, as well as the favorable results that were achieved following mechanical debridement of partial SL ligament tears.[12,13] We were also influenced by the biomechanical importance of the SL ligament for stability of the carpus and the paucity of treatment methods for carpal instability, as well as the relative ease of performing an arthroscopic shrinkage of the SL ligament.

The SL ligament is not a homogeneous structure. It is divided into three parts: dorsal, proximal, and palmar (Figure 10.1). The dorsal part is the strongest subregion of the SL ligament. It meets all criteria for the definition of an articular ligament in that it is composed of collagen fascicles surrounded by connective tissue with intertwined neurovascular bundles.[14–16] It has a thickness of 2 to 3 mm and a length of 4 to 5 mm (Figure 10.2), and it merges with the dorsal capsule (Figure 10.3).

The proximal portion is grossly anisotropic. It is composed mainly of fibrocartilaginous tissue, which is relatively

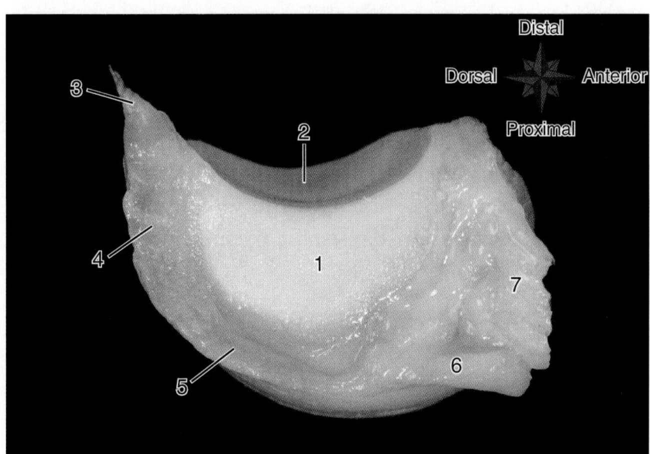

FIGURE 10.1. Lunate and SL ligament. (1) lunate, (2) midcarpal articular surface, (3) dorsal capsule, (4) SL ligament dorsal part, (5) SL ligament proximal part, (6) radioscapholunate ligament, and (7) long radiolunate ligament.

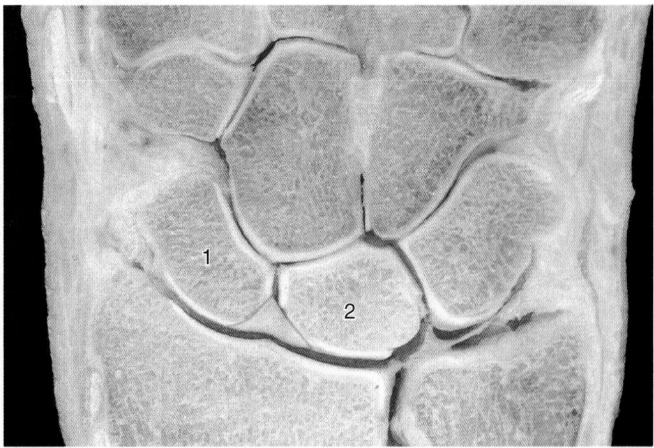

FIGURE 10.2. (1) Scaphoid, (2) lunate, (3) triangular area SL ligament.

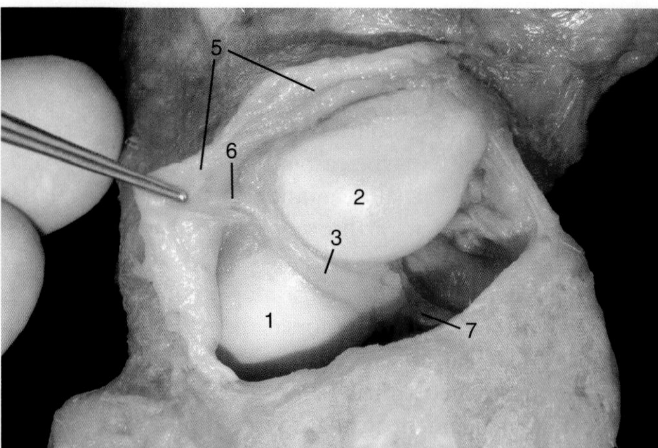

FIGURE 10.3. Dorsal part of SL ligament merges with the dorsal capsule. (1) lunate, (2) scaphoid, (3) SL ligament, (5) dorsal capsule, (6) union of SL with dorsal capsule, and (7) l. testud.

weak due to its avascularity. The transition zone between the proximal and palmar portions is marked by the radioscapholunate ligament, which inserts on the palmar aspect of the scapholunate ligament. The palmar portion is composed of thin collagen fascicles (1 mm thick) of length 4 to 5 mm. This portion is not visible through the standard dorsal arthroscopic portals in the face of an intact radioscapholunate ligament.

The three parts do not have the same tensile strength. The dorsal part is most resistant to shear forces, with an ultimate yield strength of 300 N. The palmar part fails at a load of 150 N, whereas the proximal portion can withstand only 25 to 50 N of stress. The triquetrolunate ligament, which is also divided into three parts, has the exact reverse characteristics in regard to loading failure as those of the SL ligament. Biomechanical studies have also demonstrated that the dorsal subregion of the SL ligament is responsible for controlling scaphoid flexion and the extension motion, whereas the palmar subregion controls rotational motion.[17–20]

Based on this evidence, it was apparent to us that the use of thermal shrinkage of the SL ligament was feasible and most appropriate for the dorsal part of the ligament. When considering the kinematics and the instability of the carpus in SL ligament injuries, it is important to remember the role of the dorsal radiocarpal ligaments (Figure 10.4) and the dorsal capsule (Figure 10.5). They are initimately connected with the SL ligament and must be included in the thermal shrinkage (Figure 10.6).

The aim of thermal shrinkage of the SL ligaments along with the dorsal ligaments and the dorsal capsule is to maintain the ligament and capsular shortening achieved during shrinkage, while awaiting the secondary fibroplasia and resultant thickening of the joint capsule and ligament. Another theoretical goal is the interruption of any painful

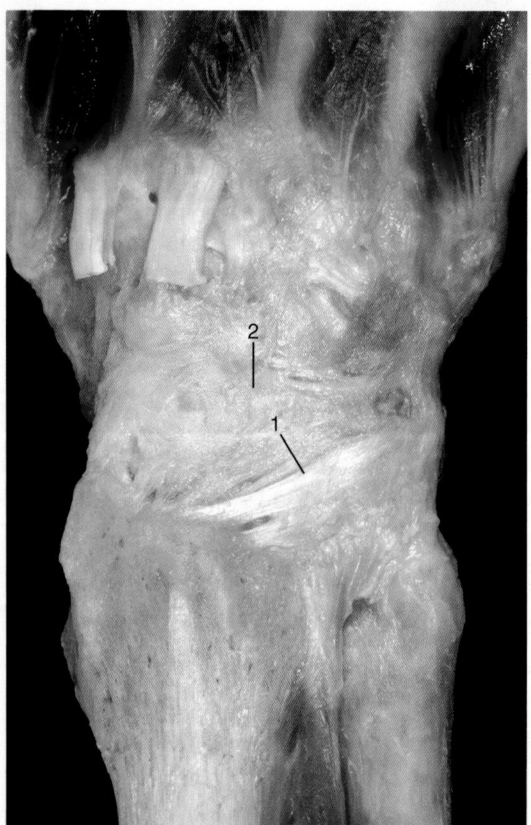

FIGURE 10.4. Dorsal radiocarpal ligament (1) with the dorsal capsule (2).

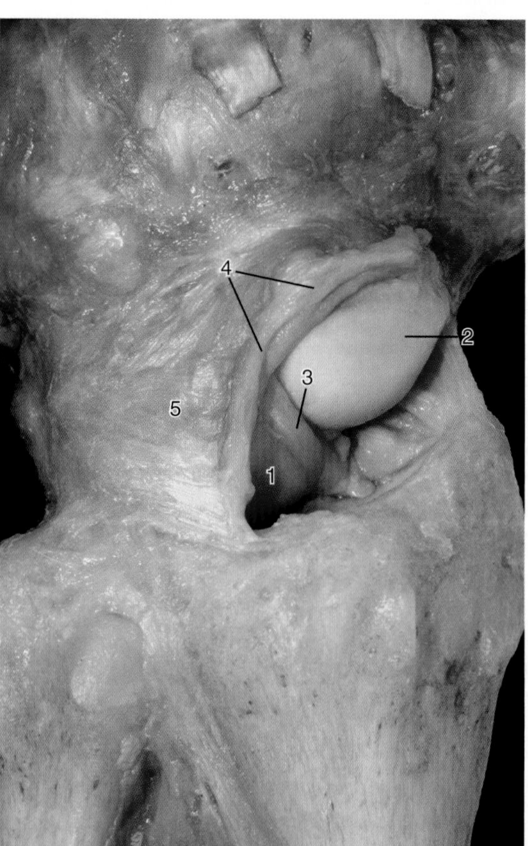

FIGURE 10.5. Anatomic photo. Dorsal capsule intimately connected with SL ligament. (1) Lunate, (2) scaphoid, (3) SL ligament, (4) dorsal capsule, and (5) dorsal radiocarpal ligament.

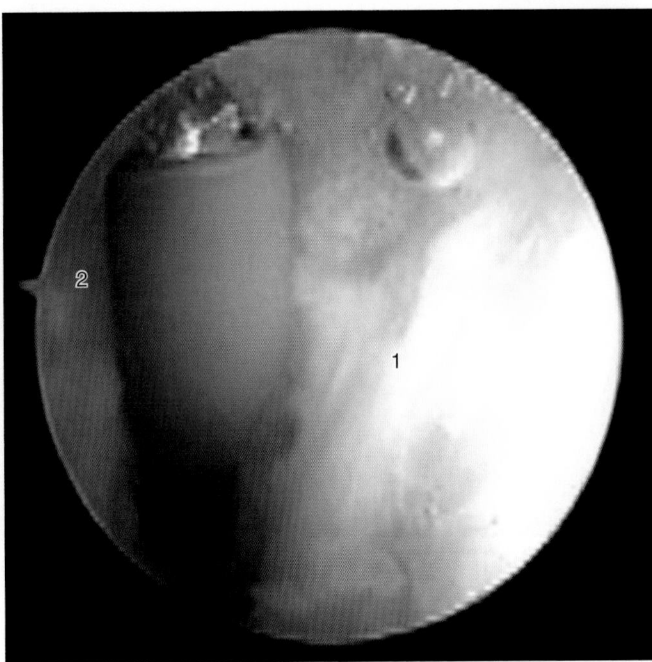

FIGURE 10.6. Arthroscopic photo. (1) SL ligament dorsal part and (2) dorsal capsule.

afferent sensory pathways through the destruction of sensory receptors.[21–23]

Technique

Wrist arthroscopy is performed using a standard technique. The arthroscopy is performed by placing the affected extremity in a distraction tower with 3 to 5 kg of distraction. The correct amount and direction of the distraction force is monitored fluoroscopically, to avoid iatrogenic injury to the carpal ligaments and to control the palmar flexion of the scaphoid. The joint is insufflated with 5 to 7 ml of normal saline, followed by the establishment of the 3-/,4 and 4-/,5 portals (respectively) as a viewing portal and working portal l (as well as establishment of a midcarpal portal).

The wrist is examined from radial to ulnar, and the stability of the SL interval is assessed by probing the transition zone between the dorsal portion of the SL ligament (which is thick and taut). The weaker proximal portion is identified by palpation. All undergo stress testing of the scapholunate ligament under direct visualization. Any ligamentous injury is classified according to the arthroscopic classification scheme described by Geissler.[24] The shrinkage of the SL ligament is performed with a 2.3-mm monopolar RF probe dedicated for shrinkage (Micro-Tacs), includiing an angled tip and a controlled temperature system.

The shrinkage is performed on the entire dorsal section of the ligament (Figures 10.7 through 10.9), extending up to its confluence with the dorsal capsule (Figure 10.10). The palmar subregion of the SL ligament is not included in the shrinkage. The SL ligament and capsular tissue are

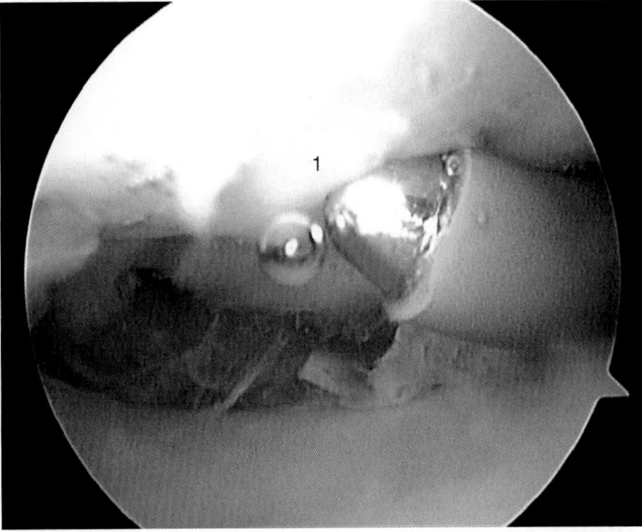

FIGURE 10.7. Arthroscopic photo. (1) SL ligament: shrinkage is performed on the entire dorsal section of the ligament.

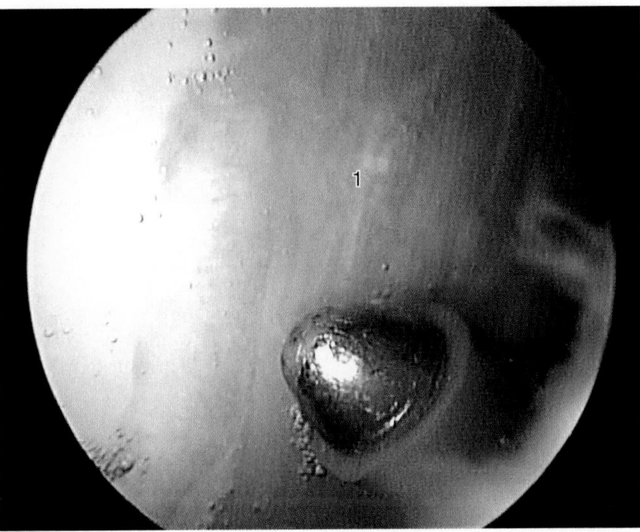

FIGURE 10.8. Arthroscopic photo. (1) SL ligament: shrinkage is performed on the entire dorsal section of the ligament.

treated with multiple single linear passes (grid pattern) to leave more viable tissue adjacent to the treated areas, which may result in faster cellular invasion and matrix formation. There is no objective way of measuring the effect of RF probes, and therefore the surgeon relies on visual assessment of the morphologic ligament tissue changes and capsular volume reduction to quantify the degree of tissue shrinkage.

Using the Geissler classification of SL ligament injuries (Table 10.1), symptomatic grade I lesions are treated with the standard technique for shrinkage. Grade II lesions that demonstrate dynamic instability (i.e., an increased scapholunate gap with loading) are treated with shrinkage in addition to Kirschner wire fixation of the scaphoid and lunate.[25,26] In grade III lesions (where there is a complete SL ligament perforation), the shrinkage is mainly performed

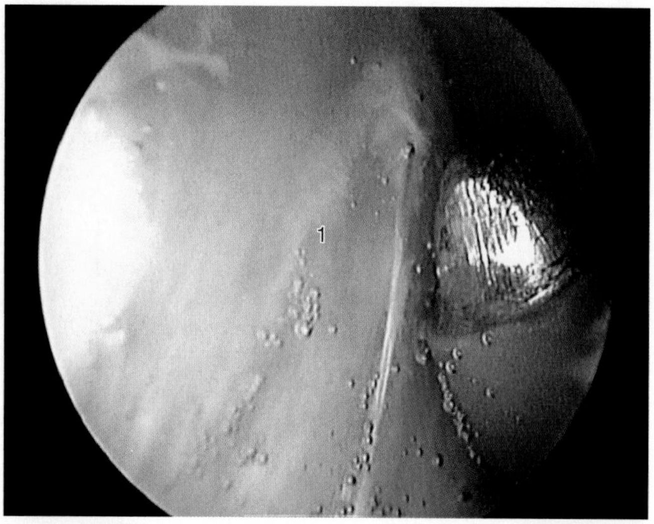

FIGURE 10.9. Arthroscopic photo. (1) SL ligament: shrinkage is performed on the entire dorsal section of the ligament.

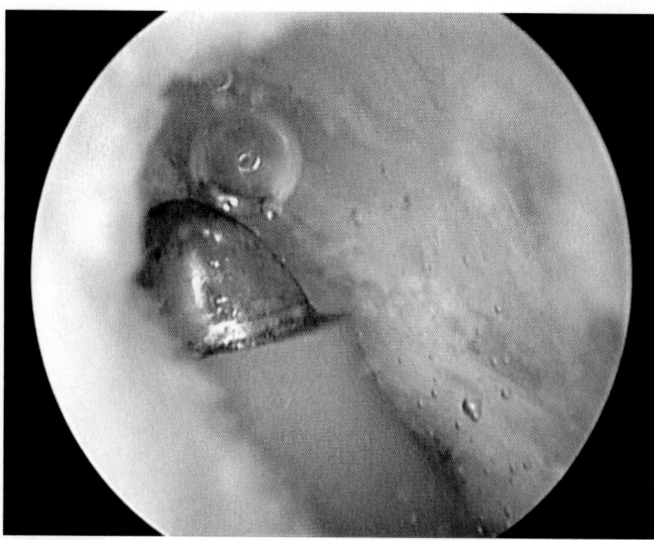

FIGURE 10.10. Arthroscopic photo. The shrinkage is extended up to confluence with the dorsal capsule.

Table 10.1.

Arthroscopic Classification of Scapholunate Ligament (SLIL) Injury

Grade	Radiocarpal SLIL	Midcarpal Instability	Step-Off
I	Hemorrhage of SLIL, no attenuation	None	None
II	Incomplete partial or full substance tear, no attenuation	Slight gap (less than width of 3-mm probe)	Midcarpal only
III	Ligament attenuation, incomplete partial or small full substance tear	Probe can be passed between carpal bones	Midcarpal and radiocarpal
IV	Complete tear	Gross instability 2.7 mm arthroscope can be passed between SL gap (drive-through sign)	Midcarpal and radiocarpal
IV	Complete tear		

Adapted from Geissler WB, Freeland AE, Savoie F, et al. Intracarpal soft-tissue lesions associated with an intra articular fracture of the distal end of the radius. J Bone Joint Surg Am 1996;78:357–64.

on the dorsal capsule and radiocarpal ligaments—with only marginal shrinkage of the torn dorsal ligament combined with Kirschner wire fixation of the scaphoid and lunate.

Acute and sub-acute grade III lesions less than four months old that demonstrate a static SL dissociation and rotational instability require an arthroscopic reduction and Kirschner wire fixation. The arthroscopic reduction is performed with the "joystick" technique: One Kirschner wire is drilled through the skin just radial to the extensor carpi radialis longus tendon into the proximal pole of the scaphoid toward the lunate but not across the scapholunate interval, and a second Kirschner wire is drilled through the dorsal skin into the lunate (with the arthroscope in the midcarpal portal). The scaphoid and lunate are reduced and aligned using the scaphoid K-wire and lunate K-wire as joysticks.

Once the reduction is achieved, one or two additional scaphoid K-wires are drilled across the articulation into the lunate (under fluoroscopic examination to ensure that the radiocarpal and midcarpal joints have not been violated). The K-wires are bent and left protruding through the skin. A thumb spica cast is worn. The cast and K-wires are removed four to six weeks postoperatively, and a cock-up splint is used intermittently between physiotherapy sessions for another four weeks.

Scientific Study

A prospective randomized clinical study was performed to determine the effectiveness of arthroscopic thermal shrinkage with radiofrequency for the treatment of symptomatic

SL ligament injuries. From 2001 to 2004, 120 patients with SL ligament injuries were treated. Inclusion criteria consisted of patients with a Geissler grade I , II, or III SL ligament injury associated with dorsoradial wrist pain unresponsive to six to eight weeks of conservative treatment. Patients with DISI deformities on plain X-rays were excluded. The patients were randomized into four treatment groups, as follows.

- *Group A:* 20 patients (12 male, 8 female), with a mean age of 34.5 years with Geissler grade I SL injuries treated with shrinkage.
- *Group B (control):* 20 patients (11 male, 9 female), with a mean age of 37.5 years with Geissler grade I injuries treated with arthroscopic debridement.
- *Group C:* 40 patients (28 male, 12 female), with a mean age of 36.5 years with Geissler grades II and III SL injuries treated with shrinkage plus pinning with K-wires.
- *Group D (control):* 40 patients (26 male, 14 female), with a mean age of 38.5 years with Geissler grades II and III SL injuries treated with arthroscopic debridement plus pinning with K-wires.

Clinical outcomes were evaluated at 3, 6, 12, and 24 months. Outcome instruments included pre- and postoperative use of the modified Mayo wrist-score range of motion; a visual analog scale for pain at rest, during everyday activity, and heavy manual work; grip strength as a percentage of the contralateral side; and standard and loading radiographs. Data from both groups as compared using the student T test for continuous variables, and the level of significance was set to $p < 0.05$.

Results

No complications were noted from the use of RF probes. The scores for overall clinical outcome demonstrated that group A had better outcomes than group B. Patients in group C had better outcomes than group D. No statistically significant changes were noted between the pre- and postoperative X-rays for groups A and B. There was a statistically significant reduction, however, in the SL interval seen on X-rays during loading for group C.

Based on these findings, we concluded that SL ligament shrinkage in patients with symptomatic predynamic and dynamic instability is a safe technique that had a good success rate at a minimum of two years of follow-up. The treatment of grade I SL injuries with shrinkage is more effective than arthroscopic debridement alone in our hands. Similarly, SL ligament shrinkage when combined with K-wire fixation is more effective than arthroscopic debridement pinning for grades II and III lesions. In the short term, arthroscopic shrinkage is a viable treatment option for SL ligament tears. Long-term studies are still needed to fully evaluate this method.

References

1. Hirsh L, Sodha S, Bozentka D, Monaghan B, Steinberg D, Beredjiklian PK. Arthroscopic electrothermal collagen shrinkage for symptomatic laxity of the scapholunate interosseous ligament. J Hand Surg 2005;30B(6):643–47.
2. Darlis NA, Weiser RW, Sotereanos DG. Partial scapholunate ligament injuries treated with arthroscopic debridement and thermal shrinkage. J Hand Surg 2005;30A:908–14.
3. Shih JT, Lee HM. Monopolar radiofrequency electrothermal shrinkage of the scapholunate ligament arthroscopy 2006; 22(5):553–57.
4. Arnoczky SP, Aksan A. Thermal modification of connective tissues: Basic science considerations and clinical implications. Journal of the American Academy of Orthopaedic Surgery 2000;5:305–13.
5. Owens BD, Stickles BJ, Busconi BD. Radiofrequency energy: Applications and basic science. Am J Orthop 2003;32:117–20.
6. Wallace AL, Hollinshead RM, Frank CB. The scientific basis of thermal capsular shrinkage. J Shoulder Elbow Surg 2000;9:354–60.
7. Medvecky MJ, Ong BC, Rokito AS, Sherman OH. Thermal capsular shrinkage: Basic science and clinical applications. Arthroscopy 2001;17:624–35.
8. Vangsness CT, Mitchell W III, Nimni M, Erlich, Saadat V, Schmotzer H. Collagen shortening: An experimental approach with heat. Clin Orthop 1997;337:267–71.
9. Berger RA, Garcia-Elias M. General anatomy of the wrist. In RA Berger, WP Cooney III (eds.), *Biomechanics of the Wrist Joint*. New York: Springer-Verlag 1991:1–22.
10. DeWal H, Ahn A, Raskin KB. Thermal energy in arthroscopic surgery of the wrist. Clinics in Sports Medicine 2002;21:727–35.
11. Vangsness CT Jr., Mitchell W III, Nimni M, Erlich M, Saadat V, Schmotzer H. Collagen shortening: An experimental approach with heat. Clinical Orthopaedics and Related Research 1997;337:267–71.
12. Lopez MJ, Hayashi K, Fanton GS, Thabit G III, Markel MD. The effect of radiofrequency energy on the ultrastructure of joint capsular collagen. Arthroscopy 1998;14:495–501.
13. Lu Y, Hayashi K, Edwards RB, Fanton GS, Thabit G, Markel MD. The effect of monopolar radiofrequency treatment pattern on joint capsular healing: In vitro and in vivo studies using an ovine model. Am J Sports Med 2000;28:711–19.
14. Wall MS, Deng XH, Torzilli PA, Doty SB, O'Brien SJ, Warren RF. Thermal modification of collagen. J Shoulder Elbow Surg 1998;8:339–44.
15. Fanton GS. Arthroscopic electrothermal surgery of the shoulder. Oper Tech Sports Med 1998;6:139–46.
16. Obrzut LS, Hecht P, Hayashi K, Fanton GS, Thabit G III, Markel MD. The effect of radiofrequency energy on the length and temperature properties of the glenohumeral joint capsule. Arthroscopy 1998;14:395–400.
17. Ruch DS, Poehling GG. Arthroscopic management of partial scapholunate and lunotriquetral injuries of the wrist. J Hand Surg 1996;21A:412–17.
18. Hayashi K, Markel MD. Thermal capsulorrhaphy treatment of shoulder instability: Basic science. Clin Orthop 2001; 390:59–72.
19. Hecht P, Hayashi K, Cooley AJ, Lu Y, Fanton GS, Thabit G III, Markel MD. The thermal effect of monopolar radiofrequency energy on the properties of joint capsule: An in vivo

histologic study using a sheep model. Am J Sports Med 1998;26:808–14

20. Berger RA. The gross and histologic anatomy of the scapholunate interosseous ligament. The Journal of Hand Surgery 1996;21A:170–78.
21. Sokolow C, Saffar P. Anatomy and histology of the scapholunate ligament. Hand Clin 2001;17:77–81.
22. Geissler WB, Haley T. Arthroscopic management of scapholunate instability. Atlas of Hand Clinics 2001;6:253–74.
23. Goldberg SH, Strauch RE, Rosenwasser MP. Scapholunate and lunotriquetral instability in the athlete. Diagnosis and management operative techniques in sports medicine. 2006;14(2):108–21.
24. Geissler WB, Freeland AE, Savoie F, et al. Intracarpal soft-tissue lesions associated with an intra articular fracture of the distal end of the radius. J Bone Joint Surg Am 1996;78:357–64.
25. Weiss APC, Sachar K, Glowacki KA. Arthroscopic debridement alone for intercarpal ligament tears. The Journal of Hand Surgery 1997;22A:344–49.
26. Whipple TL, Schengel D, Caffrey WD. Arthroscopic reduction and internal fixation of scapholunate dissociation. Arthroscopy 1992;8(3):410.

Gregory J. Hanker

CHAPTER 11

To my wonderful family who have brought me great joy.

Arthroscopic Treatment of Lunotriquetral Ligament Injuries

Introduction

An injury of the lunotriquetral interosseous ligament (LTIL) and associated dysfunction at the articulation of the lunotriquetral joint (LTJ) is a common cause of ulnar-sided wrist pain. The LTIL can be damaged to varying degrees, depending on the mechanism of injury and whether the injury is partial or complete or acute versus chronic. These LTIL injuries can be associated with a broad spectrum of ulnar-sided joint maladies: acute trauma from a sprain or a fracture; repetitive motion stress, such as ulnar impaction syndrome (UIS); degenerative joint disease with chronic attritional wear and tear; and inflammatory medical conditions that result in synovitis. LTIL injuries often exist with associated pathologic conditions, and are frequently combined with other problems involving the carpus, the triangular fibrocartilage complex (TFCC), and the distal radioulnar joint (DRUJ).

Wrist arthroscopy plays a critically important role in assessing ulnar-sided wrist pain in general, and LTJ injuries in particular. This chapter describes the current approach to the diagnosis and treatment of LTIL injuries, and the related use of wrist arthroscopy as an important extension of our clinical examination, imaging studies, and therapeutic surgical interventional tools.

Mechanism of Injury

The wrist is an extremely complex joint.[1] Its osseous and ligamentous anatomy as well as the normal carpal kinematics have been well studied.[2–5] There are intrinsic ligaments that both insert and originate on the carpal bones, and extrinsic ligaments that insert on the carpal bones but originate on the wrist outside the carpus. The LTIL is the intrinsic interosseous ligament that stabilizes the lunate to the triquetrum (i.e., the LTJ). The LTJ is found along the ulnar portion of the proximal carpal row (PCR), which consists of the scaphoid, lunate, and triquetrum.

The PCR acts as an intercalated segment (IS), providing a mechanical linkage between the distal carpal row and the distal radius and ulna. There are three distinct regions of the LTIL (Figure 11.1). The dorsal and palmar portions are thickened and provide a strong, stable connection at the LTJ. The palmar portion of the LTIL is the thickest and strongest of the three regions, and is most important in the transmission of load and strain from the triquetrum to the lunate. The central, proximal portion of the LTIL consists of a fibrocartilaginous membrane that provides minimal joint stability.[6]

Additional secondary constraints to the ulnar aspect of the PCR include intrinsic and extrinsic ligaments. The intrinsic ligaments stabilizing the midcarpal row consist of the triquetrohamate (THL) and the triquetrocapitate (TCL) ligaments. The palmar extrinsic ligaments include the ulnolunate (ULL) and the ulnotriquetral (UTL) ligaments. The dorsal extrinsic ligaments are comprised of the dorsal radiocarpal (DRCL) and the dorsal intercarpal (DICL) ligaments.

Carpal instability (CI) is the end result of a wrist ligamentous injury, which may occur from a variety of mechanisms. The failure of wrist ligaments (and the resultant carpal instability) causes pain (i.e., a symptomatic dysfunction),

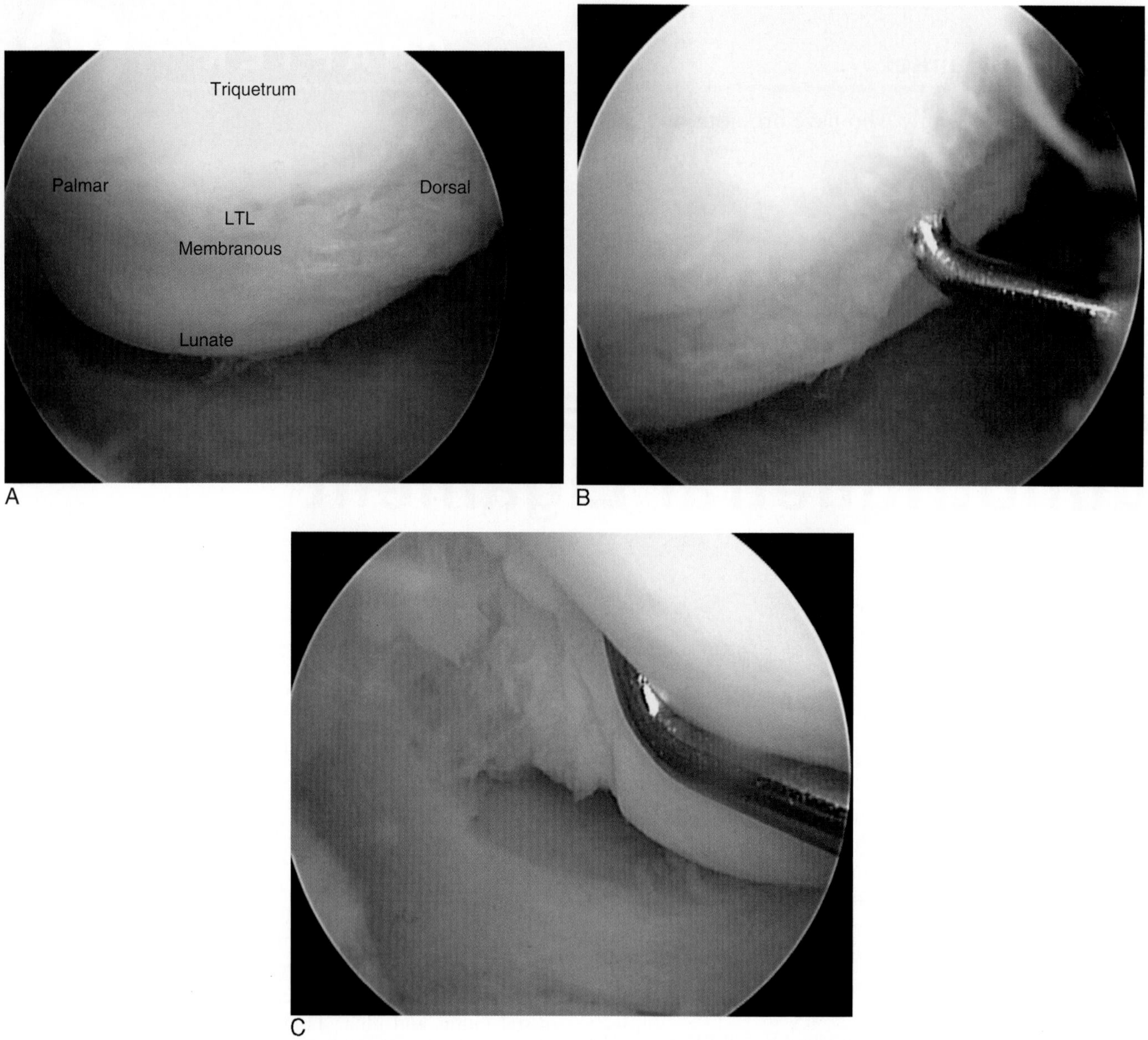

FIGURE 11.1. (A) Usual appearance of LTIL and LTJ viewed from the 6-U portal. Note that this portal allows for complete observation of the palmar central and dorsal portions of the LTIL. (B) Dorsal portion of LTIL is probed. The fraying of the dorsal ligament is consistent with a chronic grade I injury. (C) From the 6-U portal (or a volar portal), the entire palmar portion of the LTIL can be observed and probed for possible injury.

produces abnormal carpal kinetics (i.e., altered stress with the inability to bear functional loads), and abnormal joint kinematics (i.e., abnormal carpal motion).[7] The degree of instability can vary from a subtle micro-movement due to ligament attenuation to gross carpal displacement with a wide intracarpal gap and abnormal carpal alignment.[8–16]

With an injury to the LTIL, the normal kinetics and kinematics of the wrist are disturbed.[17,18] A spectrum of LTJ injuries can develop, ranging from a mild sprain with or without dynamic instability to a complete disruption with a secondary carpal instability dissociative (CID) pattern. This may culminate in a static altered carpal alignment, often referred to as volar intercalated segment instability (VISI). A static CI is characterized by a fixed dissociation between carpals that is clearly evident on imaging studies or during arthroscopy. A dynamic CI is characterized by normal routine radiographs, abnormal kinematics on stress imaging, or altered kinetics and kinematics viewed during arthroscopy.

The mechanism of LTIL tearing resulting in injury to the LTJ is somewhat controversial.[19] Perilunate and reverse perilunate injury patterns caused by dorsally and/or palmarly applied forces, fractures of the distal radius or carpals, degenerative wear from ulnar abutment, prolonged repetitive stress, and inflammatory arthritis/synovitis have all been implicated.[20,21] Furthermore, the presence of an ulnar positive variant at the DRUJ can facilitate attritional wear and tear of the LTIL.[22–24]

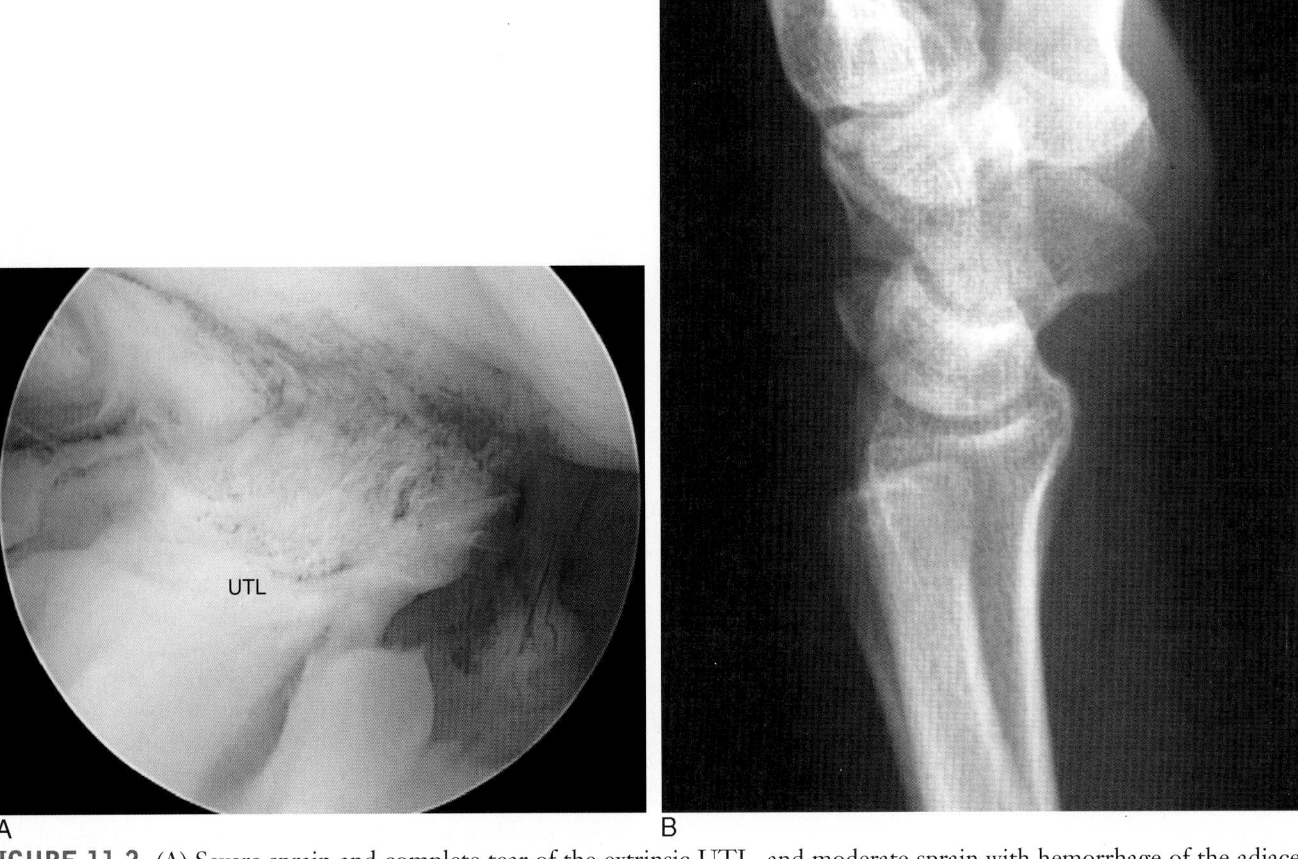

FIGURE 11.2. (A) Severe sprain and complete tear of the extrinsic UTL, and moderate sprain with hemorrhage of the adjacent ULL. (B) X-ray showing a VISI deformity from a CID.

Most investigators believe that when the LTIL is injured subtle micro-motion instability begins, which results in wrist joint synovitis and subsequent chondromalacia.[6] Some investigators would consider this early stage as a *predynamic* instability. Interestingly, damage to the intrinsic interosseous ligament alone is usually not sufficient to cause LTJ dissociation and a grossly unstable VISI. Additional tearing of the secondary constraints to the LTJ is necessary to produce a static CI (Figure 11.2).

Significant injury to either the ulnocarpal ligamentous complex (ULL and UTL) or the dorsal extrinsic ligaments (DRCL and DICL) will then result in a VISI. Secondary attenuation from prolonged cyclic loading may also play an important role.[6,15,17] Although these pathomechanics ultimately result in a VISI type of CID pattern, other carpal instabilities of the nondissociative type [i.e., CIND involving the midcarpal joint (MCJ), radiocarpal joint (RCJ), or combined MCJ/RCJ] can produce similar VISI patterns.[13,25]

Evaluation of LTJ Injuries

The differential diagnosis of ulnar-sided wrist pain is staggering. Extrinsic wrist disorders and internal wrist derangements must be taken into account during the patient history and physical examination. A careful evaluation of the painful wrist will help to differentiate ulnar-sided pain emanating from LTJ injury versus a variety of associated wrist lesions that mimic ulnar-sided wrist pain. These include TFCC injury, DRUJ injury, MCJ injury and instability, cartilage injury producing chondromalacia and degenerative joint disease, UIS, carpal fractures, dorsal extrinsic ligament sprains, pisotriquetral joint injuries, extensor carpi ulnaris (ECU) subluxation, ulnar neurovascular injuries, and inflammatory connective tissue disorders.[13,20,21]

A typical patient with an LTIL injury usually presents with a history of acute trauma or repetitive stress to the hand and wrist. Symptoms may be recent or chronic. The ulnar-sided wrist pain is usually intermittent to frequent and is worsened with activities, especially those wrist movements that require rotation and ulnar deviation. Wrist motion produces clicking or a clunk. The wrist feels stiff and the grip is weak. The physical examination usually does not reveal a palmar sag of the carpus (which is characteristic of a VISI) but often shows decreased range of motion, clicking, a clunk with movement, or especially painful ulnar deviation or rotation. There is often tenderness to palpation dorsally at the LTJ region or directly ulnarly over the carpus.

Provocative tests that stress the LTJ and reveal pain, crepitus, or joint laxity are suggestive of a ligament injury.[26–28]

Standard plain posteroanterior and lateral radiographs should be obtained on every patient with a suspected LTJ injury. Typically these radiographs are normal, but they might assist with the differential diagnosis of other wrist injuries known to cause ulnar-sided wrist pain. The plain radiographs can be scrutinized for hints of LTJ instability, such as disruptions of Gilula's lines, a relative malalignment between the lunate and capitate, or possibly a static collapse with a VISI pattern of lunate flexion and triquetral extension (Figure 11.2B). A gap or diastasis between the lunate and triquetrum is virtually never observed. If a VISI is present, the lunate and capitate are no longer colinear and the lunotriquetral axes become negative (mean value of –16 degrees) whereas the mean value is normally positive at 14 degrees.

Some investigators have advocated wrist motion or stress radiographic studies, cineradiography, three-compartment wrist arthrography, nuclear bone scans, computed tomography, and magnetic resonance imaging (MRI).[26,29] The author routinely obtains posteroanterior, lateral, and oblique radiographs of the wrist. In those select patients in whom the diagnosis of wrist pain is still indeterminate, a high-resolution 1.5-Tesla MRI is performed and read by an experienced musculoskeletal radiologist. Even though the MRI scan is neither sensitive nor specific for an LTIL tear, it may produce additional information about other associated wrist joint injuries.

Role of Wrist Arthroscopy

The arthroscopic examination of the painful wrist, especially in the evaluation of LTJ injuries, has become the definitive modality of diagnostic investigation. Wrist arthroscopy is an essential component of a thorough examination because it provides the only direct means of inspecting the integrity of the LTIL, the stability of the LTJ, and the presence of associated wrist joint pathology. Subtle LTJ instabilities that were not detected by the other previously described imaging modalities can now be accurately diagnosed with arthroscopy. Wrist arthroscopy of both the RCJ and the MCJ is now the gold standard in the diagnosis of CI based on its superior accuracy in the direct evaluation of ligamentous injuries.[19–28,30–40]

Treatment of Lunotriquetral Joint Injuries

Wrist arthroscopy plays the critical role of focusing attention on the nature and extent of the LTJ instability and the presence of associated pathology. This enables the surgeon to better plan appropriate treatment of the injured wrist. The initial procedure of therapeutic surgical intervention should be a preliminary, comprehensive, systematic diagnostic wrist arthroscopy to confirm the suspected diagnosis and to allow one to proceed with the most appropriate surgical management program. Beyond this, the treatment of LTJ instability becomes controversial. However, there are two factors that should be taken into account when planning therapeutic intervention: the elapsed period of time between injury and the initiation of treatment (i.e., acute versus chronic injuries) and whether or not the pattern of CI is dynamic and reducible or static and fixed into a VISI pattern.

The presence of associated injuries to the ulnar-sided wrist joint, especially those of degenerative cartilage changes, significantly alters the surgical options. Finally, the desires of the patient must be taken into account. A patient may not want to undergo an operation with a low likelihood of success or one with significant risk and complications, or an operation with a long period of convalescence and rehabilitation. Permanent wrist stiffness associated with carpal fusions may not be appealing to some patients.

In an attempt to minimize the surgical trauma of an open wrist operation and to accelerate the rehabilitation process, the treatment of LTJ instability by arthroscopic technique has been recently investigated.[19–28,31–50] The technique of arthroscopic ligament debridement and arthroscopic reduction of LTJ injury with internal fixation using K-wires [i.e., arthroscopic reduction and internal fixation (ARIF)] is described in material following.

In the past, treatment of stable acute and chronic LTJ injuries consisted of a period of splint or cast immobilization in conjunction with other supportive conservative measures.[10] It is highly unlikely that this approach will work successfully for any serious acute or chronic LTJ instability. Currently it is believed that only minor acute LTIL sprains respond to rest and immobilization. If symptoms do not improve within six weeks, if the clinical examination is consistent with a moderate or severe sprain of the LTIL, if a wrist MRI scan reveals a serious LTJ injury, or if LTJ instability is already present, arthroscopy should be performed. The degree of LTIL damage, degree of LTJ instability (dynamic or static), and level of associated wrist joint pathology determine whether or not to proceed with ARIF or an open surgical technique.

Direct ligament repair, ligament reconstruction with autogenous tendon graft, LTJ arthrodesis, midcarpal arthrodesis, proximal row carpectomy, and total wrist fusion are the open surgical procedures that have been advocated to restore LTJ alignment and thus the integrity of the PCR. Several investigators have recommended direct ligament repair for an acute injury whenever sufficient LTIL remains.[10,26,31,43,44] The LTIL is reattached to the triquetrum, as this is the usual site of avulsion. The repair technique is surgically demanding, and may require both dorsal and palmar approaches. Augmentation of the LTIL repair with a dorsal capsulodesis to improve the extrinsic ligament support has been suggested to be of some benefit.[45–47] The results of direct LTIL repair to restore stability of the LTJ have been satisfactory, with the Mayo Clinic reporting an 86% success rate.[31]

In patients with chronic static LTJ instability with VISI, or in the case of an arthroscopic or open surgical finding of a nonrepairable LTIL, several investigators have recommended LTIL reconstruction with autogenous tendon graft.[10,31,44] On the other hand, other investigators have argued that they prefer an LTJ arthrodesis over a tendon graft reconstruction. The technique of LTIL reconstruction utilizing a distally based strip of extensor or flexor carpi ulnaris is an extremely demanding surgical procedure, and may require significant surgical exposure via dorsal and palmar arthrotomies. Advocates of the reconstruction argue that it preserves LTJ motion and near normal carpal kinematics, as opposed to LTJ arthrodesis that entails significant loss of wrist motion. Only a small group of patients have undergone reconstruction, but the Mayo Clinic group has reported good success.[10,31]

LTJ arthrodesis is a technically less demanding surgical procedure than reconstruction, and has been shown by several investigators to be successful at reducing or eliminating wrist pain and improving function. It has been reported to have a high rate of LTJ nonunion, however, and mild to slight associated stiffness in wrist mobility.[51–55] In several comparative studies of LTJ arthrodesis versus reconstruction or repair, the later groups achieved superior results in regard to patient satisfaction, postoperative complications, and necessity for reoperation.[26,31]

It should be pointed out that in patients with a fixed VISI deformity it is also necessary to consider reconstruction of the palmar ulnocarpal ligaments or the dorsal extrinsic ligaments in order to prevent permanent rotation of the PCR into a VISI.[31,56–58] In some wrists, it may even be necessary to proceed to a midcarpal arthrodesis (i.e., lunate-triquetrum-hamate or lunate-triquetrum-hamate-capitate) if restoration of PCR alignment cannot be achieved.[20,45–48,53]

Ligamentous repair, reconstruction, or joint arthrodesis needs to take into account the presence of degenerative cartilaginous changes or findings of UIS with degeneration of the TFCC and ulnar cartilage.[10,20,21,30,31] In these circumstances, an ulnar shortening osteoplasty may also be needed. As an added benefit from an ulnar shortening, it has been shown that the procedure partially stabilizes the ulnar aspect of the wrist through an increased tension in the ulnocarpal ligament complex.[59] Furthermore, a debridement of the degenerative TFCC lesion can be performed. In selected cases, an arthroscopic wafer procedure to remove the protuberant dome of the distal ulna might be feasible in place of an ulnar shortening osteotomy.[59,60]

Arthroscopic Technique

The diagnostic wrist arthroscopy begins with a systematic and thorough examination of the RCJ via a dorsoradial (3,4) portal, dorsoulnar (4,5 or 6-R) portal, and ulnar (6-U) portal. Use of a probe is essential to palpate the internal wrist structures, especially the intrinsic and extrinsic ligaments and the TFCC. The LTIL and LTJ are difficult to visualize with the arthroscope in the dorsoradial portal. These ulnar-sided structures are best observed through the dorsoulnar portal, with the probe in the ulnar portal. Through the dorsoulnar portal, the dorsal and membranous portions of the LTIL are clearly observed and the volar portion of the LTIL can be palpated with the probe.

The ulnocarpal ligaments (ULL and UTL) are clearly seen, as is the entire TFCC and the cartilaginous surfaces of the entire PCR (Figure 11.3). The volar portion of the LTIL is best visualized through the ulnar (6-U) portal, where it can be seen in its entirety (Figure 11.1C). As an alternative, a volar wrist portal can be established that also provides excellent viewing of the volar LTIL and dorsal wrist structures such as the DRCL (Figure 11.4B). Associated injuries to the TFCC, extrinsic ligaments, cartilage,

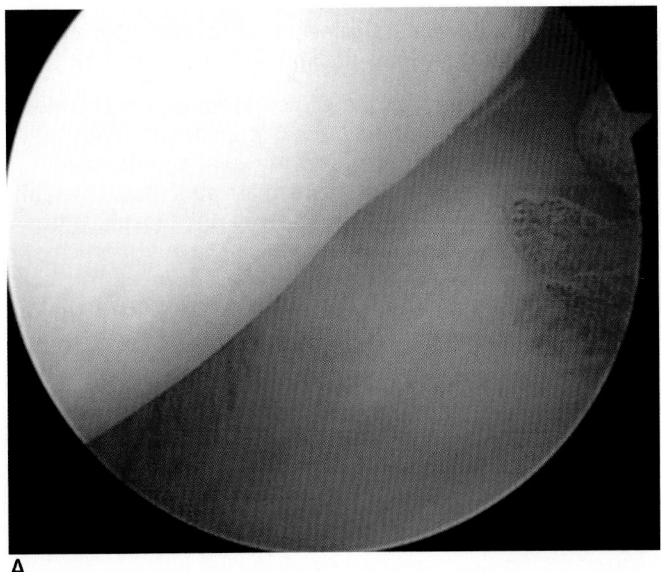
A

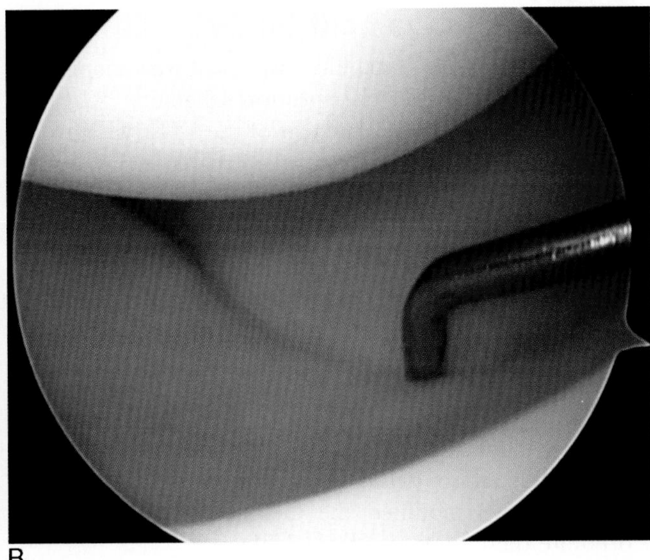
B

FIGURE 11.3. (A) Normal appearance of the LTJ viewed through the dorsoulnar wrist portal, with normal ULL and UTL in the backround and the TFCC below. (B) Normal appearance of the LTJ viewed through the MCR portal. Probe is at the LTJ line.

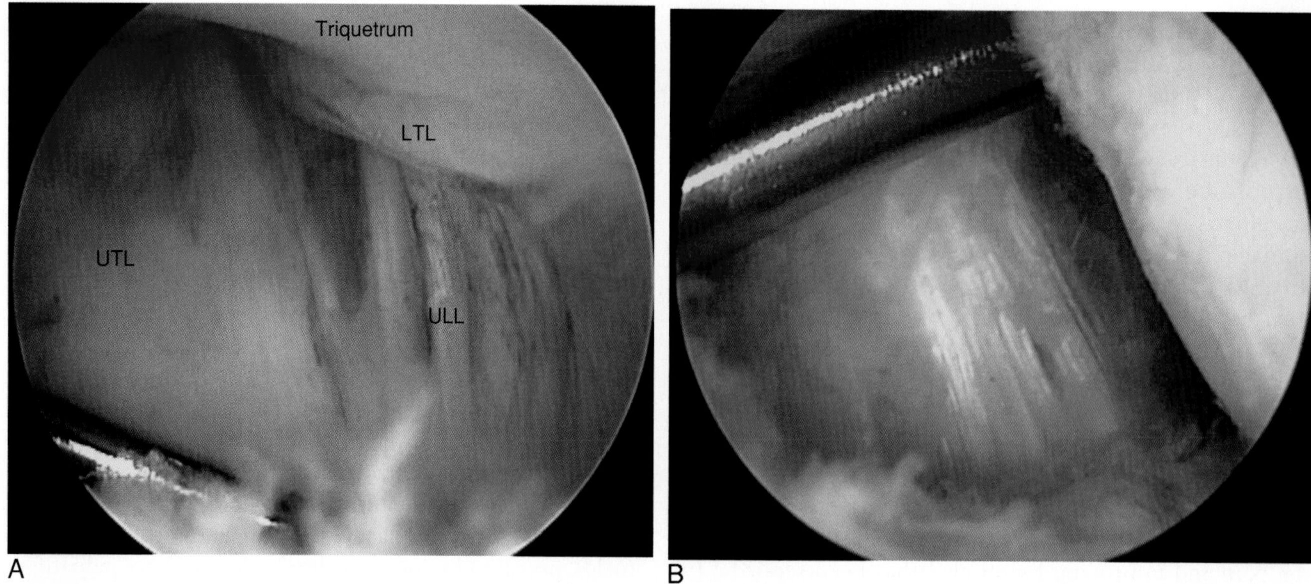

FIGURE 11.4. (A) Grade 0 sprain of LTIL. Mild hemorrhage is seen in the central membranous portion of the ligament. In the background, note mild sprains of the ulnocarpal extrinsic ligaments. (B) Sprained DRCL viewed from the ulnar-sided portal.

and capsule can be assessed with RCJ arthroscopy using a combination of these four portals.

To complete the arthroscopic evaluation of LTJ injury, it is essential to establish midcarpal portals.[61] The midcarpal-radial (MCR) portal is the best vantage point to observe the LTJ. Because the LTIL does not extend distally into the MCJ, the interval between the lunate and triquetrum can be seen clearly and instability of the LTJ can be accurately assessed (Figure 11.3). A probe placed into the midcarpal-ulnar (MCU) portal or triquetrohamate (TH) portal can then be used to assess dynamic or static instability. This instability assessment is further enhanced by stress loading the LTJ.

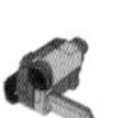

Arthroscopic Classification of Carpal Interosseous Ligament Injury

The degree of LTJ instability can be arthroscopically graded with the Geissler classification scheme.[41,62] In the author's experience, a complete tear of the LTIL with gross dissociation of the LTJ is clearly discernable arthroscopically. The most important subtle arthroscopic observation is whether or not there is attenuation of the LTIL. If attenuation is present, the possibility for instability can range from a *predynamic* condition with subtle kinetic changes to a more grossly observable dynamic instability with more obvious kinematic carpal alterations of movement. The current Geissler classification does not take into account the important distinction between an attenuated ligament (with or without subtotal tearing) and a ligament injury with no attenuation (with or without subtotal tearing). As such, I have modified the Geissler classification to incorporate these findings (Table 11.1).

The Geissler grade I interosseous ligament injury class actually comprises several separate and distinct patterns of intrinsic ligament damage. In the first pattern, the LTIL shows evidence of hemorrhage but no attenuation or laxity of its fibers that would be consistent with instability. When a mild sprain of the LTIL occurs, hemorrhage of the ligamentous fibers can be visualized arthroscopically—but as

Table 11.1.

Modified Geissler Classification of LTJ Injuries

Grade	Arthroscopic Findings
0	Hemorrhage of interosseous ligament seen in RCJ. No attenuation. No incongruency of carpal alignment in MCJ.
I	Incomplete partial or full substance tear of the interosseous ligament as seen in RCJ. No attenuation. No joint incongruency. No instability.
II	Attenuation of the interosseous ligament. Most often the central membranous portion is completely torn, and the volar and dorsal portions of the ligament are stretched. Often an incomplete partial or small full substance tear is present. There is possibly a *predynamic* or mild dynamic instability, as evidenced by excessive joint movement at the MCJ. Usually excessive scar tissue builds up and synovitis is seen in RCJ and possibly MCJ.
III	Interosseous ligament is completely torn. Probe can be easily passed through the joint, but a wide diastasis is not present. The joint is dynamically unstable but reducible. No static instability.
IV	Gross instability. Marked joint incongruency with static VISI instability. Arthroscope passes through the gap between carpals.

long as the fibers of the ligament have not been stretched beyond their plastic limit of elongation the basic integrity of the LTIL is maintained. Hemorrhage within the LTIL absent any observable attenuation of its fibers leaves the LTJ stable. This pattern of mild sprain will heal in an uneventful fashion. In the modified Geissler classification, this injury pattern would be considered a grade 0 lesion (Figure 11.4A).

The second pattern within the Geissler grade I classification consists of a partial or full substance, incomplete, subtotal tear of the LTIL. There is no attenuation of the ligamentous fibers, nor any altered carpal kinetics or kinematics. The LTJ remains stable because the integrity of the ligament is maintained (Figure 11.5). This would be a grade I lesion in the modified classication. The mechanical irritation to the wrist joint caused by the tearing of the ligamentous fibers results in pain.

When attenuation of the ligament is arthroscopically observable, this is a much more serious finding and has more serious consequences for both outcome and treatment of these injuries. Attenuation of the LTIL indicates that its fibers have been sprained or stretched beyond their plastic limit, and consequently the basic integrity of the ligament has been compromised. Arthroscopically, the attenuated LTIL appears lax or loose or wavy—but morphologically it remains basically intact and still physically connects the lunate to the triquetrum. Frequently, partial or full substance incomplete tears are present—but it is possible to have ligamentous attenuation without any tearing whatsoever (Figure 11.6).

When palpated by the intra-articular probe, the ligamentous fibers are clearly loose. In the acute stage of injury, an attenuated LTIL has the potential to produce laxity or an early stage of instability that could be considered *predynamic*

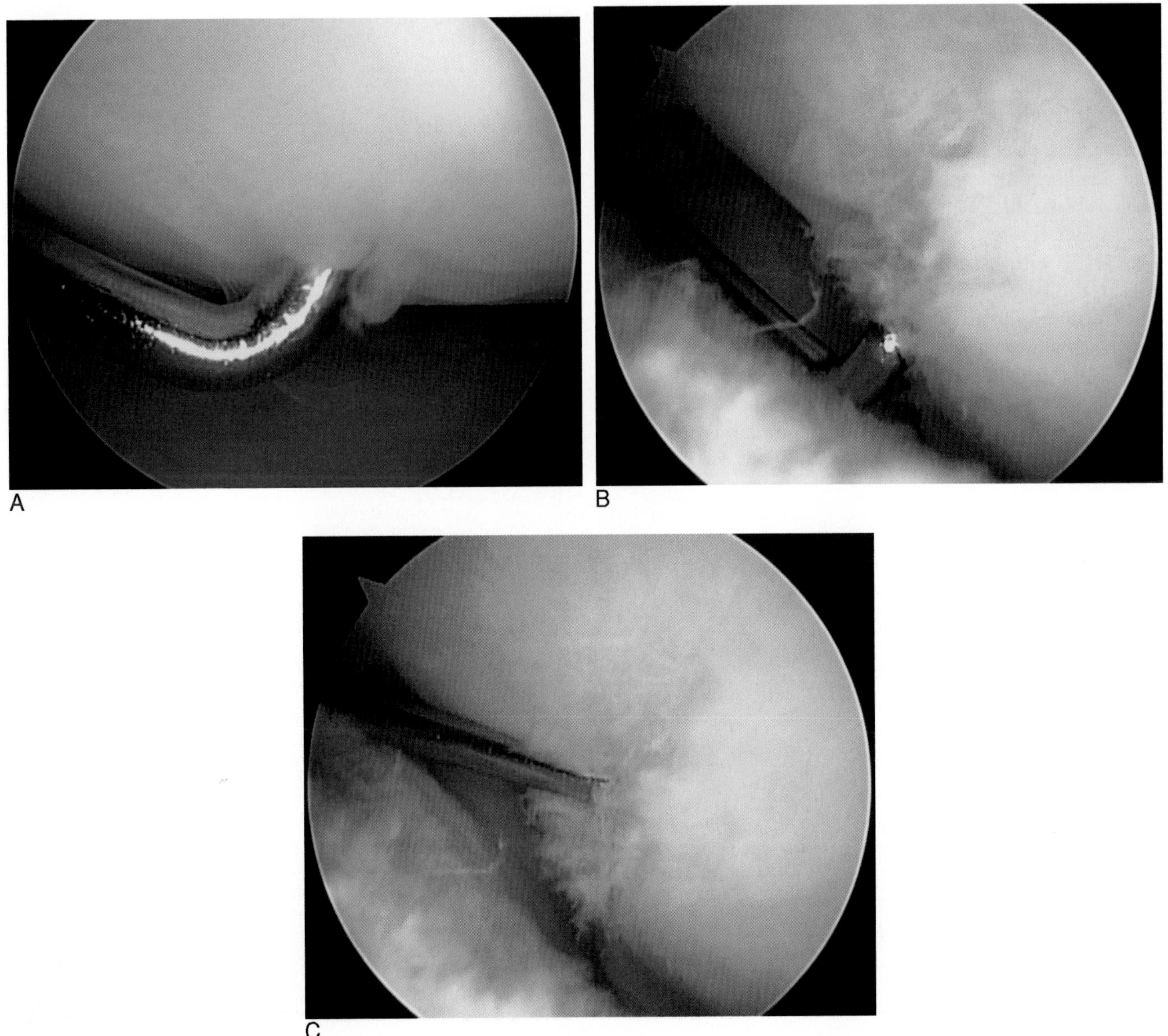

FIGURE 11.5. (A) Grade I membranous injury of LTIL with a small punctuate subtotal incomplete tear at the attachment to the lunate. There is no ligamentous attenuation or joint instability. (B) Larger grade I central tear, but no attenuation of the ligament. (C) Probe passes through the full substance central tear. No instability is present.

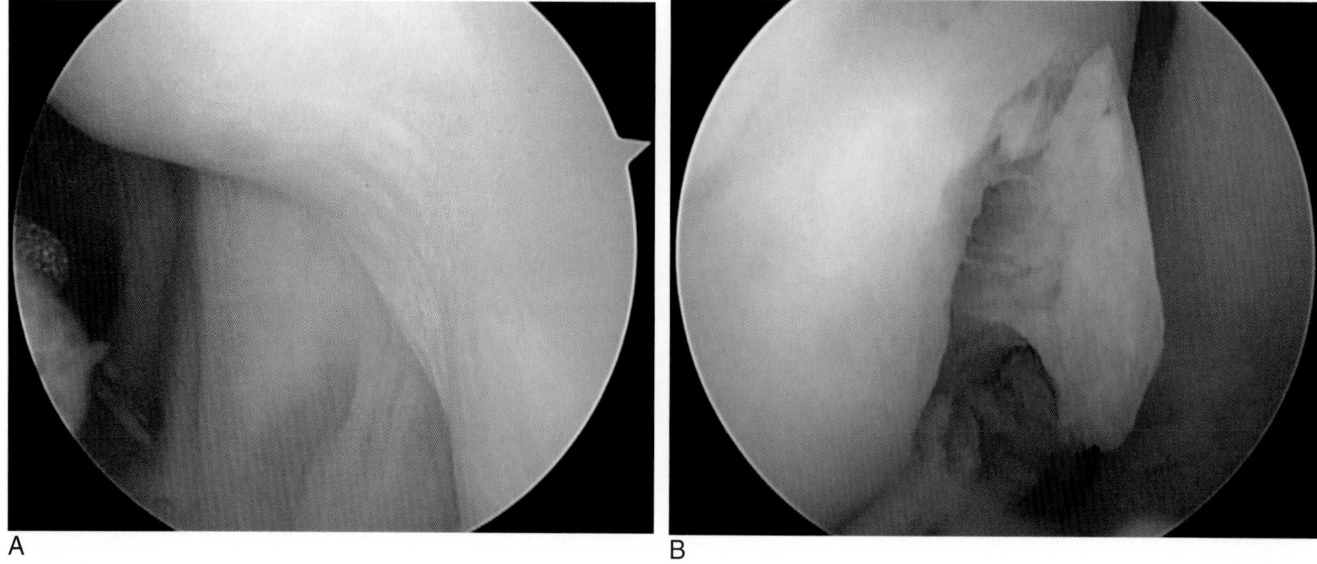

FIGURE 11.6. (A) Grade II LTIL injury with significant attenuation of the ligament, but no tearing of its fibers. (B) Grade II injury with attenuation and a subtotal partial tear of the central membranous section.

in the sense that further instability develops with time and additional joint loading. As the injury becomes chronic, cyclic loading of the attenuated LTIL can lead to dynamic and possibly static LTJ instability. In the modified classification, a grade II interosseous ligament injury is a slight sprain of the LTIL with arthroscopically observable attenuation or laxity of the LTIL, no complete disruption of the volar and dorsal ligamentous fibers, and the potential for *predynamic* or early dynamic instability of the LTJ as evidenced by excessive LTJ movement (i.e., altered kinematics) or early chondromalacia at the joint line (i.e., altered kinetics). Probing usually reveals a complete central membranous tear with stretching of the volar and dorsal portions of the LTIL; or a partial or full substance incomplete tear of the ligament (Figure 11.7).

In a Geissler grade III injury of the LTIL, complete disruption of the ligament leads to a dynamically altered relationship between the lunate and the triquetrum. Arthroscopically, an intra-articular probe can be easily passed through the LTJ—revealing an excessive abnormal carpal movement, as seen in the MCJ and often in the RCJ. There is usually much more scar tissue built up in the ulnar aspect of the RCJ adjacent to the LTJ, which is often accompanied by excessive synovitis in the RCJ and MCJ. A diastasis of the LTJ is not seen, and there is no static instability. The LTJ can be reduced with simple

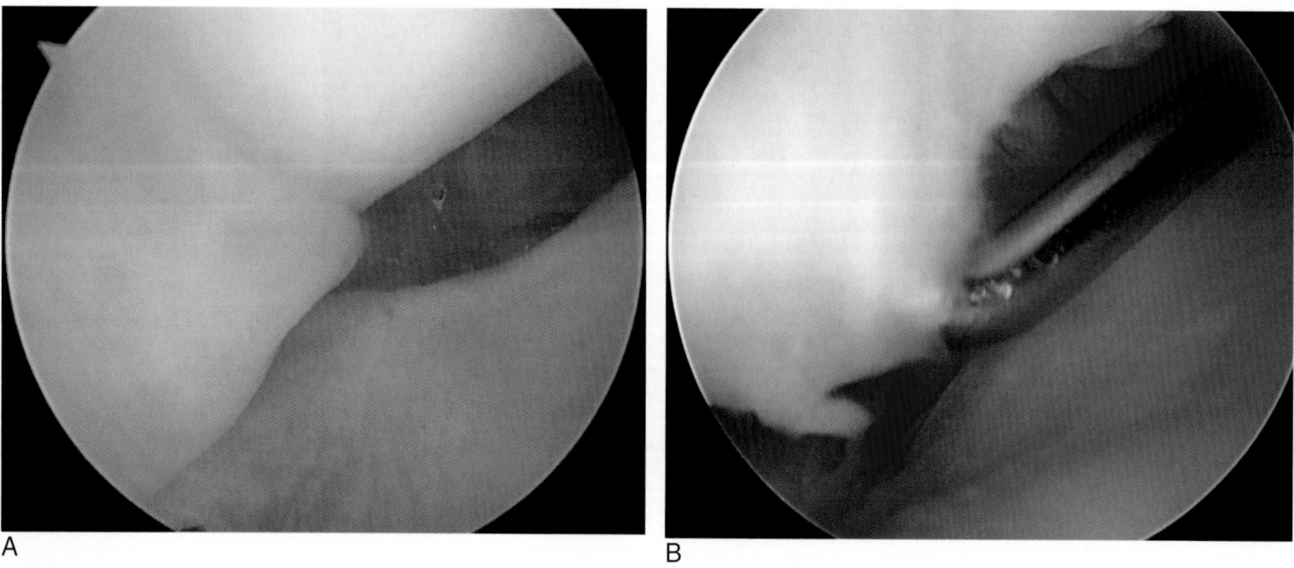

FIGURE 11.7. (A) Grade II LTIL tear. (B) Probe displays the redundancy of the torn LTIL.

Continued

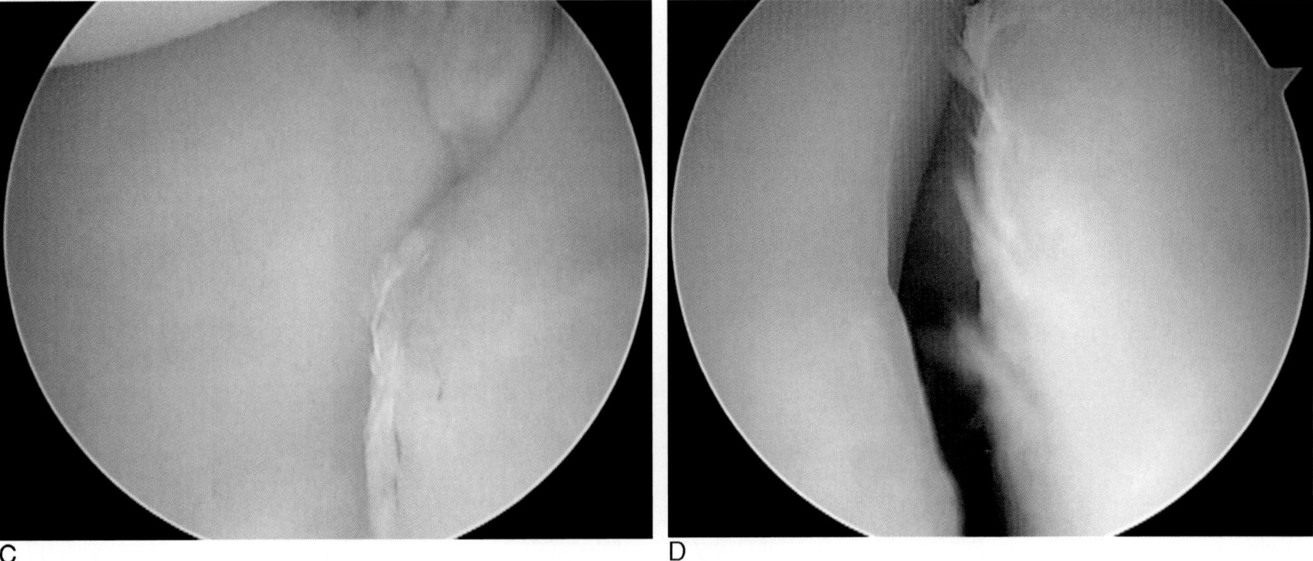

FIGURE 11.7. Cont'd (C) View of the LTJ from the MCU portal. LTJ is congruently aligned. (D) Gapping of the LTJ occurs when stress is applied to the LTJ. Note the cartilage wear on the proximal triquetrum, indicative of altered joint kinetics secondary to dynamic LTJ instability.

manipulation of the lunate and triquetrum. A VISI deformity is not present. The arthroscope cannot be passed through the LTJ because the small gap produced by the instability is not sufficient to allow this to occur (Figure 11.8). This pattern corresponds to a severe ligamentous sprain, and to a grade III interosseous ligament injury.

A grade IV injury in both classifications results from a complete disruption of the LTIL, with a static or stress-induced diastasis of the LTJ such that the arthroscope can be passed easily through the wide gap between lunate and triquetrum (Figure 11.9). The secondary ligamentous constraints (i.e., the extrinsic ligaments) are injured, and a CID pattern that usually results in VISI is present (Figure 11.10).

This arthroscopic classification of wrist interosseous ligament instability is most useful for the CID pattern of PCR instability. The revised classification scheme the author has suggested is especially germane for understanding the various classes of LTIL injury and the resultant degree of LTJ instability. As will be demonstrated in the next section, this revised arthroscopic classification scheme aids in the choice of appropriate therapeutic intervention and provides a prognosis for outcome.

Arthroscopic evaluation of the sprained wrist provides the treating physician with the unique capability to directly examine the full extent of the internal pathologic process. A thorough visual examination of both the RCJ and MCJ

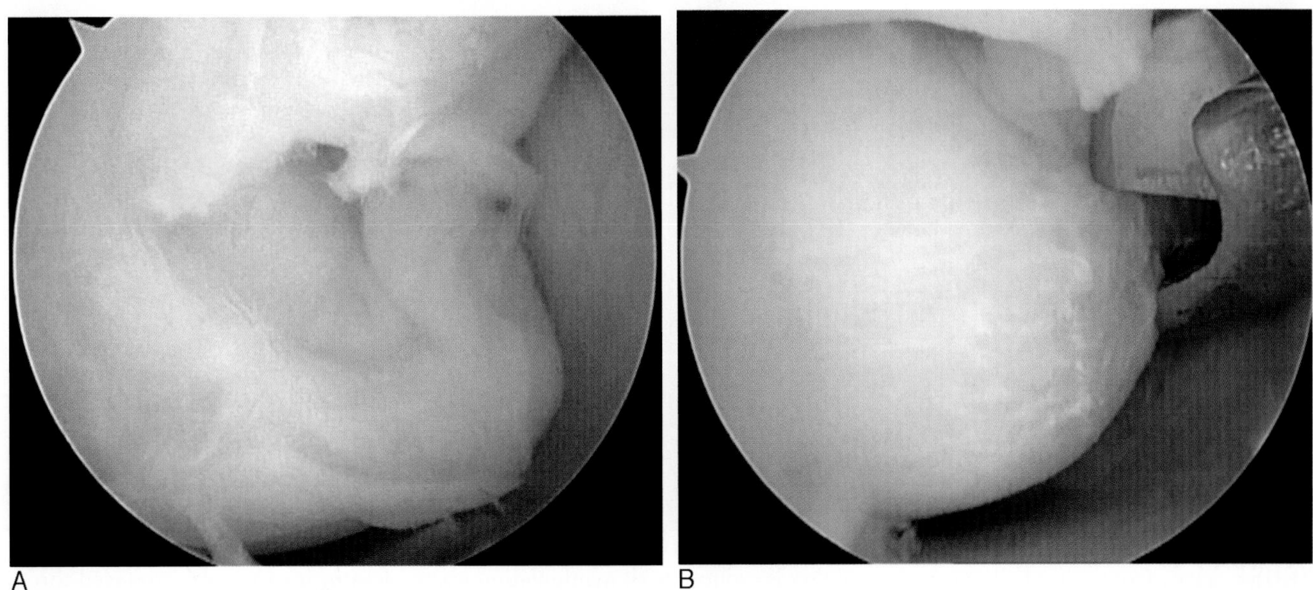

FIGURE 11.8. (A) Grade III complete tear of LTIL with dynamic instability. (B) The torn portion of the ligament is debrided.

Continued

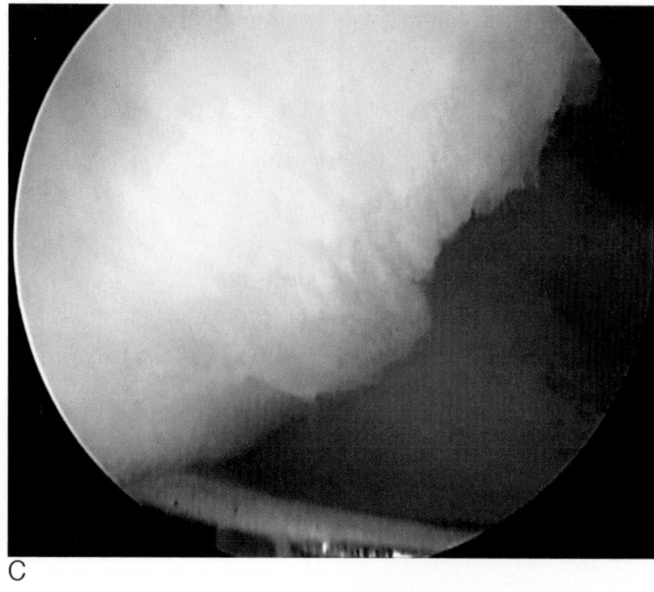

C

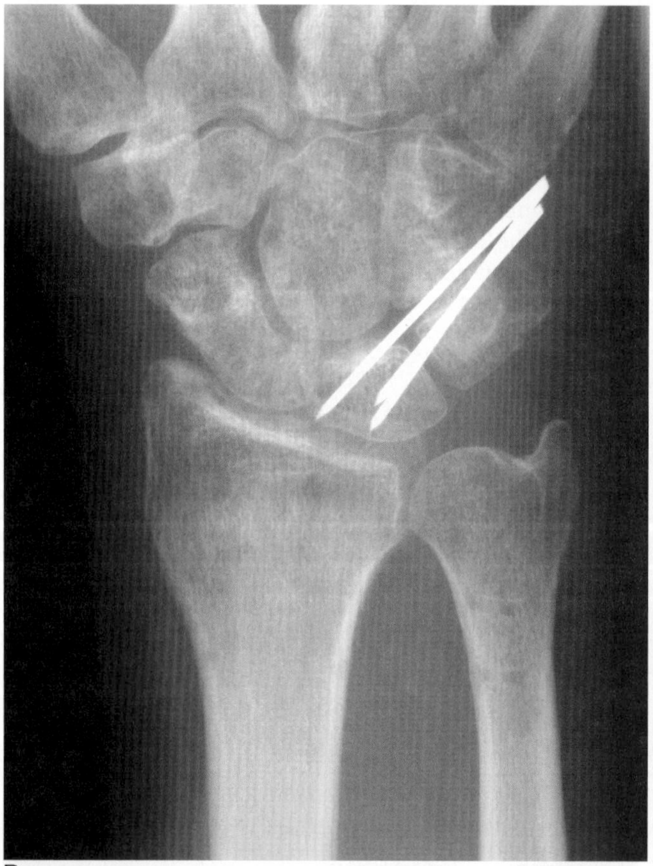

D

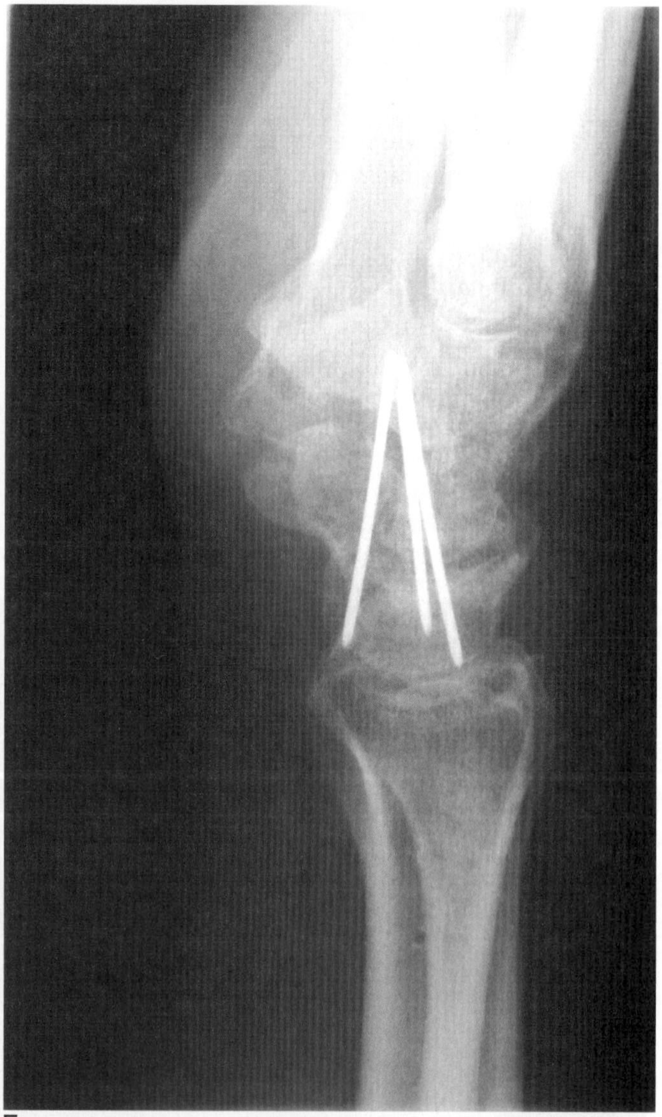

E

FIGURE 11.8. Cont'd (C) LTJ dynamic instability is reduced with manipulation via an elevator instrument introduced through the 6-U portal. (D) X-ray showing the technique of ARIF. (E) Lateral X-ray view showing the reduced LTJ placed back into congruent alignment. Percutaneous K-wires are placed across the reduced LTJ, viewing both arthroscopically and fluoroscopically.

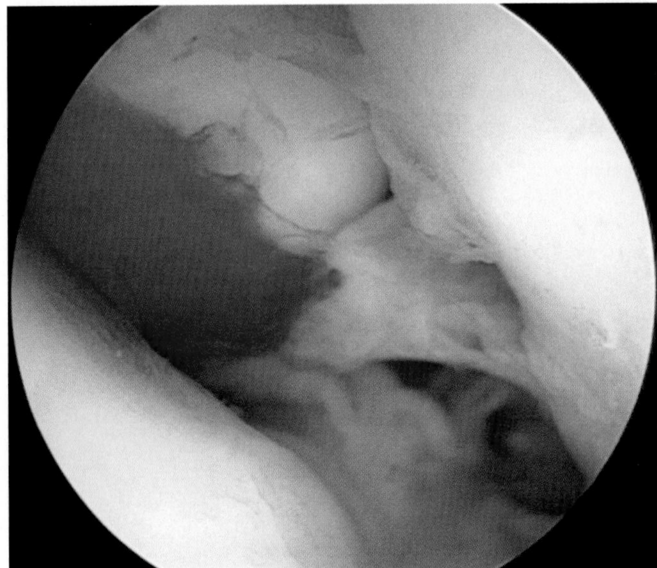

FIGURE 11.9. Grade IV LTIL tear. Note the "drive-through" sign as the arthroscope can be maneuvered into the wide diastasis between the lunate and the triquetrum. The MCJ is visible in the background.

will directly define the nature and extent of not only the ligamentous injury but significant associated osseous, cartilaginous, and fibrocartilaginous injuries.[35,36,38–40,42,61,62]

In the ulnar aspect of the RCJ, it is common to find a significant buildup of dorsal capsular scar tissue that forms from the original traumatic injury to the LTIL (Figure 11.11). This scar tissue must be debrided to fully visualize the three regions of the LTIL, the proximal cartilaginous surfaces of the lunate and triquetrum, the TFCC, the ulnocarpal ligaments, and the DRCL. If the LTJ instability is chronic, it is important to assess the ulnar aspect of the carpus for signs of UIS (Figure 11.12). If degeneration of the TFCC or cartilage is present, consideration should be given to formally treating the UIS in addition to treating the LTJ instability.[23,24,60]

The diagnostic role of arthroscopy in the MCJ is to search out additional cartilaginous and ligamentous pathology.[63] Degeneration of the cartilage on the proximal poles of the capitate and hamate, and the distal articular surfaces of the lunate and triquetrum, may be present (Figure 11.13). LTJ instability may occur in conjunction with midcarpal instability.[64] MCJ arthroscopy allows for examination of the intrinsic ligaments of the MCJ, especially the THL and TCL. Technically, these two ligaments are difficult to visualize because of the narrow constraints of the triquetrohamate articulation.

If the midcarpal ligaments have been injured, altered joint kinetics and kinematics should be evident (Figure 11.7D). The degree of instability can be assessed and classified as previously described. The arthroscopic findings of MCJ arthritis or instability enable the treating physician to alter the therapeutic intervention. Without the beneficial role of arthroscopy, there would be no reliable nonsurgical diagnostic modality to assist with classification of the CI or to aid in the discovery of ancillary pathology that would alter the treatment plan.

Author's Preferred Treatment

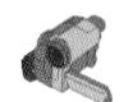

Acute ulnar-sided wrist pain suspected to have originated from an LTIL injury and that has not responded to conservative care after six weeks of treatment (and certainly by three months) should be evaluated arthroscopically. Likewise, if an MRI has been obtained and is suggestive or diagnostic of an ulnar-sided internal derangement one should proceed to arthroscopy. The wrist arthroscopy will

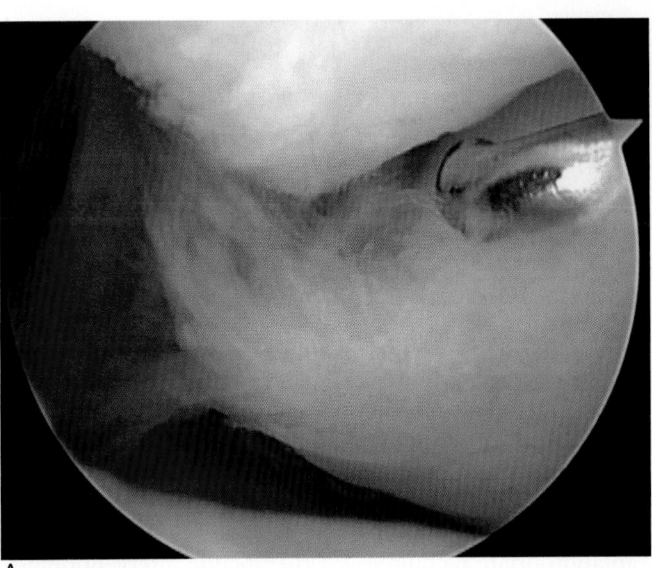

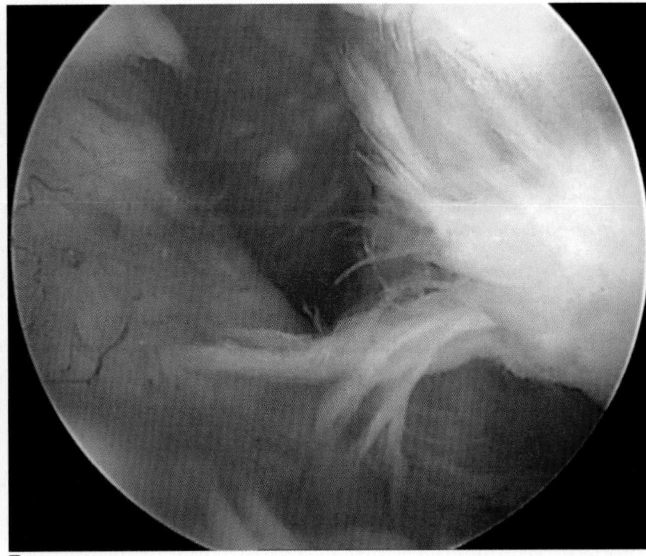

FIGURE 11.10. (A) Grade IV injury with marked static instability. (B) Severe extrinsic injury of the palmar ULL and UTL. The extrinsic ligament injury combined with the complete tear of the LTIL contributed to the VISI instability pattern.

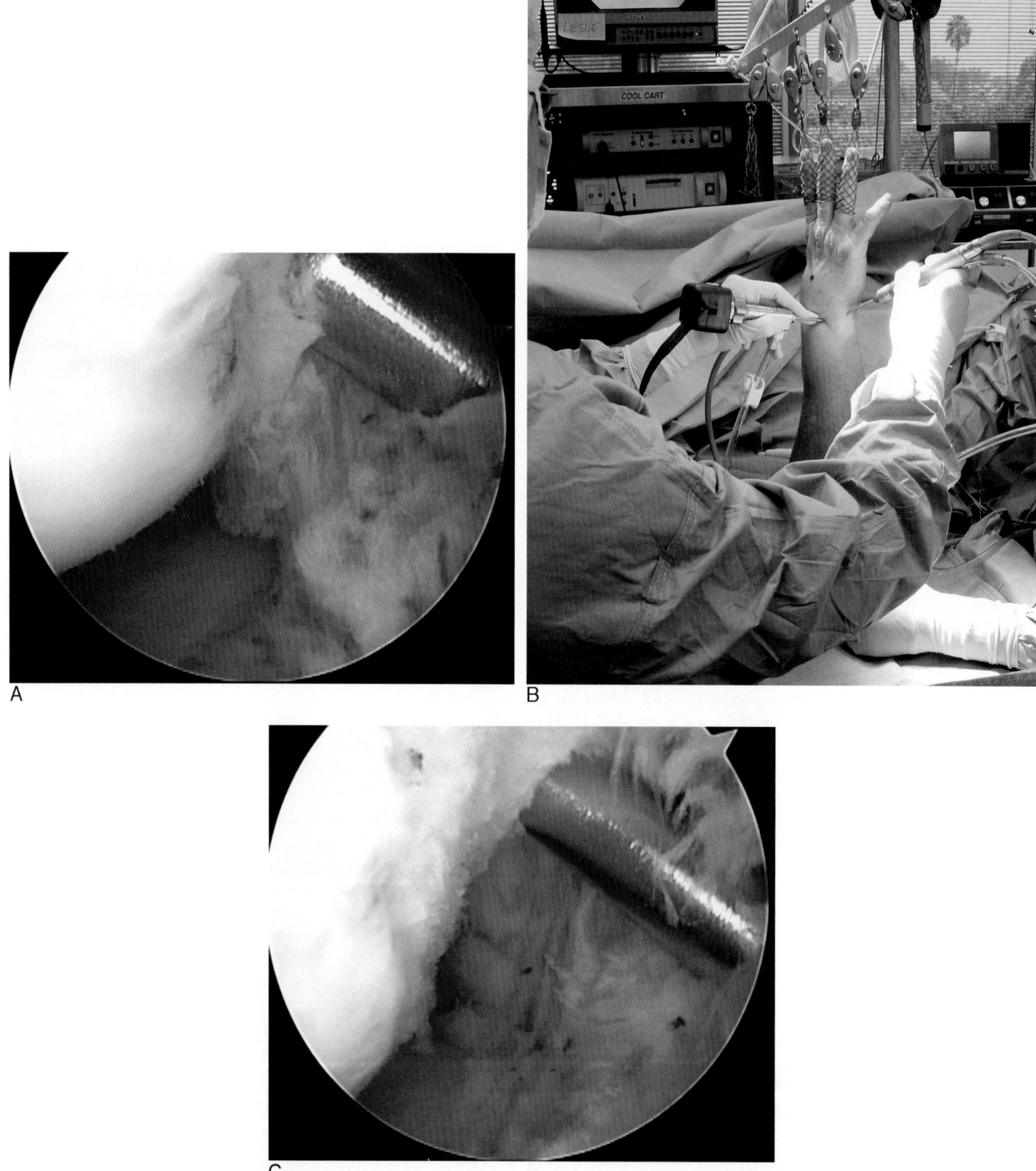

FIGURE 11.11. (A) A significant amount of scar tissue develops in the dorsoulnar aspect of the RCJ, in association with a tear of the LTIL. (B) Arthroscopic debridement is necessary to clean out the scar tissue. (C) Following debridement, the intra-articular structures about the ulnar aspect of the RCJ can now be seen, probed, and evaluated for injury.

provide valuable information unobtainable via any other diagnostic or imaging source. Arthroscopy of both the RCJ and MCJ will allow for a thorough evaluation of the LTIL, and the extent of LTJ instability. The modified classification scheme provides a helpful guide in choosing an appropriate technique for therapeutic intervention.

Grade 0 LTJ instability is a stable ligamentous injury that should be expected to heal with wrist immobilization

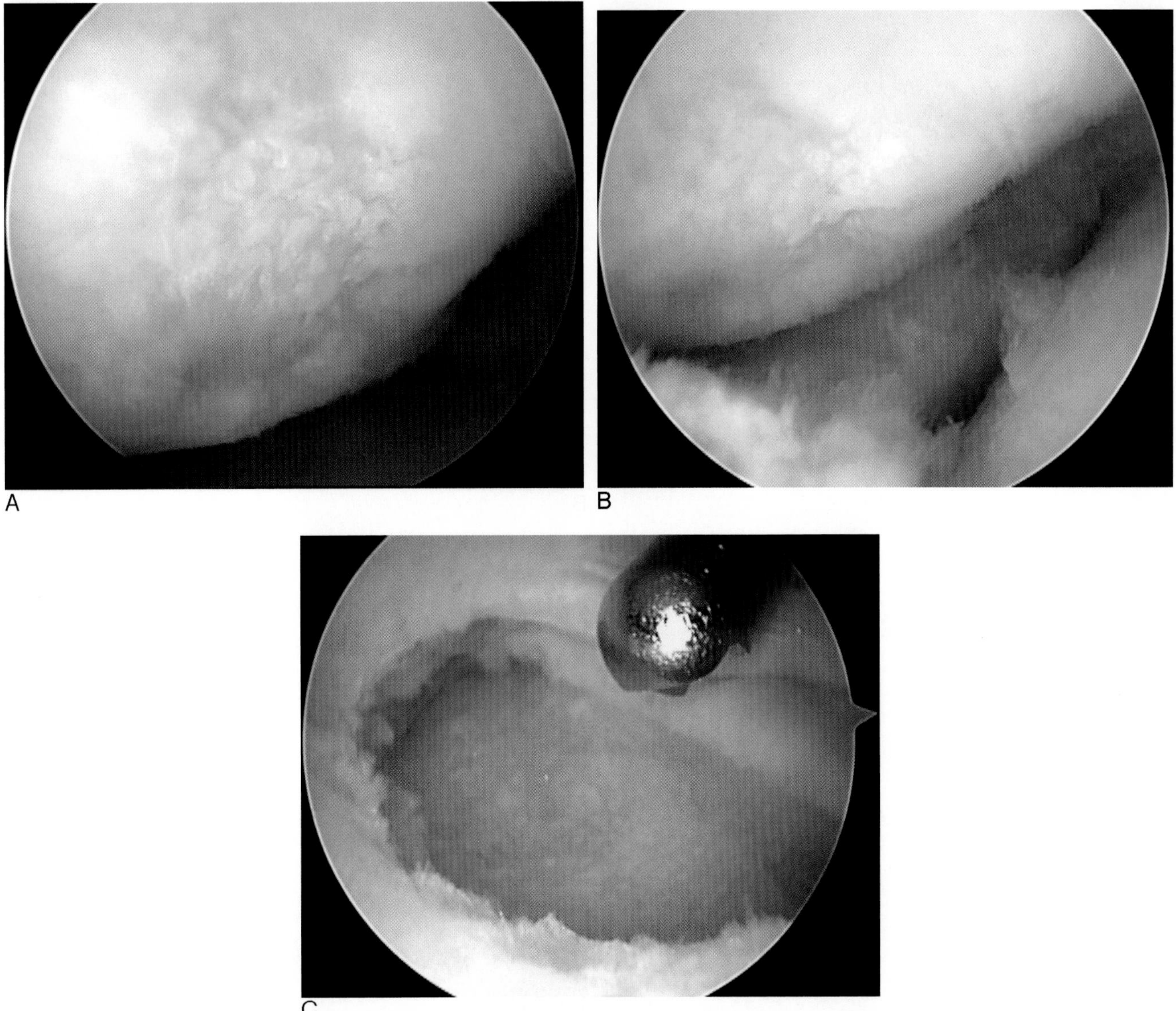

FIGURE 11.12. (A) Chronic UIS with attritional cartilage wear of the inferoulnar aspect of the lunate. (B) Abutment between the protuberant dome of the distal ulna and the degenerated lunate. (C) Arthroscopic view after an arthroscopic wafer procedure.

(Figure 11.4A). The prognosis of successful resolution of the wrist pain associated with the mild to slight sprain is excellent. Grade I LTJ instability reveals an intact LTIL with no attenuation of its fibers. There may be an incomplete partial or small full substance tear. There is no increased carpal movement between the lunate and triquetrum. The LTJ is congruent, and no altered carpal kinetics or kinematics is present during the diagnostic arthroscopy (Figure 11.5). If a small ligamentous tear is present, it should be debrided utilizing a full-radius arthroscopic shaver, suction punch, or electrothermal device (Figures 11.8B and 11.14). The wrist is immobilized for four to six weeks in a supportive splint. The prognosis of a successful outcome is excellent.

Grade II LTJ instability is characterized by significant attenuation of the LTIL. Often a partial or full substance incomplete tear of the palmar and/or dorsal portions of the LTIL is present. More frequently, there is a complete central membranous tear associated with stretching of the volar and dorsal portions of the LTIL (Figures 11.6 and 11.7). A *predynamic* instability characterized by cartilage wear and possible increased LTJ motion may be seen in the MCJ. Usually there is excessive scar tissue built up in the dorsoulnar aspect of the carpus, with synovitis (Figure 11.11). This injury pattern has the potential to lead to progression of cartilage degeneration and chronic pain. This specific injury pattern has not been adequately addressed in the literature. Treatment options would include further wrist joint immobilization, debridement of the torn interosseous ligament, ligamentous shrinkage utilizing a radiofrequency probe, LTJ percutaneous K-wire pinning for eight weeks, or a combination of these techniques.

An arthroscopic debridement of the torn LTIL flap should be done to eliminate any mechanical source of

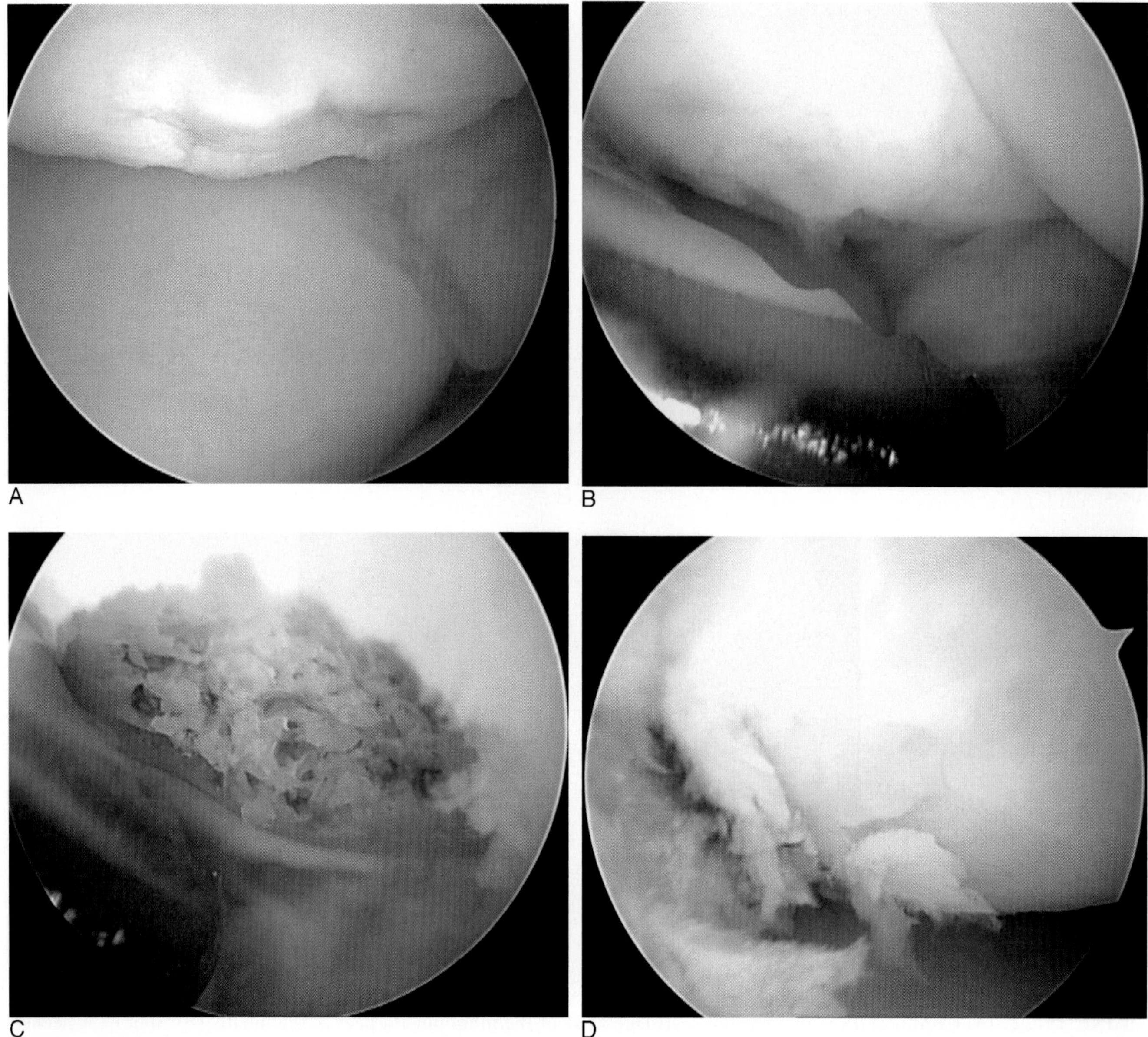

FIGURE 11.13. (A) Chondral injury of the proximal pole of the hamate with complete loss of cartilage. (B) Debridement of hamate chondral injury. (C) Arthroscopic appearance after a hamate chondroplasty. (D) Chondral injury of the proximal pole of the capitate.

joint irritability (Figure 11.8B). Several studies suggest that a debridement of the flap tear alone will produce satisfactory outcomes.[35,36,39,40] Only one very small study contradicted this finding.[37] Some authors also suggest reduction of the LTJ and percutaneous K-wire pinning for approximately eight weeks[20,35,38,48,49] (Figure 11.15 and 11.8D and E). Electrothermal ligamentous shrinkage can be performed with either a radiofrequency probe or a laser[64–67] (Figure 11.16). This relatively new technology can be applied to an attenuated LTIL, or even to the ulnocarpal extrinsic ligaments.

Biomechanically, the tensile strength of the heated collagen within the ligament decreases and does not return to normal for approximately 12 weeks. Therefore, it is important to immobilize the wrist for at least 8 weeks, and to avoid any heavy activity for 12 weeks.[66] Frequently, an excessive amount of dorsal capsular scar tissue is present in the dorsoulnar section of the RCJ. This scar tissue inhibits full visualization of the ulnar-sided wrist structures and should be arthroscopically debrided (Figure 11.11).

The author's treatment of choice for a grade II LTIL injury is an arthroscopic debridement of the central membranous tear, debridement of any partial or incomplete tears of the palmar and dorsal portions of the ligament, arthroscopic reduction of the LTJ aided by fluoroscopy, percutaneous K-wire fixation of the LTJ for a minimum of eight weeks (aided by cast immobilization), and electrothermal LTIL shrinkage utilizing a spot welding technique. In the author's experience, this combination of procedures has produced predictable good results utilizing a minimally invasive arthroscopic procedure.

Grade III LTIL injury reveals a complete tear of the LTIL (Figure 11.8). The LTJ is clearly unstable when a force is applied, but the joint is anatomically reducible.

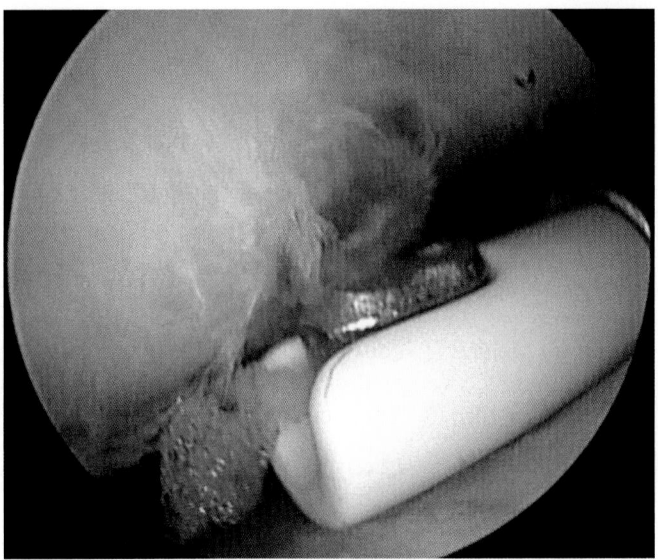

FIGURE 11.14. Electrothermal debridement of a partial substance LTIL tear.

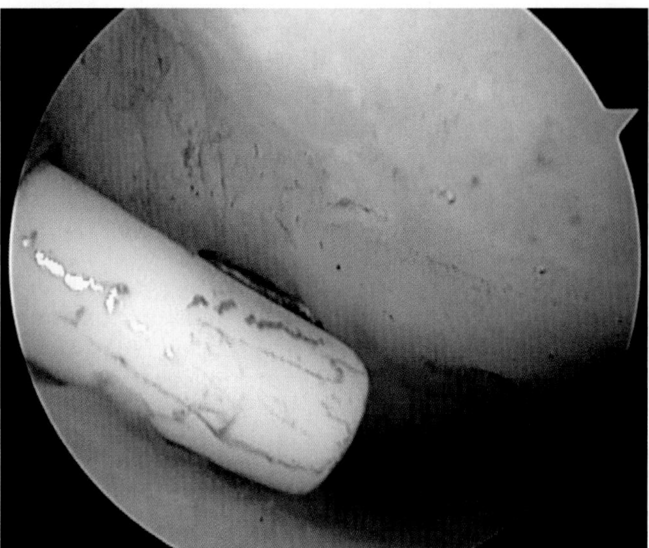

FIGURE 11.16. Electrothermal shrinkage of an attenuated LTIL.

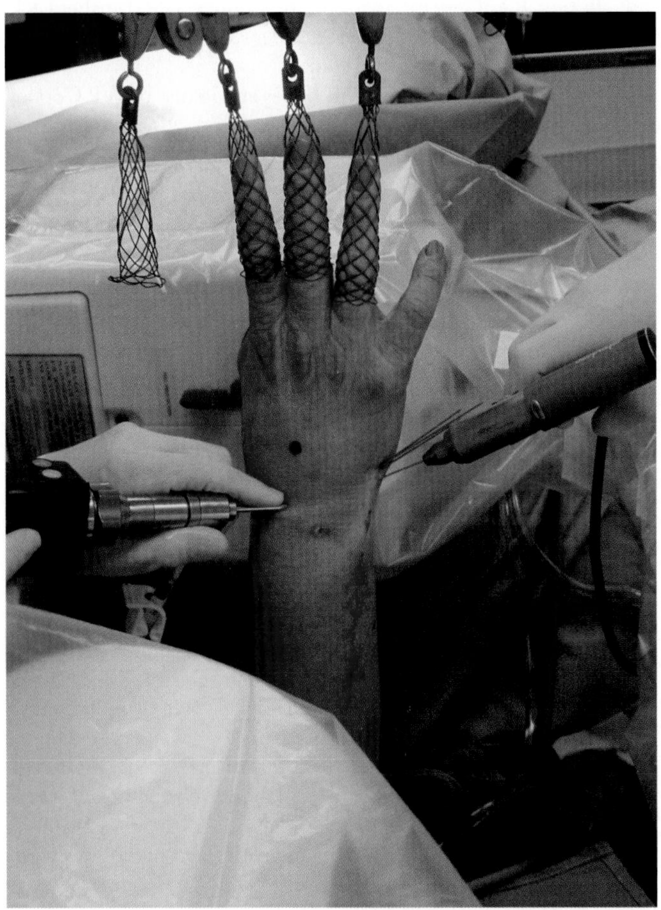

FIGURE 11.15. Arthroscopic reduction and percutaneous pin fixation of a grade III LTIL injury.

A static LTJ diastasis is not present, and injury to the secondary restraint extrinsic ligaments is not seen. A probe can be passed through the small gap present between the lunate and the triquetrum. The author recently reviewed a series of 40 patients with a grade III injury who were treated with arthroscopic debridement of the torn LTIL, arthroscopic reduction of the LTJ, and percutaneous K-wire fixation for 8 to 10 weeks.

Using the modified Mayo Wrist Score to assess outcome, it was found that 55% of the patients had a good or excellent result. However, 80% of the patients had virtually no wrist pain. The lower scores producing fair results were due to persistent wrist stiffness or grip weakness. Of the 40 patients, 23 developed LTJ grade III instability secondary to a displaced intra-articular distal radius fracture. The remaining 17 patients injured their wrists secondary to an acute sprain. Those patients with LTJ instability resulting from a distal radius fracture all scored satisfactory with arthroscopic treatment. The poorest outcomes occurred in those patients with wrist sprains that were treated six months or more after their injury.

A suitable surgical alternative to the previously described arthroscopic treatment is to proceed to an open repair of the torn LTIL as long as the ligament appears arthroscopically viable and therefore repairable. An LTIL reconstruction with tendon graft or an LTJ arthrodesis is an alternative. The author would not recommend these two procedures as the initial treatment option, but suggests they be reserved as a reconstruction option if the arthroscopic treatment or open repair of the ligament is not possible or fails.

The literature also reports satisfactory results with debridement of the torn LTIL, or debridement combined with pinning of the LTJ. However, these studies do not clearly sort out grade II from grade III ligament injuries, and may even contain a few grade IV patterns. In addition, confusing terminology such as *partial ligament tear* and *complete ligament tear* are used to describe a broad category of ligamentous injuries. This makes interpretation of the results difficult.

An alternative arthroscopic surgical procedure would be a ligament plication of the ulnocarpal ligaments and pinning of the LTJ. Early results with this technique of arthroscopic plication have been promising.[57] A tenodesis of the LTJ using a distally based segment of the ECU tendon has been successful in a recent report.[58] The author does not have any direct experience with either of these surgical techniques.

A chronic grade III LTIL injury that is over six months old will not likely do well with only arthroscopic treatment. An open delayed primary repair, ligament reconstruction, capsulodesis or tenodesis, or LTJ arthrodesis would be better treatment options. The author favors a delayed direct repair of the LTIL if this is still possible. The author has had no personal experience with tendon reconstruction, tenodesis, or capsulodesis but has had good success with an LTJ arthrodesis.

Acute grade IV LTIL injuries present with a severe alteration of carpal alignment, incongruency of the LTJ, and gross instability (Figure 11.10). It is possible to manage these with an ARIF before a fixed VISI occurs. If the LTJ is arthroscopically reducible, it may be pinned. The triquetrum should also be pinned to the hamate to maintain its anatomical alignment between the distal radius and ulna, and the distal carpal row to allow for healing of the torn extrinsic ligaments. Cast and pin immobilization should continue for a minimum of eight weeks. The author has had some success with this technique of ARIF, even as long as one year following LTIL injury.

A chronic grade IV LTIL injury is usually beyond arthroscopic management. The fixed rigidity of the CI, and the high association of TFCC injuries with possible secondary cartilage degenerative changes, limits our reconstructive surgical options. A fixed, irreducible LTJ instability is best managed with an intercarpal arthrodesis such as a lunate-triquetral-capitate-hamate fusion (which will then stabilize the PCR to the distal row).

If the chronic instability is still reducible, ligament reconstruction or LTJ arthrodesis in conjunction with a dorsoulnar capsulodesis or ECU tenodesis may be of benefit. The usefulness of arthroscopy in the treatment of chronic instability is to assess the wrist joint for associated pathology. The findings of cartilage degeneration within the RCJ, MCJ, or DRUJ; SLL injury and SLJ instability; MCJ ligamentous injury and midcarpal instability; TFCC injury; and UIS with positive ulnar variance will significantly affect the choice of surgical procedure.

Summary

The role of wrist arthroscopy in the treatment of LTIL injury and LTJ instabilities is diagnostic and therapeutic. Diagnostic arthroscopy of both the RCJ and MCJ is the most essential tool in accurately assessing the extent of the injury and in classifying the grade of interosseous ligament instability. It also aids in the discovery of any associated pathology that would change the choice of surgical alternatives. Based on these arthroscopic findings, treatment can be appropriately planned.

Even though the therapeutic surgical options for treatment of LTJ instability remain somewhat controversial, the technique of arthroscopic reduction of LTJ instability with percutaneous K-wire fixation (ARIF) is a viable alternative for the acute modified grade I, II, and select grade III injuries. The feasibility and practicality of ARIF should be weighed against the established success of ligament repair, ligament reconstruction, or LTJ arthrodesis.

References

1. Patterson RM, Nicodemus CL, Viegas SF. High-speed, three-dimensional kinematic analysis of the normal wrist. J Hand Surg 1998;23:446–53.
2. Berger RA. General anatomy. In Cooney WP, Linsheid RL, Dobyns JH (eds.), *The Wrist: Diagnosis and Operative Treatment*. St. Louis: Mosby 1998.
3. Garcia-Elias M, Dobyns JH. Bones and joints. In WP Cooney, RL Dobyns, JH Dobyns (eds.), *The Wrist: Diagnosis and Operative Treatment*. St. Louis: Mosby 1998.
4. Berger RA. Ligament anatomy. In WP Cooney, RL Linsheid, JH Dobyns, (eds.), *The Wrist: Diagnosis and Operative Treatment*. St. Louis: Mosby 1998.
5. Mastella DJ, Zelouf DS. Anatomy of the lunotriquetral joint. DS Ruch (ed.), *Atlas of the Hand Clinics*. Philadelphia: W.B. Saunders 2004.
6. Ritt MJ, Bishop AT, Berger RA, et al. Lunotriquetral ligament properties: A comparison of three anatomic subregions. J Hand Surg 1998;23:425–31.
7. The Anatomy and Biomechanics Committee of the International Federation of Societies for Surgery of the Hand. Position statement: Definition of carpal instability. J Hand Surg 1999;24:866–67.
8. Linscheid RL, Dobyns JH, Beabout JW, et al. Traumatic instability of the wrist: Diagnosis, classification and pathomechanics. J Bone Joint Surg 1972;54:1612–32.
9. Mayfield JK, Johnson RP, Kilcoyne RK. Pathomechanics and progressive perilunar instability. J Hand Surg 1980;5:226–41.
10. Reagan DA, Linsheid RL, Dobyns JH. Lunotriquetral sprains. J Hand Surg 1984;9:502–14.
11. Lichtman DM, Schneider JR, Swafford AR, et al. Ulnar midcarpal instability: Clinical and laboratory analysis. J Hand Surg 1981;6:515–23.
12. Freeland AE, Geissler WB. Kinematics and pathophysiology of carpal instability. In WB Geissler (eds.), *Wrist Arthroscopy*. New York: Springer 2005.
13. Weber ER. Wrist mechanics and its association with ligamentous instability. In DM Lichtman, AH Alexander (eds.), *The Wrist and Its Disorders*. Philadelphia: W.B. Saunders 1988.
14. Trumble TE, Bour CJ, Smith RJ, et al. Kinematics of the ulnar carpus related to the volar intercalated segment instability pattern. J Hand Surg 1990;15:384–92.
15. Viegas SF, Patterson RM, Peterson PD, et al. Ulnar-sided perilunate instability: An anatomic and biomechanic study. J Hand Surg 1990;15:268–78.

16. Horii E, Garcia-Elias M, An KN, et al. A kinematic study of luno-triquetral dissociations. J Hand Surg 1991;16:355–62.
17. Ritt MJ, Linsheid RL, Cooney WP, et al. The lunotriquetral joint: Kinematic effects of sequential ligament sectioning, ligament repair, and arthrodesis. J Hand Surg 1998;23:432–45.
18. Garcia-Elias M, Ritt JP. Lunotriquetral dissociation: Pathomechanics. In DS Ruch (ed.), *Atlas of the Hand Clinics*. Philadelphia: W.B. Saunders 2004.
19. Bednar JM, Osterman AL. Carpal instability: Evaluation and treatment. J Am Acad Orthop Surg 1993;1:10–17.
20. Butterfield WL, Joshi AB, Lichtman DM. Lunotriquetral injuries. J Am Soc Hand Surg 2002;2:195–203.
21. Moran SL, Shin AY. Open treatment options for lunotriquetral instability and dissociation. In DS Ruch (ed.), *Atlas of the Hand Clinics*. Philadelphia: W.B. Saunders 2004.
22. Bindra DS, Slade JF III. Lunotriquetral arthritis and ulnar impaction syndrome. In DS Ruch (ed.), *Atlas of the Hand Clinics*. Philadelphia: W.B. Saunders 2004.
23. Hanker GJ. Arthroscopic management of ulnar impaction syndrome. In WB Geissler (ed.), *Techniques in Wrist Arthroscopy*. New York: Springer-Verlag 2003.
24. Hanker GJ. Arthroscopic management of ulnar impaction syndrome. In WB Geissler (ed.), *Wrist Arthroscopy*. New York: Springer 2005.
25. Dobyns JH, Cooney WP. Classification of carpal instability. In WP Cooney, RL Linsheid, JH Dobyns (eds.), *The Wrist: Diagnosis and Operative Treatment*. St. Louis: Mosby 1998.
26. Shin AY, Battaglia MJ, Bishop AT. Lunotriquetral instability: Diagnosis and treatment. J Am Acad Orthop Surg 2000; 8:170–79.
27. Kalainov DM, Hartigan BJ, Cohen MS. Lunotriquetral instability: Clinical findings. In DS Ruch (ed.), *Atlas of the Hand Clinics*. Philadelphia: W.B. Saunders 2004.
28. Atzei A, Luchetti R. Clinical approach to the painful wrist. In WB Geissler (ed.), *Wrist Arthroscopy*. New York: Springer 2005.
29. Michalko K, Allen S, Akelman E. Evaluation of the painful wrist. In WB Geissler (ed.), *Wrist Arthroscopy*. New York: Springer 2005.
30. Cooney WP, Berger RA. Interosseous ligamentous injuries of the wrist. In JB McGinty (ed.), *Operative Arthroscopy, Third Edition*. Philadelphia: Lippincott Williams and Wilkins 2003.
31. Bishop AT, Reagon DA. Lunotriquetral sprains. In WP Cooney, RL Linsheid, JH Dobyns (eds.), *The Wrist: Diagnosis and Operative Treatment*. St. Louis: Mosby 1998.
32. Cassidy C, Ruby LK. Carpal instability. Instr Course Lect 2003;52:209–20.
33. Pillukat T, Van Schoonhoven J, Lanz U. Ulnar instability of the carpus. Orthopade 2004;33(6):676–84.
34. Bottcher R, Mutze S, Lautenbach M, et al. Diagnosis of lunotriquetral instability. Handchir Mikrochir Plast Chir 2005;37(2):131–36.
35. Ritter MR, Chang DS, Ruch DS. The role of arthroscopy in the treatment of lunotriquetral ligament injuries. Hand Clin 1999;15(3):445–54.
36. Ruch DS, Bowling J. Arthroscopic assessment of carpal instability. Arthroscopy 1998;14(7):675–81.
37. Westkaemper JG, Mitsionis G, Giannakopoulos PN. Wrist arthroscopy for the treatment of ligament and triangular fibrocartilage complex injuries. Arthroscopy 1998;14:479–83.
38. Osterman AL, Seidman GD. The role of arthroscopy in the treatment of lunotriquetral ligament injuries. Hand Clin 1995;11:41–50.
39. Ruch DS, Poehling GG. Arthroscopic management of partial scapholunate and lunotriquetral injuries of the wrist. J Hand Surg 1996;21:412–17.
40. Weiss AP, Sachar K, Glowacki KA. Arthroscopic debridement alone for intercarpal ligament tears. J Hand Surg 1997;22:344–49.
41. Geissler WB , Freeland A , Savoie FH III, et al. Intraarticular soft-tissue lesions associated with an intraarticular fracture of the distal end of the radius. J Bone Joint Surg 1996; 78:357–65.
42. Gupta R, Bozentka DJ, Osterman AL. Wrist arthroscopy: Principles and clinical applications. J Am Acad Orthop Surg 2001;9:200–09.
43. Palmer AK, Dobyns JH, Linsheid RL. Management of post-traumatic instability of the wrist secondary to ligament rupture. J Hand Surg 1978;3:507–32.
44. Shin A, Weinstein L, Berger R, et al. Treatment of isolated injuries of the lunotriquetral ligament. J Bone Joint Surg 2001;83:1023–28.
45. Watson HK, Black DM. Instabilities of the wrist. Hand Clin 1987;3:103–11.
46. Kirschenbaum D, Coyle M, Leddy J. Chronic lunotriquetral instability: Diagnosis and treatment. J Hand Surg 1993; 18:1107–12.
47. Pin P, Young V, Gilula L, et al. Management of chronic lunotriquetral ligament tears. J Hand Surg 1989;14:77–83.
48. Alexander CE, Lichtman DM. Triquetrolunate instability. In DM Lichtman, AH Alexander (eds.), *The Wrist and Its Disorders, Second Edition*. Philadelphia: W.B. Saunders 1997.
49. Whipple TL. Intrinsic ligaments and carpal instability. *Arthroscopic Surgery: The Wrist*. Philadelphia: J.B. Lippincott 1992.
50. Schadel-Hopfner M. Therapy of acute triquetrum fractures and LT ligament injuries. Kongressbd Dtsch Ges Chir Kongr 2001;118:395–98.
51. Nelson D, Manske P, Pruitt D, et al. Lunotriquetral arthrodesis. J Hand Surg 1993;18:1113–20.
52. Sennwald GR, Fischer M, Mondi P. Lunotriquetral arthrodesis: A controversial procedure. J Hand Surg [Br] 1995; 20:755–60.
53. Trumble T, Bour C, Smith R, et al. Intercarpal arthrodesis for static and dynamic volar intercalated segment instability. J Hand Surg 1988;13:384–90.
54. Guidera PM, Watson HK, Dwyer TA, et al. Lunotriquetral arthrodesis using cancellous bone graft. J Hand Surg 2001;26:422–36.
55. Novak V, Weisler EA. Lunotriquetral arthrodesis. In DS Ruch (ed.), *Atlas of the Hand Clinics*. Philadelphia: W.B. Saunders 2004.
56. De Smet L, Janssens I, van de Sande W. Chronic lunotriquetral ligament injuries: Arthrodesis or capsulodesis. Acta Chir Belg 2005;105(1):79–81.
57. Moskal MJ, Savoie FH III. Management of lunotriquetral instability. In WB Geissler (ed.), *Wrist Arthroscopy*. New York: Springer 2005.
58. Shahane SA, Trail IA, Takwale VJ, et al. Tenodesis of the extensor carpi ulnaris for chronic, post-traumatic lunotriquetral instability. J Bone Joint Surg Br 2005;87(11):1512–15.
59. Smith B, Short W, Werner F, et al. The effect of ulnar shortening on lunotriquetral motion and instability: A biomechanical study. Presented at the American Society for Surgery of the Hand, Annual Fellow and Residents Meeting, 1994.

60. Geissler WB. Combined lunotriquetral and triangular fibrocartilage complex ligamentous injuries. In DS Ruch (ed.), *Atlas of the Hand Clinics*. Philadelphia: W.B. Saunders 2004.
61. Hofmeister EP, Dao KD, Glowacki KA, et al. The role of midcarpal arthroscopy in the diagnosis of disorders of the wrist. J Hand Surg 2001;26:407–14.
62. Hanker GJ. The role of wrist arthroscopy in the diagnosis and treatment of lunotriquetral joint injuries. In DS Ruch (ed.), *Atlas of the Hand Clinics*. Philadelphia: W.B. Saunders 2004.
63. Dautel G, Merle M. Chondral lesions of the midcarpal joint. Arthroscopy 1997;13:97–102.
64. Sweet A, Weiss L. Applications of electrothermal shrinkage in wrist arthroscopy. Atlas Hand Clin 2001;6(2):203–10.
65. Frostick SP. Thermal capsulorrhaphy: Basic science. In J McGinty (ed.), *Operative Arthroscopy, Third Edition*. Philadelphia: Lippincott Williams and Wilkins 2003.
66. Nagle DJ. Lasers and electrothermal devices. In WB Geissler (ed.), *Wrist Arthroscopy*. New York: Springer 2005.
67. Darlis NA, Weiser RW, Sotereanos DG. Partial scapholunate ligament injuries treated with arthroscopic debridement and thermal shrinkage. J Hand Surg 2005;30:908–14.

Jason W. Levine, Felix H. Savoie III, and Michael J. Moskal

CHAPTER 12

To Terry Whipple, Jim Roth, and Gary Poehling, who all taught me wrist arthroscopy.

Arthroscopic Plication of Lunotriquetral Ligament Tears

Introduction

Injuries to the ulnar side of the wrist may be difficult to diagnose and to treat. Ulnar-sided wrist pain can occur from acute injuries, such as rotation and hyperextension, or from repetitive injuries. These injuries can result in tears of the lunotriquetral interosseous ligament (LTIOL), triangular fibrocartilage complex (TFCC), the palmar ulnocarpal ligaments, or a combination of these structures. Lunotriquetral (LT) joint injuries often exist with associated pathologic conditions such as TFCC injuries and may represent a continuum of injury severity involving the ulnar-sided wrist structures.

Arthroscopy of the wrist has been promoted as an important adjunct to the diagnosis of subtle ligamentous instability because of the ability to directly view the interosseous ligaments, secondary articular cartilage changes, and intra-articular pathology.[1] With the development of advanced techniques and improved instrumentation, wrist arthroscopy is also becoming an important tool in the treatment of complex injuries (including carpal instability).

Normal lunotriquetral kinematics are dependent on the integrity of the lunotriquetral interosseous ligament, ulnolunate ligament (UL), ulnotriquetral ligament (UT), and the dorsal radiocarpal and scaphotriquetral ligaments. The LTIOL is thick both palmarly and dorsally, with a membranous proximal portion. Injury to the LTIOL results in instability between the lunate and triquetrum.

History and Physical Exam

The initial evaluation of the wrist begins with the patient's history, specifically reviewing mechanism of injury, hand dominance, athletic participation, work history, and recent activities. Areas of swelling, tenderness, and crepitation should be identified. Ballottement or shuck testing is often helpful in diagnosing intercarpal instability.[2] To perform this maneuver, stabilize the lunate or triquetrum and feel for increased motion of the LT joint during palmar and dorsal stressing. Important physical findings are tenderness over the LT joint and/or the TFCC, increased translation of the lunate with respect to the triquetrum, and crepitation with pain during pronation, supination, or ulnar deviation.

Radiographic evaluation of a painful wrist should include a zero rotation posteroanterior,[3,4] true lateral, and oblique views of the wrist. Ulnar variance, lunotriquetral interval, greater and lesser arc continuity, and the radiolunate and scapholunate angles are assessed. In cases where the physical examination findings are equivocal, an arthrogram or MRI can be obtained.

Ulnar Ligamentous Anatomy

Our approach to LT injuries had evolved from the anatomical concepts of the ulnar ligaments in relationship to the lunotriquetral joint and the TFCC. The lunotriquetral interosseous ligament is thicker both volarly and dorsally[5] with a membranous central portion. Normal lunotriquetral kinematics is imparted from the integrity of the LTIOL,[6] ulnolunate, ulnotriquetral,[6–8] dorsal radiotriquetral (RT), and scaphotriquetral (ST) ligaments.[6,7,9] Severe instability such as a volar intercalated segmental instability (VISI) requires damage to both the dorsal RTand ST ligaments.[6,7,9]

The TFCC is the primary stabilizer of the distal radioulnar joint via the dorsal and volar radioulnar ligaments.[10,11]

This helps to stabilize the ulnar carpus, and transmits axial forces to the ulna.[12,13] The TFCC originates from the ulnar aspect of the lunate fossa of the radius and inserts on the base of the ulnar styloid and distally on the lunate, triquetrum, hamate, and fifth metacarpal base. The integrity of the triangular fibrocartilage, volar radiocarpal, and dorsal radiocarpal ligaments is visible at arthroscopy. TFCC compromise is often a part of more extensive ulnar-sided injuries.[14] The volar and dorsal aspects of the lunotriquetral ligament merge with the ulnocarpal extrinsic ligaments volarly and the dorsal radiolunotriquetral ligament dorsally, anchoring the triquetrum.[15]

The ulnocarpal volar ligaments are composed of the ulnolunate (also known as the disc-lunate), the ulnotriquetral (UT)—also known as the disc-triquetral ligaments—and the ulno-capitate. The ulnolunate and ulnotriquetral ligaments originate on the volar triangular fibrocartilage complex (TFCC) and insert on the volar lunate and volar triquetrum (respectively) as well as the LT ligament.[14,16,17] Just palmar lies the ulno-capitate ligament, providing a direct attachment from the ulna to the palmar ulnar ligamentous complex.

The arthroscopic approach to symptomatic LT instability is based on the contributing factors of the ulnar carpal ligaments to lunotriquetral joint stability. Suture plication of the ulnar ligaments serves to shorten the disc-carpal ligaments and augment the palmar capsular tissue as part of the arthroscopic reduction and internal fixation.

Ligament plication has been implemented to manage capitolunate instability.[18] The central portion of the volar radiocapitate ligament was tethered to the radiotriquetral ligament by a volar approach. UT-UL ligament plication, developed by one of the authors (FHS), mimics this technique. It has been used in treating those injuries that do not severely destabilize the LT joint, such as those producing a VISI deformity that requires functional compromise of the dorsal extrinsic ligaments (dorsal radiotriquetral and scaphotriquetral). Arthroscopic volar ulnar ligament plication both reduces surgical trauma and allows concurrent assessment of its effect while viewing through the radiocarpal and midcarpal joints.

Arthroscopic Operative Technique

The following is a general approach to arthroscopic stabilization of ulnar-sided instability. It can be used in conjunction with associated pathology such as ulnar abutment syndrome and TFCC tears when associated with an LTIOL tear. 3-/,4, 6-R, volar 6-U, and the radial and ulnar midcarpal portals are used during arthroscopic capsulodesis and arthroscopic reduction and internal fixation.

An arthroscopic video system should be positioned to allow a clear view of the monitor by the surgeon and assistant. After the limb is exsanguinated, a traction tower is used and 8 to 10 pounds of traction are applied through finger traps with the arm strapped to the hand table. A complete diagnostic radiocarpal and midcarpal diagnostic arthroscopy is performed, typically utilizing the 3-/,4 and 6-R radiocarpal portals and the radial and ulnar midcarpal portals. Diagnostic radiocarpal arthroscopy should include visualization from the 6-R portal to ensure complete visualization of the LTIOL from dorsal to palmar. The LTIOL should be debrided as necessary. Depending on each unique case, the addition of a 4-/,5 portal as either the working or viewing portal can be helpful.

Midcarpal assessment begins with the arthroscope inserted into the radial midcarpal portal and the ulnar midcarpal portal as the working portal. The lunotriquetral joint is assessed for congruency and laxity of the triquetrum.

Congruency

- The lunate and triquetrum should be co-linear. If the view of the lunotriquetral joint from the midcarpal radial portal is blocked by a separate lunate facet,[19] place the arthroscope in the midcarpal ulnar portal to gain visualization. Under these conditions, the radial articular edge of triquetrum should be aligned with the most ulnar articular edge of the hamate facet of the lunate.
- Although congruent, the LT joint may be unstable due to excessive laxity.

Laxity

- Assuming it is normal, the scapholunate (SL) joint can be used as a reference. Laxity should be assessed both upon triquetral rotation and separation from the lunate.
- Upon midcarpal arthroscopic assessment of an unstable LT joint, the dorsal portion of the triquetrum is often rotated such that its articular surface is distal to the lunate. The triquetrum can be translated to a reduced state in which the articular surfaces of the triquetrum and lunate are co-linear.
- An unstable LT joint may have co-linear articular surfaces. However, the triquetrum can be ulnarly translated so as to "gap open" the LT joint. The normal SL joint can be used as a reference.

The final midcarpal assessment of the LT joint is the dorsal capsular structures. The dorsal radiocarpal and dorsal intercarpal ligaments attach in part to the lunate and triquetrum. In certain cases, avulsions of the dorsal capsuloligamentous structures have been observed.

After the confirmation of LT instability, the arthroscope is placed in the 3-4 portal during disc-lunate to ulno-capitate to disc-triquetral ligament plication. The volar 6-U (v6-U) is established. The v6-U portal is located in the soft spot adjacent to the prestyloid recess, dorsal to the volar disc carpal ligaments. It is established via spinal needle localization utilizing an outside-in technique. Care is taken to avoid injury to the dorsal sensory branches of the ulnar nerve during placement.

The interval between the disc-lunate and disc-triquetral ligament identifies the lunotriquetral joint and interosseous ligament. The LTIOL is gently debrided (Figure 12.1). Through the v6-U portal, an 18-gauge spinal needle is passed just volar to the disc-triquetral, ulno-capitate, and disc-lunate—entering the radiocarpal joint at the radial edge of the UL ligament just distal to the articular surface of the radius. A #2–0 PDS suture is placed through the needle into the joint. The suture is retrieved either sequentially through the 6-R and then through the v6-U or directly through the v6-U—using a wire loop suture retriever. It is then tagged as the first plicating suture (Figure 12.2).

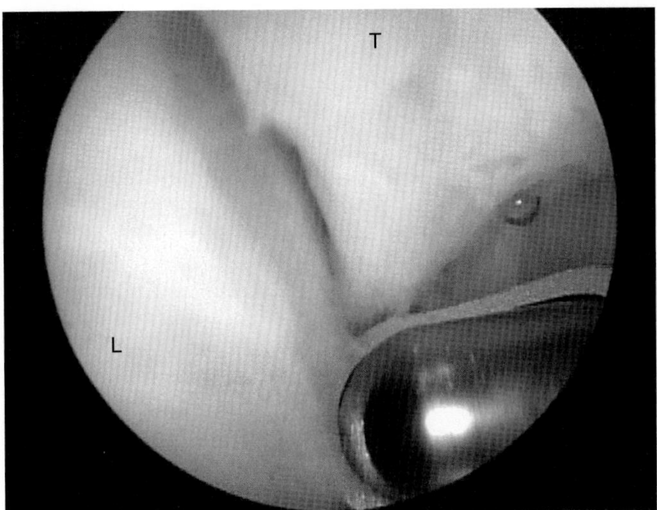

FIGURE 12.1. The tear in the lunotriquetral interosseous ligament is visualized. A motorized shaver is used to remove the frayed tissues.

In likewise fashion, a second plicating suture is placed approximately 5 mm distal to the first so that the suture loops are parallel to the lunate and triquetrum and tagged as the second plicating suture (Figure 12.3). Tension on the first stitch often facilitates a second needle passage through the ulnolunate and ulnotriquetral ligaments. The adequacy of the plication should be assessed by applying tension to the stitch and observing its effect on the LT interval after each suture passage.

Finally, through the v6-U portal a spinal needle and then a suture are passed through the volar aspect of the capsule at the pre-styloid recess and then through the peripheral rim of the TFCC. The wire retriever is introduced through the ulnar capsule and the suture is brought out the v6-U portal to tighten the ulnar capsule. The three sets of sutures are tied at the termination of the procedure after

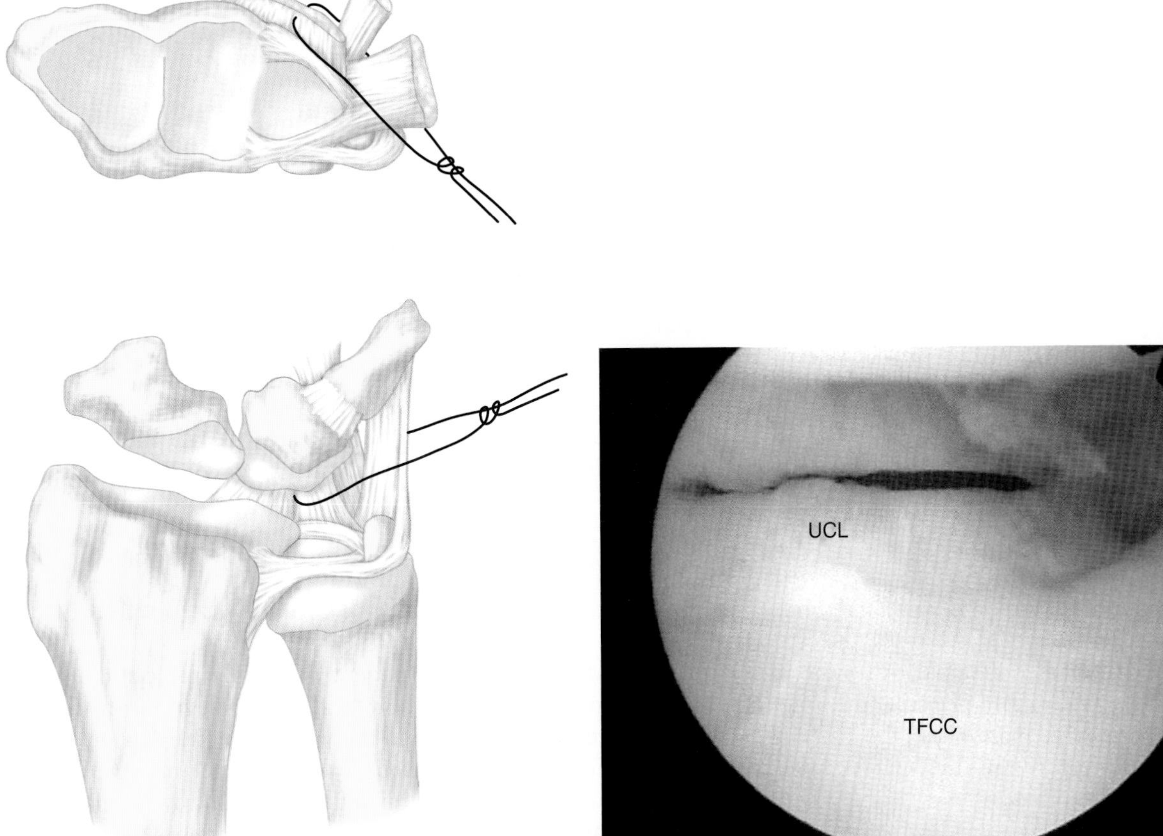

FIGURE 12.2. (A) Diagram depicting first plication suture encompassing the UL ligament. *(Courtesy of the Christine M. Kleinert Institute for Hand and Microsurgery).* (B) View from the 3-4 portal of the first plication suture.

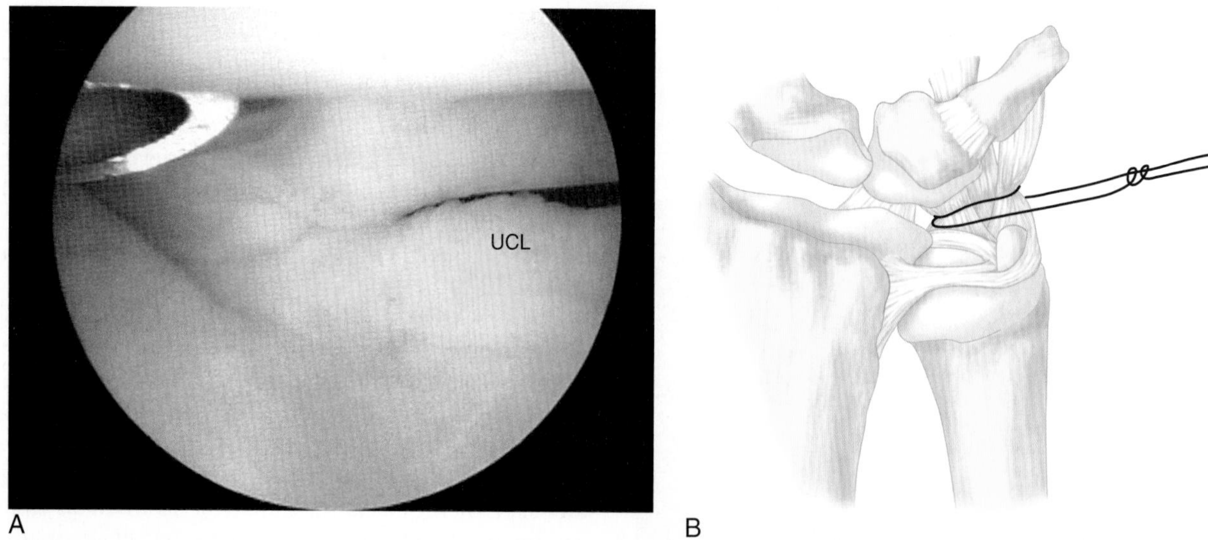

FIGURE 12.3. (A) Placement of spinal needle superficial to the UL ligaments in preparation for passage of the second plication suture. (B) Diagram of second plication suture. *(Courtesy of the Christine M. Kleinert Institute for Hand and Microsurgery.)*

the lunotriquetral joint has been congruently reduced and stabilized with K-wires.

While viewing through the midcarpal radial portal, a midcarpal-ulnar (MCU) portal is created. A probe is used to assess lunotriquetral joint incongruity and mobility, and to reduce the lunotriquetral joint (Figure 12.4). A spinal needle can be placed in the midpalmar space from ulnar to radial across the distal aspect of the LT joint and used as a guide for percutaneous pin placement into the triquetrum. The triquetrum is reduced congruent with the lunate articular cartilage by applying traction to the plication sutures and firm pressure on the triquetrum.

The initial K-wire should be inserted 2 to 3 millimeters proximal to the spinal needle. Two 0.045 smooth K-wires are placed percutaneously across the lunotriquetral joint (Figure 12.5). The first pin is advanced across the lunotriquetral interval from ulnar to radial under fluoroscopic guidance, and the second pin is placed using the first pin as a guide to placement. After satisfactory reduction of the lunotriquetral joint, traction is released, the forearm is held in neutral rotation, and the plication stitches are tied at the 6-U portal (with the knots placed below the skin; Figure 12.6). The K-wires are either cut subcutaneously or bent outside the skin.

LTIOL tears can be seen in combination with TFCC pathology, such as traumatic peripheral tears and degenerative tears seen in isolation or as part of an ulnar abutment syndrome. In degenerative TFCC tears, the central avascular portion is debrided to a stable rim prior to plication. In traumatic tears, the suture placement through the ulnar capsule and peripheral margin can be extended dorsally to simultaneously repair the TFCC tear after the initial plication sutures are placed.

Patients with lunotriquetral ligament tears often have a positive ulnar variance.[2,20,21] In an extension of the initial treatment group, patients with ulnar abutment syndrome (with associated lunate chondromalacia, TFCC tears, and LTIOL tears) have been treated by LT plication stabilization in conjunction with an arthroscopic wafer procedure.

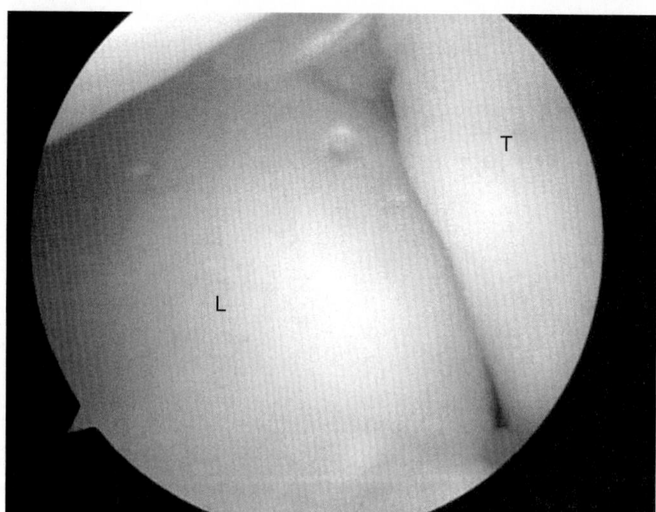

FIGURE 12.4. View of the lunotriquetral joint from the midcarpal portal.

Postoperative Care

After surgery the patient is initially placed in a long arm splint, with the elbow flexed at 90 degrees, the forearm in neutral rotation, and the wrist in neutral flexion and extension. At approximately one week after surgery, a Muenster cast is applied—with the forearm and wrist in neutral rotation and flexion, respectively. At approximately six weeks after surgery, the K-wires are removed. A removable Muenster cast is used for an additional two weeks to allow daily gentle wrist flexion, extension, pronation, and supination

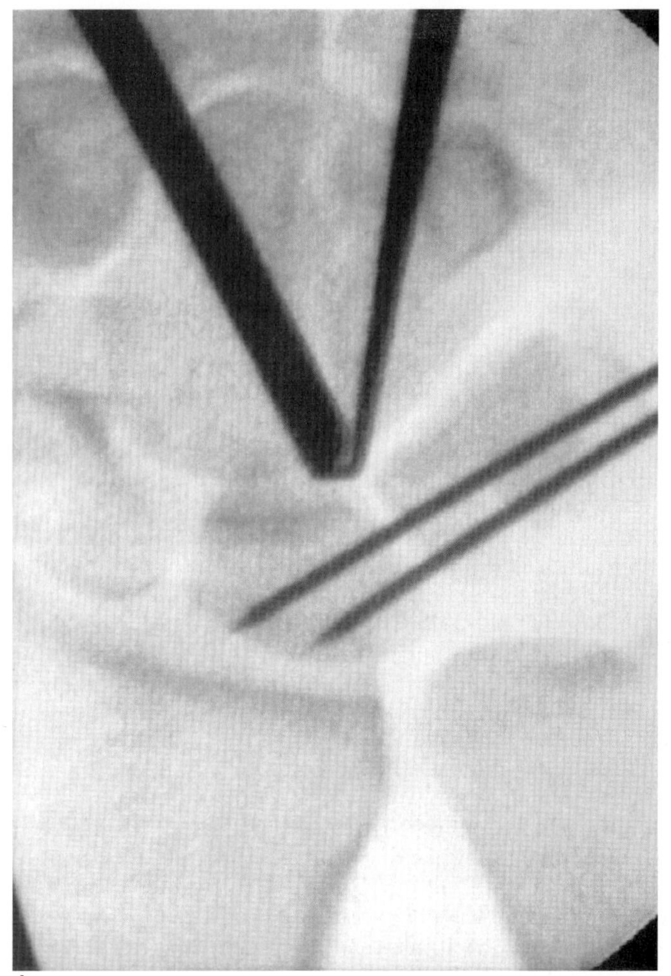

A

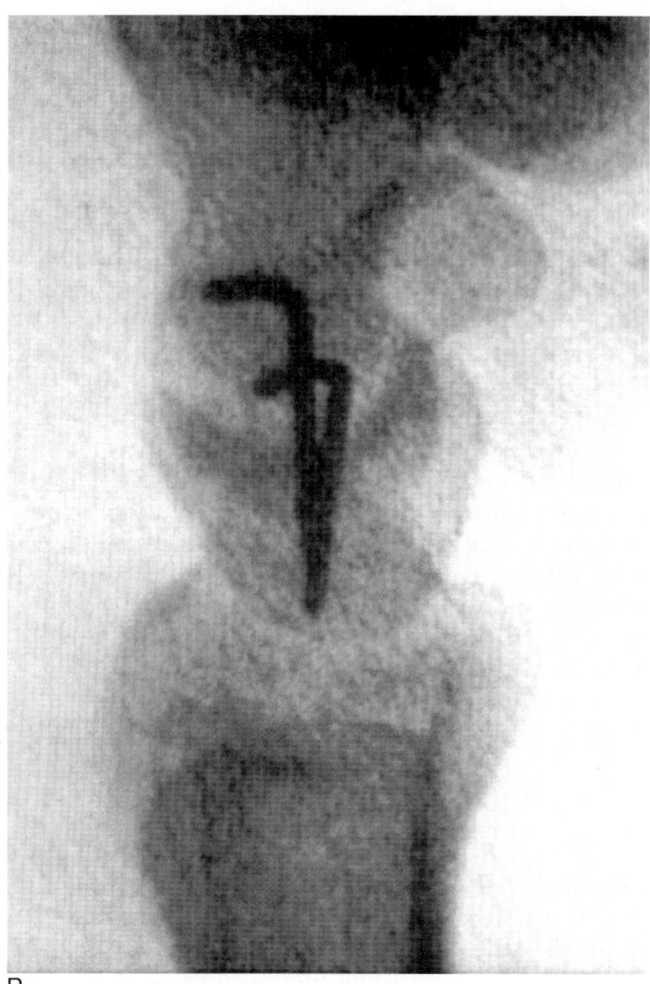

B

FIGURE 12.5. (A) PA of the wrist after reduction of the lunotriquetral joint and stabilization with two 0.045 K-wires. Note: probe used to aid reduction. (B) Lateral of the wrist after reduction of the lunotriquetral joint and stabilization with two 0.045 K-wires.

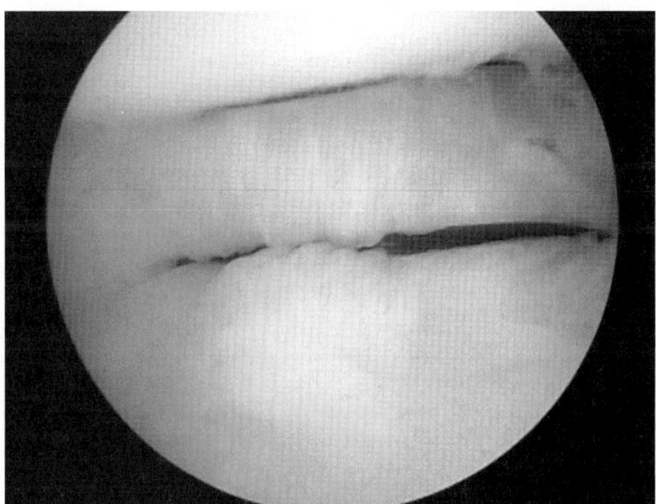

FIGURE 12.6. View of UL ligament after plication sutures have been tied.

within a painless arc of motion. Eight weeks after surgery, strengthening exercises are instituted and work hardening can begin slowly over 8 to 24 weeks postoperatively.

Results

In a case series, we looked at a group of 21 patients, including 7 who were treated as workman's compensation claimants and 4 patients were competitive athletes who sustained their injury during sport. All patients complained of ulnar-sided wrist pain, which was invariably increased by use of the wrist. The mean time between the onset of symptoms and treatment was 2.5 years (range 1 week to 5.5 years). Seventeen patients recalled a specific injury (hyperextension 12, twisting 2, unknown 3), and four noted a gradual onset of symptoms. Three patients had additional significant injuries to the affected extremity: elbow dislocation, humeral shaft fracture, and anterior shoulder dislocation.

The patients were uniformly tender over the lunotriquetral joint. Provocative tests for lunotriquetral instability—such as the lunotriquetral ballotement, TFCC grind, ulnocarpal shuck, and midcarpal instability evaluation—were specifically positive in nine and for TFCC in six. Crepitus was produced with pronosupination or ulnar deviation in 10 patients. A VISI instability pattern was not present. The average preoperative Mayo wrist score was 50 and increased to an average postoperative score of 88 at a mean of 3.1 years after surgery.

Range of motion was equal to the opposite side upon final follow-up. Nineteen of 21 patients had excellent and good results, whereas 2 patients had fair results. The average postoperative score for the 7 workman's compensation claimants or litigants was slightly lower than the overall group. Three patients had complications, which included prolonged tenderness along the extensor carpi ulnaris. One patient had a persistent neuritis of the dorsal branches of the ulnar nerve.

Summary

Symptomatic lunotriquetral interosseous ligament tears have been managed by simple arthroscopic debridement, ligamentous repair, and intercarpal arthrodesis. Ligamentous repair or reconstruction with a tendon graft requires an extensile approach. Lunotriquetral joint fusion limits flexion and extension and radioulnar deviation by 14 and 25%, respectively.[22] Arthroscopic ulnocarpal ligament plication in addition to LT joint reduction and stabilization is designed to augment the volar aspect of the LT joint. LT ligament tears are often associated with other pathology, notably ulnar-carpal ligament tears and disruption of the distal radioulnar joint.[23] Suture plication of the ulnocarpal ligaments shortens their length, which acts as a check-rein to excessive lunotriquetral motion (perhaps similar to ulnar shortening procedures). Suture plication of the peripheral rim of the TFCC is thought to increase tension in the ulnar DRUJ capsule.

Postoperative improvement in comfort and function is common following the described approach for lunotriquetral instability. The use of arthroscopy allowed for a comprehensive evaluation of the injured structures, and in many cases facilitated the treatment of multiple concurrent injuries. Arthroscopic stabilization of the lunotriquetral joint is a useful technique for the treatment of LTIOL tears, with minimal loss of wrist motion and limited surgical exposure.

References

1. Kulick M, Chen C, Swearingen P. Determining the diagnostic accuracy of wrist arthroscopy. Annual meeting of the American Society for Surgery of the Hand, Toronto, 1990.
2. Reagan D, Linscheid R, Dobyns J. Lunatotriquetral sprains. J Hand Surg 1984;9A:502–14.
3. Palmer A, Glisson R, Werner F. Ulnar variance determination. J Hand Surg 1982;7:376.
4. Gilula L. Posteroanterior wrist radiography: Importance of arm positioning. J Hand Surg 1987;12A:504–08.
5. Bednar J, Osterman A. Carpal instability: Evaluation and treatment. J Am Acad Orthop Surg 1993;1:10–17.
6. Horii E, Garcias-Elias M, An KN, et al. A kinematic study of luno-triquetral dissociations. J Hand Surg 1991;16A:355–62.
7. Viegas S, Peterson P, et al. Ulnar-sided perilunate instability: An anatomic and biomechanical study. J Hand Surg 1990; 15A:268.
8. Trumble T, Bour C, Smith R, et al. Kinematics of the ulnar carpus to the volar intercalated segment instability pattern. J Hand Surg 1990;15A:384.
9. Reagan DS, Linscheid RL, Dobyns JH. Lunotriquetral sprains. J Hand Surg 1984;9A:502–14.
10. Cooney W, Dobyns J, Linscheid R. Arthroscopy of the wrist: Anatomy and classification of carpal instability. Arthroscopy 1990;6:113–40.
11. Mayfield J. Patterns of injury to carpal ligaments: A spectrum. Clin Orthop 1984;187:36.
12. Palmer A, Werner F. Triangular fibrocartilage complex of the wrist: Anatomy and function. J Hand Surg 1981;6:153.
13. Werner F, Palmer A, Fortino M, et al. Force transmission through the distal ulna: Effect of ulnar variance, lunate fossa angulation, and radial and palmar tilt of the distal radius. J Hand Surg 1992;17A:423.
14. Melone C Jr., Nathan R. Traumatic disruption of the triangular fibrocartilage complex, pathoanatomy. Clin Orthop 1992;275:65–73.
15. Green D. Carpal dislocation and instabilities. In D Green (ed.), *Operative Hand Surgery.* New York: Churchill Livingston 1988: 878–79.
16. Palmer A, Werner F. Biomechanics of the distal radioulnar joint. Clin Orthop 1984;187:26.
17. Garcias-Elias M, Domenech-Mateu J. The articular disc of the wrist: Limits and relations. Acta Anat 1987;128:51.
18. Johnson R, Carrera G. Chronic capitolunate instability. J Bone Joint Surg 1986;68A:1164–76.
19. Viegas S, Wagner K, Patterson R, et al. Medial (hamate) facet of the lunate. J Hand Surg 1990;15A:564–71.
20. Pin P, Young V, Gilula L, et al. Management of chronic lunatotriquetral ligament tears. J Hand Surg 1989;14A:77–83.
21. Osterman A, Sidman G. The role of arthroscopy in the treatment of lunatotriquetral ligament injuries. Hand Clin 1995;11:41–50.
22. Seradge H, Sterbank P, Seradge E, et al. Segmental motion of the proximal carpal row: Their global effect on the wrist motion. J Hand Surg 1990;15A:236–39.
23. Ambrose L, Posner M. Lunate-triquetral and midcarpal joint instability. Hand Clin 1992;8:653–68.

David J. Slutsky

CHAPTER 13

Arthroscopic Dorsal Radiocarpal Ligament Repair

Introduction

In recent years, various investigators have highlighted the role of the dorsal radiocarpal ligament (DRCL) in maintaining carpal stability.[1–4] Tears of the DRCL have been linked to the development of both volar and dorsal intercalated segmental instabilities and may be implicated in the development of midcarpal instability.[5–7] The existence of a DRCL tear when combined with a scapholunate interosseous ligament (SLIL) tear connotes a greater degree of carpal instability. This has been acknowledged by some authors, who have advocated an open SLIL repair versus arthroscopic pinning when there is an associated DRCL tear.[8] An isolated tear of the dorsal radiocarpal ligament can also be a source of chronic wrist pain.[9]

In most series, the DRCL is overlooked during the typical arthroscopic examination of the wrist. It is difficult to visualize a DRCL tear through the standard dorsal wrist arthroscopy portals because the torn edge of the DRCL tends to float up against the arthroscope while viewed through the 3/-,4 portal and 4/-5 portals, which makes both identification and repair of the DRCL tear cumbersome. It can be seen obliquely through the 1/-,2 or 6-U portals, but visualization of the DRCL across the radiocarpal joint may be laborious in a tight or small wrist—especially if synovitis is present. Wrist arthroscopy through a volar radial portal (VR) is the ideal way to assess the dorsal radiocarpal ligament due to the straight line of sight[10–12] (see chapter on arthroscopic portals).

Indications

A classification system for DRCL tears was devised based on the presence or absence of associated carpal pathology (Table 13.1). Each successive stage denotes a longer-standing and/or more severe condition that negatively impacts the prognosis.

An arthroscopic DRCL repair is indicated for stage I, or isolated DRCL tears due to the favorable outcomes that can be achieved.[9,13,14] Geissler grade I and II SLIL and/or LTIL ligament injuries are still amenable to arthroscopic treatment. DRCL repairs are also indicated in Geissler grade I and II injuries since repair of a secondary stabilizer may augment the coronal plane stability (Table 13.2). Thermal shrinkage of the ST ligaments can theoretically augment sagittal plane stability of the scapholunate joint. This can be accomplished arthroscopically and is currently under investigation, but no data is available to recommend this procedure as yet. Grade III ligament injuries represent a relative gray area. They can be successfully treated with thermal shrinkage and pinning, which should be augmented with a DRCL repair, but if this is combined with instability of the ulnocarpal joint due to a large TFCC tear and/or Geissler III ligament tear there is a high risk of failure following arthroscopic treatment alone. Grade IV ligament injuries are beyond the realm of arthroscopic treatment and require open repair or reconstruction. Due to the frequent association of DRCL tears when there is a TFCC tear, I would also recommend a DRCL repair if the TFCC tear is treated arthroscopically.

Contraindications

When the treatment of an SLIL tear or dynamic scapholunate instability includes some type of dorsal capsulodesis, the dorsal incision followed by the creation of a

Table 13.1.

Classification of Dorsal Radiocarpal Ligament Tears

Stage I	Isolated DRCL tear
Stage II	DRCL tear with associated SLIL ± LTIL (Geissler I/II) ± TFCC tear
Stage IIIA	DRCL tear with associated SLIL ± LTIL (Geissler III) ± TFCC tear
Stage IIIB	DRCL tear with associated SLIL ± LTIL (Geissler IV) ± TFCC tear
Stage IV	Chondromalacia with widespread carpal pathology

The ligament with the highest Geissler grade determines the stage.
DRCL – dorsal radiocarpal ligament
SLIL – scapholunate interosseous ligament
LTIL – lunotriquetral interosseous ligament
TFCC – triangular fibrocartilage complex

Table 13.2.

Algorithm for Treatment of DRCL Tears

Stage I	Arthroscopic DRCL repair
Stage II	Arthroscopic DRCL repair, SLIL or LTIL debridement ± shrinkage, TFCC repair/debridement
Stage IIIA	Arthroscopic DRCL repair, SLIL/LTIL shrinkage + pinning, TFCC repair/debridement ± wafer (consider STT shrinkage)
Stage IIIB	Open SLIL repair/reconstruction ± capsulodesis, LTIL repair/reconstruction, TFC repair/debridement ± wafer/ulnar shortening
Stage IV	Partial carpal fusion vs. PRC

DRCL – dorsal radiocarpal ligament
SLIL – scapholunate interosseous ligament
LTIL – lunotriquetral interosseous ligament
PRC – proximal row carpectomy

dorsal capsular check-rein to restrain palmar flexion of the scaphoid renders any separate treatment of the DRCL tear unfeasible. When the DRCL tear is seen in association with palmar midcarpal instability (MCI), a soft-tissue repair of the dorsal ligaments will not by itself correct the MCI.[15,16]

Contraindications to a DRCL repair would also include those that preclude wrist arthroscopy in general, such as any cause of marked swelling that distorts the topographic anatomy, large capsular tears that can lead to extravasation of irrigation fluid, neurovascular compromise, bleeding disorders, or infection. Unfamiliarity with the regional anatomy is a relative contraindication.

Clinical Studies

A retrospective chart review was performed of patients who underwent diagnostic wrist arthroscopy with the use of a volar radial portal.[13,14] This identified 53 patients (56 wrists) over a six-year period. Additional pathology was seen in 24 patients that was not visible from the standard dorsal portals. This included 22 patients with tears of the dorsal radiocarpal ligament. Static wrist radiographs were obtained for all patients. Radiographs included a neutral-rotation posteroanterior view and a lateral view. None of the wrists showed a static carpal instability pattern. Magnetic resonance imaging was performed under the direction of the referring physician in six patients. Preoperative arthrograms were performed as a part of the diagnostic work-up for wrist pain in 20 patients.

None of the DRCL tears in this series was identified with preoperative arthrography or MRI. A preoperative MRI in one patient with a DRCL tear was misinterpreted as representing a dorsal wrist ganglion. There were no specific historical or physical findings that were helpful in making the diagnosis preoperatively, especially in cases of isolated DRCL tears. Specifically, there was no consistent dorsal wrist tenderness over the DRCL. The concomitant wrist pathology was largely responsible for any positive physical findings. The Watson test was positive in cases where there was coexisting scapholunate ligament pathology. Similarly, there was lunotriquetral or ulnar capsule tenderness and/or crepitus in patients with ulnar-sided wrist pathology.

There were 6 men and 16 women. The average patient age was 40 years (range 25 to 62 years). All patients failed a trial of conservative treatment with wrist immobilization, cortisone injections, and work restrictions. The average length of conservative treatment was seven months. The time interval between injury and surgical intervention averaged 25 months (range 8 to 53 months). At the time of arthroscopy, four patients were found to have an isolated DRCL tear that was solely responsible for their wrist pain. The remaining 17 patients had additional ligamentous pathology, summarized in Table 13.3. A dorsal capsulodesis was performed in seven patients as the primary treatment for derangements of the SLIL.

Thirteen of the 21 patients underwent an arthroscopic DRCL ligament repair and/or thermal shrinkage (repair = 5, repair + shrinkage = 6, shrinkage = 2), as described in material following. Ten of these patients underwent ancillary procedures for treatment of the coexisting wrist pathology. Lunotriquetral tears were treated with debridement and pinning. Triangular fibrocartilage tears were debrided or repaired. Scapholunate ligament tears or instability was treated with capsulodesis ± repair. One patient had generalized arthrofibrosis (MG), which precluded a

Table 13.3.

Associated Pathology/Conditions

Patient	DRCL Tear	SLIL Tear/ Instability	LTIL Tear	TFC Tear	CHIL Tear	MCI	Other
MA	+	—	—	—	—	—	—
DA	+	—	—	—	—	—	CTS
ND	+	—	—	—	—	—	CTS
MR	+	—	—	—	—	—	—
BM	+	Complete	—	—	—	—	—
DL	+	Partial	—	—	—	—	—
SC	+	Partial	—	+	—	—	—
MJ	+	Dynamic	—	—	—	—	CTS
BL	+	Dynamic	—	—	—	—	—
VB	+	Dynamic	—	—	—	—	De Quervain's
CE	+	Dynamic	—	—	—	—	De Quervain's
MB	+	Dynamic	+	—	—	—	—
HS	+	—	+	—	—	—	CTS, lunate chondromalacia
MG	+	—	+	+	—	—	Arthrofibrosis
MRO	+	—	+	+	—	—	—
AD	+	—	+	+	—	—	—
JP	+	—	+	+	—	—	—
GJ	+	—	+	+	—	—	Lunate, hamate chondromalacia
YB	+	—	—	+	—	—	—
ML	+	—	—	+	—	—	CTS
GN	+	—	—	—	+	—	—
RF	+	—	Dynamic	—	—	+	—

DRCL = dorsal radiocarpal ligament
SLIL = scapholunate interosseous ligament
LTIL = lunotriquetral interosseous ligament
CHIL = capitohamate interosseous ligament
TFC = triangular fibrocartilage
MCI = midcarpal instability
CTS = carpal tunnel syndrome

DRCL repair. Concomitant nerve entrapment was a common finding, which was treated at the same time.

The average duration of the follow-up period was 16 months (range 7 to 41 months), with one patient lost to follow-up at four weeks. Pain was graded as none, mild, moderate, and severe.[17] Wrist extension, wrist flexion, radial deviation, ulnar deviation, and grip strength were assessed. Wrist range of motion was compared with presurgical values. Grip strength was compared with the contralateral side at follow-up evaluation.

Patient outcomes are summarized in Table 13.4. The four patients who underwent an isolated DRCL repair were satisfied with the outcome of surgery and would repeat the surgery again because it improved their symptoms. All four patients graded their pain as none or mild. None of these patients were taking pain medications. All returned to their previous occupations without restriction. Their wrist motion was unchanged compared to the preoperative status. Grip strengths were 90 to 130% of the opposite side. The wide variety of ancillary procedures in the remaining patients and the small numbers in each subgroup precluded any statistical analysis of the possible influence of the DRCL repair on wrist motion and grip strengths.

Table 13.4.

Procedures/Outcomes

Patient	DRCL Tear	SLIL Tear/ Instability	LTIL Tear	TFC Tear	CHIL Tear	Other	Pain
MA	Repair	—	—	—	—	—	Occ., mild
DA	Repair	—	—	—	—	CTR	None
ND	Repair + shrinkage	—	—	—	—	CTR	None
MR	Repair + shrinkage	—	—	—	—	—	None
BM	—	SLIL repair Capsulodesis	—	—	—	—	Chronic, severe
DL	—	Capsulodesis	—	—	—	—	Occ., mild
SC	—	Capsulodesis	—	Debrided	—	—	Chronic, moderate
MJ	—	Capsulodesis	—	—	—	CTR	Occ., mild
BL	—	Capsulodesis	—	—	—	—	None
VB	—	Capsulodesis	—	—	—	1st extensor release	Chronic, moderate
CE	—	Capsulodesis	—	—	—	1st extensor release	Chronic, moderate
MB	—	Capsulodesis	Debrided	—	—	—	Chronic, moderate
HS	Repair	—	Debrided + pinned	—	—	CTR	Chronic, moderate
MG	—	—	Debrided	Debrided + wafer	—	—	Chronic, moderate
MRO	Shrinkage	—	—	Debrided + wafer	—	Cubital tunnel release	Occ., mild
AD	Repair + shrinkage	—	Debrided	Repair	—	—	Lost to f/u
JP	Repair	—	Debrided + pinned	Debrided	—	—	Occ., mild
GJ	Repair + shrinkage	—	Debrided	Debrided + ulnar shortening	—	—	Chronic, moderate
YB	Shrinkage	—	—	Debrided	—	—	Chronic, moderate
ML	Repair	—	—	Repair	—	CTR	Chronic, moderate
GN	Repair	—	—	—	Pinned	—	Chronic, moderate
RF	Repair + shrinkage	—	Ppinned	—	—	—	Occ., mild

DRCL = dorsal radiocarpal ligament
LTIL = lunotriquetral interosseous ligament
TFC = triangular fibrocartilage
CTR = carpal tunnel release

A dorsal capsulodesis was performed as the primary treatment for an SLIL tear or a dynamic scapholunate instability in seven patients instead of a DRCL repair. This remains a popular treatment method for both static and dynamic scapholunate instability. The presence of a DRCL tear did not preclude a good result (none or mild pain) in 3/7 patients. The capsulodesis was ineffective in controlling pain in the remaining four patients, three of whom had additional wrist pathology. This is consistent with other studies, which have demonstrated that although pain is improved it does not completely resolve following a dorsal capsulodesis in the majority of cases.[18]

Cadaver studies suggest that dynamic scaphoid instability results from an isolated injury to the SLIL without damage to the dorsal intercarpal and DRCL ligaments.[4] The author has found the corollary to hold true in that 4/7 patients with dynamic scapholunate instability had a DRCL tear but an intact scapholunate ligament. The diagnosis of dynamic carpal instability in these patients hinged upon the demonstration of the abnormal kinematics and increased motion at the scapholunate joint. This easily allowed insertion of a 3-mm probe between the scaphoid and the lunate when viewed from the midcarpal joint (i.e., Geissler grade III[19]), yet there was no apparent scapholunate ligament tear while probing from the radiocarpal joint.

The remaining 10 patients had a DRCL tear in combination with ulnar-sided pathology. One patient (AD) was lost to follow-up. Of these nine patients, six had chronic residual pain (with three of these patients showing arthroscopic evidence of osteoarthritis). Soft-tissue procedures alone were ineffective in controlling their symptoms. There was a trend toward a worse outcome when there was coexisting ulnar-sided carpal pathology, which may reflect more severe or longer-standing carpal instability. This was not invariable, however, because 2/9 patients in this group had only occasional mild pain after treatment. The final patient in this subgroup had an associated palmar midcarpal instability with laxity of the lunotriquetral joint (LT). Although a DRCL repair and lunotriquetral joint pinning improved his symptoms, they did not correct the midcarpal instability (which remained mildly symptomatic).

The volar radial portal has been used in 80 patients since 1998. Excluding distal radius fractures and staging for OA, 64 patients were scoped for the investigation and treatment of wrist pain that was unresponsive to conservative treatment. There were 35/64 patients/wrists with DRCL tears, for an overall incidence of 55%. The marked association of DRCL tears in the presence of ligament and TFCC tears was quite surprising. The average age of the patients with DRCL tears was 41 years (range: 19–62 years). The average duration of wrist pain prior to treatment was 20 months (range 4–60 months). In 5 patients an isolated DRCL tear alone was responsible for chronic dorsal wrist pain. Thirteen patients in this series had an SLIL instability and/or tear: 7/13 (54%) also had a DRCL tear. Of this subgroup 4 had a Geissler I/II grade and 3 had a Geissler III/IV grade. Seven patients had an LTIL instability and/or tear: 2/7 (28%) also had a DRCL tear. Of this subgroup 1 had a Geissler I/II grade and 1 had a Geissler III/IV grade. Two patients had a capitohamate ligament tear: 1 of these patients also had a DRCL tear. There were 7 patients with a solitary TFCC tear: 6/7 (86%) were in association with a DRCL tear. One patient had a chronic ulnar styloid nonunion and a DRCL tear. There was TFCC fraying but no tear or detachment. Two or more lesions were present in 23 patients; DRCL tears were present in 12 patients (52%). Of note was that 62% of the combined lesions that were associated with a DRCL tear also included a TFCC tear. One case involved a 24 year old male with a 6 year old ulnar styloid nonunion. Arthroscopy of the distal radioulnar joint established that the deep fibers of the TFCC were well attached to the fovea hence the patient underwent an ulnar styloid excision along with a DRCL repair.

Clinical Relevance

The true incidence of dorsoradiocarpal ligament tears is not known. It is difficult to detect a DRCL tear with nonoperative methods. It is possible that a number of patients presenting with dorsal wrist pain may be misidentified as having dorsal wrist syndrome[20] or an occult dorsal wrist ganglion. DRCL tears are poorly seen through an open approach. Although seven patients who underwent a dorsal capsulodesis for scapholunate instability were found to have a DRCL tear during wrist arthroscopy, none of these tears could be identified through a dorsal capsulotomy. This may be partly because the capsular ligaments are best seen from within the wrist joint, or that the DRCL is divided during the surgical approach for a dorsal capsulodesis.

DRCL tears appear to be part of a spectrum of radial and ulnar-sided carpal instability. It is instructive to consider the wrist as having a number of primary and secondary stabilizers. The SLIL, LTIL, and TFC are the primary stabilizers. The capsular ligaments (including the radioscaphocapitate, radiolunotriquetral, ulnolunate, ulnotriquetral, dorsal radiocarpal, and dorsal intercarpal ligaments) can be thought of as secondary stabilizers. A chronic tear of a primary stabilizer may culminate in the attenuation or tearing of the secondary stabilizer. This is seen in patients with long-standing triquetrolunate dissociation of more than six months duration. Arthroscopy in these cases often reveals fraying of the ulnolunate ligaments and ulnotriquetral ligaments.[21] In the previously referenced series, there was a frequent association of a DRCL tear with either an SLIL or LTIL/TFC tear.

Injury to the DRCL has been implicated in palmar midcarpal instability (MCI).[5,6,15] Soft-tissue repairs of the dorsal ligaments alone appear to be insufficient to correct this type of carpal instability.[15,16] Goldfarb et al. reported on one patient with palmar MCI in whom a diffuse tear involving the dorsal ligaments was shown on a preoperative MRI. A repair of the dorsal ligaments failed to relieve the patient's symptoms and a midcarpal fusion was ultimately performed.[17] Palmar MCI was seen in one patient in the author's series, which did not resolve following LTIL pinning and a DRCL repair.

The cause of wrist pain with isolated capsular ligament tears is not entirely clear. In nondissociative carpal instability the pain is believed to be due to dynamic joint incongruity.[22] Chronic impingement of a detached ulnar sling on the triquetrum has been implicated as a cause of wrist pain.[23] It is plausible that tears of the DRCL may cause pain through their deleterious effects on carpal stability or through impingement of the torn edge of the DRCL against the lunate. Repair of an isolated tear of a capsular ligament can alleviate wrist pain. This has been demonstrated with repairs of ulnolunate ligament tears.[24,25] All four of the patients with an isolated DRCL tear also had a favorable response to arthroscopic repair. Slater et al. demonstrated that the dorsal wrist ligaments have a constant blood supply.[26] The implication of their work is that tears of the DRCL have the potential to heal. This provides a rationale for arthroscopic repair of a DRCL tear.

Arthroscopic ligament plication for combined LTIL and TFC tears has been previously reported.[27] The DRCL repair as described stabilizes the torn edge by plicating it to the dorsal capsule, but it does not necessarily restore the integrity of the ligament per se. Its ameliorating effect on wrist pain may act by forestalling impingement on the lunate or by normalizing carpal kinematics, but there is a lack of biomechanical data to support these theories. Thermal shrinkage was added in some patients in an effort to shorten a voluminous DRCL when sutures alone were ineffective.

Shrinkage by itself was used as a primary treatment modality in only two cases, with mixed results (MRO, YB). It was hence abandoned as a solitary procedure. From the previously cited findings, it is apparent that the results of the DRCL repairs are greatly influenced by and partly determined by the outcomes of treatment for the coexisting wrist pathology. What is not known is how much of a poor outcome is attributable to the coexistence of a DRCL tear. It is evident that any type of soft-tissue procedure is inadequate when there are frank degenerative changes.

Equipment and Implants

Required

In general, a 2.7-mm 30-degree angled arthroscope and a camera attachment are necessary. A fiberoptic light source, video monitor, and printer are also standard equipment. Newer digital systems provide superior video quality compared to analog cameras and allow direct writing to a CD. A 3-mm hook probe is needed for palpation of intracarpal structures. Some method of overhead traction is useful. This may include a traction from the overhead lights or a shoulder holder along with 5- to 10-pound sandbags attached to an arm sling. A traction tower such as the Linvatec tower (Conmed - Linvatec Corporation, Largo, FL) or the ARC wrist traction tower designed by Dr. William Geissler (Arc Surgical LLC, Hillsboro, OR) greatly facilitates instrumentation.

The use of a motorized shaver and suction punch forceps is useful for debridement. Some type of diathermy unit, such as the Oratec radiofrequency probe (Smith and Nephew, NY), is needed in cases where augmentation of the repair with capsular shrinkage is desired. A variety of curved and straight 18-gauge spinal needles are used for passage of an absorbable 2–0 suture for the outside-in repair. A suture lasso or grasper is needed to retrieve the suture ends. If an inside-out repair is performed, a standard knee meniscal repair kit can be adapted for the wrist. These should include a swedged on 2–0 suture on 4-inch double-armed straight meniscal repair needles with a variety of arthroscopic cannulas, such as the Zone specific II Meniscal Repair System (Conmed - Linvatec Corporation, Largo, FL).

Optional

There are a variety of commercially available suture repair kits, including the InteqTFCC repair kit (Conmed - Linvatec, Largo, FL) and the Arthrex TFCC repair kit (Arthrex, Inc., Naples, FL).

Surgical Technique

An inside-out arthroscopic repair technique of the DRCL is performed through a volar radial (VR) wrist arthroscopy portal that allows a direct line of sight with the dorsal radiocarpal ligament (Figure 13.1a). A 2-cm longitudinal incision is made in the proximal wrist crease, exposing the

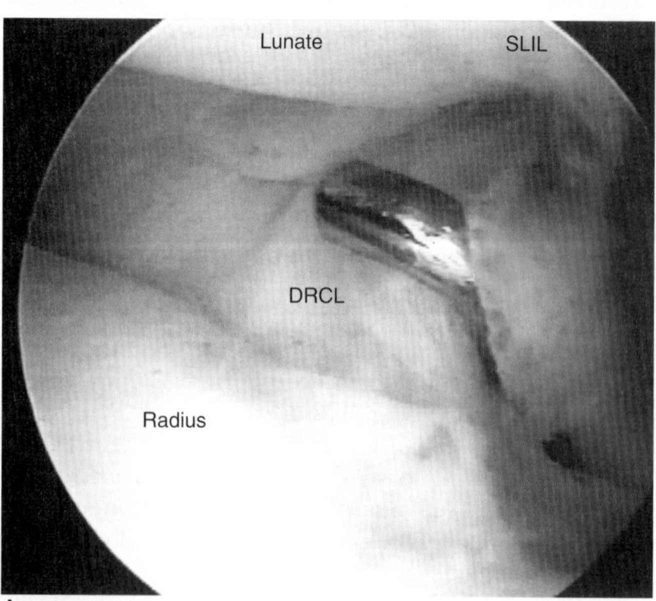

FIGURE 13.1. Inside-out two-cannula DRCL repair. (A) View of an intact dorsoradiocarpal ligament (DRCL) from the VR portal. The hook probe is in the 3/-,4 portal.

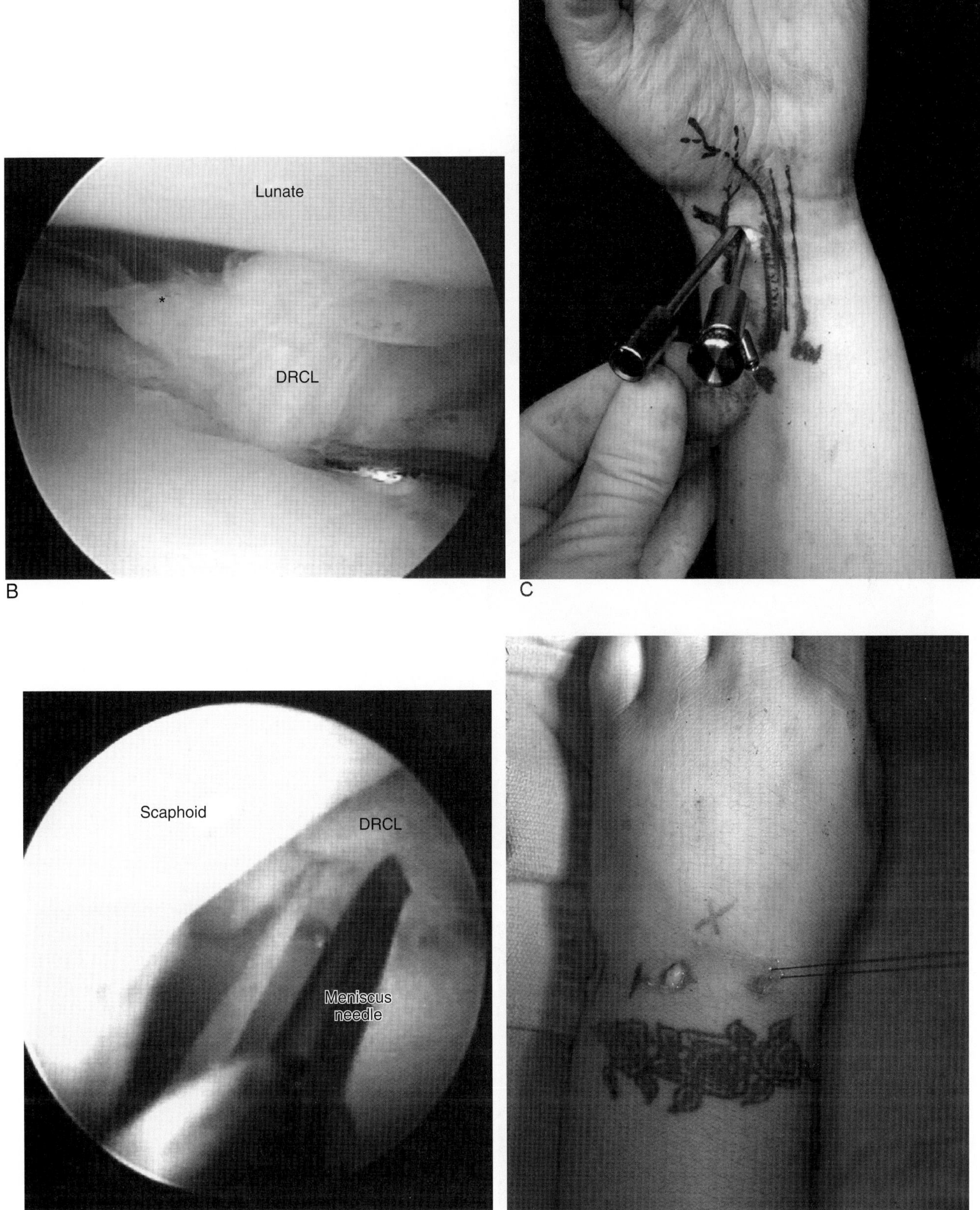

FIGURE 13.1. Cont'd (B) Dorsal radiocarpal ligament tear (*). (C) Two-cannula repair technique. (D) Insertion of second suture with meniscal repair needle. (E) Suture exiting dorsally prior to tying. *(From Slutsky, DJ. Arthroscopic repair of dorsal radiocarpal ligament tears. Arthroscopy: The Journal of Arthroscopic and Related Surgery 2002;18(9):E49, with permission.)*

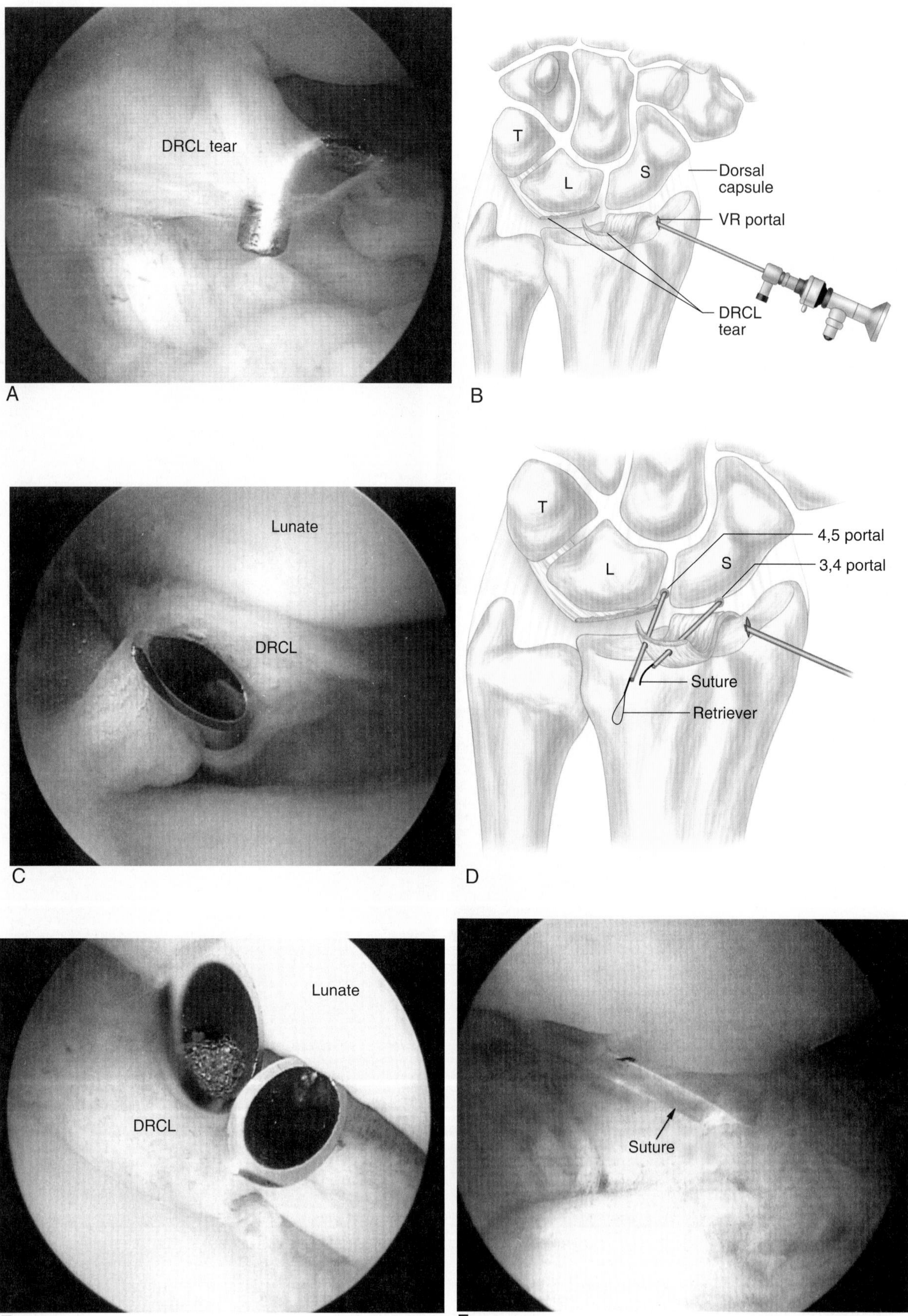
DRCL tear
A
T
L
S
Dorsal capsule
VR portal
DRCL tear
B
Lunate
DRCL
C
T
L
S
4,5 portal
3,4 portal
Suture
Retriever
D
Lunate
DRCL
E
Suture
F

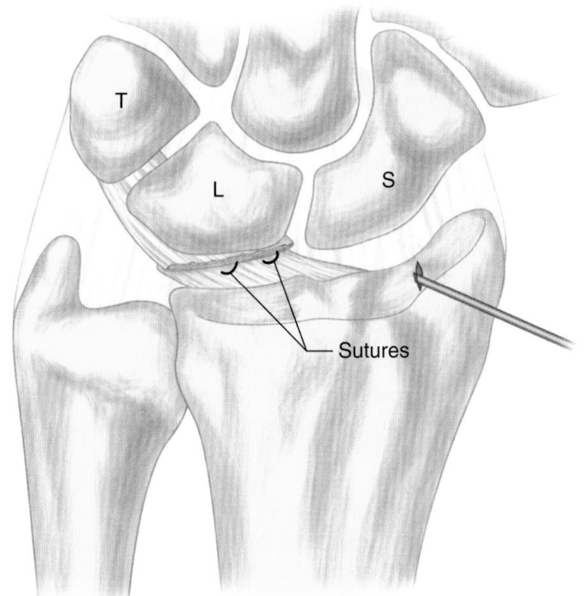

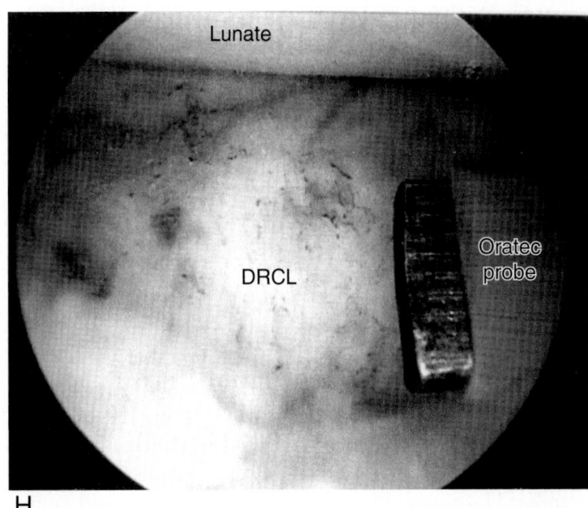

G H

FIGURE 13.2. Outside-in DRCL repair technique. (A) Arthroscopic view of DRCL tear from the VR portal. (B) Drawing of DRCL tear. (C) Insertion of curved spinal needle through edge of DRCL tear. (D) Drawing of outside-in technique using two spinal needles and a suture retriever. (E) Insertion of second spinal needle. (F) Arthroscopic view of suture loop prior to tying. (G) Drawing of completed repair. (H) Repair augmented with thermal shrinkage after suture has been tied. *(Figures A, C, E, F, and H from Slutsky, DJ. Clinical applications of volar portals in wrist arthroscopy. Techniques in Hand and Upper Extremity Surgery 2004;8(4):229–38, with permission. Figures B, D, and G from Slutsky, DJ. Arthroscopic repair of dorsal radiocarpal ligament tears. Arthroscopy: The Journal of Arthroscopic and Related Surgery 2005;21(12):1486e1–86e8, with permission.)*

flexor carpi radialis (FCR) tendon sheath. The sheath is divided and the FCR tendon retracted ulnarly. The radiocarpal joint space is identified with a 22-gauge needle and the joint inflated with saline. A blunt trochar and cannula are introduced through the floor of the FCR sheath, which overlies the interligamentous sulcus between the radioscaphocapitate ligament and the long radiolunate ligament.

A 2.7-mm 30 degree arthroscope is inserted through the cannula. A meniscus repair cannula is then inserted adjacent to the arthroscope. In a small wrist, the capsular intervals on either side of the long radiolunate ligament can be used. While visualizing the DRCL tear through the VR portal, a 2–0 absorbable suture on double-armed straight needles is introduced through the meniscal repair cannula. The needles are passed across the radiocarpal joint through the torn edge of the DRCL, exiting through the floor of the fourth extensor compartment (Figure 13.1b through e). One or two horizontal mattress sutures are inserted in this fashion. A small dorsal incision is made to retrieve the sutures before tying, to ensure there is no extensor tendon entrapment.

An outside-in repair is technically easier and has been used more recently. The repair is performed by spearing the radial side of the DRCL tear with a curved 21-gauge spinal needle placed through the 3/-,4 portal while viewing through the arthroscope, which is inserted in the VR portal. A 2–0 absorbable suture is threaded through the spinal needle and retrieved with a grasper or suture snare inserted through the 4/-,5 portal (Figure 13.2a through f). A curved hemostat is used to pull either end of the suture underneath the extensor tendons, and the knot is tied either at the 3/-,4 or 4/-,5 portal. The repair is augmented with thermal shrinkage if the torn edge of the DRCL is voluminous and still protrudes into the joint after the sutures are tied (Figure 13.2g).

Rehabilitation

Following the repair, the patient is placed in a below-elbow splint with the wrist in neutral rotation. Finger motion and edema control are instituted immediately. At the first postoperative visit, the sutures are removed and the patient is placed in a below-elbow cast for a total immobilization time of six weeks. Wrist motion with use of a removable splint for comfort is instituted after cast removal. Gradual strengthening exercises are added after eight weeks. Dynamic wrist splinting is instituted at 10 weeks if needed.

Summary

DRCL tears are more common than previously suspected. The ideal method of detection at this point remains arthroscopy. The arthroscopist must be diligent in recognizing this condition, but ongoing research into the ideal method of treatment is needed.

References

1. Mitsuyasu H, Patterson RM, Shah MA, et al. The role of the dorsal intercarpal ligament in dynamic and static scapholunate instability. J Hand Surg [Am] 2004;29:279–88.
2. Short WH, Werner FW, Green JK, Weiner MM, Masaoka S. The effect of sectioning the dorsal radiocarpal ligament and insertion of a pressure sensor into the radiocarpal joint on scaphoid and lunate kinematics. J Hand Surg [Am] 2002;27:68–76.
3. Viegas SF, Yamaguchi S, Boyd NL, Patterson RM. The dorsal ligaments of the wrist: Anatomy, mechanical properties, and function. J Hand Surg [Am] 1999;24:456–68.
4. Ruch DS, Smith BP. Arthroscopic and open management of dynamic scaphoid instability. Orthop Clin North Am 2001;32:233–40.
5. Horii E, Garcia-Elias M, An KN, et al. A kinematic study of luno-triquetral dissociations. J Hand Surg [Am] 1991;16: 355–62.
6. Viegas SF, Patterson RM, Peterson, PD, et al. Ulnar-sided perilunate instability: An anatomic and biomechanic study. J Hand Surg [Am] 1990;15:268–78.
7. Moritomo H, Viegas SF, Elder KW, et al. Scaphoid non-unions: A 3-dimensional analysis of patterns of deformity. J Hand Surg [Am] 2000;25:520–28.
8. Ruch DS, Poehling GG. Wrist arthroscopy: Ligamentous instability. In RN Hotchkiss, WC Pederson (eds.), *Green's Operative Hand Surgery, Fourth Edition*. Philadelphia: Churchill Livingstone 1999: 200–06.
9. Slutsky DJ. Arthroscopic repair of dorsal radiocarpal ligament tears. Arthroscopy 2002;18:E49.
10. Slutsky DJ. Wrist arthroscopy through a volar radial portal. Arthroscopy 2002;18:624–30.
11. Slutsky DJ. Volar portals in wrist arthroscopy. Journal of the American Society for Surgery of the Hand 2002;2:225–32.
12. Slutsky DJ. Clinical applications of volar portals in wrist arthroscopy. Tech Hand Up Extrem Surg 2004;8(4):229–38.
13. Slutsky DJ. Arthroscopic repair of dorsoradiocarpal ligament tears. The Journal of Arthroscopic and Related Surgery 2005;21:1486e1–86e8.
14. Slutsky DJ. Management of dorsoradiocarpal ligament repairs. Journal of the American Society for Surgery of the Hand 2005;5:167–74.
15. Lichtman DM, Bruckner JD, Culp RW, Alexander CE. Palmar midcarpal instability: Results of surgical reconstruction. J Hand Surg [Am] 1993;18:307–15.
16. Wright TW, Dobyns JH, Linscheid RL, Macksoud W, Siegert J. Carpal instability non-dissociative. J Hand Surg [Br] 1994;19:763–73.
17. Goldfarb CA, Stern PJ, Kiefhaber TR. Palmar midcarpal instability: The results of treatment with 4-corner arthrodesis. J Hand Surg [Am] 2004;29:258–63.
18. Moran SL, Cooney WP, Berger RA, Strickland J. Capsulodesis for the treatment of chronic scapholunate instability. J Hand Surg [Am] 2005;30:16–23.
19. Geissler WB, Freeland AE, Savoie FH, McIntyre LW, Whipple TL. Intracarpal soft-tissue lesions associated with an intra-articular fracture of the distal end of the radius. J Bone Joint Surg Am 1996;78:357–65.
20. Watson HK, Weinzweig J. Physical examination of the wrist. Hand Clin 1997;13:17–34.
21. Zachee B, De Smet L, Fabry G. Frayed ulno-triquetral and ulno-lunate ligaments as an arthroscopic sign of longstanding triquetro-lunate ligament rupture. J Hand Surg [Br] 1994;19:570–71.
22. Bednar JM, Osterman AL. Carpal instability: Evaluation and treatment. J Am Acad Orthop Surg 1993;1:10–17.
23. Watson HK, Weinzweig J. Triquetral impingement ligament tear (tilt). J Hand Surg [Br] 1999;24:321–24.
24. Osterman AL. Wrist arthroscopy: Operative procedures. In RN Hotchkiss, WC Pederson (eds.), *Green's Operative Hand Surgery, Fourth Edition*. Philadelphia: Churchill Livingstone 1999: 207–22.
25. Mooney JF, Poehling GG. Disruption of the ulnolunate ligament as a cause of chronic ulnar wrist pain. J Hand Surg [Am] 1991;16:347–49.
26. Slater RR Jr., Safian CC, Laubach JE. Vascular anatomy of the dorsal wrist ligaments. Presented at the Fifty-fifth Annual Meeting of the American Society for Surgery of the Hand, Seattle, Washington, 2000.
27. Moskal MJ, Savoie FH III, Field LD. Arthroscopic capsulodesis of the lunotriquetral joint. Clin Sports Med 2001;20: 141–53.

David M. Lichtman, Randall W. Culp, Eric S. Wroten, and David J. Slutsky

CHAPTER 14

Even if you're on the right track, you'll get run over if you just sit there.

—Will Rogers

From David Lichtman: This chapter is dedicated to a pair of fine young thespians: Spencer and Miranda, my grandchildren.

From all of the authors: This chapter is dedicated to Leslie Ristine of the Philadelphia Hand Center, in appreciation for her diligence and endless labors in bringing this chapter to completion.

The Role of Arthroscopy in Midcarpal Instability

Introduction

The concept of midcarpal instability (MCI) has evolved slowly since it was first described in 1934. Many investigators have contributed to our understanding of this condition over the years, which led to the consolidated classification by the senior author (DML) (Table 14.1).[1] It appears that MCI represents several distinct clinical entities differing in the cause and direction of subluxation but sharing the common characteristic of abnormal force transmission at the midcarpal joint. The following discussion centers on intrinsic MCI. Extrinsic MCI due to a dorsally mal-united distal radius fracture is treated by a distal radius osteotomy and hence falls outside the scope of this discussion.

Pathomechanics

The mechanism of the clunk in palmar midcarpal instability (PMCI) has been described in detail by Lichtman et al.[2] The palmar arcuate ligament complex is comprised of a radial arm that is confluent with and distal to the radioscaphocapitate (RSC) ligament and an ulnar arm or the triquetro-hamate-capitate ligament (TCL) (Figure 14.1). In the normal situation, the proximal carpal row moves smoothly from a flexed position when the wrist is in radial deviation to extension when the wrist is in ulnar deviation. This is due to the progressive tightening effect of the arcuate ligament as it stretches out to length (which incrementally pulls the mid-carpal row into extension) and to the carpal bone geometry, which causes the triquetrum to translate dorsally along the helicoidal facet of the hamate. When the arcuate ligament is attenuated, this synchronous motion is lost.

Studies by Trumble et al.[3] and Viegas and coauthors[4] have shown that sectioning either the TCL or the dorsal radiocarpal (i.e., dorsal radiotriquetral ligament) can produce a volar intercalated segmental instability (VISI) deformity and simulate PMCI. More recently, Lichtman showed in vivo that tightening the DRCL alone can stabilize the proximal carpal row and eliminate the clunk of PMCI—emphasizing the potential importance of dorsal ligament laxity in the pathogenesis of this disorder.[5] The senior author now believes that PMCI is caused by laxity of both the TCL and the DRCL, which allows an excessive palmar sag of the heads of the capitate and hamate at the midcarpal joint. This produces a VISI pattern of the proximal row in the nonstressed wrist. This sag results in a loss of joint contact across the midcarpal joint, which manifests clinically as a loss of the smooth transition of the proximal row from flexion to extension as the wrist deviates ulnarward.

The proximal carpal row thus stays in a flexed position until the terminal extent of ulnar deviation, when the helicoidal shape of the hamate facet suddenly forces the triquetrum dorsally. This snaps the lunate and subsequently the scaphoid into extension, causing a sudden reversal of the VISI. This sudden proximal row extension is responsible for the painful and rapid catch-up clunk that occurs. As the wrist moves back to neutral, the triquetrum translates down the hamate facet—which allows the proximal row to drop back into VISI while the distal row again settles palmarly into its slightly subluxated starting point (Figure 14.2a and b).

Table 14.1.

Classification of Midcarpal Instability

Intrinsic	Extrinsic
A. Palmar	A. Distal radius mal-union
B. Dorsal	
C. Combined	

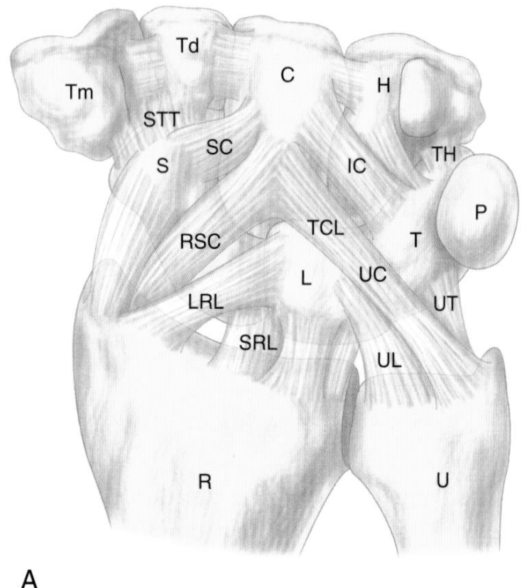

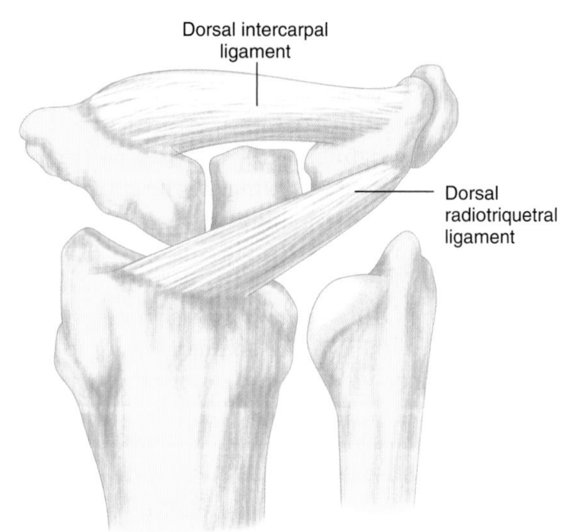

FIGURE 14.1. (A) Line drawing of the volar ligaments. (B) Line drawing of the dorsal ligaments. Ligaments: TCL, triquetrohamate-capitate ligament; RSC, radioscaphoid ligament; LRL, long radiolunate ligament; SRL, short radiolunate ligament; UL, ulnolunate ligament; UC, ulnocapitate ligament; UT, ulnotriquetral ligament; SC, scaphocapitate ligament; STT, scaphotrapezial trapezoidal ligament; TH, triquetrohamate ligament; IC, intercarpal ligament Bones: R, radium; U, ulna; S, scaphoid; L, lunate; C, capitate; T, triquetrum;H, hamate; P, pisiform; Tm, trapezium; Td, trapezoid.

The dorsal pattern of MCI has not been studied as extensively. It appears that laxity of the radial arm of the palmar arcuate ligament permits the capitate and hamate to translate dorsally to an excessive degree, especially with ulnar deviation of the wrist.[6,7] It is of note that in both the palmar and dorsal patterns the proximal row always moves into extension and the distal row translates dorsally with ulnar deviation. It is the timing and force of this movement that differentiate the two patterns.

In PMCI, the distal carpal row starts out in palmar subluxation with the wrist in neutral. As the wrist moves into ulnar deviation, the subluxation suddenly corrects. In dorsal MCI, the wrist starts out in a reduced position in neutral. Dorsal subluxation of the distal row then occurs with ulnar deviation. In either case, the instability is caused primarily by laxity of the selected extrinsic carpal ligaments that support the proximal row—which prevents them from controlling the complex kinematic relationships between the articular surfaces across the midcarpal joint.

Diagnosis

Clinical Findings

In PMCI the patient presents with a history of clunking of the wrist. Patients can often reproduce the clunk on both sides because generalized ligamentous laxity frequently coexists. However, the patient may have a trivial injury that accentuates this normal laxity—resulting in a painful clunk. Upon physical examination, close inspection will reveal a sag of the midcarpal joint with the wrist in radial deviation—which is reduced with active or passive ulnar deviation (Figure 14.3a and b). The clunk may be reproduced by performing the midcarpal shift test.[2] This test is performed by placing the patient's wrist in neutral with the forearm in pronation. A palmar force is then applied to the hand at the level of the distal capitate. The wrist is simultaneously loaded and deviated ulnarly. The test result is positive if a painful clunk occurs that reproduces the patient's symptoms.

In dorsal MCI, a history of an extension injury may be present. Patients complain of post-traumatic chronic pain, weakness, and wrist clicking. Tight grasping (especially in supination) aggravates the symptoms. A dorsal capitate displacement test is performed by applying dorsal pressure to the scaphoid tuberosity while longitudinal traction and flexion are applied to the wrist. There is an associated painful click as the lunate is abruptly shifted dorsally and ulnarly.

Imaging

Static X-rays are typically normal, but occasionally reveal a mild VISI pattern with the wrist in the neutral position. Arthrograms are normal, unless there are associated

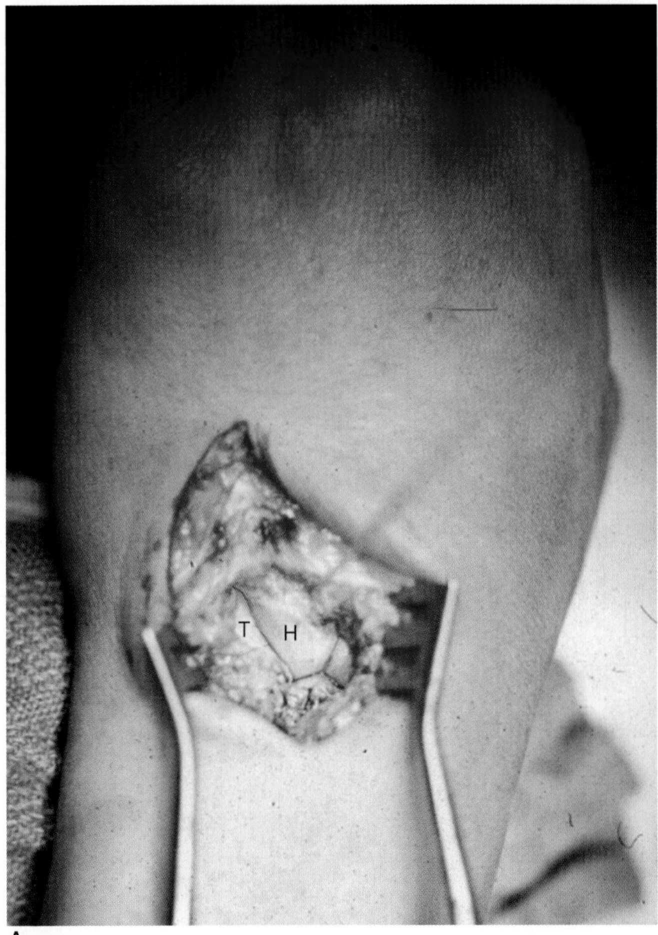

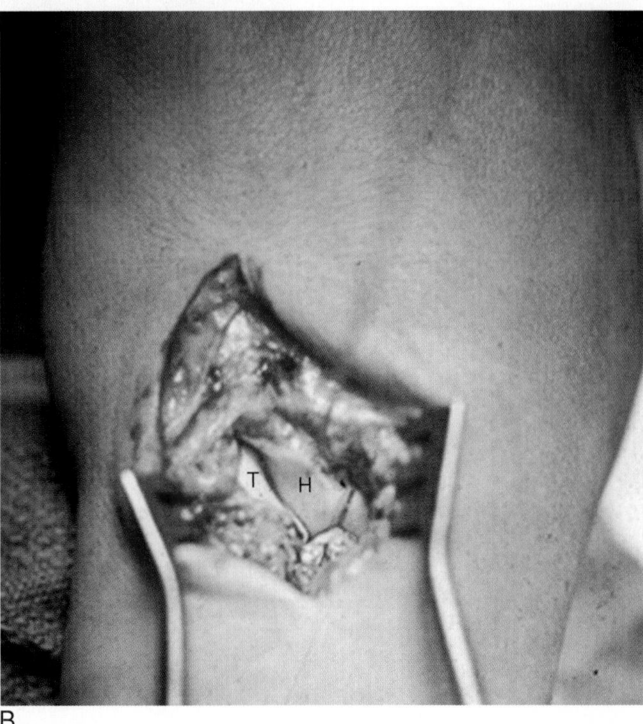

A B

FIGURE 14.2. Dorsal exposure of the midcarpal joint in a left wrist. (A) Triquetrohamate joint with the proximal row reduced. (B) Subluxed triquetrohamate joint with volar sag of the proximal row (T = triquetrum, H = hamate).

intracarpal or triangular fibrocartilage (TFC) tears. MRI findings are nonspecific. Videofluoroscopy provides the hallmarks for diagnosis of this condition. With normal wrist kinematics, the proximal carpal row rotates synchronously from flexion to extension as ulnar deviation of the wrist is achieved. With PMCI, the proximal row maintains a volar flexed position until terminal ulnar deviation is reached—at which point it suddenly snaps into extension.

In dynamic dorsal MCI, X-rays are usually normal. In chronic cases, X-rays often show a volar intercalated segmental instability (VISI) pattern (Figure 14.4a and b). The capitolunate displacement test shows dorsal subluxation of the proximal carpal row in addition to dorsal subluxation of the capitate from the lunate (Figure 14.5a and b).[8] This led Louis and colleagues to coin the term *capitolunate instability pattern* (CLIP) *wrist*.[9]

Arthroscopic Findings

There are no arthroscopic findings that are diagnostic of MCI. Inspection of the radiocarpal joint may reveal a nonspecific synovitis. One of us has seen an associated tear of the dorsal radiocarpal ligament (DJS). In this case, an arthroscopic DRCL repair failed to correct the MCI.[10] Inspection of the midcarpal row may demonstrate erosive lesions along the matching surfaces of the triquetrum and the hamate. Laxity of the lunotriquetral ligament may be seen, although this is not invariable. Midcarpal arthroscopy may reveal laxity of the triquetrohamate-capitate ligament, but this is difficult to gauge. More commonly, synovitis obscures the view of the ligament.

Nonoperative Treatment

Nonsurgical treatment consists of activity modification, NSAIDs, and splinting.[11] Various pisiform support splints have been described. They work based on the observation that applying dorsally directed pressure under the pisiform reduces the carpal sag along with the VISI position of the carpal row. Applying this principle, a three-point dynamic splint may maintain the reduction while permitting wrist motion in milder cases (Figure 14.6). The splint may be worn full time for six to eight weeks to reduce the midcarpal synovitis, and then be worn as needed.

The senior author has observed that active co-contraction of the extensor carpi ulnaris, flexor carpi ulnaris, and

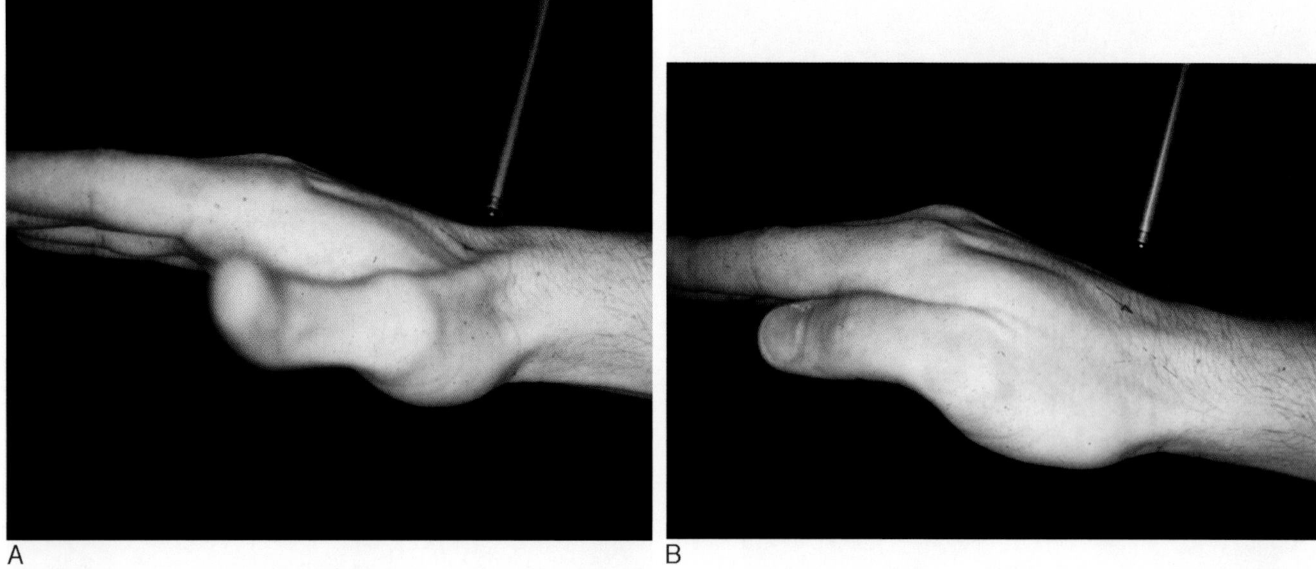

FIGURE 14.3. Palmer MCI. (A) Note the sag in the midcarpal joint with the wrist in radial deviation. (B) The carpus is reduced in ulnar deviation and the sag disappears.

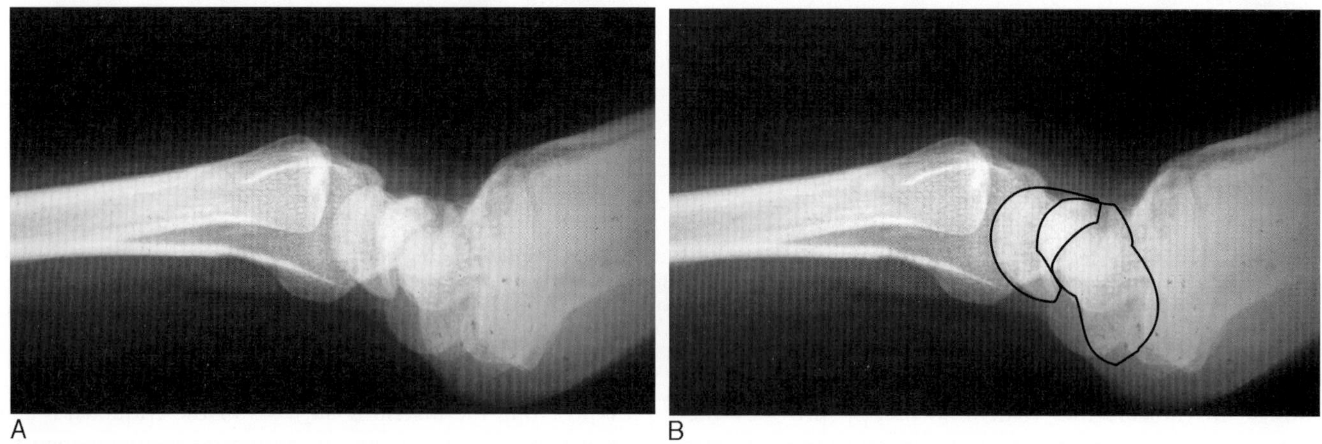

FIGURE 14.4. Volar intercalated segmental instability. (A) Lateral X-ray demonstrating volar tilting of the lunate and extension of the scaphoid. (B) Same view with the lunate and scaphoid outlined for clarity.

hypothenar muscles can reduce the sagging of the midcarpal joint. In fact, some patients can eliminate the catch-up clunk by contracting these muscles before ulnar deviation of the wrist. Patients are taught this isometric muscle contraction as part of the therapy program. Definitive treatment of this condition, however, ultimately requires surgical treatment.

Surgical Treatment

Initial efforts by the senior author were directed at soft-tissue reconstruction by rerouting of the extensor carpi ulnaris to stabilize the triquetrohamate joint.[2] The long-term results were disappointing. This evolved to a direct advancement and tightening of the arcuate ligament complex. Reefing of the DRCL is now preferred. This was based on the observation that temporarily reefing the DRCL by plicating it with a clamp significantly reduced the clunking during the midcarpal shift test. In severe cases, midcarpal arthrodesis is still preferred over soft-tissue procedures (Figure 14.7a and b).[12–14]

Dorsal Reefing of the DRCL (DML)

The patient is positioned in the supine position, with the arm abducted and lying on an arm board. The procedure is performed under tourniquet control after limb exsanguination. An 8-cm dorsal longitudinal incision is made centered over Lister's tubercle. The skin is elevated from the extensor retinaculum, and then the extensor pollicis longus is elevated from its groove and retracted radially. The fourth extensor compartment is elevated along with the finger extensor tendons and retracted ulnarward to expose

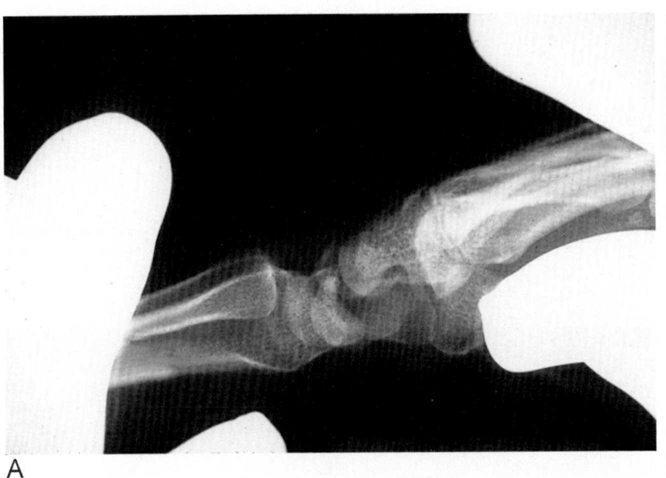

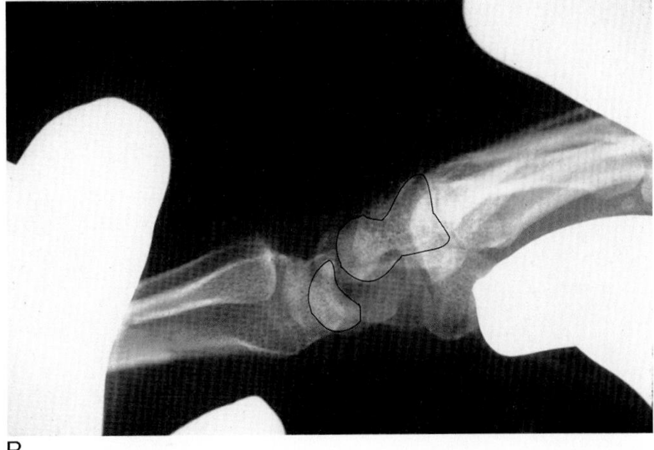

FIGURE 14.5. Capitolunate displacement test. (A) Lateral X-ray demonstrating dorsal subluxation of the capitate on the lunate. (B) Same view with the lunate and capitate outlined for clarity.

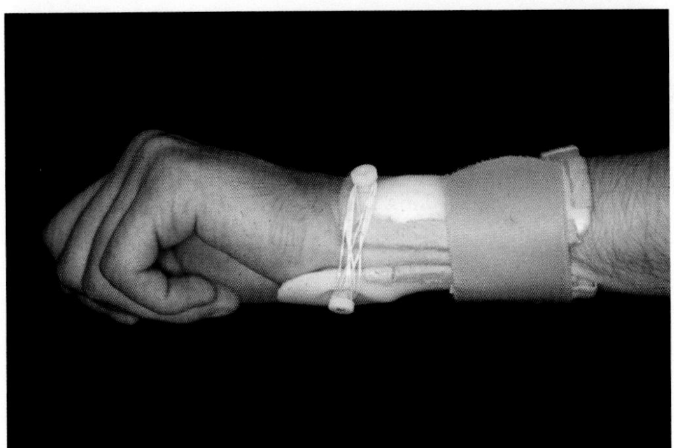

FIGURE 14.6. Three-point fixation with a dynamic splint.

the dorsal capsule. The DRCL is identified as it courses from its origin just ulnar to Lister's tubercle to its insertion on the dorsal aspect of the triquetrum. The DRCL is divided by making a 3-cm transverse incision in the dorsal capsule approximately 1 cm distal to the end of the radius, with the wrist distracted (Figure 14.8a through d).

The distal edge of the capsular flap is pulled proximally, which corrects the volar rotation of the lunate and the proximal carpal row. Fluoroscopy is used to check that there is a neutral alignment of the proximal row and that the capitate and lunate and radius are co-linear. A percutaneous 0.45-mm K-wire is then drilled from the triquetrum to the capitate to maintain this midcarpal alignment. Next, two rows of sutures are placed in a pants-over-vest fashion to shorten the dorsal capsule and maintain the tension on the proximal carpal row.

Postoperative Care

The patient is placed in a short arm cast, with the wrist in neutral. Finger motion begins immediately. The cast is discontinued and the pins are removed at eight weeks, followed by a removable splint. Gentle active wrist motion exercises are instituted at 12 weeks. Strengthening exercises follow.

Arthroscopic Capsular Shrinkage (RWC)

Thermal capsular shrinkage has not enjoyed great success in the shoulder. However, its role in the treatment of wrist disorders remains promising.[15,16] Thermal energy unwinds the collagen triple helix in capsular and ligamentous structures, with subsequent healing in a shortened or tightened position. The biomechanical properties of the tissue do not appear to be detrimentally altered if shrinkage is limited and if ablation or excess focal treatment is avoided.[17] This concept has led to the use of these techniques as a treatment option for midcarpal instability of the wrist.

The patient is placed in a supine position on the operating table. After exsanguination, the tourniquet is inflated to 250 mmHg. A 2.7-mm 30E-angle arthroscope along with a fiberoptic light source and camera setup are used. Some type of diathermy unit is used for the thermal shrinkage. Large-bore outflow cannulas are desirable to provide rapid joint irrigation in order to minimize the risk of chondral damage through heat necrosis. Using a tower, 10 pounds of traction is applied to the index and long fingers. The radiocarpal joint is inflated 1 cm distal to Lister's tubercle at the 3-/,4 portal and the 2.7 arthroscope is introduced. Outflow is established through the 6-R portal.

The standard dorsal portals, including a 3-/,4 and 4-/,5 portal, are used for an arthroscopic survey. Any associated triangular fibrocartilage tears or lunotriquetral ligament tears are noted and treated by debridement or repair. The ulnar extrinsic ligaments are assessed for laxity. If laxity is noted, a 1.5-mm electrothermal probe (Arthrocare, Sunnyvale, CA; or Oratec, Menlo Park, CA) is introduced through the 6-R portal. The ulnolunate and ulnotriquetral ligaments are painted with the probe using a stripe technique, leaving sections of untouched ligament between. The correction of any associated VISI deformity is assessed using a combination of arthroscopy and fluoroscopy.

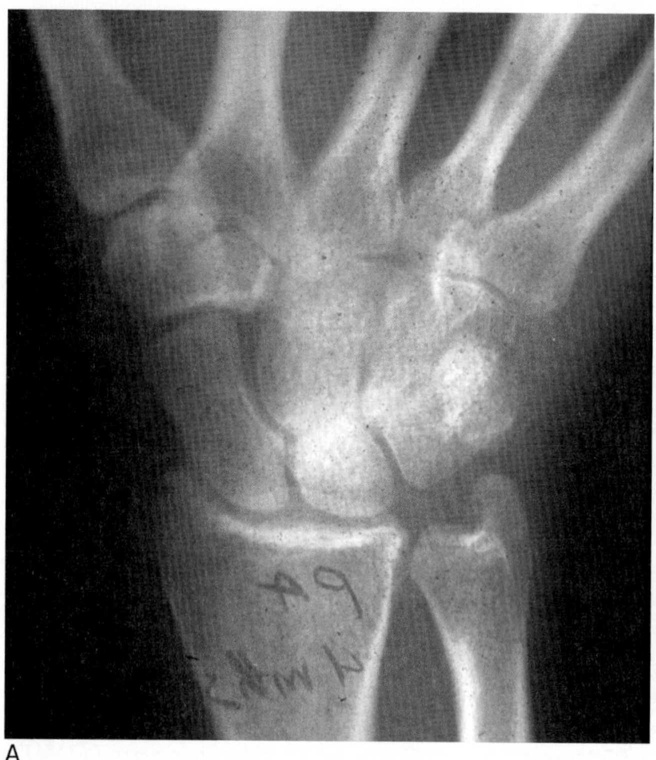

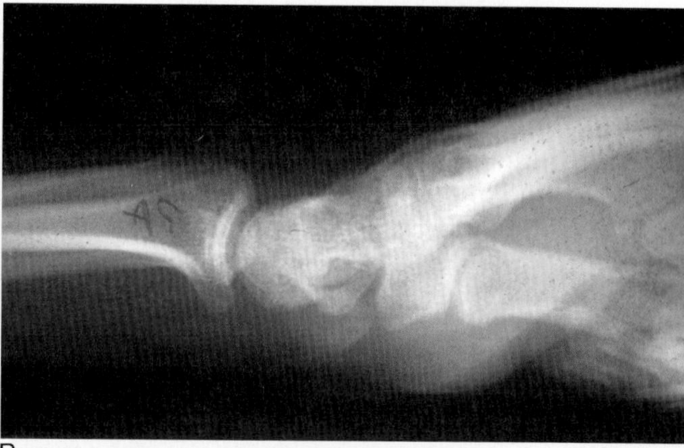

FIGURE 14.7. (A) AP X-ray following a capitolunate fusion. (B) Lateral X-ray of the same patient.

A midcarpal radial portal is then established. The scapholunate and lunotriquetral joints are inspected and probed for laxity. The TCL is identified as it runs obliquely from the triquetrum, across the proximal corner of the hamate, to the palmar neck of the capitate. A midcarpal ulnar portal is established and used for introduction of the thermal probe. The TCL is then shrunk while again adjusting the tension with correction of any VISI deformity.

A volar radial portal is now established. The arthroscope is reintroduced through the 3-/,4 portal and advanced palmarly until it abuts the sulcus between the radioscaphocapitate and long radiolunate ligaments. The arthroscope is removed and replaced by a switching stick. A small palmar incision is made to retract the FCR and protect the neurovascular structures. The switching stick is advanced and brought out volarly though the FCR sheath, at the level of the proximal wrist crease.

A cannula is placed over the switching stick from volar to dorsal, followed by the arthroscope. The dorsal radiocarpal ligament is then assessed. When laxity is present, the electrothermal probe is introduced through the 6-R portal and used to shrink the DRCL—again in a striped fashion. The tension of the DRCL can be adjusted by correcting any VISI deformity with a K-wire in the lunate under fluoroscopic control. At the end of the procedure, 0.045-mm K-wires are used to pin the triquetrum to the capitate and hamate in a neutral and reduced position.

Postoperative Care

The patient is placed in a short arm cast. The cast and K-wires are removed at four weeks, followed by home range-of-motion exercises and gradual strengthening.

Results

In 1993, Lichtman et al. published a review of 13 patients who underwent 15 surgical procedures for MCI, at an average follow-up of 48 months.[12] Nine patients had one of several soft-tissue procedures. The first patient had a triquetrohamate ligament reconstruction using the extensor carpi ulnaris tendon, two patients had a palmar capsular reefing, one patient had a dorsal radiocarpal capsulodesis, and five patients underwent a distal advancement of the ulnar arm of the arcuate ligament. Two patients required repeat surgery due to failure. Six patients underwent a limited midcarpal arthrodesis. It was clear that midcarpal arthrodesis was the most reliable procedure. Only two of the patients with an arcuate ligament advancement and the patient with the dorsal capsulodesis had a satisfactory outcome compared to all six of the midcarpal fusions.

The results of dorsal capsular reefing are unpublished. Thus far, patients who have undergone this procedure have done well with no reported incidents to date of recurring clunk. It must be stressed that this procedure is only performed in mild to moderate cases, meaning that the clunk can be prevented with mild to moderate dorsally directed pressure on the pisiform. Should the clunk recur postoperatively, a midcarpal arthrodesis can be performed through the same incision.

In 2003, Culp et al. reported their experience of five patients who underwent an arthroscopic capsular shrinkage.[5] Eight patients to date have now undergone this procedure. The average age was 33 (range 29 to 57) years. Follow-up has averaged 9 months (range 3 to 18) months. The midcarpal clunk has resolved in six of the eight

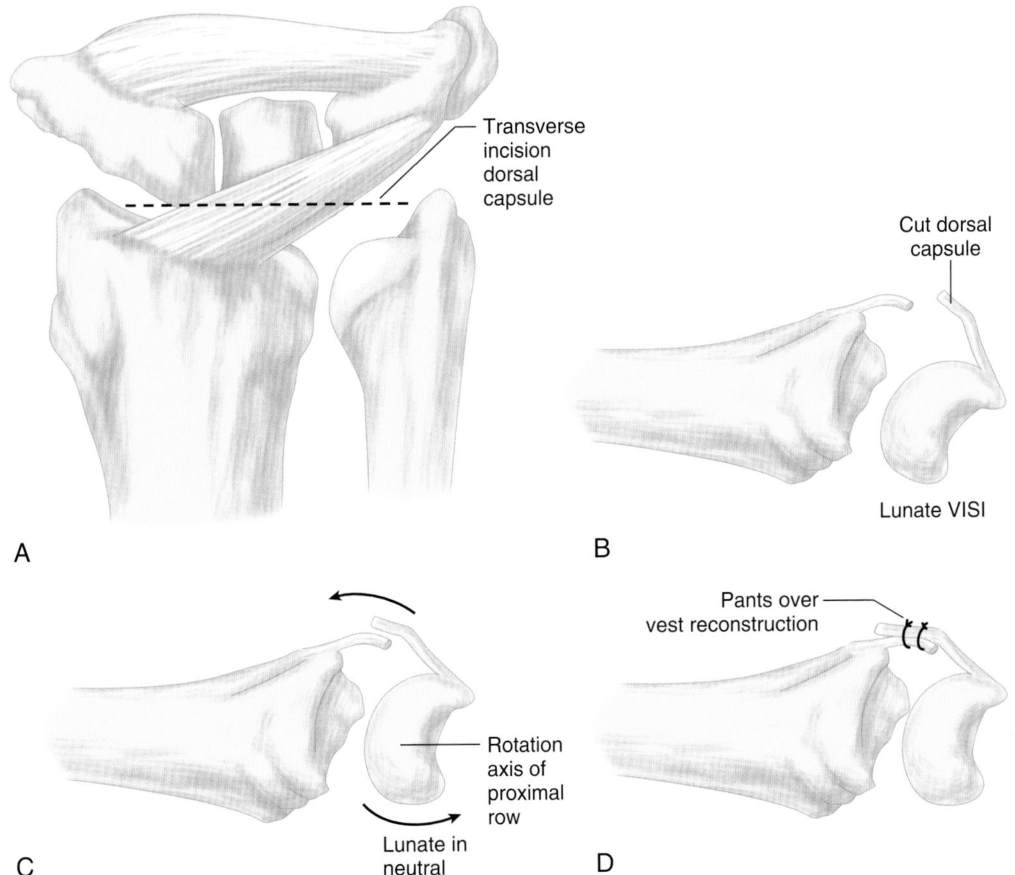

FIGURE 14.8. Reefing of the dorsal radiocarpal ligament. (A and B) Location of the incision in the dorsal capsule and dorsal radiocarpal ligament (DRCL). (C) Volar intercalary segmental instability deformity can be corrected by pulling proximal distal flap of capsule and DRCL. This rotates the proximal row around its axis. (D) Two rows of sutures (pants-over-vest) are placed to maintain capsular tightening.

patients with pain resolution. Range of motion has decreased 20% in the flexion/extension plane, and grip strengths have increased by an average of 15%. Long-term follow-up is still needed to assess the efficacy of this procedure.

References

1. Lichtman DM, Wroten ES. Understanding midcarpal instability. J Hand Surg [Am] 2006;31:491–8.
2. Lichtman DM, Schneider JR, Swafford AR, Mack GR. Ulnar midcarpal instability: Clinical and laboratory analysis. J Hand Surg [Am] 1981;6:515–23.
3. Trumble TE, Bour CJ, Smith RJ, Glisson RR. Kinematics of the ulnar carpus related to the volar intercalated segment instability pattern. J Hand Surg [Am] 1990;15:384–92.
4. Viegas SF, Patterson RM, Peterson PD, et al. Ulnar-sided perilunate instability: An anatomic and biomechanic study. J Hand Surg [Am] 1990;15:268–78.
5. Lichtman DM, Culp RW, Joshi, A. Palmar midcarpal instability. In EM [last name] (ed.), *Operative Arthroscopy, Third Edition.* Philadelphia: Lippincott Williams & Wilkins 2003: 737–42.
6. Johnson RP, Carrera GF. Chronic capitolunate instability. J Bone Joint Surg Am 1986;68:1164–76.
7. Apergis EP. The unstable capitolunate and radiolunate joints as a source of wrist pain in young women. J Hand Surg [Br] 1996;21:501–06.
8. White SJ, Louis DS, Braunstein EM, Hankin FM, Greene TL. Capitate-lunate instability: Recognition by manipulation under fluoroscopy. AJR Am J Roentgenol 1984;143:361–64.
9. Louis DS, Hankin FM, Greene TL. Chronic capitolunate instability. J Bone Joint Surg Am 1987;69:950–51.
10. Slutsky D. Arthroscopic repair of dorsoradiocarpal ligament tears. The Journal of Arthroscopic and Related Surgery 2005;21:1486e1–1486e8.
11. Lichtman DM, Pollock GR. Midcarpal and proximal carpal instabilities. In DM Lichtman, AH Alexander (eds.), *The Wrist and Its Disorders.* Philadelphia: W.B. Saunders 1997: 316–28.
12. Lichtman DM, Bruckner JD, Culp RW, Alexander CE. Palmar midcarpal instability: Results of surgical reconstruction. J Hand Surg [Am] 1993;18:307–15.
13. Goldfarb CA, Stern PJ, Kiefhaber TR. Palmar midcarpal instability: The results of treatment with 4-corner arthrodesis. J Hand Surg [Am] 2004;29:258–63.

14. Rao SB, Culver JE. Triquetrohamate arthrodesis for midcarpal instability. J Hand Surg [Am] 1995;20:583–89.
15. D'Alessandro DF, Bradley JP, Fleischli JE, Connor PM. Prospective evaluation of thermal capsulorrhaphy for shoulder instability: Indications and results, two- to five-year follow-up. Am J Sports Med 2004;32:21–33.
16. Hayashi K, Markel MD. Thermal capsulorrhaphy treatment of shoulder instability: Basic science. Clin Orthop Relat Res 2001;390:59–72.
17. Medvecky MJ, Ong BC, Rokito AS, Sherman OH. Thermal capsular shrinkage: Basic science and clinical applications. Arthroscopy 2001;17:624–35.

Daniel J. Nagle

CHAPTER 15

To my daughter Claire

Capsular Shrinkage in the Treatment of Wrist Instability

Basic Science

What is old is new again. Capsular shrinkage was used by Hippocrates 2,400 years ago to stabilize dislocated shoulders. Luckily, anesthetic techniques and thermal delivery methods have improved during the past two millennia. Recently (comparatively speaking), the biology of capsular shrinkage has been extensively studied in animal models. These studies have shown that the triple helix of collagen "unwinds" and "shrinks" when heated to 60° C, maximum shrinkage being achieved between 65 and 75° C (Figures 15.1 and 15.2). The hydrogen bonds that maintain the 3D configuration of the type I collagen triple-helix rupture as the collagen is heated beyond 60° C. The denatured collagen can potentially shorten to 50% of the resting length of the untreated collagen. The shortened denatured collagen acts as scaffolding onto which new collagen is deposited.[1] The new collagen fibers maintain this shortened conformation, thus assuring the long-term maintenance of the shortening.

Biomechanical studies have demonstrated that the tensile strength of heated collagen decreases rapidly and does not return to normal values for 12 weeks.[2] The tensile strength returns to nearly 80% normal by six weeks after heating (Figure 15.3). This transient loss of tensile strength would suggest that the application of stress to recently heated collagen is contraindicated. Premature loading of the shrunk collagen will lead to a lengthening of the collagen. This has been verified in an animal model.[3,4] Based on this data, it would seem reasonable to recommend at least six to eight weeks of joint immobilization after capsular shrinkage. Clearly heavy loading of the joint should be avoided for 12 weeks.

Indications and Contraindications

Capsular shrinkage can be used to treat mild forms of carpal instability. Patients with symptomatic Geissler type I and II scapholunate and mild midcarpal instability would be considered good candidates. Greater degrees of carpal instability associated with disruption or severe attenuation of the interosseous ligaments will not respond to capsular shrinkage. Lunotriquetral instability is the manifestation of a spectrum of pathology. The following are three possible LT instability scenarios.

- Isolated LT interosseous ligament *attenuation* without gross LT instability.
- Isolated LT interosseous ligament *disruption* without gross instability.
- LT interosseous ligament disruption associated with DIC and/or DRC and/or ulnocarpal ligament disruption *with gross instability*.

The first two scenarios lend themselves to capsular shrinkage because the integrity of the LT stabilizers, although compromised, is maintained. Shrinkage in the third scenario will be ineffective due to the extensive disruption of the LT stabilizers.

Technique

Generalities

Shrinkage requires very low energy settings. The RF devices must be adjusted to heat the tissue to a temperature of

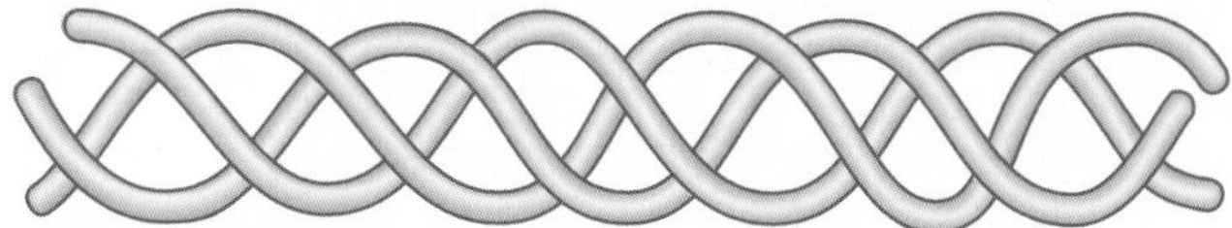

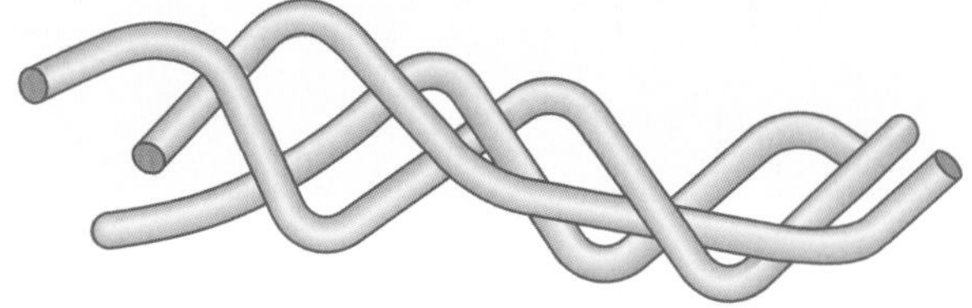

FIGURE 15.1. Thermally induced unraveling of collagen triple helix.

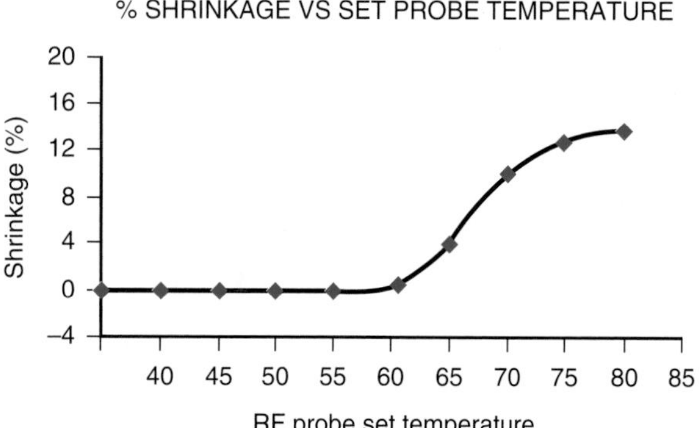

FIGURE 15.2. Shrinkage versus RF probe temperature.

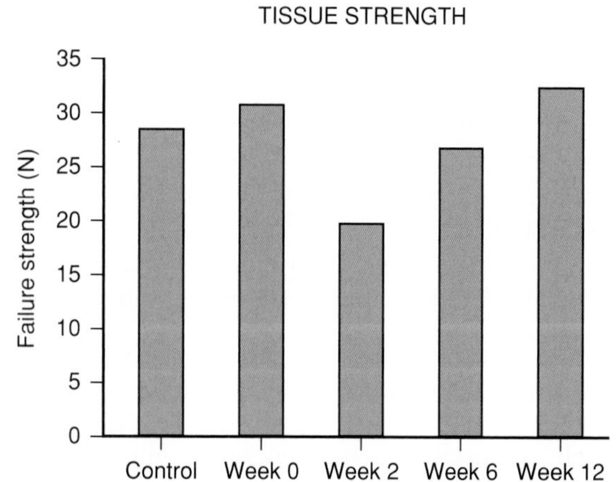

FIGURE 15.3. Post-shrinkage tensile strength versus time.

between 65 and 75° C. It is wise to start at low energy and slowly increase the energy output until the desired shrinkage is observed. If a laser is used, it should be set to very low energy [i.e., 0.2 to 0.5 Joules at 15 pulses per second (3 to 7.5 Watts)]. The laser is held away from the target ligament and slowly advanced until the ligament is seen to shrink.

Once the shrinkage has stopped, continued heating will only further weaken the ligament without increasing the shrinkage. The color of the ligament changes from white to light yellow during the shrinkage. Lu et al. have suggested that a cross-hatching shrinkage pattern optimizes the in-growth of healthy tissue and hastens the recovery of the ligament.[5] During the shrinkage, the traction on the wrist should be reduced as much as possible to permit optimal shrinkage.

Scapholunate Instability

The question is what should or can be shrunk to stabilize the scapholunate axis. The SL interosseous ligament is a heterogenous structure. Its central portion is composed of fibrocartilage that is not shrinkable (Figure 15.4). The dorsal and palmar portions of the SL ligament are composed of type I collagen and are, however, shrinkable (Figure 15.5). The arthroscope and thermal wand can be placed in either the 3-4 or 4-5 portal. The 70-degree side-firing laser probe and 90-degree RF probe can be placed in the 4-5 portal, with the scope placed in the 3-4 portal. If the zero-degree probes are used, the scope should be placed in the 4-5 portal and the wand passed through the 3-4 portal. Extreme caution is exercised so as to avoid injury to normal hyalin cartilage. Good fluid inflow and outflow are critical because the arthroscopy fluid removes the excess thermal energy generated by the probes.

Capsular shrinkage of the dorsal intercarpal (DIC) ligament could potentially reinforce the stabilizing effect of SL ligament shrinkage. The DIC is attached to the distal dorsal aspect of the scaphoid and the dorsal triquetrum[6,7] (Figure 15.6). Shrinkage of this ligament could simulate the tensioning of this ligament noted during open capsulodesis.[8] To accomplish this, the scope and laser/RF angled

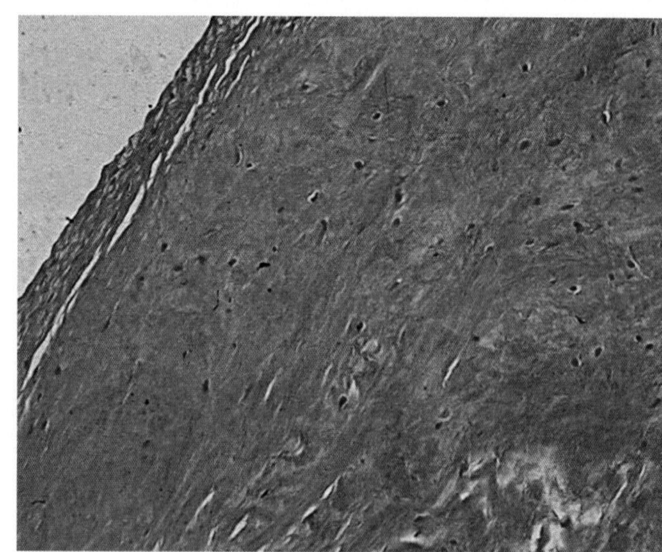

FIGURE 15.4. Histology of central fibrocartilaginous portion of the scapholunate ligament. *(Taken from Berger RA. [chapter title]. WP Cooney, RL Lilnscheid, JH Dobyns (eds.), The Wrist Diagnosis and Operative Treatment. St. Louis: Mosby 1998.)*

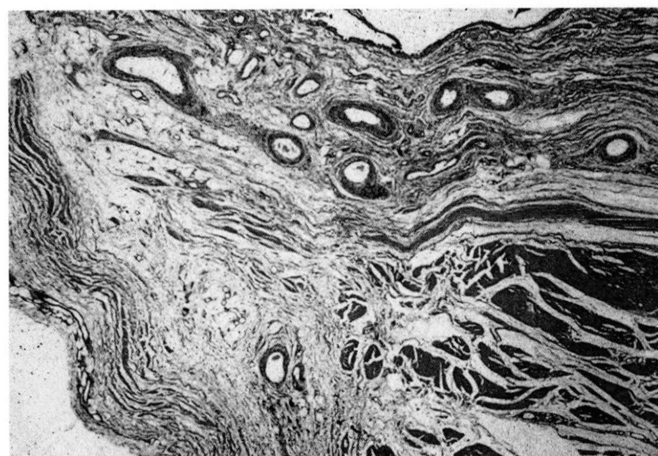

FIGURE 15.5. Histology of capsule demonstrating loose collagen (CF) in a fibrous stratum (FS). *(Taken from Berger RA. [chapter title]. WP Cooney, RL Lilnscheid, JH Dobyns (eds.), The Wrist Diagnosis and Operative Treatment. St. Louis: Mosby 1998.)*

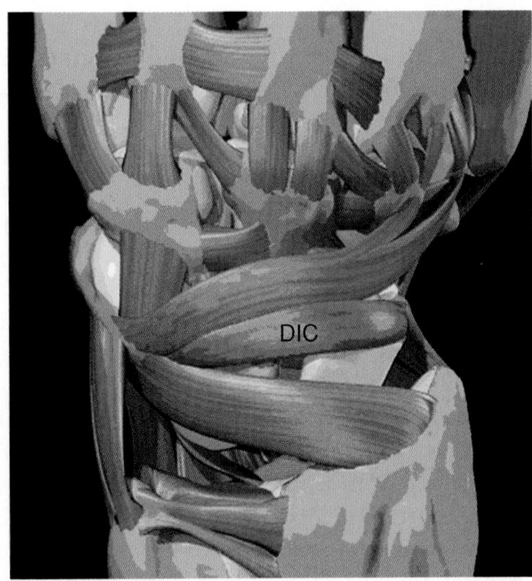

FIGURE 15.6. Dorsal intercarpal ligament. *(Reproduced with permission from D.A. McGrouther, Interactive Hand 2000. Primal Pictures, Ltd. www.primalpictures.com.*

probes would be placed in the radial and ulnar midcarpal portals. Alternatively, the scope can be placed in the midcarpal joint via the radial midcarpal volar portal described by Slutsky,[9] with the thermal probes passed through the ulnar midcarpal portal.

Lunotriquetral and Ulnocarpal Instability

Mild forms of lunotriquetral instability can be treated with ulnocarpal ligament shrinkage. The author has applied this technique in a limited number of cases with satisfying results. This procedure takes advantage of the anatomy of the ulnotriquetral and ulnolunate ligaments. These ligaments form a V as they diverge from their origin on the palmar distal radioulnar ligament and insert on the palmar aspect of the lunate or triquetrum (Figure 15.7).

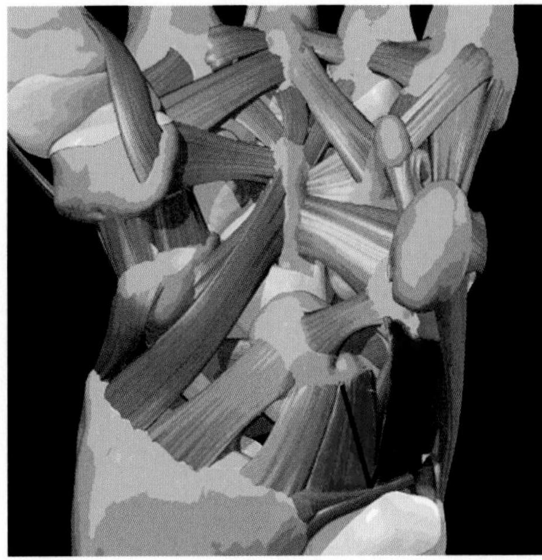

FIGURE 15.7. Palmar view of ulnocarpal ligaments demonstrating V configuration. *(Reproduced with permission from D.A. McGrouther, Interactive Hand 2000. Primal Pictures, Ltd. www.primalpictures.com.*

As the ligaments are shrunk, the arms of the V shorten and approximate the lunate to the triquetrum (thus stabilizing the LT joint). This stabilization can be further reinforced with the shrinkage of the LT interosseous ligament. The LT ligament histology is similar to that of the SL ligament and can therefore undergo dorsal and palmar (but not central) shrinkage. Isolated ulnocarpal ligament instability can also be treated with ulnocarpal ligament shrinkage. Ulnocarpal shrinkage is accomplished with the arthroscope in the 3-4 portal and the laser in the 4-5 or 6-U portal.

Midcarpal Instability

It is tempting to apply capsular shrinkage to the treatment of midcarpal instability. Midcarpal instability is associated with attenuation of the ulnar arcuate ligament, triquetrohamate ligament, dorsal intercarpal, and radiocarpal ligaments. All of these ligaments can be shrunk. To access the ulnar arcuate ligament and triquetrohamate ligament, the arthroscope would be placed in the radial midcarpal portal and the zero-degree laser/RF probe placed in the ulnar midcarpal portal. To access the fibers of the dorsal radiocarpal and dorsal intercarpal ligaments, the angled laser/RF probes are placed in the ulnar midcarpal portal.

Results

Few capsular shrinkage clinical trials have been reported. Table 15.1 lists three such trials. They all deal with the treatment of mild SL instability. They all suggest that capsular shrinkage has been very helpful for the majority of the patients treated. In addition to these results, Dr. Battistalla discusses his results in Chapter 10.

Table 15.1.

Results of Capsular Shrinkage for Scapholunate Instability

Author	Patients	SL Lesions	Follow-Up	Excellent Good	Results	Fair	Poor
Darlis[a]	16	G I and II	19 months	8	6	1	1
Hirsh[b]	10	G II	28 months	9			1
Shih[c]	19	Dynamic and predynamic	28 months	15			4

[a]Darlis NA, Weiser RW, Sotereanos DG. Partial scapholunate ligament injuries treated with arthroscopic debridement and thermal shrinkage. J Hand Surg [Am] 2005;30(5):908–14.
[b]Hirsh L, Sodha S, Bozentka D, Monaghan B, Steinberg D, Beredjiklian PK. Arthroscopic electrothermal collagen shrinkage for symptomatic laxity of the scapholunate interosseous ligament. J Hand Surg [Br] 2005;30(6):643–47 (E-pub 2 Sept. 2005).
[c]Shih JT, Lee HM. Monopolar radiofrequency electrothermal shrinkage of the scapholunate ligament. Arthroscopy 2006;22(5):553–57.

There are no clinical studies reporting the outcome of capsular shrinkage for lunotriquetral, ulnocarpal, or midcarpal instability. The author has found ulnocarpal ligament shrinkage for ulnocarpal ligament laxity, mild TFCC laxity, and mild lunotriquetral instability to be rewarding in the 12 patients so treated. He has used shrinkage to treat mild midcarpal instability in just two cases. Both patients are better, although one remains somewhat symptomatic when she applies heavy stress to the wrist.

References

1. Lopez MJ, Hayashi K, Vanderby R Jr., Thabit G III, Fanton GS, Markel MD. Effects of monopolar radiofrequency energy on ovine joint capsular mechanical properties. Clin Orthop 2000;374:286–97.
2. Hecht P, Hayashi K, Lu Y, Fanton GS, Thabit G III, Vanderby R Jr., Markel MD. Monopolar radiofrequency energy effects on joint capsular tissue: Potential treatment for joint instability. An in vivo mechanical, morphological, and biochemical study using an ovine model. Am J Sports Med 1999;27(6):761–71.
3. Naseef GS III, Foster TE, Trauner K, Solhpour S, Anderson RR, Zarins B. The thermal properties of bovine joint capsule: The basic science of laser- and radiofrequency-induced capsular shrinkage. Am J Sports Med 1997;25(5):670–74.
4. Hayashi K, Markel MD. Thermal capsulorrhaphy treatment of shoulder instability: Basic science. Clin Orthop 2001; 390:59–72.
5. Lu Y, Hayashi K, Edwards RB III, Fanton GS, Thabit G III, Markel MD. The effect of monopolar radiofrequency treatment pattern on joint capsular healing: In vitro and in vivo studies using an ovine model. Am J Sports Med 2000;28(5):711–19.
6. Mitsuyasu H, Patterson RM, Shah MA, Buford WL, Iwamoto Y, Viegas SF. The role of the dorsal intercarpal ligament in dynamic and static scapholunate instability. J Hand Surg [Am] 2004;29(2):279–88.
7. Viegas SF, Yamaguchi S, Boyd NL, Patterson RM. The dorsal ligaments of the wrist: Anatomy, mechanical properties, and function. J Hand Surg [Am] 1999;24(3):456–68.
8. Szabo RM, Slater RR Jr., Palumbo CF, Gerlach T. Dorsal intercarpal ligament capsulodesis for chronic, static scapholunate dissociation: Clinical results. J Hand Surg [Am] 2002;27 (6):978–84.
9. Slutsky DJ. Clinical applications of volar portals in wrist arthroscopy. Tech Hand Up Extrem Surg 2004;8(4):229–38.

SECTION 4

Wrist and Carpal Fractures

Joseph F. Slade III and Greg Merrell

CHAPTER 16

Arthroscopically Assisted Reduction and Percutaneous Fixation of Scaphoid Fractures Using a Simple External Targeting System

Rationale

Percutaneous screw fixation is recognized as an effective treatment of acute nondisplaced scaphoid fractures.[1–9] These techniques result in rapid healing, with minimal complications. Displaced fractures have traditionally required open reduction. Several authors have reported good results in small case series using arthroscopic-assisted reduction of displaced fractures, but achieving reduction and stable fixation with these techniques can be challenging.[10,11]

This chapter describes our technique in a step-by-step manner. That technique is the use of arthroscopy and percutaneous reduction rather than an open exposure to achieve reduction and fixation of acute displaced scaphoid fractures. A new technique for targeting the central axis is described, which simplifies the process of achieving reduction and fixation. Using these techniques, the authors have achieved 100% union of all acute displaced scaphoid fractures (without complications).

Indications

This technique is recommended for any acute closed scaphoid fracture. It has been used successfully for fractures at the proximal pole, waist, and distal third position. Either angular or translational displacement is usually correctable percutaneously. Fractures with delayed presentation or with delayed union from cast treatment have also been treated successfully with this technique. In addition, one can address combined injuries such as trans-scaphoid perilunate dislocations or combined distal radius and scaphoid fract4ures.

Contraindications

As with any new surgical technique, we recommend starting with more straightforward nondisplaced waist fractures to develop the skill set needed to approach more difficult acute displaced or proximal pole fractures. A pediatric tubercle fracture is a relative contraindication because these heal with casting.

Surgical Technique

Critical Equipment

Critical equipment involved in the surgical technique is as follows.

- Mini-fluoroscope
- Traction tower
- Wire driver with .045 and .062 double-cut K-wires
- Acutrak screw, standard size
- Wrist arthroscope

Imaging

The injured wrist is imaged with a mini-fluoroscope to identify fracture displacement and ligament injury. Imaging is used to identify the fracture plane and position. This may impact the location and size of implant. Imaging may also identify other carpal or radius fractures not appreciated using standard radiographs, which require treatment. Excessive gapping between the carpal bones may suggest ligament injuries and will direct arthroscopic inspection.

Scaphoid imaging includes locating the central scaphoid axis. This is accomplished by pronating the wrist until the scaphoid poles are aligned, and flexing the wrist approximately 45 degrees until the cylinder of the scaphoid becomes a circle (Figure 16.1). A perpendicular placed at the center of the circle represents the central axis of the scaphoid. This perpendicular is the longest distance a straight line can be placed through the scaphoid, the central scaphoid axis. Along the central axis, the longest screw can be placed without violating the scaphoid cartilage envelope. Biomechanically, the longest screw distributes and reduces the bending forces—which act to displace the scaphoid. Finally, clinical reports confirm that screws placed along the central axes achieve faster healing than those placed eccentrically.[12]

Scaphoid displacement can occur either as lateral displacement visualized on a posterior-anterior view as a step-off (Figure 16.2) or as forward flexion of the distal fragment on the proximal fragment displaying a V separation of the dorsal cortex on lateral or oblique views (Figure 16.3)—a future humpback deformity. On the PA view, this displacement appears as a foreshortened scaphoid. At the completion of this survey, two decisions must be made. First, is the scaphoid grossly aligned or not? Second, are there other injuries that need to be addressed?

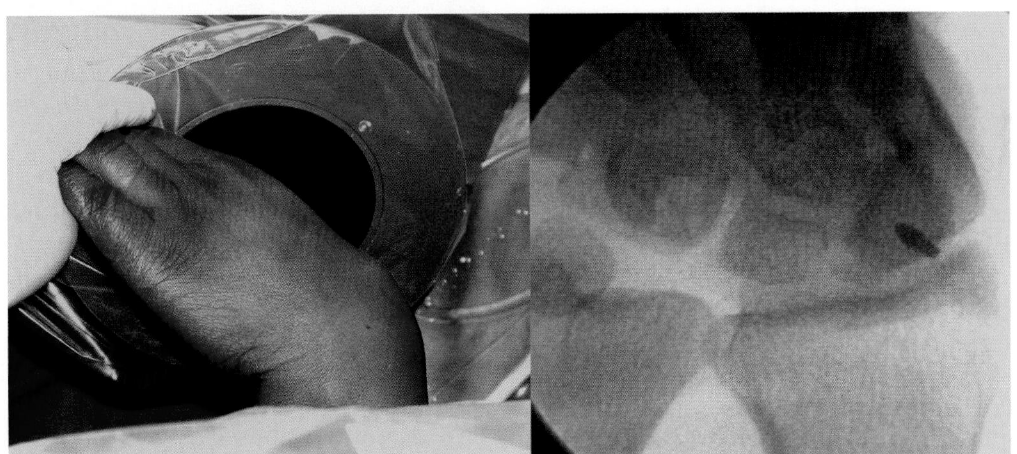

FIGURE 16.1. Images demonstrating the position of the hand and central axis of the scaphoid.

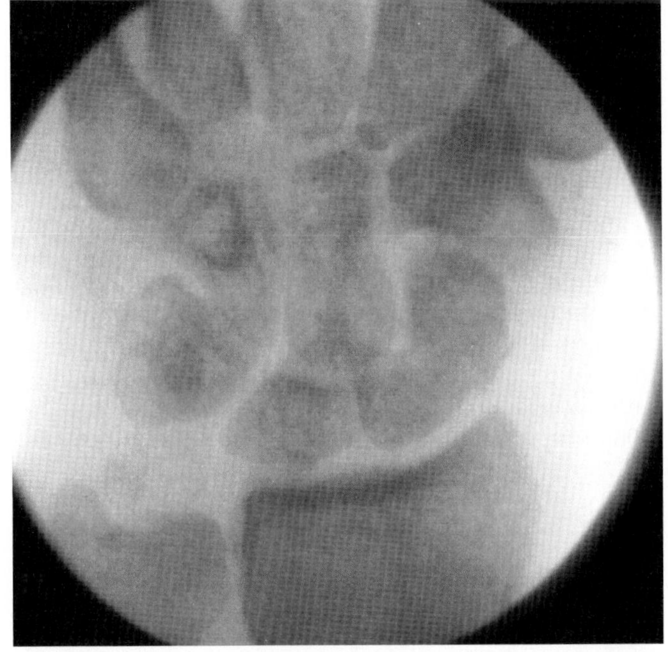

FIGURE 16.2. Translational displacement of the scaphoid.

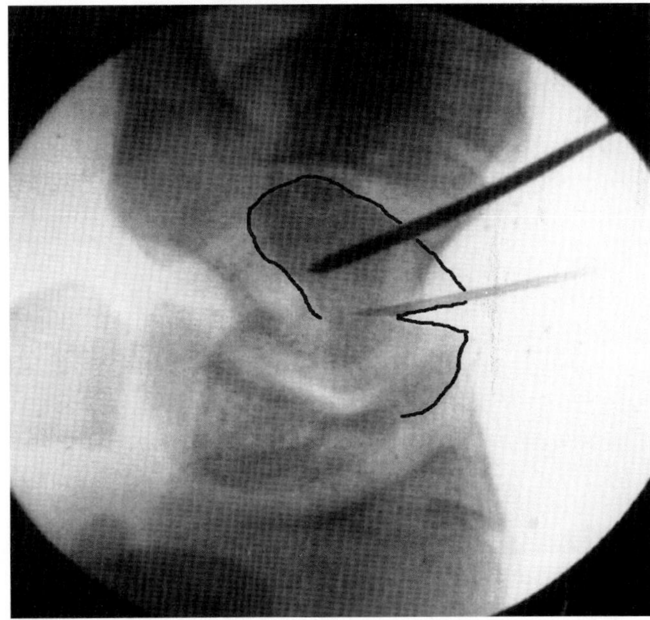

FIGURE 16.3. Flexion deformity of an acute scaphoid fracture.

Fracture Reduction and Guide-Wire Placement: A New Technique

Grossly Aligned Scaphoid

With minimal (<1 mm) or no displacement on imaging, the next step is to place a guide wire down the central scaphoid axis. For a variety of reasons, it might be difficult to visualize the central axis. A simple technique we now use is an "external cross K-wire scaphoid guide," which permits external sighting of the distal scaphoid by percutaneously placed perpendicular K-wires. It does not require continuous imaging to drive the wire along the central axis. Imaging is only used to set up the targeting system. This guide requires the placement of two K-wires in the distal scaphoid in the same axial plane, perpendicular to the scaphoid and offset in a 90-degree arc. One wire is driven dorsal to volar in the PA plane of the distal scaphoid (Figure 16.4) and a second wire in the lateral scaphoid radial to ulnar (Figure 16.5).

These wires cross at the distal scaphoid central axis and form a crosshair target for guide-wire placement (Figure 16.6a through c). To place the dorsal wire, the wrist must be ulnar deviated. This will extend the distal scaphoid fragment and will make the percutaneous perpendicular placement of the wire easier. With the wrist extended and ulna deviated, PA imaging of the dorsal scaphoid wire (if correctly perpendicular to the bone axis) will appear as a single dark point. The lateral radial wire is introduced also perpendicular to the distal scaphoid and driven toward and across the dorsal wire as it appears on image as a single point. A lateral fluroscopic image will confirm that the lateral wire has been placed in the mid-axis of the distal scaphoid.

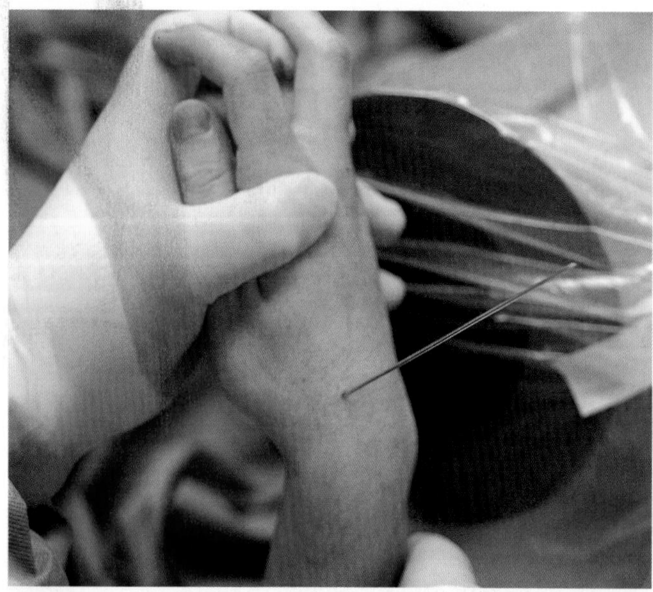

FIGURE 16.4. First .062-inch targeting wire placed dorsal to volar in the distal scaphoid with the wrist in ulnar deviation to extend the scaphoid.

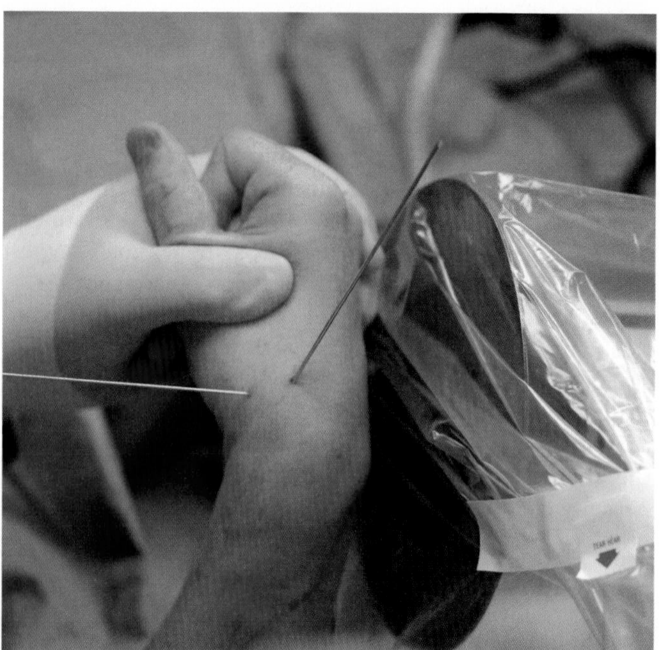

FIGURE 16.5. Second .062-inch targeting wire placed radial to ulnar in the midlateral position of the distal scaphoid.

Next, the 3,4 arthroscopic portal is identified and marked using a 19-gauge needle (Figure 16.7a and b). The 3,4 arthroscopic portal is located 1 cm distal to Lister's tubercle and can be easily imaged using a mini-fluoroscopic unit. This is the location of the proximal scaphoid pole and the starting point for the central axis guide wire to be driven from dorsal to volar in the flexed wrist.

A .045-inch double-cut K-wire is placed in the 3-4 portal and impaled into the proximal scaphoid pole (Figure 16.8). Its position is confirmed fluoroscopically. Next, as the wire is driven toward the thumb base the direction is checked using the dorsal and radial guide wires (Figure 16.9). If the central axis guide wire is in the plane of both targeting wires, it will intersect the cross wires in the distal scaphoid in the central axis. This wire is usually driven through the trapezium because the scaphoid and trapezium are colinear. The wire is withdrawn volarly until the trailing end clears the radiocarpal joint, allowing the wrist to be extended (Figure 16.10).

Imaging is now used to confirm the position of the wire and the scaphoid fracture alignment (Figure 16.11a and b). If satisfactory, the next step is an arthroscopic inspection of the joint. If placing the central axis scaphoid wire results in an incorrect path due to multiple incorrect passes, a correct path can be difficult to establish using a 0.045 wire. A stouter 0.062 wire, with its increased stiffness, can be used to establish the correct track. Once the correct path is established, the 0.062 wire can be exchanged for the 0.045 guide wire.

Grossly Displaced Scaphoid Fracture

To grossly align the scaphoid, the external cross K-wire scaphoid guide is assembled as described previously. Once

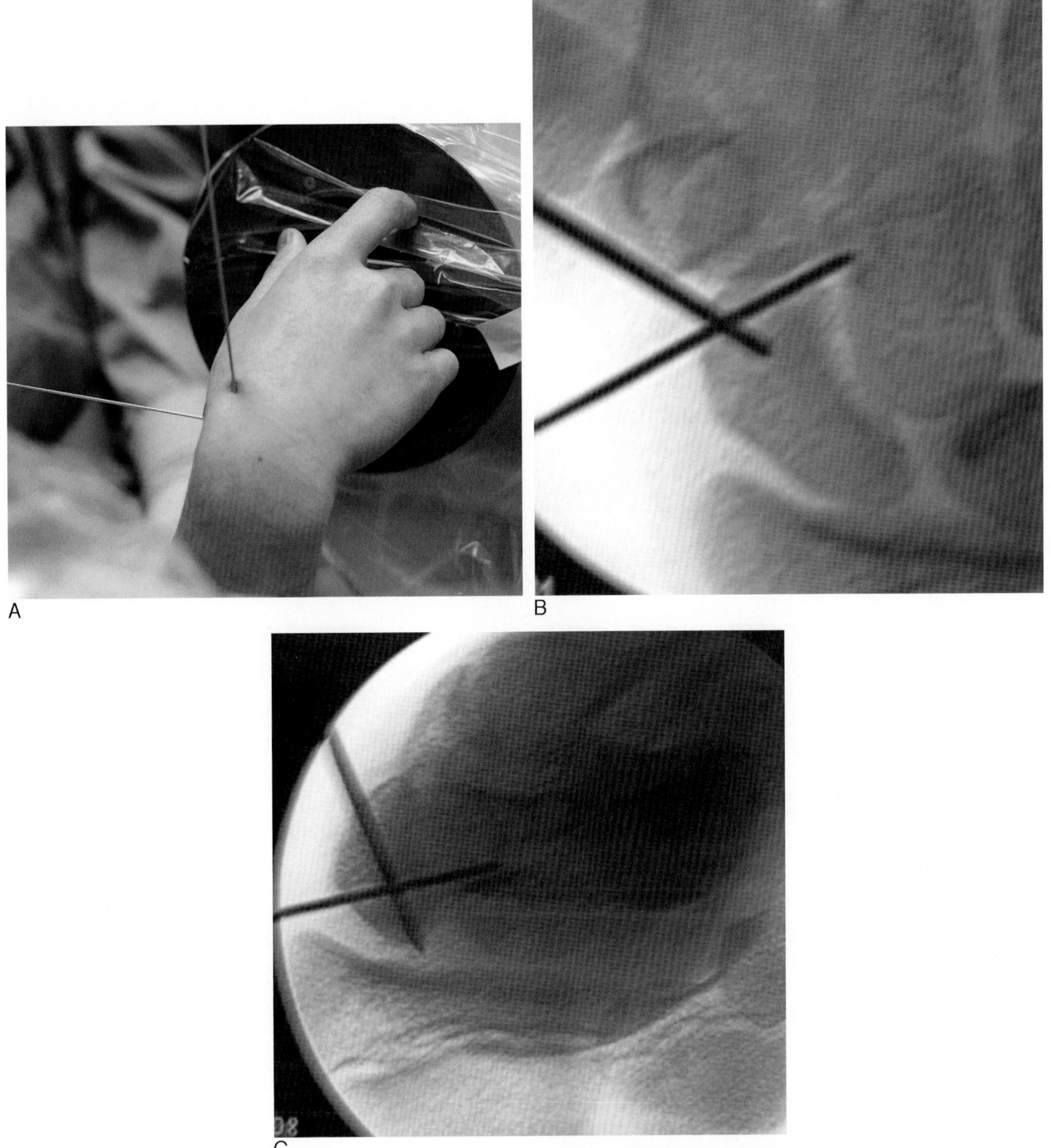

FIGURE 16.6. (A) Cross K-wire guides for targeting of central axis guide wire. (B) AP fluoroscopic imaging of the targeting system. (C) Pronated ulnarly deviated view of the central axis with the targeting system guide wires in place.

the external cross K-wire scaphoid guide is assembled, a PA image is obtained and the fracture site is identified. A 19-gauge needle is inserted through the skin into the fracture site. The distal central scaphoid axis is identified. Because the distal scaphoid fracture fragment is commonly flexed (exposing the dorsal intramedullary canal of the scaphoid), a K-wire can easily be introduced into the fracture site and driven through the distal scaphoid intramedullary canal. The external cross K-wire scaphoid guide will provide direction as the wire is driven from dorsal to volar.

The position of the proximal fragment at this time is irrelevant, but will later be reduced. The wire is withdrawn volarly until the trailing edge of the wire is at the fracture site. Next, a .062 K-wire joystick is placed dorsal

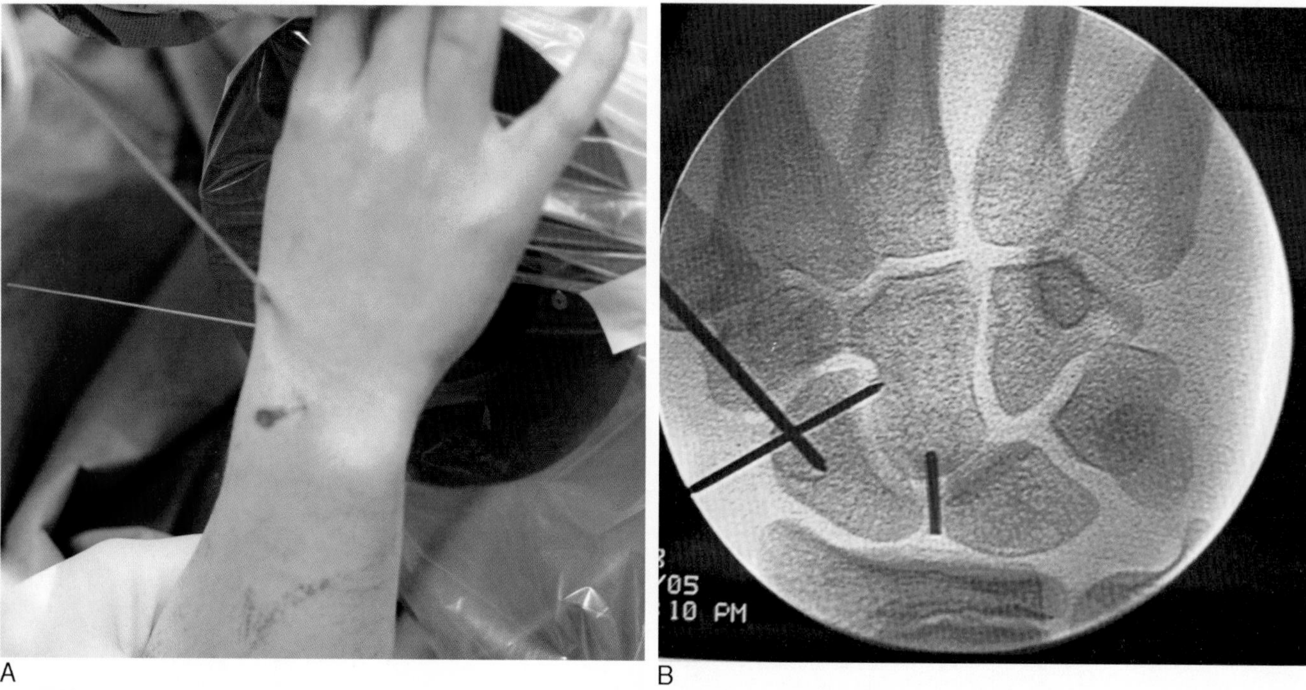

FIGURE 16.7. (A and B) Localization of 3-4 portal and entry site for central axis wire.

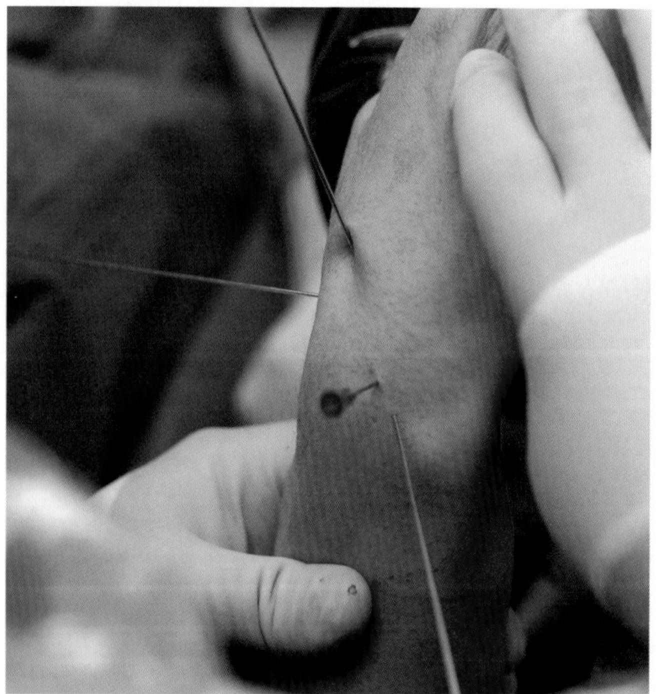

FIGURE 16.8. Impaling of proximal scaphoid using 3-4 portal guide.

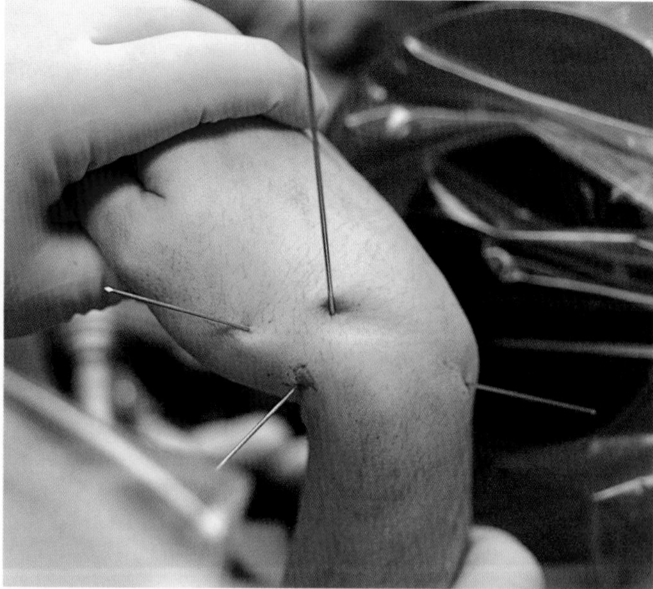

FIGURE 16.9. Driving central axis wire using cross K-wire targeting system.

to volar into the proximal scaphoid fragment. With the wrist extended in a neutral position, the wrist is imaged as the two dorsal joysticks (one in the distal fragment and one in the proximal scaphoid fragment) are manipulated until fracture alignment is obtained (Figure 16.12a through d). The concave scaphoid surface is used as the key reference for fracture reduction. Fracture reduction is captured by driving the volar wire dorsally across the fracture site.

Once reduction and provisional fixation of the grossly displaced fracture has occurred, the next step is placement of the central axis scaphoid guide wire (as described previously). This wire will provide direction for both scaphoid reaming and screw implantation. With the wrist partially flexed, a mini-fluroscopic unit is used to locate the proximal scaphoid pole at the scapholunate interosseous ligament. This is the starting point for the central axis

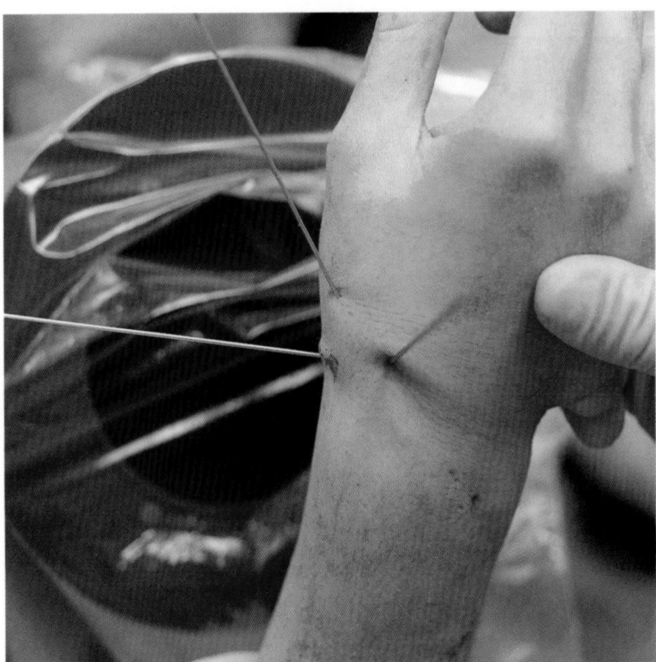

FIGURE 16.10. Central axis wire withdrawn volarly to allow wrist extension for imaging.

scaphoid guide wire, which will be driven from dorsal to volar with the wrist flexed. As the central axis wire is driven toward the thumb base, its direction is corrected using the external distal scaphoid K-wires (the dorsal wire provides radial ulna guidance and the lateral K-wire provides dorsal/volar orientation).

A successfully placed central axis scaphoid wire will hit the crossing wires in the distal scaphoid, the location of the central axis. The wire is driven volarly past this intersection, through the trapezium, and exits at the thumb base in a zone devoid of neurovascular structures. The wire is withdrawn until the trailing edge crosses the radiocarpal joint and the wrist can be safely extended without bending the wire. There are now two K-wires down the length of the scaphoid: one used to capture the initial reduction and the second placed down the long axis (Figure 16.13). The use of two K-wires limits bending forces and acts as an anti-rotation construct during scaphoid reaming and screw placement. Imaging is now used to confirm the position of the wire and the scaphoid fracture alignment. If satisfactory, the next step is an arthroscopic inspection of the joint.

If a DISI deformity is present due to extreme scaphoid flexion at the fracture site, fracture reduction can be achieved

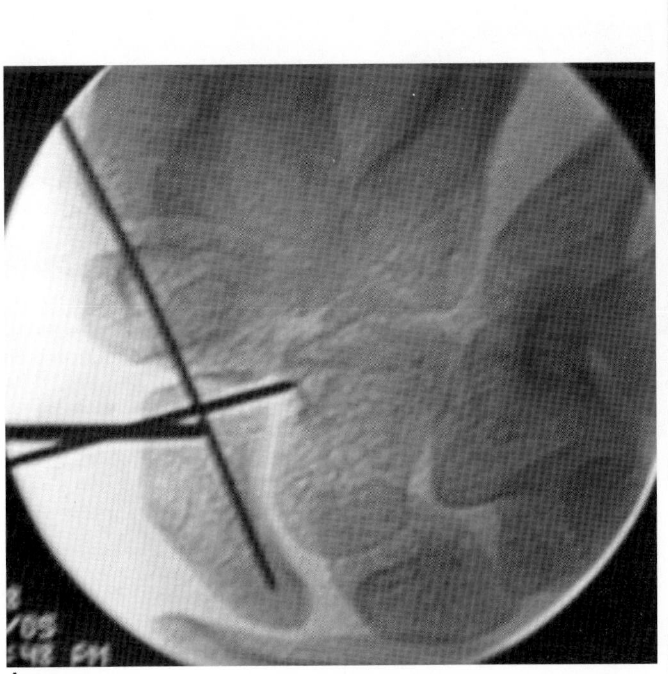

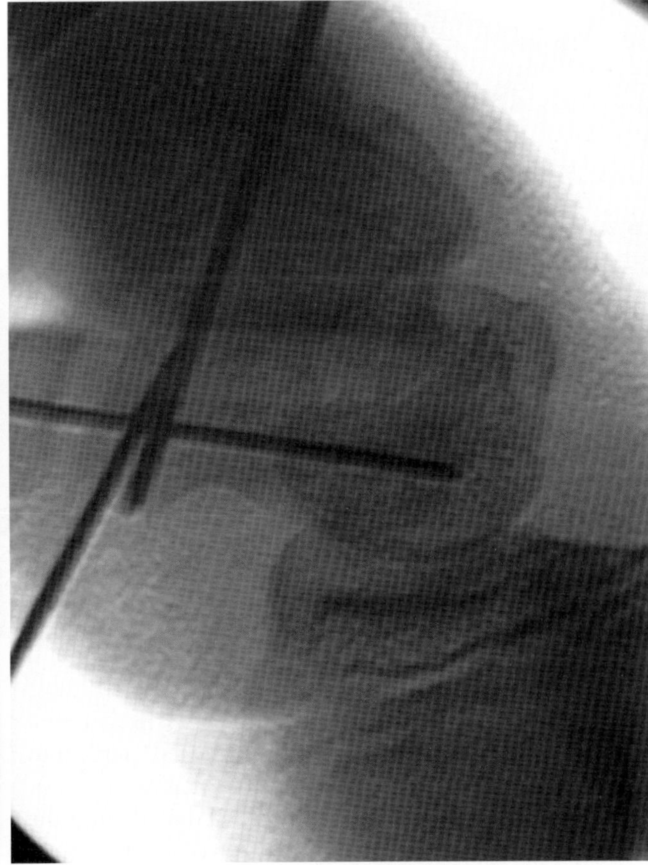

A B

FIGURE 16.11. (A and B) Guide wire correctly placed down the central axis on AP and lateral imaging.

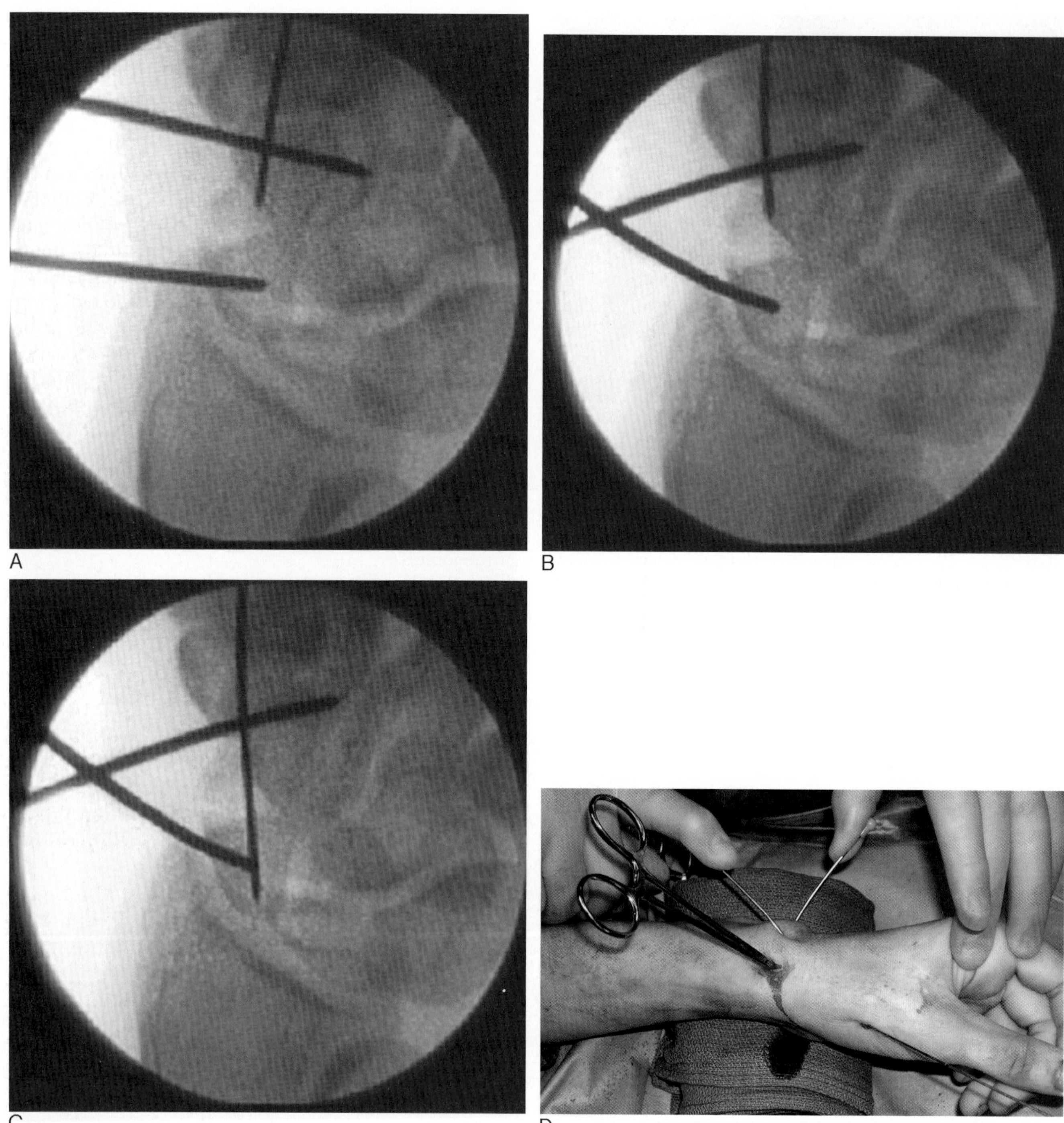

FIGURE 16.12. (A) Displaced scaphoid fracture with .062-inch joysticks in place prior to reduction. (B) Fluoroscopic image of fracture reduction using joysticks. (C) Capturing the reduction with the central axis wire. (D) Demonstration of reduction technique. Occasionally, for additional leverage a percutaneous snap can be introduced to assist with reduction.

by hyperflexion of the wrist until the lunate is in a neutral position and a wire is driven through the distal radius into the lunate—securing it provisionally in a neutral position. Alternatively, the wire can be placed dorsal directly into the lunate in a neutral position. As long as an intact scapholunate interosseous ligament exists, the reduction force is transferred from the lunate to the scaphoid (Figure 16.14).

Arthroscopy

After positioning the guide wire and confirming fracture alignment using fluoroscopy, an arthroscopic survey is performed. The goal of arthroscopy here is to identify and treat ligament injuries and to directly inspect the quality of the reduction.

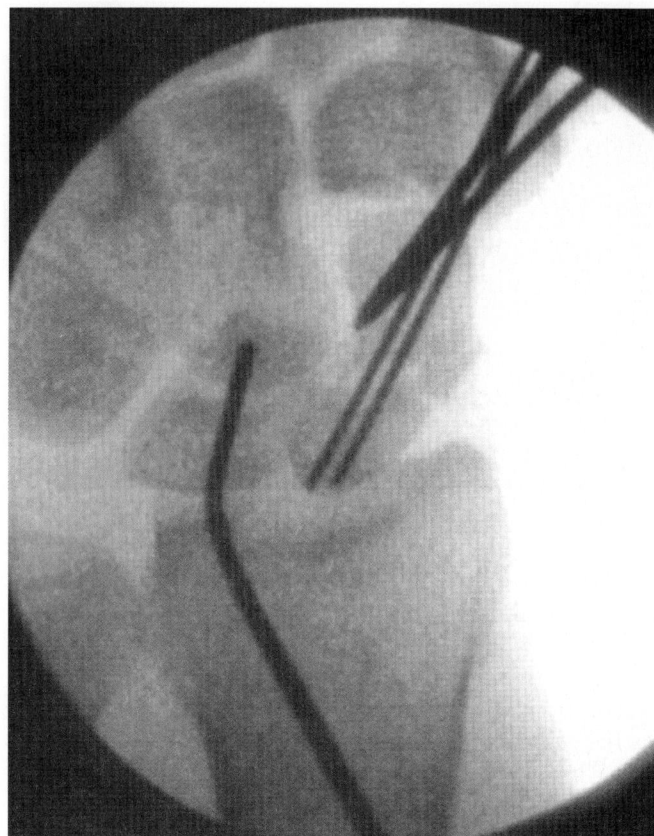

FIGURE 16.13. Two .045-inch K-wires placed in a reduced fracture.

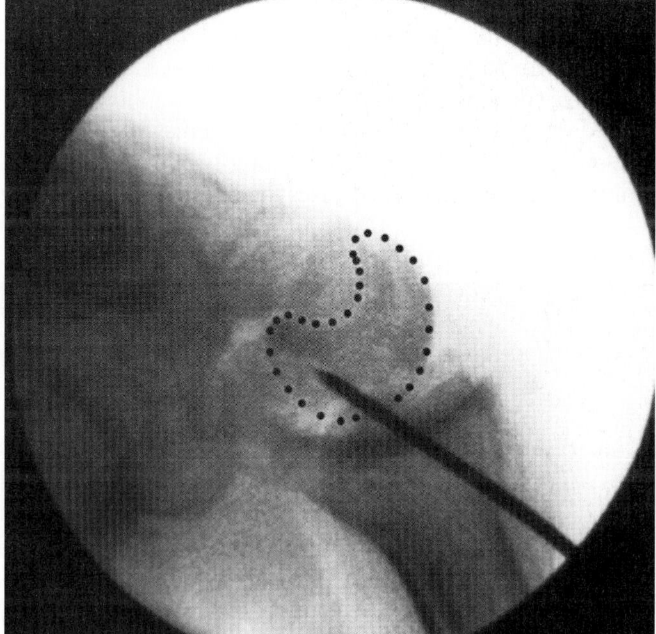

FIGURE 16.14. Wire to control DISI deformity of the lunate.

With the patient in a supine position, the arm is exsanguinated, the elbow is flexed, and the wrist is positioned upright in a spring-scale-driven traction tower. Twelve pounds of traction is distributed between four finger traps to reduce the possibility of a traction injury. A fluoroscopy unit is placed horizontal to the floor and perpendicular to the wrist as the radiocarpal and midcarpal joints are identified with imaging. Nineteen-gauge needles are introduced into the wrist joint to identify the radiocarpal and midcarpal portals. This maneuver limits iatrogenic injury to the joint, which can result from multiple attempts to introduce a blunt trocar blindly.

Once the portals have been successfully located and marked, the imaging unit is removed and the skin alone incised. A small curved blunt hemostat is used to separate the soft tissue and enter the wrist joint. A blunt trocar is placed at the radial midcarpal portal and a small-joint angled arthroscope is introduced. Additional 19-gauge needles are inserted to establish outflow. A probe is introduced at the ulna midcarpal portal and the competency of the carpal ligaments is evaluated by directly stressing their attachments to detect partial and complete tears. The probe is also placed in the 3-4 portal, immediately proximal to the radial midcarpal portal.

With arthroscopy, the sulcus (which defines the scapholunate ligament) can be identified and probed. With partial tears, the probe will be visualized by the arthroscope in the midcarpal portal as it passes from the radiocarpal joint into the midcarpal joint through a tear in the SLIO (scapholunate interosseous) ligament. Any carpal ligament injuries detected are graded using the Geissler grading system.[13] Grade I and II ligament injuries are treated with debridement and shrinkage alone. Grade III injuries are treated with debridement, and after fracture repair carpal pinning for six weeks. Grade IV ligament injuries require open repair of the dorsal SLIO ligament with bone anchors and carpal pinning. The need for the addition of a dorsal capsulodesis tether is determined by the quality of the acute repair after scaphoid fixation. Tears of the triangular fibrocartilage complex are classified using the Palmer classification and treated accordingly.[14]

During arthroscopy, with the wrist in traction, imaging can quickly confirm the location of arthroscopic portals and pathology. Wrist arthroscopy requires that both the camera and shaver be maintained in a plane perpendicular to the wrist. This can be a tedious task, which can result in bending and/or breakage of the shaver or scope. One way to reduce this upper extremity strain is by using 1/4-inch penrose drains, which are secured around the camera head with a small hemostat. The penrose's length is adjusted until the camera is supported perpendicular to the wrist. The drain is then attached to the traction tower. This way, no hands are required to support either the camera or shaver as surgical adjustments are made during an operation.

Scaphoid Length

At completion of arthroscopy, with fracture reduction and guide-wire position confirmed, the screw size must now be selected. To accomplish this, the scaphoid length must

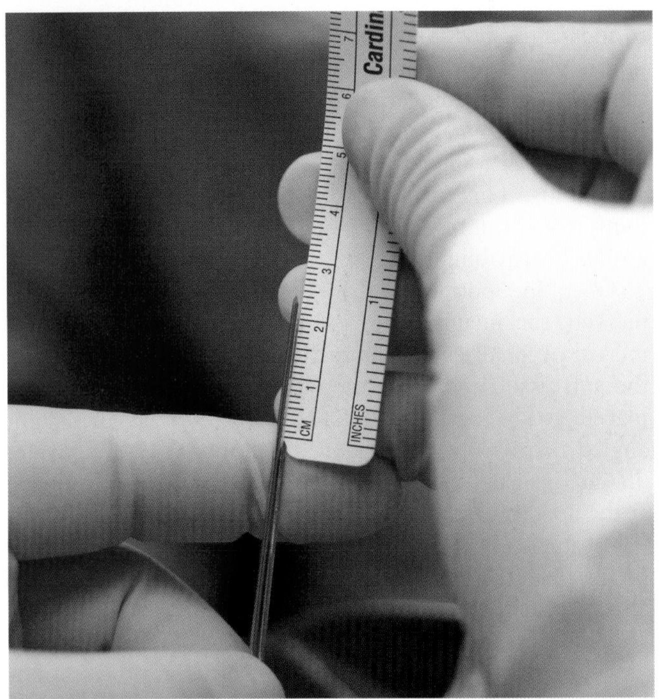

FIGURE 16.15. Measurement of the length of the scaphoid.

be determined. The wrist is flexed and the central axis scaphoid guide wire at the base of the thumb is driven dorsally. The wire is adjusted until the trailing end is in the subchondral bone of the distal scaphoid pole. A second wire of equal length is placed percutaneously at the proximal scaphoid pole and parallel to the guide wire. The difference in length between the trailing end of each wire is the scaphoid length (Figure 16.15).

The screw length selected should be 4 mm less than the scaphoid length. This permits 2 mm of clearance of the screw at each end of the scaphoid, thus ensuring complete implantation without screw exposure. The most common reported complication of percutaneous screw scaphoid fixation is implantation of a screw that is too long.[2]

Rigid Fixation with Headless Cannulated Screw

Once the scaphoid is correctly aligned and its length has been determined, with the wrist maintained in a flexed position the central axis guide wire is adjusted so that its ends are equally exposed between the dorsal wrist and volar radial thumb. This prevents the wire from becoming dislodged during bone reaming and screw implantation (Figure 16.16). It is critical that the wrist maintains a flexed position to prevent the wire from bending. Otherwise, drilling and screw placement will be difficult.

Dorsal implantation of a headless compression screw is recommended for scaphoid fractures of the proximal pole and volar implantation for distal pole fractures because this permits maximum fracture compression. Fractures of the waist may be fixed from a dorsal or volar approach as long as the screw is implanted along the central scaphoid axis. Volar implantation often requires reaming through the trapezium, because this is the central axis. Our experience has been that smooth holes in articular surfaces heal without difficulty. Blunt dissection along the guide wire exposes a tract to the dorsal wrist capsule and scaphoid base (Figure 16.17).

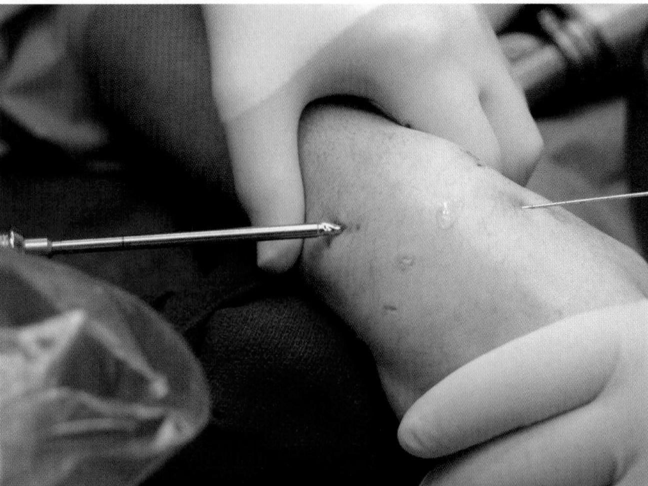

FIGURE 16.16. Reaming of scaphoid with wrist in flexed position and wire advanced equally on either side to prevent bending or dislodging of the central axis wire.

The scaphoid is prepared by drilling a path 2 mm short of the opposite scaphoid cortex with a cannulated hand drill. Newer self-drilling screws have reduced the need for extensive drilling, but drilling of the scaphoid should include at least several millimeters across the fracture site—the concern being that in young bone with increased bone density as the screw crosses the fracture site the screw

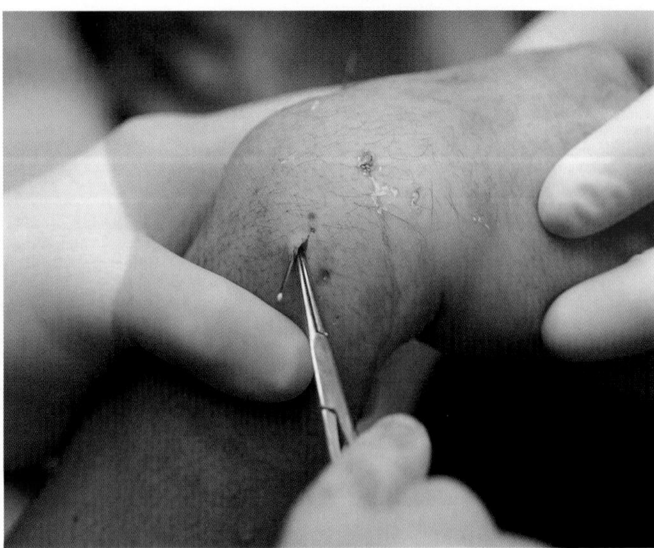

FIGURE 16.17. Clearing soft tissue to make a path for reaming and screw placement.

may be unable to cut and penetrate the opposite bone fragment and force fracture separation (even with self-drilling screws).

The implantation of a headless screw 4 mm shorter greatly reduces the chance that the screw will penetrate the scaphoid cartilage envelope. It is critical to use fluoroscopy to check the position and depth of the drill during reaming. The scaphoid should never be reamed to the opposite bone cortex (over-drilling). This reduces fracture compression and increases the risk of motion at the fracture site. A standard Acutrak screw is advanced under fluoroscopic guidance down the central scaphoid axis to within 1 to 2 mm of the opposite cortex (Figure 16.18). If the screw is advanced to the distal cortex, attempts to advance the screw further will force the fracture fragments to gap and separate.

With unstable or displaced fractures, a counterforce must be applied to maintain compression at the fracture site during reaming and screw implantation. This is accomplished by using a dorsal K-wire in the distal scaphoid bone fragment to compress against the proximal scaphoid bone fragment during reaming and screw implantation.

Unstable fractures may not achieve rigid fixation with screw implantation alone because fracture comminution reduces the strength of the construct. Other temporary fixations may be required to achieve a rigid construct, until healing has occurred. The distal scaphoid pole acts as a long lever arm to the proximal scaphoid pole and proximal carpal row during wrist motion. Proximal pole fractures have only a few threads crossing the fracture line. Wrist motion results in continuous rocking at the fracture site.

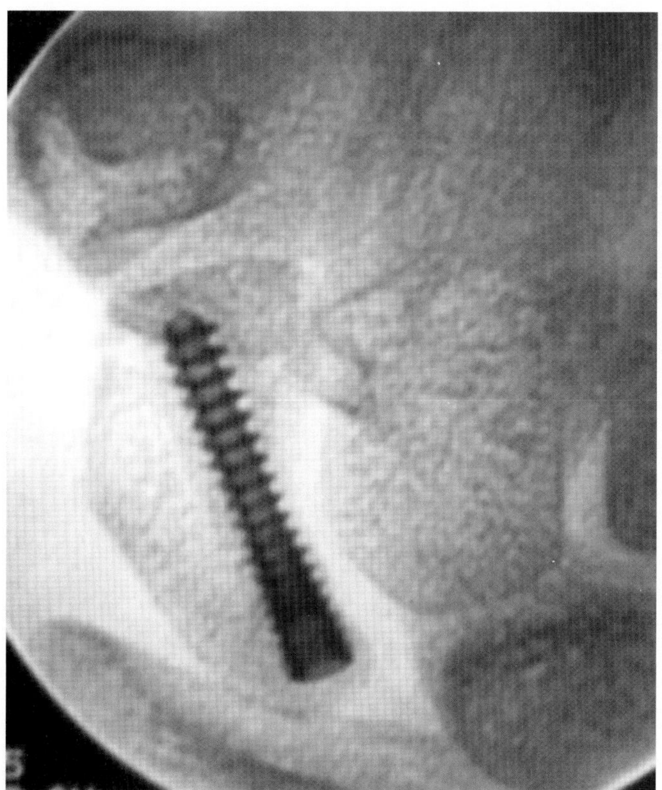

FIGURE 16.18. Screw down the central axis of the scaphoid.

The forces concentrated here are significant and can result in reduction of compression and loosening of fixation. These bending forces can be balanced by the placement of a 0.062-inch K-wire or headless compression screw from the scaphoid into the capitate. These implants temporarily block midcarpal motion and reduce forces acting on the scaphoid fracture site. Another mechanical block is a 0.062-inch K-wire placed between the II or III web space into the capitate and the lunate. After healing has been confirmed with CT scan, these mechanical blocks are removed percutaneously.

Severe comminution at the fracture site may make rigid fixation impossible. In these cases, alignment of the scaphoid fracture fragments with multiple K-wires down the central axis, and an additional provisional stabilization of the capitolunate joint with K-wires may be required. After one month, these provisional fixation wires are removed. Dorsal percutaneous bone grafting of the scaphoid and rigid fixation of the scaphoid with a headless compression screw can then be accomplished.

Postoperative Care and Scaphoid Healing

Immediate postoperative care includes a bulky compressive hand dressing and a volar splint. The patient is encouraged to initiate early finger exercises to reduce swelling. At the first postoperative visit, the therapist fashions a removable volar splint that holds the wrist and hand in a functional position. The patient is started on an immediate strengthening program. The purpose of the strengthening program is to axially load the fracture site now secured with an intramedullary screw to stimulate healing.

This early motion also decreases swelling and permits an early return of hand function. Patients with ligament injuries or proximal pole fractures are restricted from wrist motion until CT scan confirms bridging bone at the fracture site six weeks postoperatively. Postoperative radiographs are obtained with the first postoperative visit and at six-week intervals. CT scans with 1-mm cuts and sagittal and coronal reconstructions are used to evaluate bridging bone at the fracture site. CT scans are ordered at six-week intervals until final union is established.

Standard radiographs at three months have been demonstrated to be unreliable in determining scaphoid healing.[15] It is important to understand that patients are often pain free prior to CT evidence of healing. Contact sports and heavy labor are restricted until fracture healing is confirmed by CT. If bridging bone is not identified by 12 weeks, one must consider aggressive treatment (including percutaneous bone grafting). Delay in treatment for early nonunions delays healing. We do not routinely cast our scaphoid fractures postoperatively, but candidates for additional protection are evaluated on a case-by-case basis.

Summary

Percutaneous techniques have provided a powerful tool for limiting iatrogenic injuries and speeding healing and recovery. Fluoroscopic imaging and arthroscopy are modalities useful in restoration of the injured extremity. Over the past 10 years percutaneous fixation of nondisplaced scaphoid fractures has resulted in a high union rate, and early return of hand function with minimal complications. Using these same tools and the external cross K-wire scaphoid guide, displaced scaphoid fractures can be reduced and rigidly fixed—permitting rapid healing and an early return of hand function. Development of small-joint arthroscopic skills is one of the cornerstones of mastering this method of scaphoid fracture treatment.

References

1. Adolfsson L, Lindau T, Arner M. Acutrak screw fixation versus cast immobilisation for undisplaced scaphoid waist fractures. J Hand Surg [Br] 2001;26(3):192–95.
2. Bond CD, Shin AY, McBride MT, et al. Percutaneous screw fixation or cast immobilization for nondisplaced scaphoid fractures. J Bone Joint Surg [Am] 2001;83-A(4):483–88.
3. Haddad FS, Goddard NJ. Acute percutaneous scaphoid fixation: A pilot study. J Bone Joint Surg [Br] 1998;80(1):95–9.
4. Inoue G, Shionoya K. Herbert screw fixation by limited access for acute fractures of the scaphoid. J Bone Joint Surg [Br] 1997;79(3):418–21.
5. Ledoux P, Chahidi N, Moermans JP, Kinnen L. Percutaneous Herbert screw osteosynthesis of the scaphoid bone. Acta Orthop Belg 1995;61(1):43–7.
6. Taras JS, Sweet S, Shum W, Weiss LE, Bartolozzi A. Percutaneous and arthroscopic screw fixation of scaphoid fractures in the athlete. Hand Clinics 1999;15(3):467–73.
7. Slade JFIII, Grauer JN, Mahoney JD. Arthroscopic reduction and percutaneous fixation of scaphoid fractures with a novel dorsal technique. Orthop Clin North Am 2001;32 (2):247–61.
8. Schadel-Hopfner M, Bohringer G, Gotzen L. Percutaneous osteosynthesis of scaphoid fracture with the Herbert-Whipple screw: Technique and results. Handchirurgie, Mikrochirurgie, Plastische Chirurgie 2000;32(4):271–76.
9. Yip HS, Wu WC, Chang RY, So TY. Percutaneous cannulated screw fixation of acute scaphoid waist fracture. J Hand Surg [Br] 2002;27(1):42–6.
10. Shih JT, Lee HM, Hou YT, Tan CM. Results of arthroscopic reduction and percutaneous fixation for acute displaced scaphoid fractures. Arthroscopy 2005;21(5):620–26.
11. Slade JF, Merrell G, Lozano-Caldron S, Ring D: Arthroscopic Assisted, Percutaneous Reduction and Fixation of Displaced Scaphoid Fractures. Poster, ASSH Annual Meeting, September 2005.
12. Trumble TE, Gilbert M, Murray LW, Smith J, Rafijah G, McCallister WV. Displaced scaphoid fractures treated with open reduction and internal fixation with a cannulated screw. J Bone Joint Surg [Am] 2000;82(5):633–41.
13. Geissler WB, Freeland AE, Savoie FH, McIntyre LW, Whipple TL. Intracarpal soft-tissue lesions associated with an intra-articular fracture of the distal end of the radius. J Bone Joint Surg [Am] 1996;78(3):357–65.
14. Palmer AK. Triangular fibrocartilage complex lesions: A classification. J Hand Surg 1989;14A:594–606.
15. Dias JJ. Definition of union after acute fracture and surgery for fracture nonunion of the scaphoid. J Hand Surg [Br] 2001;26(4):321–25.

William B. Geissler

CHAPTER 17

The Role of Wrist Arthroscopy in Intra-Articular Distal Radius Fracture Management

Introduction

Displaced intra-articular fractures of the distal radius are a unique subset of radius fractures. These fractures are usually the result of a high-energy injury and are usually associated with intra-articular soft-tissue injuries. These fractures are traditionally unstable, and are less amenable to closed manipulation and casting.

Lafontaine has described several radiographic features that signify when a fracture of the distal radius is unstable.[1] These include initial dorsal angulation greater than 20 degrees, extensive dorsal comminution, associated ulnar styloid fracture, significant intra-articular involvement, and older patients greater than the age of 60.

The prognosis for intra-articular fractures of the distal radius has been shown to depend on numerous factors.[2] These include the amount of radial shortening, residual extra-articular angulation, articular congruity of both the radiocarpal and radioulnar joints, and associated intra-articular soft-tissue injuries. Trumble et al., in their review of 52 intra-articular fractures, noted that factors that strongly correlated with a successful outcome included the amount of residual radial shortening and intra-articular congruity.[3]

The use of wrist arthroscopy as an adjunct in the management of displaced intra-articular distal radius fractures takes advantage of its ability to view the articular surface with bright light and magnified conditions with minimal surgical morbidity.[4] Fracture hematoma and debris may be arthroscopically lavaged, which potentially can improve the patient's final range of motion[5] (Figure 17.1). In addition, associated intra-articular soft-tissue injuries may be detected and managed at the same sitting[6] (Figure 17.2). Pathology not readily identified on plain radiographs is frequently discovered during arthroscopic-assisted reduction and internal fixation of distal radius fractures. In most instances, it is much easier to manage an acute soft-tissue injury that occurs with a distal radius fracture than chronic pathology. The purpose of this chapter is to review the rationale and technique in the application of wrist arthroscopy as a useful adjunct in the management of displaced intra-articular fractures of the distal radius.

Two millimeters of articular displacement has over the past several years become a well-established critical threshold for articular incongruity of the distal radius. Knirk and Jupiter, in their classic article, demonstrated the importance of an articular reduction within 2 mm or less.[7] A patient whose articular reduction is greater than 2 mm at final follow-up visit has a significantly higher incidence of degenerative changes within the wrist. Bradway and Amadio further substantiated these findings in their study.[8]

In their series of 40 patients, Fernandez and Geissler noted that the critical threshold may be as low as 1 mm or less.[9] They reported in their study that the incidence of complications was substantially lower and articular reduction was within 1 mm or less.

Edwards et al. described the advantage of viewing intra-articular reduction by wrist arthroscopy compared to monitoring under fluoroscopy alone.[10] In their series, 15 patients underwent arthroscopic evaluation of the articular surface of the distal radius following reduction and stabilization under fluoroscopy. They found that 33% of the

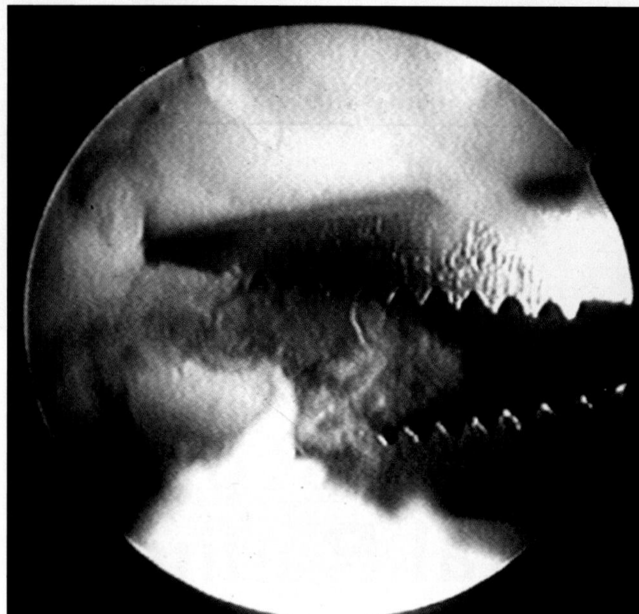

FIGURE 17.1. Loose bodies are frequently seen during arthroscopic-assisted reduction of distal radius fractures, which are not readily apparent on plain radiographs. Removal of these loose fragments and cartilage debris may improve the patient's final prognosis.

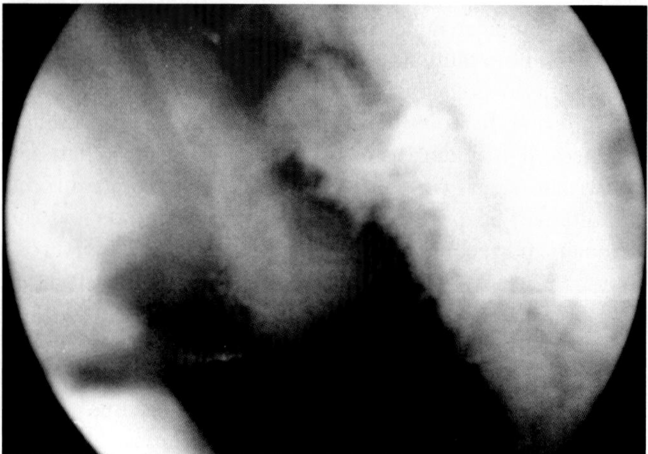

FIGURE 17.2. Partial and complete tears to the interosseous ligaments are frequently identified during the wrist arthroscopic procedure. Management of acute tears to the interosseous ligaments may have a better prognosis compared to chronic injuries.

patients had an articular step-off of 1 mm or more as viewed arthroscopically. Frequently, the fragment was rotated. Wrist arthroscopy is particularly useful in judging the rotation of fracture fragments, which is not readily identifiable under fluoroscopy. Edwards et al. concluded that utilizing wrist arthroscopy as an adjunct may detect residual gapping not previously identified under fluoroscopy alone.

A high incidence of associated intra-articular soft-tissue injuries involving the triangular fibrocartilage complex and the interosseous ligaments has been shown by several studies of displaced intra-articular fractures of the distal radius.[11] Mohanti and Fontes, in two separate wrist arthrogram studies, noted a high incidence of tears of the triangular fibrocartilage complex associated with distal radius fractures. Fontes, in his series, noted a 66% incidence of tears of the triangular fibrocartilage complex in 58 patients.[12] Similarly, Mohanti noted an injury of the triangular fibrocartilage complex in 45% of 60 patients in his series.[13]

Several recent arthroscopic studies have documented incidences of associated intercarpal soft-tissue injuries with fractures of the distal radius. In three recent published studies, an injury to the triangular fibrocartilage complex seems to be the most common associated intra-articular soft-tissue injury. Geissler et al. reported their experience in 60 patients with displaced intra-articular fractures of the distal radius undergoing arthroscopic-assisted reduction and evaluation.[14] The criterion for surgical stabilization in his series was an intra-articular fracture displaced 2 mm or more that cannot be reduced by closed manipulation. In Geissler et al.'s series, 49% of the patients had a tear of the triangular fibrocartilage complex. An injury to the interosseous ligaments was less common. Tears to the scapholunate interosseous ligament were present in 32% of patients, and injury to the lunotriquetral interosseous ligament was identified in 15%.

Lindau, in a similar arthroscopic study of 50 patients, noted that tears of the triangular fibrocartilage complex were present in 78% of patients, injuries to the scapholunate ligament were identified in 54% of patients, and tears of the lunotriquetral interosseous ligament were less common and seen in 16% of patients.[15] Hanker, in a series of 65 patients, noted that tears of the triangular fibrocartilage complex were very common and were present in 55% of the patients in his series.[16] Although it is clearly documented that associated soft-tissue injuries are common with displaced intra-articular fractures of the distal radius, how they may affect the final outcome in patients is still unknown.

Geissler et al. described an arthroscopic classification of an interosseous ligament injury based on their work on arthroscopic management of fractures of the distal radius.[14] They noted that a spectrum of injury may occur to the interosseous ligament. The ligament attenuates, and then eventually tears, and the degree of rotation between the carpal bones increases. The scapholunate interosseous ligament appears to tear from volar to dorsal. This arthroscopic classification of carpal instability is based on observation of interosseous ligaments from both the radiocarpal and midcarpal spaces (Table 17.1).

The normal scapholunate and lunotriquetral interosseous ligaments have a concave appearance between the carpal bones as viewed from the radiocarpal space. The scapholunate ligament is best seen with the arthroscope in the 3-4 portal. The lunotriquetral interosseous ligament is best observed with the arthroscope placed in either the 4-5 or 6-R portal. The lunotriquetral interval will not be adequately seen with the scope in the 3-4 portal alone.

Table 17.1.

Geissler Arthroscopic Classification of Carpal Instability

Grade	Description	Management
I	Attenuation/hemorrhage of interosseous ligament as seen from the radiocarpal joint. No incongruency of carpal alignment in the midcarpal space.	Immobilization
II	Attenuation/hemorrhage of interosseous ligament as seen from the radiocarpal joint. Incongruency/step-off as seen from midcarpal space. A slight gap (less than width of a probe) between the carpal bones may be present.	Arthroscopic reduction and pinning
III	Incongruency/step-off of carpal alignment is seen in both the radiocarpal and midcarpal space. The probe may be passed through gap between the carpal bones.	Arthroscopic/open reduction and pinning
IV	Incongruency/step-off of carpal alignment is seen in both the radiocarpal and midcarpal space. Gross instability with manipulation is noted. A 2.7-mm arthroscope may be passed through the gap between the carpal bones.	Open reduction and repair

In the midcarpal space, the scapholunate interval should be tight and congruent without any articular step-off. Similarly, the lunotriquetral interval should be congruent, but usually a 1-mm step-off or slightly increased play may be seen between the lunate and triquetrum as observed from the radial midcarpal space. A probe or needle may be inserted in the ulnar midcarpal space to evaluate the amount of play between the carpal bones.

In Geissler grade I injuries, there is a loss of the normal concave appearance between the carpal bones as the interosseous ligament attenuates and becomes convex (as seen in the radiocarpal space). Hemorrhage may be seen within the ligament itself in acute situations. However, in the midcarpal space the interval between the carpal bones will still be tight and congruent (with no step-off).

In Geissler grade II injuries, the interosseous ligament continues to become attenuated and becomes convex (as seen in the radiocarpal space, similar to grade I injuries). There is no gap between the carpal bones. However, in the midcarpal space the interval between the involved carpal bones is no longer congruent and a step-off is present. With scapholunate instability, there is slight palmar flexion of the dorsal edge of the scaphoid compared to the lunate. In lunotriquetral instability, the interosseous ligament again becomes attenuated as seen from the radiocarpal space with the arthroscope in the 6-R portal. In the radial midcarpal space, increased play will be seen between the lunate and triquetrum as palpated with a probe.

In Geissler grade III injuries, the interosseous ligament now starts to tear from volar to dorsal as seen with the arthroscope in the radial midcarpal space. A probe is frequently helpful to demonstrate the gap between the involved carpal bones. In the midcarpal space, a 2-mm probe may be placed between the carpal bones and twisted. The dorsal portion of the interosseous ligament is still intact, and complete separation of the carpal bones is not seen.

In Geissler grade IV injuries, the interosseous ligament is completely detached and the arthroscope may be passed freely from the radiocarpal space through the tear to the midcarpal space. This is the so-called "drive-through sign."

It is felt that Geissler grade I injuries are consistent with a wrist sprain and usually respond to immobilization over a period of weeks. In Geissler grade II and grade III tears, these may be arthroscopically reduced and pinned in the acute situation. Pinning is not recommended for chronic injuries of the interosseous ligaments. In Geissler grade IV injuries, where there is complete detachment of the interosseous ligament, it is felt that open repair will have the best prognosis in an acute situation.

Large-joint instrumentation is not appropriate for arthroscopically assisted reduction of distal radius fractures. Smaller-joint arthroscopic instrumentation is essential. The small-joint arthroscope is approximately 2.7 mm, and even smaller scopes may be utilized if desired. When the arthroscope is initially placed in the wrist, it is usually full of fracture debris and hematoma. It is useful to irrigate out the fracture debris and utilize the shaver (3.5 mm or less) to clear the remaining hematoma to improve visualization, particularly to judge the rotation of the fracture fragments.

A traction tower is very useful in the arthroscopic-assisted management of intra-articular fractures of the distal radius. A traction tower allows the surgeon to flex, extend, and radial and ulnar deviate the wrist to help reduce the fracture fragments while maintaining constant traction to allow visualization. A new traction tower was designed to allow the surgeon to simultaneously evaluate arthroscopically the articular reduction and to monitor the reduction under fluoroscopy (Figure 17.3). The traction bar is uniquely placed at the side of the wrist rather than at its center, so that it does not block fluoroscopic evaluation and the surgeon does not need to work around a central bar. In addition, by having the traction bar at the side rather than centrally allows the surgeon to simultaneously arthroscope the wrist and stabilize the fracture while obtaining access through a standard volar approach.

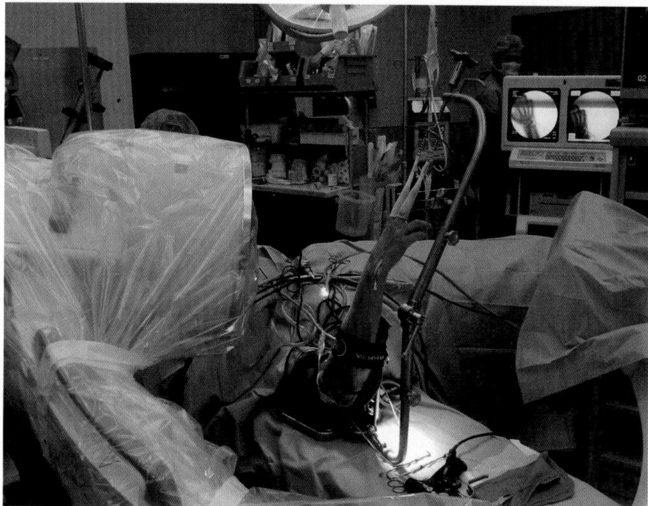

FIGURE 17.3. A new traction tower was developed to allow for simultaneous arthroscopic reduction of the distal radius fracture and fluoroscopic examination. This greatly simplifies the procedure.

The surgeon can fluoroscopically evaluate the position of the plate and screw insertion during stabilization. This new traction tower allows a surgeon to perform arthroscopic-assisted fixation in both the vertical and/or horizontal planes, depending on the surgeon's preference. (Figure 17.4). If a traction tower is not available, the wrist may be suspended with finger traps attached to a weight over the end of a hand table in the horizontal position, or with a shoulder holder in the vertical position. A small bump is useful to place under the wrist if weights are being utilized over the end of the table to maintain the wrist in slight flexion.

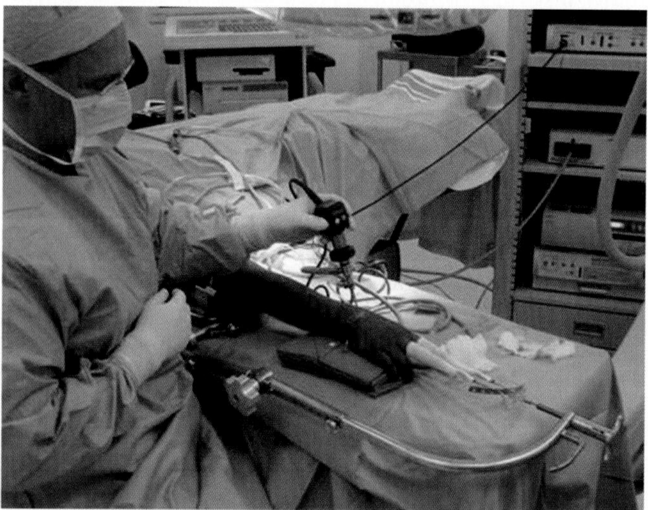

FIGURE 17.4. The new tower may be placed in a vertical or horizontal position for arthroscopic-assisted reduction of distal radius fractures, depending on the surgeon's preference.

Thorough irrigation of the joint is necessary to wash out the fracture hematoma to improve visualization. Inflow is usually provided through a 14-gauge needle through the 6-U portal. In addition, it is important to provide outflow to limit fluid extravasation into the soft tissues. Outflow is provided through the arthroscope cannula. An intervenous extension tubing is connected to the arthroscope cannula, which drains then into a basin to limit fluid extravasation and not onto the surgeon's lap or floor. It is felt that a separate inflow and outflow is necessary to improve irrigation of the joint rather than inflow through arthroscope cannula alone. The small-joint cannula in wrist arthroscopy does not allow much space between the cannula and the arthroscope itself, and this limits the amount of fluid irrigation through the arthroscope cannula. For this reason, it is felt that it is best to have a separate inflow through the 6-U portal.

A fracture of the distal radius wrist is frequently swollen. Because of this reason, it is fairly difficult to palpate the traditional extensor tendon landmarks for wrist arthroscopy. However, the bony landmarks can usually still be palpated and marked. These bony landmarks include the bases of the metacarpals, the dorsal lip of the radius, and the ulnar head. The traditional viewing portal is the 3-4 portal, which is made between the third and fourth dorsal extensor compartments. The 3-4 portal is made in line with the radial border of the long finger.

Precise portal placement is mandatory for arthroscopic-assisted reduction of distal radius fractures. If the portal is placed too proximal, the arthroscope may be placed within the fracture pattern itself. If it is placed too distally, it can injure the articular surface of the carpus. It is very useful to place an 18-gauge needle into the proposed location of the 3-4 portal prior to making a skin incision. The portal is made by pulling the skin with the surgeon's thumb against the tip of a number 11 blade.

Blunt dissection is then continued with the hemostat to the level of the joint capsule, and the arthroscope with a blunt trocar is introduced into the 3-4 portal. The 3-4 portal is the primary viewing portal in wrist arthroscopy. The fracture hematoma and debris are then washed out to improve visualization with the inflow in the 6-U portal. A working portal is then made in the 6-R or 4-5 portal and the remaining hematoma is debrided out. Similarly to making the 3-4 portal, a needle is placed and viewed arthroscopically prior to making a skin incision for the working portal.

Ideal timing for arthroscopic-assisted reduction of distal radius fractures appears to be between 3 and 10 days. Earlier attempts at arthroscopic fixation may result in troublesome bleeding. Fractures that are over 10 days post-injury are more difficult to disimpact and elevate with arthroscopic-assisted reduction.

Fractures without extensive metaphysial comminution are most ideal for arthroscopic-assisted management. Radial styloid fractures, die punch fractures, three-part

T fractures, and four-part fractures are all amenable to arthroscopic-assisted reduction and internal fixation.[17] Some three-part fractures and most four-part fractures are managed through a combination of open reduction and arthroscopic-assisted fixation. In these instances, the fracture is stabilized by a volar plate through a volar approach (but the joint capsule is not incised). Articular reduction may be arthroscopically fine-tuned, and the distal screws inserted to stabilize the fracture. Associated soft-tissue injuries are detected and managed in the same sitting.

Radial Styloid Fractures

A radial styloid fracture is an ideal fracture pattern to manage arthroscopically, particularly if one is just beginning to gain experience in arthroscopic-assisted fixation of distal radius fractures. Several techniques are possible. A closed reduction and percutaneous fixation of the radial styloid fragment may be attempted under fluoroscopy. The fracture can be provisionally stabilized anatomically as possible as viewed under fluoroscopy.

The fracture then may be placed in traction, and the wrist arthroscopically evaluated. This allows the fracture hematoma and debris to be washed out and assessment made for any associated intra-articular soft-tissue injuries. The arthroscope is initially placed in the 3-4 portal, and the reduction of the radial styloid fracture is observed. However, the best portal to view rotation of the fracture fragment is by looking across the wrist. Therefore, it is best to place the arthroscope in either the 4-5 or 6-R portal to look across the wrist to judge the reduction of the radial styloid fragment and its rotation. Frequently, the articular reduction may look anatomical under fluoroscopy. However, the radial styloid fragment may still be slightly rotated as viewed arthroscopically.

If the radial styloid fragment is mal-rotated, the guide wires are then backed out of the radial shaft (leaving them only in the radial styloid fragment). They are then utilized as joysticks controlling the rotation of the fracture fragment and then advanced across the fracture site once the reduction is judged anatomical as viewed arthroscopically. In addition, a trocar may be introduced through the 3-4 portal to provide additional control of the radial styloid fragment as it is being manipulated with the joysticks and observed with the arthroscope in the 6-R portal. The positions of the guide wires are then checked under fluoroscopy. If the guide wires are appropriate, a cannulated screw may be placed over the guide wire through the radial styloid fragment into the radial shaft to stabilize the fracture fragment.

Early on in the author's experience, only Kirschner wires were utilized to stabilize the radial styloid fragment. The author's patients had to be further stabilized with a splint. In addition, the protruding Kirschner wires irritated the skin and potentially hampered rehabilitation. Now the author prefers headless cannulated screws, which limit any metal protruding from the skin and/or bone. New self-drilling headless screws have been recently introduced (Acutrak II, Hillsboro, OR), which eliminates a step of drilling and even further simplifies the procedure. The decrease in metal prominence exiting from the bone significantly decreases irritation of the thumb extensor tendons and promotes earlier range of motion and rehabilitation.

An alternative technique is to advance the guide wire or Kirschner wire under fluoroscopy into the radial styloid fragment alone, and not across the fracture site (Figure 17.5). The position of the guide wire in the radial styloid fragment and its angle in relation to the fracture is viewed directly under fluoroscopy. The wrist is then suspended in the traction tower and the standard wrist arthroscopy portals are made. Similar to before, the best view to judge rotation and reduction of the radial styloid fragment is through the 6-R portal. The previously placed Kirschner wires are then used as joysticks and the fracture is manipulated under direct observation and anatomically reduced to the distal radius (Figures 17.6 and 17.7).

The guide wires are than advanced across the fracture site once the reduction is judged to be anatomical. It is vital to make a small skin incision over the radial styloid to insert the guide wires through a 14-gauge needle or through a cannula to prevent injury to the dorsal sensory branch of the radial nerve. An alternative technique is utilizing an oscillating drill to insert the guide wires. By use of an oscillating drill, the cutaneous nerves will not wrap around the Kirschner wire as it is being inserted. Once the position of the guide wires is checked under

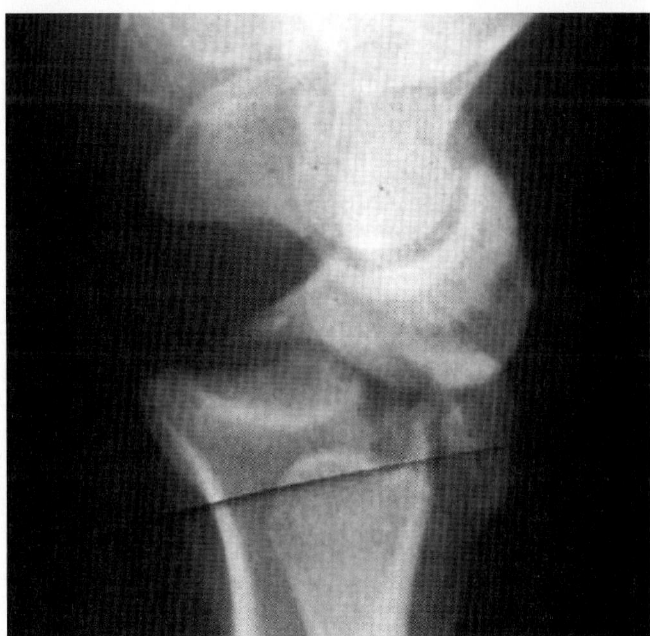

FIGURE 17.5. Lateral view of a fracture dislocation of the distal radius involving the radial styloid.

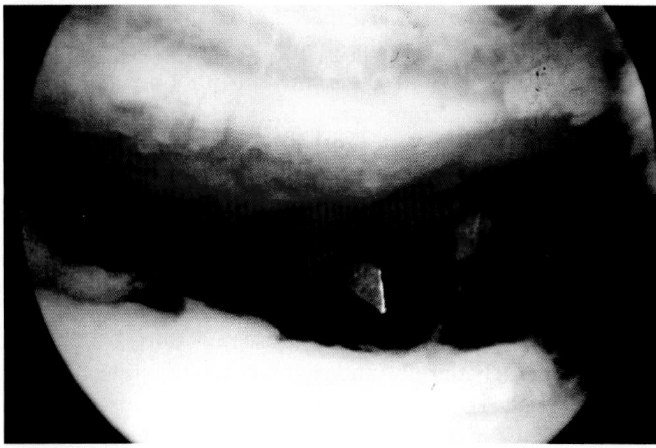

FIGURE 17.6. Arthroscopic view with the arthroscope in the 6-R portal looking across the wrist in the displaced radial styloid fragment. A guide wire has been placed into the radial styloid fragment to act as a joystick.

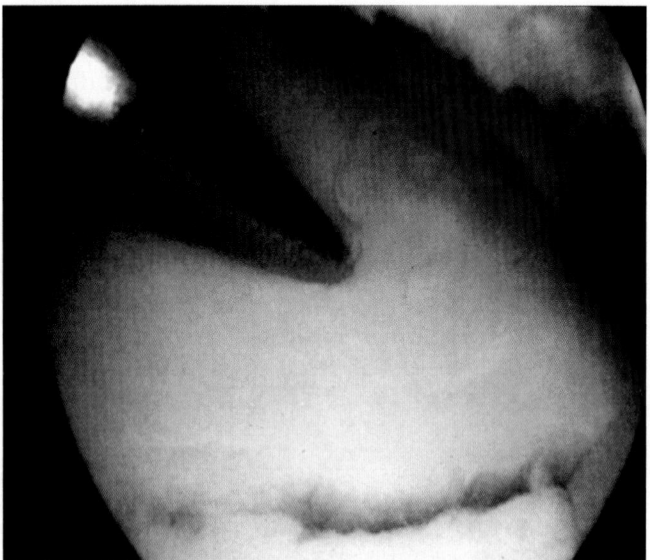

FIGURE 17.7. Arthroscopic view of the radial styloid fragment as it is being reduced. A combination of the joystick into the radial styloid fragment and a trocar inserted into the 3-4 portal helps control the rotation and reduction of the displaced radial styloid fragment.

fluoroscopy, a headless cannulated screw may be inserted (Figures 17.8 and 17.9).

It is important to remember that radial styloid fractures have a high incidence of injury to the scapholunate interosseous ligament[18] (Figures 17.10 through 17.12). The zone of injury may pass through the fracture and distally into the scapholunate interosseous ligament. Following arthroscopic reduction to the radial styloid fracture, the arthroscope is placed back in the 3-4 portal to evaluate the integrity of the scapholunate interosseous ligament (Figures 17.13 and 17.14). The arthroscope should also be placed in the radial midcarpal portal to evaluate the scapholunate interval from the midcarpal space. The potential for carpal instability should be thoroughly evaluated from both the radiocarpal and midcarpal spaces. In addition, the occasional loose body may be seen in the midcarpal space, which cannot be detected on plain radiographs. Loose bodies are usually associated with a fracture involving the lunate facet and arise from the hamate.

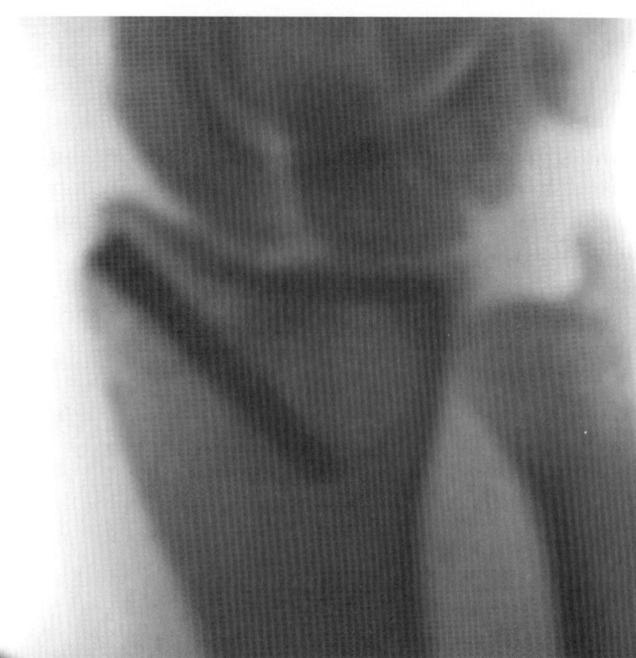

FIGURE 17.8. Fluoroscopic view of the reduced radial styloid fragment.

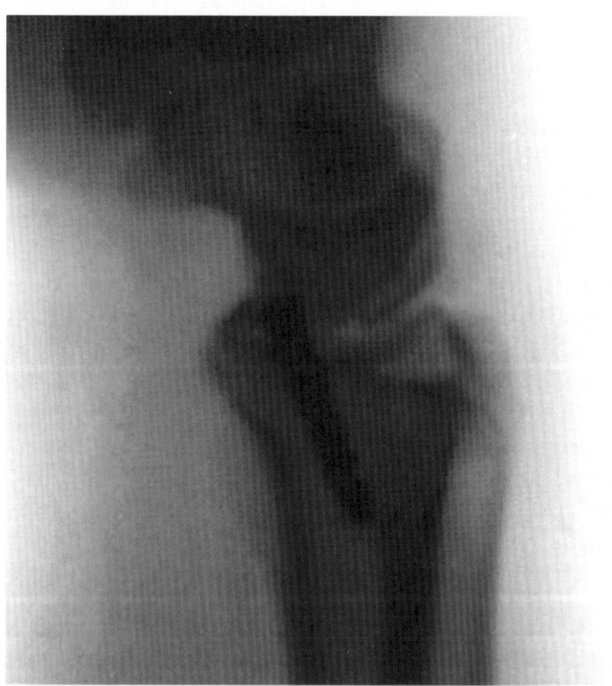

FIGURE 17.9. Lateral fluoroscopic view showing the radial styloid fragment and carpus to be anatomically reduced.

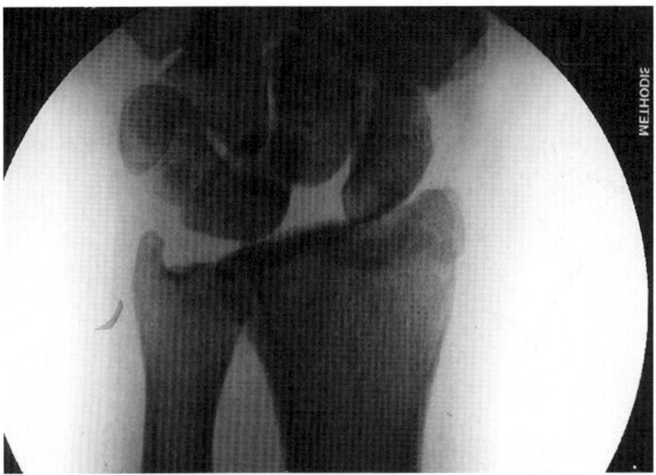

FIGURE 17.10. PA radiograph of an impacted fracture involving the scaphoid facet. In addition, a tear of the scapholunate interosseous ligament is apparent on plain radiographs.

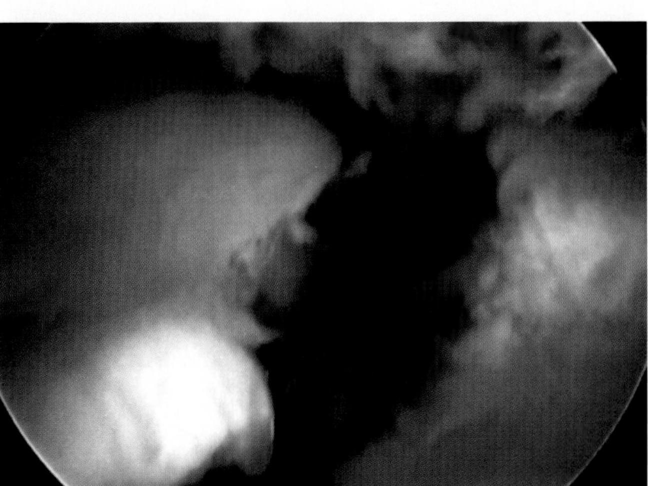

FIGURE 17.11. Arthroscopic view of the impacted scaphoid facet fracture.

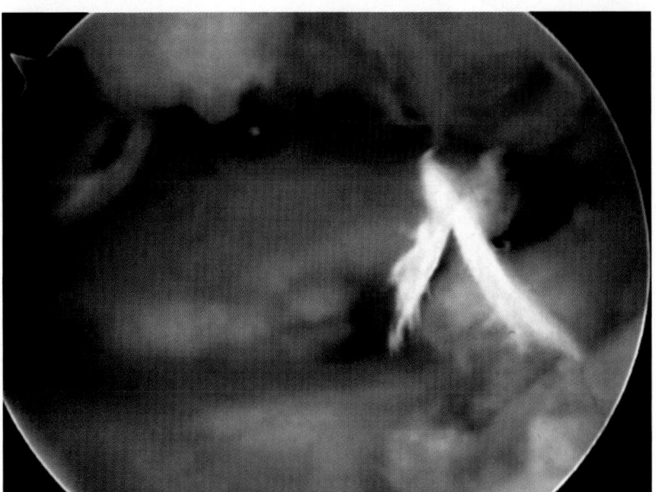

FIGURE 17.12. The impacted fracture of the scaphoid facet is elevated with a trocar in the 3-4 portal as viewed with the arthroscope in the 6-R portal.

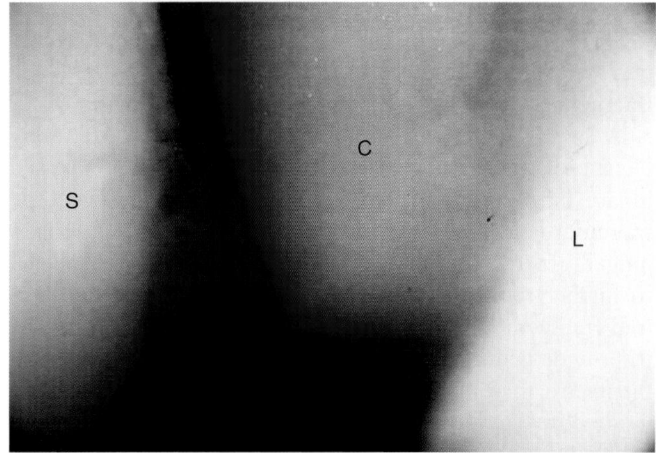

FIGURE 17.13. A complete tear of the scapholunate interosseous ligament is identified arthroscopically. This is the Geissler "drive-through sign," whereby the capitate is easily identified between the gap of the scapholunate as seen in the radial carpal space.

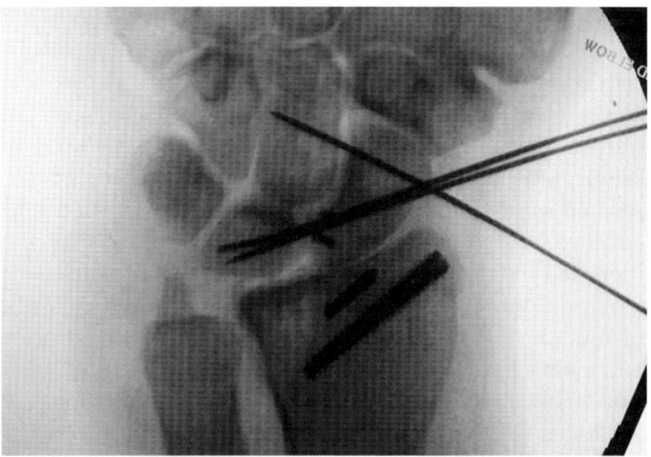

FIGURE 17.14. Anterior posterior view showing anatomical restoration of the joint surface from the impacted scaphoid facet fracture. A small open reduction was performed to repair the complete tear of the scapholunate interosseous ligament. It is felt that in complete Geissler grade IV tears open repair is preferable to arthroscopic reduction.

Three-Part Fractures

Three-part fractures involve a displaced fracture of the radial styloid and lunate facet. The radial styloid fracture may be closed reduced and percutaneously stabilized under fluoroscopic guidance. Again, it is vital to place the guide wires through a small incision to protect the dorsal sensory branch of the radial nerve when stabilizing the radial styloid fragment. The radial styloid fragment is then utilized as a landmark to which the depressed lunate facet fragment is reduced. Following percutaneous reduction and stabilization of the radial styloid fragment under fluoroscopic guidance, the wrist is suspended in the traction tower. The fracture debris and hematoma are then evacuated, and the depressed lunate facet fragment is best observed with the arthroscope in the 3-4 portal. An 18-gauge needle may be placed percutaneously directly over the depressed fragment and viewed arthroscopically as a landmark.

A large Steinmann pin is then placed approximately 2 cm proximal to the 18-gauge needle into the depressed lunate facet fragment, which is then elevated. Once the fragment is elevated back to the radial styloid fragment as judged arthroscopically, a bone tenaculum may be placed to further reduce the fracture gap between the radial styloid fragment and the depressed lunate facet fragment and to provide provisional stabilization. Once the fracture fragments are anatomically reduced as viewed arthroscopically, guide wires are placed transversely from the radial styloid subchondrally into the lunate facet fragment. If a dorsal die punch fragment is present, it is important that the guide pins be aimed dorsally to capture this fragment. Once the transverse pins are placed, it is important to pronate and supinate the wrist to ensure that the transverse pins have not violated the distal radioulnar joint.

Because of the concave nature of the distal radioulnar joint, the pins may appear under fluoroscopy to have not penetrated into the joint when in fact they have mechanically protruded into the joint. For this reason, pronate and supinate the wrist to evaluate the placement of the transverse pins. Previously, Kirschner wires were used to stabilize the fracture fragments alone. Now, headless cannulated screws are utilized if at all possible—not only to stabilize the radial styloid fragment but to stabilize the impacted lunate facet fragment. This decreases soft-tissue irritation during rehabilitation and promotes earlier range of motion. If extensive metaphysial comminution is present, a bone graft may be placed through a small dorsal incision between the fourth and fifth dorsal compartments to avoid late settling of the fracture fragments.

A volar plate may be utilized if metaphysial comminution is present. In this scenario, a standard volar approach is made over the radial side of the flexor carpi radialis. Dissection is continued down through the sheath where the flexor pollicis longus is identified and retracted ulnarly. The pronator quadratus is released off its radial border, exposing the fracture. The radial styloid fragment can be anatomically reduced back to the shaft as viewed directly through the incision. The lunate fracture fragment may be seen through the volar approach, and can be anatomically reduced and pinned through the volar approach. In this incidence, a volar plate is placed and the fracture is provisionally pinned through the plate. The wrist is then suspended in traction, and the articular reduction is viewed arthroscopically.

If the articular reduction is not anatomical, the pins may then be removed from the plate and the reduction may be fine-tuned as viewed arthroscopically. Once this reduction is felt to be anatomical, the pins are placed back through the plate to provisionally stabilize the fracture. The most distal screws are then placed through the plate into the distal articular fragment. In die punch fractures, it is particularly helpful to view the reduction while the distal screws are being placed through the plate (Figures 17.15 through 17.17). In this way, the dorsal die punch fragment can be arthroscopically viewed to be anatomical and the can

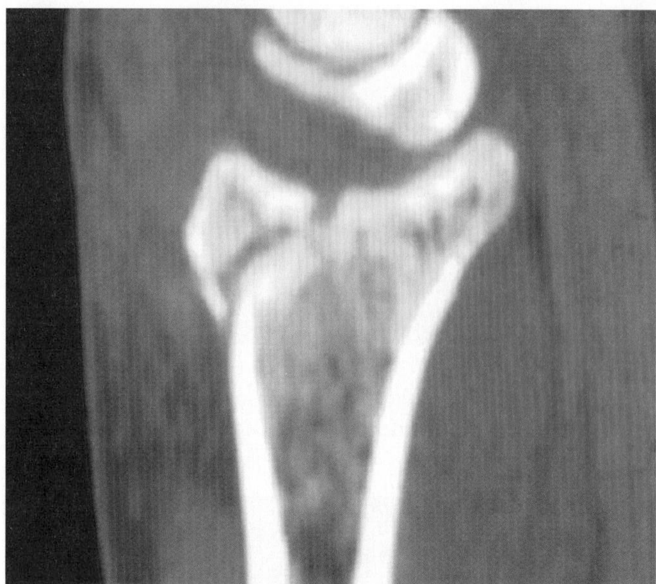

FIGURE 17.15. CT scan showing an unstable dorsal lip fracture of the distal radius.

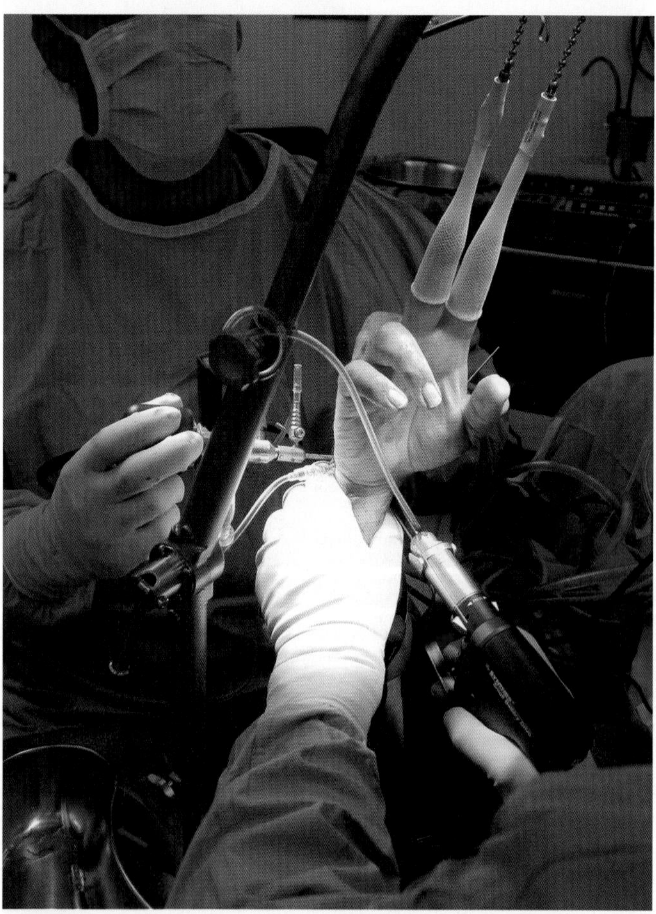

FIGURE 17.16. These fractures are typically difficult to reduce through a volar approach. However, the plate may be placed on the volar aspect and the reduction easily viewed arthroscopically.

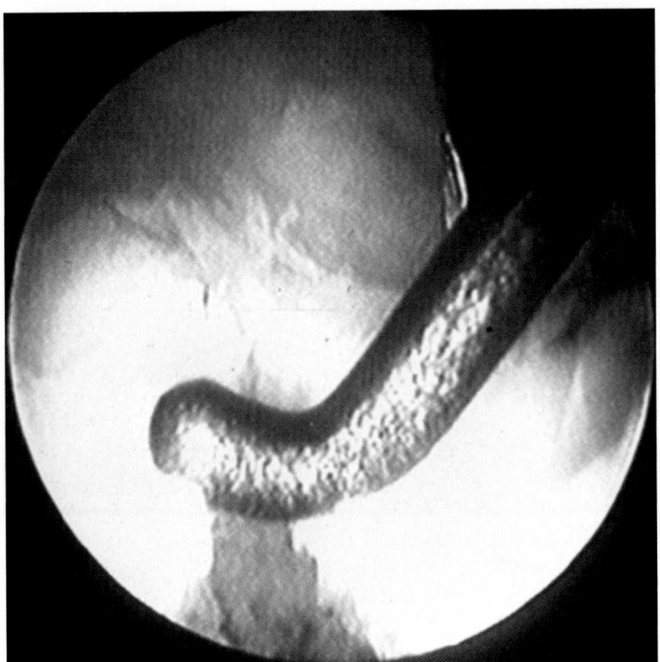

FIGURE 17.17. Arthroscopic view of the reduction of the dorsal lip fragment. The very distal pins in the plate may be viewed directly arthroscopically as they capture the dorsal lip fragment. Direct arthroscopic observation ensures that the pins are capturing the dorsal lip fragment.

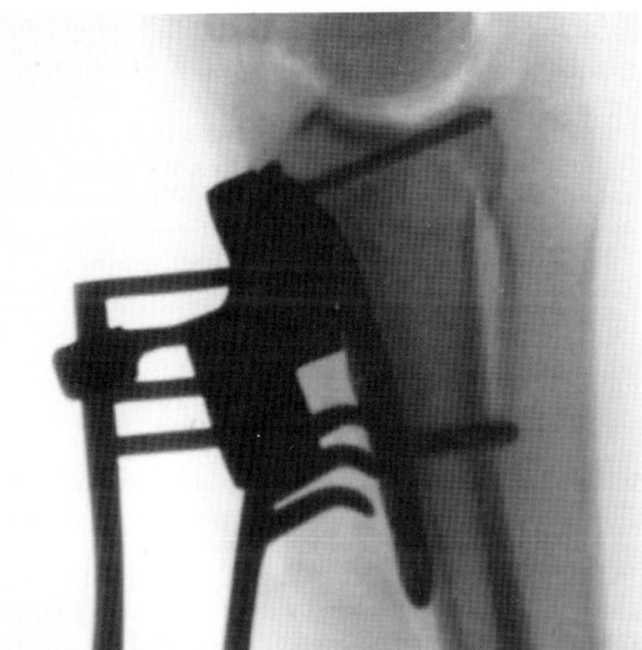

FIGURE 17.18. Fluoroscopic view confirming that the pin is capturing the small dorsal lip fragment through the volar distal radius plate.

be seen inserting into the fragment for stability (Figures 17.18 and 17.19).

The dorsal die punch fragment is best seen with the scope in the 6-R portal, or through a volar radial portal as promoted by Slutsky. In this instance, a previous volar incision has been made and the arthroscope may be placed between the radioscaphocapitate ligament and the long radiolunate ligament.[19] Particularly if any metaphysial comminution is present, plate stabilization is preferred. Volar plate fixation is very stable, and allows for earlier rehabilitation and range of motion.

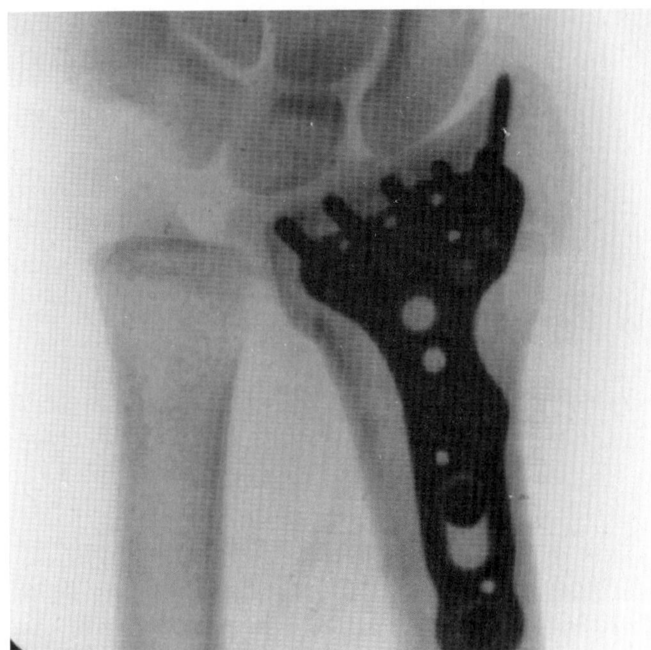

FIGURE 17.19. PA radiograph showing stabilization of the dorsal fragment.

Four-Part Fractures

In four-part fractures, the lunate facet is divided into volar and dorsal fragments (Figures 17.20 and 17.21). The volar ulnar fragment is unable to be reduced by closed manipulation. Traction on the volar wrist capsule rotates the volar ulnar fragment, causing it to be unable to be reduced by closed manipulation. The radial styloid fragment is again reduced by closed manipulation and is temporarily stabilized with Kirschner wires. A standard volar approach to the distal radius is performed as described previously. The reduction of the radial styloid fragment may be fine-tuned by direct observation of the fracture fragment and keying it into the shaft of the distal radius.

The volar ulnar fragment is then reduced under direct observation by reducing it back to the shaft and into the radial styloid fragment. It is then pinned provisionally transversely. The position of the reduction of the radial styloid and volar ulnar fragment provisionally stabilized is viewed under fluoroscopy. A volar distal radius plate is then utilized to stabilize the volar bone fragments (Figure 17.22). An initial screw is placed in the proximal portion of the plate to adjust the proximal-distal alignment of the plate in relation to the fracture fragments. The plate is then

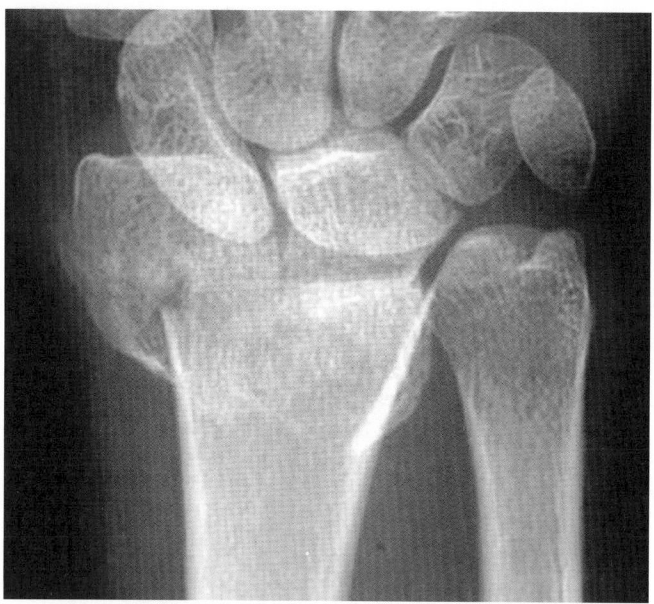

FIGURE 17.20. Comminuted metaphysial fractures with intra-articular involvement are best stabilized by a combination of arthroscopic-assisted reduction and plate stabilization.

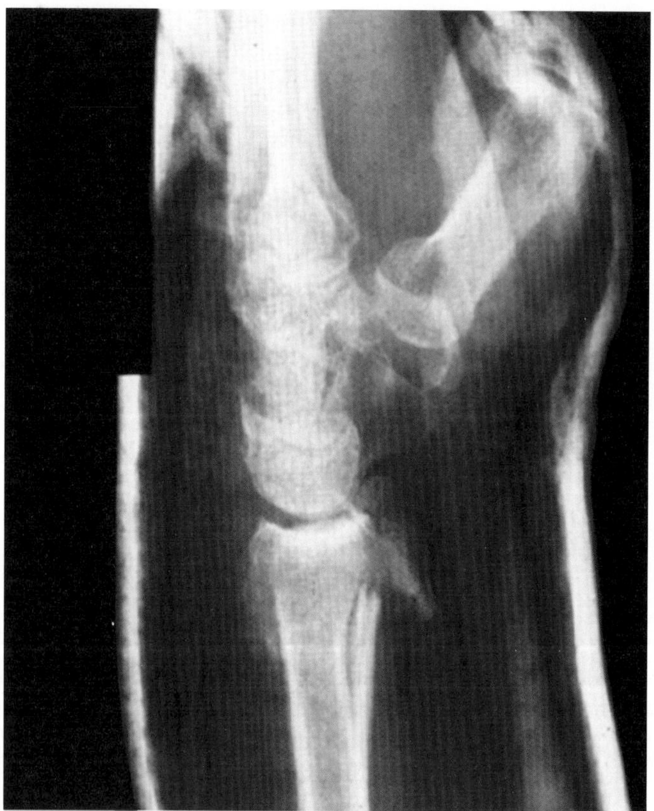

FIGURE 17.21. Similarly, four-part fractures with a large volar ulnar fragment are best stabilized by a combination of open reduction through a volar approach and confirmation of the articular reduction by arthroscopy.

provisionally pinned to the articular fragments through the holes in the plate.

The wrist is suspended in the traction tower and the arthroscope is placed in the 3-4 portal. Usually, the dorsal

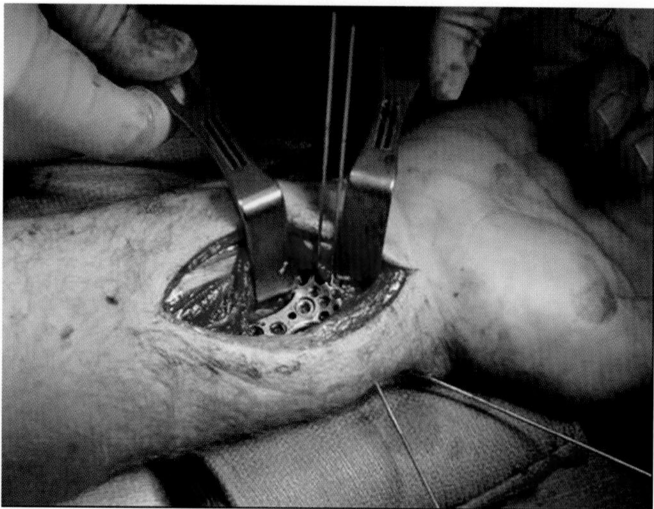

FIGURE 17.22. A standard volar approach is made to the distal radius and a volar plate is provisionally placed to stabilize the fracture. The fracture is provisionally stabilized with pins inserted through the plate.

ulnar fragment is best viewed with the arthroscope in the 6-R portal or through the volar portal as described by Slutsky. The dorsal ulnar fragment is then percutaneously elevated back to the radial styloid and reduced to the volar ulnar fragment, which is utilized as a landmark (Figures 17.23 through 17.25). The distal screws may be inserted into the plate to stabilize the articular surface (*once articular reduction of the distal radius is judged to be anatomical as viewed by the arthroscope*). It is helpful that the first screw placed is a non-locking screw, which helps reduce the fragments back through the anatomically shaped distal radius plate. Particularly in small dorsal fragments, it is helpful to view the placement of the screws arthroscopically as they are seen inserted into these fragments to provide stability (Figure 17.26).

Ulnar Styloid Fractures

Stabilization of an associated ulnar styloid fragment is usually controversial. Wrist arthroscopy provides some rationale as to when to stabilize an associate ulnar styloid fragment. Following anatomical reduction of the distal radius fracture, the tension of the articular disc is palpated arthroscopically. The arthroscope is placed in the 3-4 portal, and a probe is inserted through the 6-R portal. If there is good tension to the articular disc, the majority of the fibers of the triangular fibrocartilage complex is still attached to the base of the ulna and the ulnar styloid fragment is not stabilized. If the articular disc is lax by palpation, a peripheral tear of the triangular fibrocartilage complex is suspected. This may be covered with hematoma. It is important to debride the hematoma to obtain direct visualization of the periphery of the articular disc. A peripheral tear is then repaired arthroscopically if it is

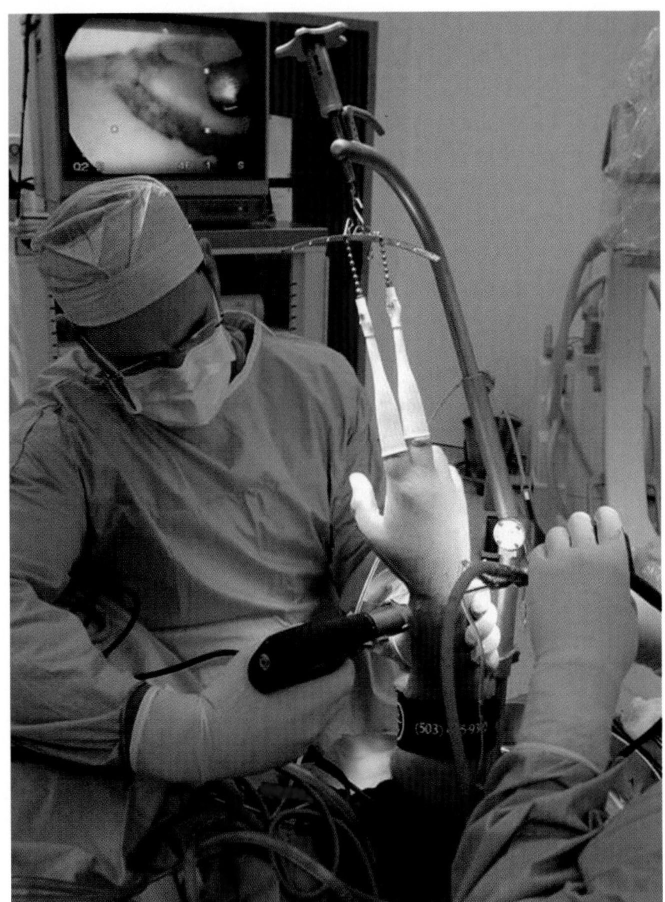

FIGURE 17.23. The wrist is then arthroscopically evaluated. Articular reduction can then be fine-tuned as viewed directly arthroscopically.

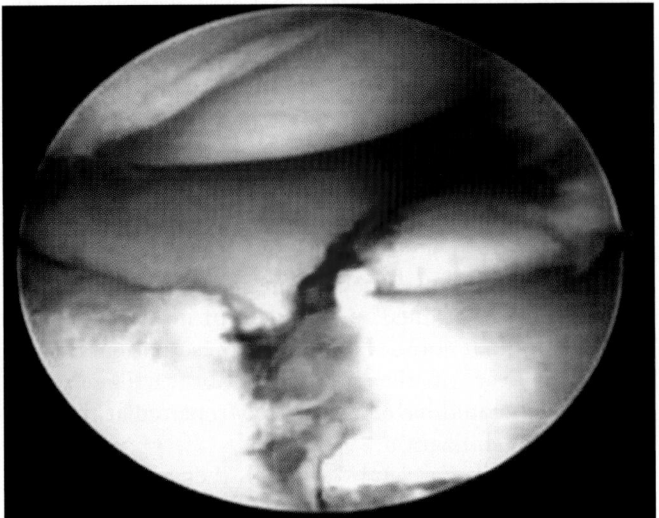

FIGURE 17.24. The comminuted intra-articular fracture is anatomically reduced as confirmed arthroscopically with the arthroscope in the 6-R portal.

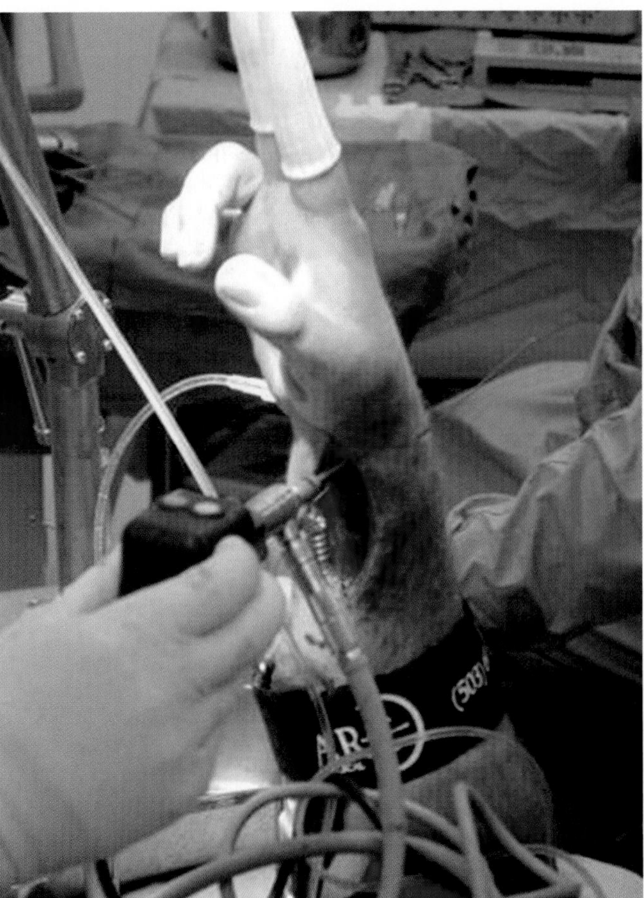

FIGURE 17.25. The reduction of the dorsal lip fragment may be viewed with the arthroscope in the 6-R portal, or through the volar portal as popularized by Slutsky.

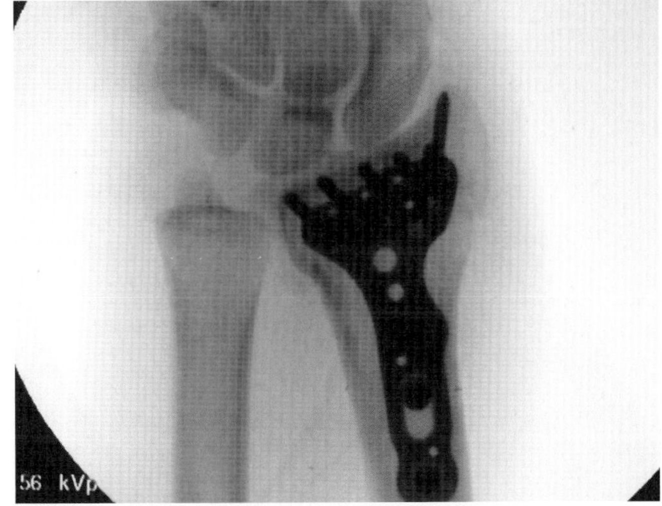

FIGURE 17.26. PA radiograph showing anatomical restoration to the joint surface of the four-part fracture.

identified (Figure 17.27). The articular disc is repaired utilizing an outside-in technique to the base of the ulna with suture anchors.

Stabilization of a large ulnar styloid fragment is considered when the articular disc is lax when palpated and no peripheral tear is identified (Figure 17.28). In this incidence, the majority of the fibers of the articular disc is attached to the displaced ulnar styloid fragment. A small incision is then made between the interval of the extensor carpi ulnaris and flexor carpi ulnaris. Blunt dissection is carried down to protect the dorsal sensory branch of the ulnar nerve, which is running just volar to the incision. The ulnar styloid fragment is then cleared of fracture debris, and is stabilized by either tension band, Kirschner wire, or preferably by a small headless cannulated screw.

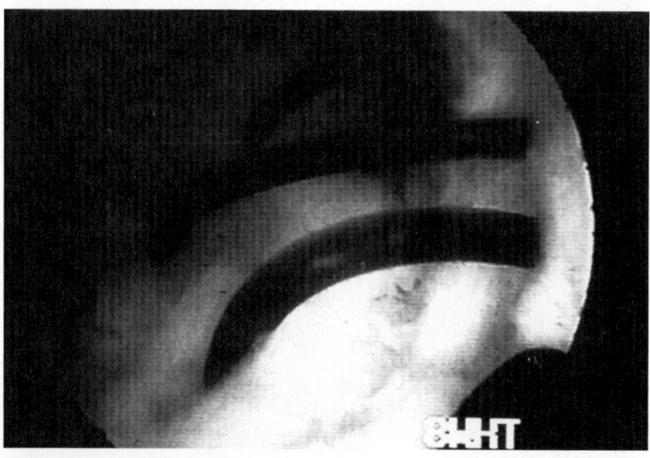

FIGURE 17.27. Wrist arthroscopy also allows for rationale of when to stabilize the ulnar styloid fragment. Following reduction of the distal radius fracture, the articular disc is palpated. In this incidence, a peripheral tear was identified and repaired arthroscopically following the reduction to the distal radius.

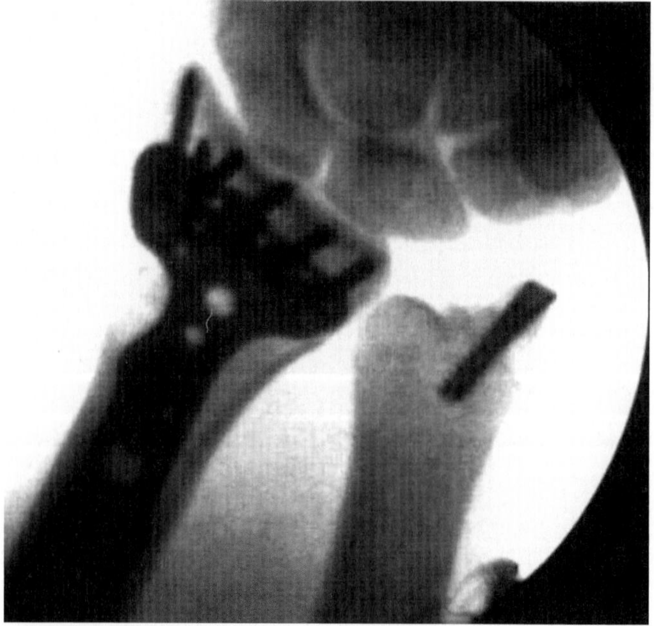

FIGURE 17.28. The patient had a large associated ulnar styloid fragment. Arthroscopic evaluation to the wrist showed laxity to the articular disc, and a peripheral tear of the triangular fibrocartilage complex was not seen. The ulnar styloid fragment was then stabilized by open reduction and internal fixation with a micro headless cannulated screw.

Discussion

The literature is relatively sparse regarding the results of arthroscopic-assisted fixation of displaced intra-articular fractures of the distal radius. Stewart et al. presented a comparison study of 12 open and 12 arthroscopic-assisted reductions of comminuted fractures of the distal radius.[20] These fractures were comminuted and were classified as AO type VII and VIII. In the arthroscopic group, they had five excellent, six good, and one fair result. The open group noted no excellent results. The authors concluded that the arthroscopic group had a significantly increased range of motion compared to the group that underwent open stabilization.

Similarly, Doi et al. reported their results in a comparison study of 38 patients who underwent arthroscopic-assisted fixation in comparison to those patients who underwent open reduction.[21] The author similarly found that the arthroscopic group had improved range of motion compared to the open group.

Ruch reported his result of a comparison study of 15 patients who underwent arthroscopic-assisted reduction and 15 patients who underwent closed reduction and were stabilized by external fixation under fluoroscopy.[22] In the 15 patients who underwent arthroscopic reduction, 10 patients had a tear of the triangular fibrocartilage complex. Seven of those tears were peripheral and underwent arthroscopic repair. No patients in the arthroscopic group had any signs of distal radioulnar joint instability at final follow-up visit. In the 15 patients who underwent closed reduction and external fixation, four patients continued to complain of instability of the distal radioulnar joint. Potentially, these patients had a peripheral tear of the triangular fibrocartilage complex—which could have been acutely repaired at the time of fracture stabilization.

Geissler and Freeland reviewed their results of 33 patients who underwent arthroscopic-assisted reduction of comminuted intra-articular fractures of the distal radius.[23] Their criteria were those fractures displaced 2 mm or more following a closed reduction. In their series, at final follow-up visit 25 patients had an anatomical reduction and eight patients had a 1-mm articular step-off. The patients were evaluated utilizing the modified Mayo wrist score and there were 20 excellent, 10 good, and 3 fair results in their series.

Simple articular fractures had a better result compared to complex fracture patterns.

In addition, they analyzed their results based on associated soft-tissue injuries. They found when a Geissler grade II scapholunate interosseous ligament was present it did not affect the final prognosis. Geissler grade II injuries were evenly distributed throughout the patients' series, and did not correlate with the final prognosis. However, when a Geissler grade III or IV tear was present in an AO type C fracture it significantly affected the final results. In the five patients with an AO type C fracture without an interosseous ligament tear, all five patients had an excellent result. However, in the five patients with an AO type C fracture with a Geissler grade III or IV interosseous ligament tear there were four good results and one fair result. It appeared that the presence of a Geissler grade III or IV interosseous ligament tear significantly affected the final prognosis in their study in AO type C fractures.

Summary

Wrist arthroscopy is a valuable adjunct in the management of displaced intra-articular fractures of the distal radius. It allows for evaluation of the articular reduction under bright light and magnified conditions. It has been previously reported that restoration of the articular surface is important and affects the patient's final prognosis. Particularly, arthroscopy allows for detection of mal-rotation of fracture fragments—which is very difficult to judge under fluoroscopy. In addition, the washing out of fracture hematoma and debris may allow for improved range of motion (as shown by the comparison studies of Stewart and Doi).

Wrist arthroscopy also allows for the detection and management of associated intra-articular soft-tissue injuries, which have been shown to occur with a high incidence with intra-articular fractures of the distal radius. Arthroscopic detection of soft-tissue injuries allows for acute stabilization. It is felt that management of acute soft-tissue injuries has a better prognosis as compared to chronic reconstruction. Tears of the triangular fibrocartilage complex have been shown to be the most frequent associated soft-tissue injury with fractures of the distal radius. In addition, chondral defects or loose bodies that would not normally be seen with plain radiographs are frequently identified arthroscopically and can be removed from both the radiocarpal and midcarpal spaces.

Associated intra-articular soft-tissue injuries or loose bodies not detected on plain radiographs may be an explanation why some patients continue to complain of pain (particularly on the ulnar side of the wrist) for several months post-injury despite anatomical restoration of the fracture as seen on plain radiographs.[24] Last, wrist arthroscopy provides a rationale of when and when not to stabilize the displaced ulnar styloid fragment when it is associated with a fracture of the distal radius.

References

1. Lafontaine M, Hardy D, Delince P. Stability assessment of distal radius fractures. Injury 1989;20:208–10.
2. Short WH, Palmer AK, Werner FW, et al. A biomechanical study of distal radial fractures. J Hand Surg 1987;12A:529–34.
3. Trumble TE, Schmitt SR, Vedder NB. Fractures affecting functional outcome of displaced intra-articular distal radius fractures. J Hand Surg [Am] 1994;19A:325–40.
4. Geissler WB, Savoie FH. Arthroscopic techniques of the wrist. Mediguide to Orthopedics 1992;11:1–8.
5. Geissler WB. Intra-articular distal radius fractures: The role of arthroscopy? Hand Clin 2005;11:407–16.
6. Geissler WB. Arthroscopically assisted reduction of intra-articular fractures of the distal radius. Hand Clin 1995; 11:19–29.
7. Knirk JL, Jupiter JB. Intra-articular fractures of the distal end of the radius in young adults. J Bone Joint Surg 1986;68A:647–58.
8. Bradway JK, Amadio PC, Cooney WP. Open reduction and internal fixation of displaced comminuted intra-articular fractures of the distal end of the radius. J Bone Joint Surg 1989;71A:839–47.
9. Fernandez DL, Geissler WB. Treatment of displaced articular fractures of the radius. J Hand Surg 1991;16:375–84.
10. Edwards CC, III, Harasztic J, McGillivary GR, Gutow AP. Intra-articular distal radius fractures: Arthroscopic assessment of radiographically assisted reduction. J Hand Surg 2001;26:A1036–A41.
11. Hixon ML, Fitzrandolph R, McAndrew M, et al. Acute ligamentous tears of the wrist associated with Colles fractures. Proceedings, American Society for Surgery of the Hand, Baltimore, 1989.
12. Fontes D, Lenoble E, DeSomer B, et al. Lesions ligamentaires associus aux fractures distales du radius. Ann Chir Main 1992;11:119–25.
13. Mohanti RC, Kar N. Study of triangular fibrocartilage of the wrist joint in Colles fracture. Injury 1979;11:311–24.
14. Geissler WB, Freeland AE, Savoie FH, et al. Carpal instability associated with intra-articular distal radius fractures. Proceedings, American Academy Orthopedic Surgeons Annual Meeting, San Francisco, 1993.
15. Lindau T. Treatment of injuries to the ulnar side of the wrist occurring with distal radial fractures. Hand Clin 2005;21: 417–25.
16. Hanker GJ. Wrist arthroscopy in distal radius fractures. Proceedings, Arthroscopy Association North America Annual Meeting, Albuquerque, NM, 1993.
17. Melone CP. Articular fractures of the distal radius. Orthop Clin North Am 1984;15:217–35.
18. Mudgal CS, Jones WA. Scapholunate diastasis: A component of fractures of the distal radius. J Hand Surg 1990;15B: 503–05.
19. Levy HJ, Glickel SZ. Arthroscopic assisted internal fixation of intra-articular wrist fractures. Arthroscopy 1993;9: 122–23.
20. Stewart NJ, Berger RA. Comparison study of arthroscopic as open reduction of comminuted distal radius fractures. Presented at the 53rd Annual Meeting of the American Society for Surgery of the Hand [programs and abstracts]. January 11, 1998, Scottsdale, AZ.
21. Doi K, Hatturi T, Otsuka K, Abe T, Tamamoto H. Intra-articular fractures of the distal aspect of the radius arthroscopically

assisted reduction compared with open reduction and internal fixation. J Bone Joint Surg 1999;81A:1093–110.
22. Ruch DS, Vallee J, Poehling GG, Smith BP, Kuzma GR. Arthroscopic reduction versus fluoroscopic reduction of intra-articular distal radius fractures. Arthroscopy 2004;20: 225–30.
23. Geissler WB, Freeland AE. Arthroscopically assisted reduction of intra-articular distal radial fractures. Clin Orthop 1996;327:125–34.
24. Hollingworth R, Morris J. The importance of the ulnar side of the wrist in fractures of the distal end of the radius. Injury 1976;7:223.

Francisco del Piñal

CHAPTER 18

Correction of Mal-United Intra-Articular Distal Radius Fractures with an Inside-Out Osteotomy Technique

Rationale and Basic Science Pertinent to the Procedure

The benefits of early correction of mal-united extra-articular distal radius fractures are well known.[1] Obviously, when the mal-union affects also the joint surface the altered mechanics[2] will lead to rapid radiocarpal osteoarthritis in young active individuals.[3–5] Although this articular disruption calls for immediate correction, there are just a few papers that deal with the problem.[4,6–8] Recently, Ring et al.[8] reported good results by using a direct open approach. The technique is difficult, however, and there is a risk of causing additional damage due to the limited access to the joint space through a capsulotomy incision. Furthermore, devascularization of the fracture fragments due to detachment from their soft-tissue attachments is possible.

We have performed an open osteototomy for correction of mal-united intra-articular distal radius fractures several times. We have been limited to performing relatively simple osteotomies (i.e., single longitudinal or coronal osteotomy, or simple transverse) due to the previously described difficulties. Our main concern, however, was the difficulty in visualizing the articular reduction. In effect, once the mal-united fragment was reduced (elevated) the narrow radiocarpal space prevented an adequate assessment of the joint congruity without extreme manipulation of the wrist. The surgeon must solely rely on fluoroscopy to assess the reduction, even though fluoroscopy has been shown to be unreliable with regard to evaluating any articular gap or step-off under the best of circumstances.[9]

Bearing in mind these limitations, we sought a method of assessing the status of the articular cartilage in the area of mal-union that would at the same time allow us to accurately identify fracture lines. This would allow us to carry out the osteotomy under direct visual control, which would provide an unimpeded and magnified view of the quality of the reduction. Our initial attempts with the classic (wet) arthroscopic techniques were frustrating due to fluid extravasation through the portals and air bubble formation that continually impaired the view.

Inspired by the experience with laparoscopy, in which carbon dioxide is used in place of fluid—and by the invaluable informal comments by other colleagues who were performing parts of arthroscopic ganglion resection without fluid irrigation (personal communication, doctors Atzei and Luchetti of Italy and doctors Zaidemberg and Perotto of Argentina)—we were inspired to perform wrist arthroscopy without infusing fluid (i.e., the dry technique).[10] This proved to be crucial to the execution of the technique described in this chapter. An intra-articular inside-out osteotomy[11] of distal radius mal-unions hinges on use of the "dry" arthroscopic technique, which is therefore also presented in detail (along with some technical tips).

Indications

The procedure is indicated for nascent mal-unions (i.e., less than three months) of intra-articular fractures of the distal radius. It allows one to define each cartilage containing fragment and to recreate the original articular fracture line without fear of creating new fracture lines. The technique can be used in cases with irregularly defined fracture fragments that are not amenable to conventional osteotomy techniques. With this technique, there is minimal interference with the ligament attachments and hence with the blood supply of the osteotomized fragment.

Contraindications

There are no absolute contraindications to this technique, provided the cartilage is not worn out.[11] We have no experience with osteotomies older than three months. It is possible that the presence of cartilage degeneration or arthrofibrosis might impede the arthroscopic procedure, but we have no data to support or refute this. A loss of articular cartilage would preclude this operation, in which case we would then opt for an osteochondral graft[12] or a partial wrist arthrodesis.[13,14] We would therefore recommend a diagnostic arthroscopy in cases older than three months prior to proceeding with an osteotomy.

Surgical Technique

The surgical technique is similar to a standard wrist arthroscopy save that irrigation fluid is not used during the procedure. It is of note, however, that this technique is more cumbersome and complicated than the average wrist arthroscopy. First, it requires an open exposure of the distal radius for plate fixation of the fragments in addition to the arthroscopic-assisted osteotomy. Second, it requires alternating the hand from a suspended position to flat on the operating table. Third, fluoroscopy is used periodically during the procedure—which is facilitated by placing the hand flat. The osteotomes and probes used need to be sturdier than the average arthroscopic instruments (Figure 18.1).

Finally, the assistance of another experienced surgeon is integral to the procedure (Figure 18.2). It is important that everyone on the surgical team be prepared and familiar with their assigned role in order to minimize operating time. It is helpful for the surgeon to preplan the osteotomies beforehand based on a review of the preoperative X-rays and if possible of the original fracture films. The author has found a good-quality preoperative CT scan to be invaluable, since the intraoperative view of the joint can be quite confusing due to the disruption (Figure 18.3).

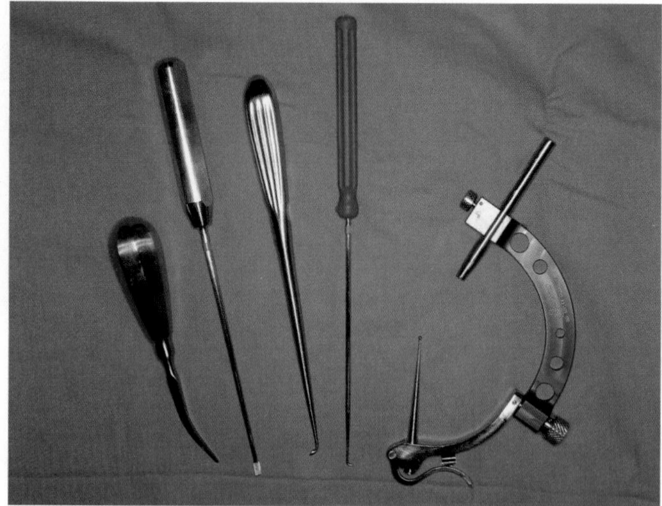

FIGURE 18.1. Instrumentation required for the procedure (from left to right): impactor, osteotome, strong-angled curette, shoulder probe, and small-joint arthroscopic guide.

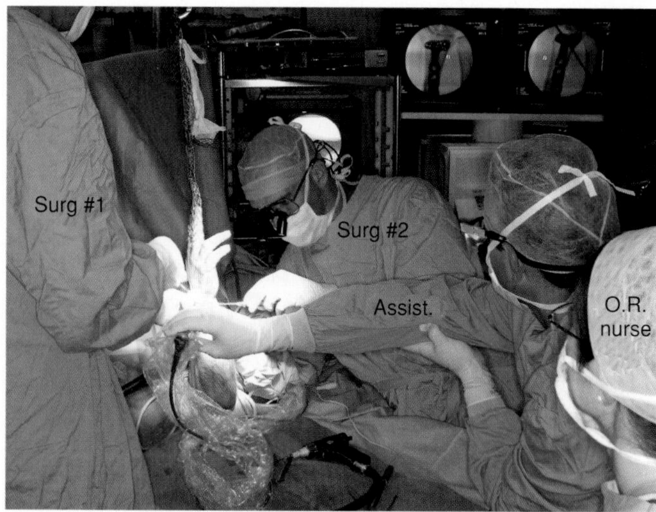

FIGURE 18.2. Set-up. The first surgeon is controlling the reduction, and the second surgeon is stabilizing the reduction by introducing the distal pegs on the plate. (A) Resident is holding the camera (assistant). The first surgeon has in front the arthroscopic tower and the fluoroscopy display.

The arm is exsanguinated with an Esmarch bandage and the tourniquet elevated to 250 mmHg. Prior to suspending the hand, the skin incisions for the proposed site of plate fixation are prepared with the arm lying on the hand table. A limited volar ulnar incision is used for a volar ulnar shearing type of intra-articular mal-union. A limited Henry approach is used in the case of a mal-united radial styloid fragment or multifragmented mal-union. A plate is then pre-placed and held in position with a single screw through its stem.

The hand is then placed on traction from a bow with a custom-made system that allows one to easily change the hand from a horizontal to a vertical position while

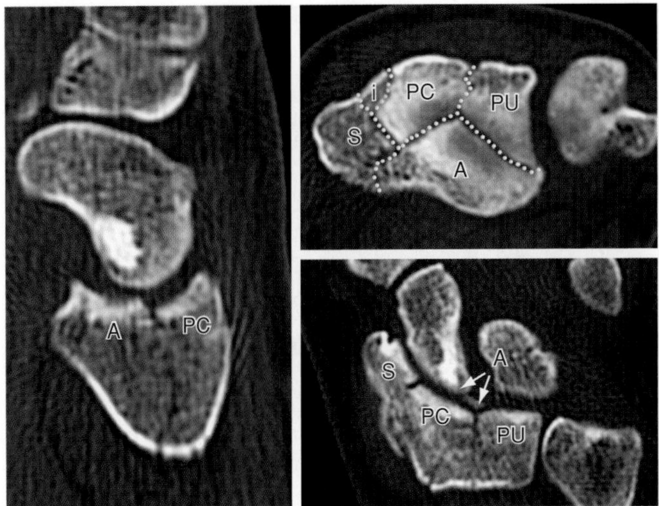

FIGURE 18.3. Preoperative CAT scan of a C3.1 fracture. (A) A 3.5-mm step-off on the scaphoid fossa (A = anterior fragment; PC = postero-central). (B) Corresponding axial view of the same case, showing a multipiece fracture. The styloid (S), postero-central (PC), and a small (I) intermiddle fragment are depressed, in relation to the anterior fragment (A) and the postero-ulnar fragment (PU) (see C). (C) Coronal CAT scan showing the depression of the styloid (S) and postero-central (PC) in relation to the postero-ulnar (PU) and anterior (A) fragments. Only the former will require correction. (*From Piñal F, et al. Dry arthroscopy of the wrist: surgical technique. J Hand Surg 2007;32A:119–23.*)

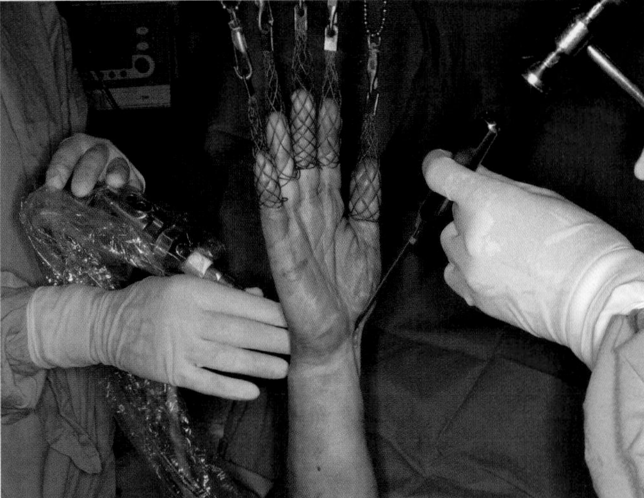

FIGURE 18.4. The osteotomy is being performed through the volar radial portal while the assistant is holding the camera. Often at the same time surgeon 2 is directing the osteotomy through a dorsal 3-4 portal.

maintaining a sterile field.[11] The standard 3-/,4 and 6-R portals are developed. Transverse 1-cm skin incisions are preferred on the dorsum of the wrist because they heal with a minimal scar. To avoid lacerating any nerve or tendon, a superficial skin incision is made with a #15 blade. A hemostat is used to widen the portal to permit the smooth entrance of the osteotomes and other necessary instruments (Figure 18.1). Apart from dorsal portals, a volar radial (VR) portal is always used. If a Henry incision is planned, the portal is developed as recommended by Levy and Glickel.[15] Otherwise, we follow the technique of Doi et al. or of Slutsky[16,17] (Figure 18.4). The quality of the articular cartilage over the adjacent scaphoid and lunate is assessed along with exploration of the midcarpal joint if there is any doubt as to the integrity of the interosseous ligaments.

Initially, a 2.7-mm scope is introduced through the 3-/,4 portal and the joint palpated (for this we prefer the stronger shoulder probe). The consistency of the cartilage, and the presence and location of steps are assessed. A shaver can be helpful to remove the synovitis and fibrin, which is always present and obscures the view (2.9-mm incisor blade; 2.9-mm barrel abrader, Dyonics, Smith & Nephew, Inc., Andover, MA, USA). Air should flow freely into the joint when the suction of the synoviotome or bur is working. Otherwise, the suction will suck the capsule in and obscure the view. Sufficient air enters through the side tube of the arthroscope's sheath. The surgeon *should keep the valve open* throughout the procedure.

Once major cartilage destruction has been ruled out, and the fragments to be mobilized are defined, the scope is moved to the 6-R portal (the 3-/,4 and VR portals are used for instrumentation). For cutting the fragments, we use periosteal elevators that are commercially available for shoulder surgery (Artrex AR-1342–30 degrees and AR-1342–15 degrees, Artrex, Naples, FL, USA). These elevators have a width of 4 mm and are strong enough to cut the fragments by gently tapping with a hammer. Recently, we have incorporated straight and curved osteotomes (Artrex AR-1770 and AR-1771) that can also be helpful because their different shapes are ideally suited to following the irregular shape of fracture lines. To avoid the risk of lacerating extensor tendons when introducing the osteotomes through the 3-/,4 portal, the blade of the osteotome should be gently introduced parallel to the tendon under direct visual control and then rotated while inside the joint. Gentle maneuvers are necessary, as there is a risk of cutting tendons if plunging volarly or dorsally.

The displaced fragments are fully mobilized by carefully prying them apart with the osteotome. In most cases, the fragments are disimpacted and easily elevated by hooking them with a strong shoulder probe and pulling upward. On one occasion, we have had to resort to elevation of a fragment from the outside with the use of a Steinmann pin introduced into the exact spot and advanced through a small arthroscopic guide (Ref 4291, Dyonics, Smith & Nephew, Inc., Andover, MA, USA).

Often, scar and new bone formation between the fragments impede reduction. This early granulation tissue should be resected with the help of small curettes or burs introduced through the portals. Once the reduction is acceptable (Figure 18.5), one surgeon maintains the position of the fragments while the assistant inserts the distal locking pegs in the plate. This step may be difficult because the flexor carpi radialis (FCR) and digital flexors are under

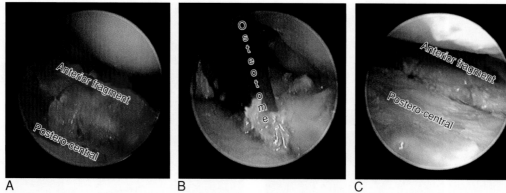

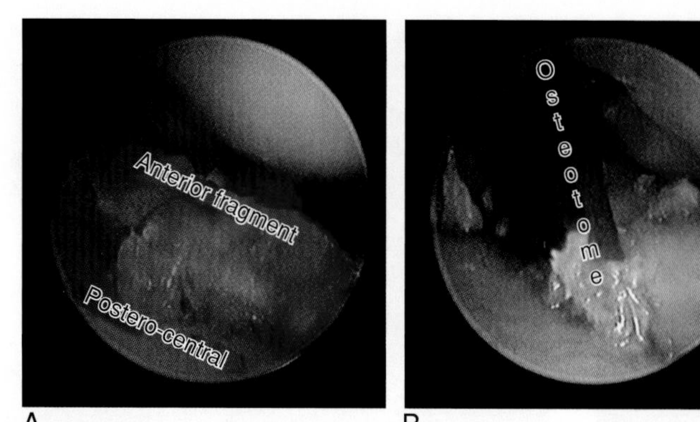

FIGURE 18.5. Correction of a step-off in the patient shown in Figure 18.2. In the right wrist, the arthroscope is in 6-R (at the very far upper left corner is the styloid). (A) Step-off on the scaphoid fossa. (B) The osteotome (entering the joint through the volo-radial portal) is separating the mal-united fragments. (C) Corresponding view after reduction. (*From Piñal F, et al. Dry arthroscopy of the wrist: surgical technique. J Hand Surg 2007;32A:119–23.*)

tension (due to the traction) and impede insertion of any ulnar screws in the plate. This step is facilitated by backing off the wrist traction sufficiently to allow tendon retraction by insertion of a Farabeuf retractor. A compromise must be made in order to prevent a complete collapse of the radiocarpal space.

Once the articular fragments have been secured under arthroscopic control, the hand is laid flat on the operating table and the rest of the screws are inserted in the plate. The type of fixation depends on the configuration of the mal-union. In one case, we used a single screw to secure a volar ulnar fragment. In another, a 2.7-mm buttress plate was used to stabilize a styloid fragment. In the most common situation (in which there are four or more fragments), a plate with locking distal pegs is preferred (DVR, Hand Innovations, Miami, FL, USA).

The hand is again suspended under traction for a final inspection of the articular surface. The joint is then irrigated with 10 to 30 cc of saline introduced through the scope's side tube, and a shaver is used to remove all debris. Fluoroscopy can be used repeatedly throughout the procedure by releasing the hand from the traction bow.[11] Some authors find it easier to perform wrist arthroscopy with the hand lying flat on the table, but we have no experience with this technique.[18]

The portals are closed with paper tape or a single stitch, and the wrist is placed in a removable splint. In all our cases the fixation was sufficiently stable as to start protected range of motion on the first postoperative visit (48 hours).

Practical Tips

The entire operation can be carried out in less than 2 hours of tourniquet time, provided the surgeon is familiar with the "dry" technique of wrist arthroscopy and the assistants are well prepared and efficient. Presently, we perform virtually all of our arthroscopic procedures (such as ulnar head recession and ganglion removal) without fluid. The advantages are many: no fluid extravasation through the portals, no air bubbles or sudden loss of vision, no risk of compartment syndrome, less postoperative swelling, and presumably less pain.

From a practical point of view, the lack of extravasated fluid allows one to easily define the tissue planes during an open approach to the distal radius. One disadvantage is the learning curve that comes with mastering any new technique. A frequent frustration of the dry technique is the frequent loss of vision from blood or soft-tissue splashes. Valuable time is lost by removing the scope for cleaning each time this occurs. There are several tricks to maintaining visual access that should be kept in mind.[10,11]

- The first recommendation is to avoid getting too close with the tip of the scope when working with burs or ostetomes in order to avoid splashes that might block your vision. It is preferable to first inspect the area of interest and then slightly pull the scope back prior to inserting your working instrument. For the same reason, avoid touching the tip of the scope with your instruments (probe, synoviotomes, and so on).
- If you get a minor splash at the tip of your scope, you can remove it by gently rubbing the tip of the scope on the local soft tissue (capsule, fat, and so on). This maneuver will clear the view sufficiently.
- If there is blood or blood clots (as after a fracture), you can clear any debris by wetting with 10 or 20 cc of saline through the side valve of the scope and then aspirating with the synoviotome. In general, this should provide a sufficiently dry field.
- It is ideal to have an absolute dry field, and for this we use small (13 x 13 mm) or medium (25 x 25 mm) surgical patties [Ref. 800–04000, size 1/2 inch x 1/2 inch; Ref. 800–04003, size 1 ft x 1 ft (25 x 25 mm) Neuray, Xomed, Jacksonville, FL, USA]. The small patty can be directly rolled and directly introduced into the joint by a grasper. The large patties have to be slightly modified by cutting them into the shape of a triangle, which facilitates

removal from the joint. If the patties become entangled, they can be removed pulling on the tail or by retrieval with a grasper.

- One must understand that much of the time vision will not be completely clear but still sufficient to safely accomplish the goals of the procedure. Having a completely clear field except for specific times during the procedure is unnecessary and wastes valuable time.
- The synoviotome, bur, or any other instruments connected to a suction machine can clog because the aspirated debris dries out. This requires frequent clearing by injecting saline through the tubing. This can be minimized by periodic saline aspiration from an external basin.

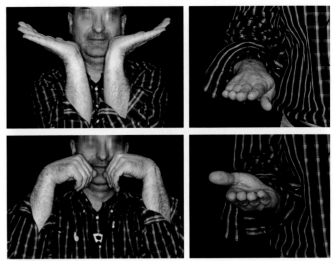

FIGURE 18.7. Results of the same patient after six months.

Results

The technique presented in this paper is drawn from experience in four patients with nascent intra-articular malunions of relatively short duration (five weeks to three months), with a follow-up of 18 days to 6 months. Two patients had a single fragment mobilized (one anteromedial fragment, one styloid fragment). The other two patients had two or more fragments mobilized (both C31 fractures of the AO classification) (Figures 18.6 and 18.7). Gaps of less than 1 mm were unavoidable after the operation due to a preexisting loss of cartilage and early granulation tissue, but intra-articular steps were reduced to 0 mm (from a maximum of 5 mm).

It may be argued that fragments may be more easily defined early on by simply breaking the external callus. Based on the experience of our group and others, however, impacted cartilage containing fracture fragments is soundly healed by as early as three to four weeks and needs to be redefined with the use of an osteotome.[19,20] Piecemeal fragmentation can occur if the mobilization is not done carefully. Herein lies the advantage of the procedure. The arthroscope allows us to follow the exact line of chondral fracture under magnification, and to restore the anatomy of the cartilaginous surface.

The inside-out technique is a minimally invasive technique that allows full assessment of the articular deformity, a more precise osteotomy, and mobilization of the displaced fracture fragments. Even irregular fragments, not amenable to other techniques, can be dealt with by this procedure. Correction of step-offs was achieved in every case with an accuracy of 0 mm. Residual gaps of about 1 mm were common due to cartilage loss, interposition of newly formed bone, and presumably cartilage destruction from the original injury. The procedure can be incorporated easily by any surgeon familiar with arthroscopy.

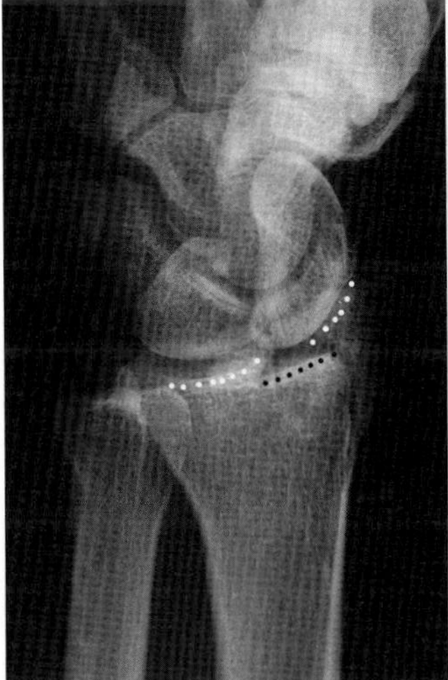

A

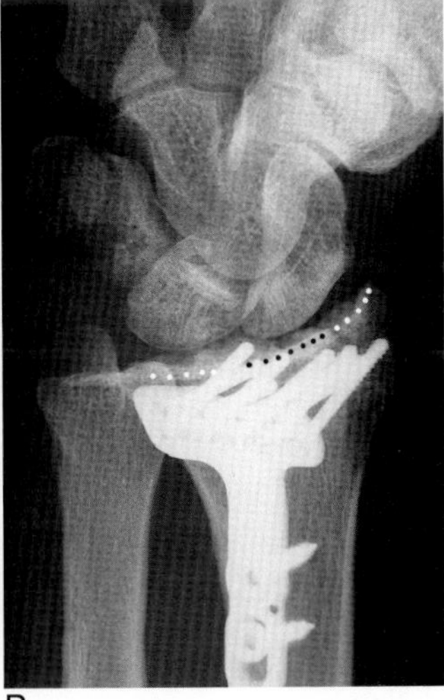

B

FIGURE 18.6. Same patient as in Figures 18.2 and 18.3. (A) Preoperative X-ray (depressed fragments highlighted by black dots). (B) Restoration of the articular line (six weeks). *(From Piñal F, et al. Dry arthroscopy of the wrist: surgical technique. J Hand Surg 2007;32A:119–23.)*

Acknowledgments

Gratitude goes to Mr. Robert Jenkins for help with the English translation of this chapter.

References

1. Jupiter JB, Ring D. A comparison of early and late reconstruction of malunited fractures of the distal end of the radius. J Bone Joint Surg 1996;78A:739–48.
2. Wagner WF Jr., Tencer AF, Kiser P, Trumble TE. Effects of intra-articular distal radius depression on wrist joint contact characteristics. J Hand Surg 1996;21A:554–660.
3. Knirk JL, Jupiter JB. Intra-articular fractures of the distal end of the radius in young adults. J Bone Joint Surg 1986; 68A:647–59.

4. Fernandez DL. Reconstructive procedures for malunion and traumatic arthritis. Orthop Clin North Am 1993;24:341–63.
5. Trumble TE, Schmitt SR, Vedder NB. Factors affecting functional outcome of displaced intra-articular distal radius fractures. J Hand Surg 1994;19A:325–40.
6. González del Piño J, Nagy L, González Hernandez E, Bartolome del Valle E. Osteotomías intraarticulares complejas del radio por fractura. Indicaciones y técnica quirúrgica. Revista de Ortopedia y Traumatología 2000;44:406–17.
7. Thivaios GC, McKee MD. Sliding osteotomy for deformity correction following malunion of volarly displaced distal radial fractures. J Orthop Trauma 2003;17:326–33.
8. Ring D, Prommersberger KJ, González del Piño J, Capomassi M, Slullitel M, Jupiter JB. Corrective osteotomy for malunited articular fractures of the distal radius. J Bone Joint Surg Am 2005;87:1503–09.
9. Edwards CC II, Haraszti CJ, McGillivary GR, Gutow AP. Intra-articular distal radius fractures: Arthroscopic assessment of radiographically assisted reduction. J Hand Surg 2001;26A:1036–41.
10. Piñal F del, Garcia-Bernal FJ, Pisani D, Regalado J, Ayala H. The dry technique for wrist arthroscopy. J Hand Surg 2007;32A:119–23.
11. Piñal F del, Garcia-Bernal FJ, Delgado J, Sanmartín M, Regalado J. Correction of malunited intra-articular distal radius fractures with an inside-out osteotomy technique. J Hand Surg 2006;31A:1029–34.
12. Piñal F del, García-Bernal JF, Delgado J, Regalado J, Sanmartín M. Reconstruction of the distal radius facet by a free vascularized osteochondral autograft: Anatomic study and report of a case. J Hand Surg 2005;30A:1200–10.
13. Saffar P. Radio-lunate arthrodesis for distal radial intraarticular malunion. J Hand Surg 1996;21B:14–20.
14. Garcia-Elias M, Lluch A, Ferreres A, Papini-Zorli I, Rahimtoola ZO. Treatment of radiocarpal degenerative osteoarthritis by radioscapholunate arthrodesis and distal scaphoidectomy. J Hand Surg 2005;30A:8–15.
15. Levy HJ, Glickel SZ. Arthroscopic assisted internal fixation of volar intraarticular wrist fractures. Arthroscopy 1993; 9:122–24.
16. Doi K, Hattori Y, Otsuka K, Abe Y, Yamamoto H. Intra-articular fractures of the distal aspect of the radius: Arthroscopically assisted reduction compared with open reduction and internal fixation. J Bone Joint Surg 1999;81A:1093–110.
17. Slutsky DJ. Clinical applications of volar portals in wrist arthroscopy. Tech Hand Up Extrem Surg 2004;8:229–38.
18. Huracek J, Troeger H. Wrist arthroscopy without distraction: A technique to visualise instability of the wrist after a ligamentous tear. J Bone Joint Surg 2000;82B:1011–12.
19. Marx RG, Axelrod TS. Intraarticular osteotomy of distal radius malunions. Clin Orthop 1996;327:152–57.
20. Piñal F del, Garcia-Bernal FJ, Delgado J, Sanmartin M, Regalado J. Results of osteotomy, open reduction, and internal fixation for late-presenting malunited intra-articular fractures of the base of the middle phalanx. J Hand Surg 2005; 30:1039–50.

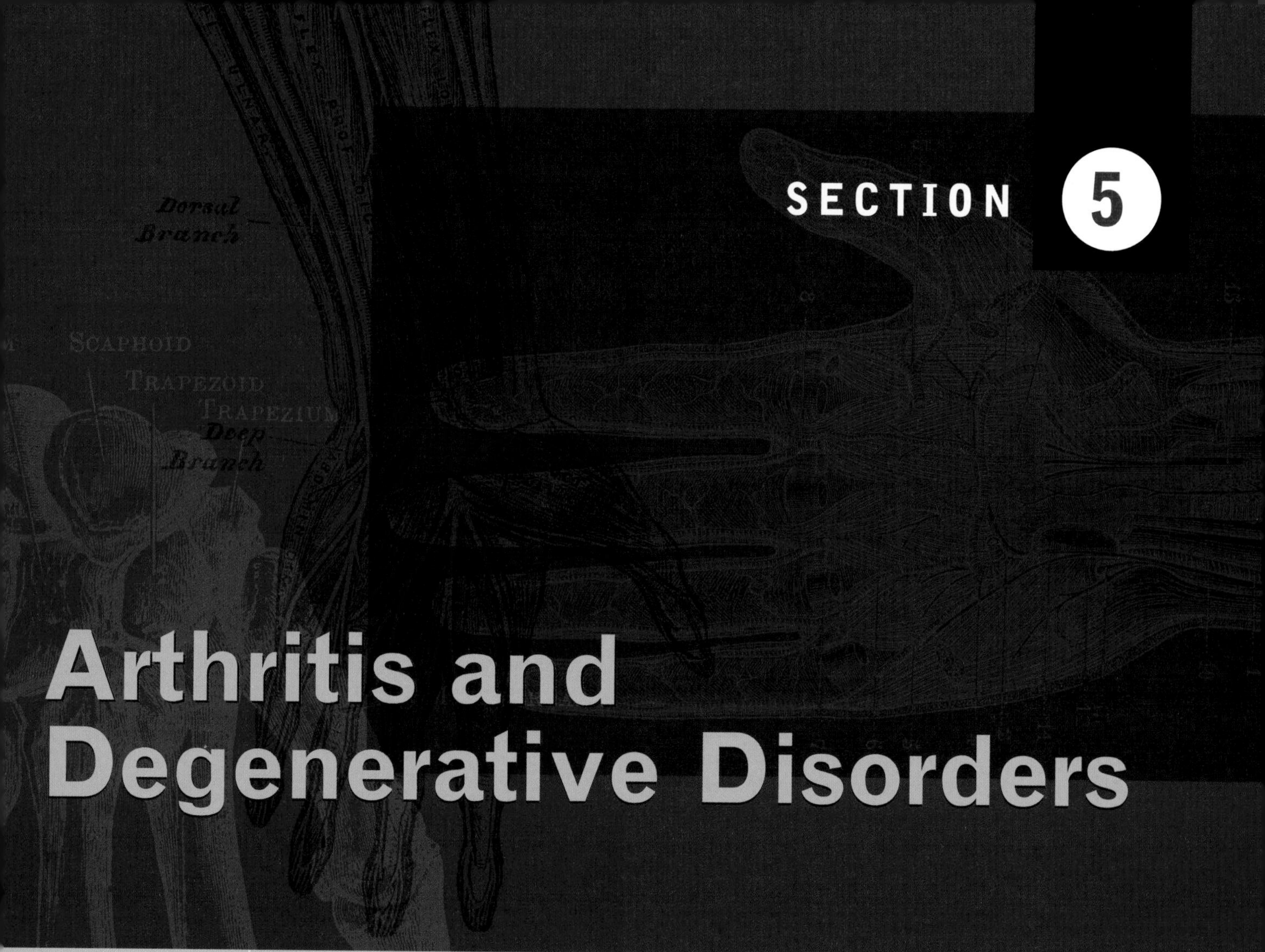

SECTION 5

Arthritis and Degenerative Disorders

David J. Slutsky

CHAPTER 19

Arthroscopic Wrist Capsulotomy

Introduction

Wrist contractures can occur following any type of wrist injury, but are most prevalent following distal radius fractures. Ganglion excision, carpal dislocation or fracture, previous wrist surgery, reflex sympathetic dystrophy, and prolonged immobilization may all lead to a loss of wrist motion. Watson has previously described a release of the volar and dorsal wrist capsule through open capsulotomies.[1] A similar approach has been described for the distal radioulnar joint.[2] Arthroscopic release of wrist contractures has been reported by a number of authors, with encouraging results.[3–5]

Indications

A biomechanical study performed by Palmer et al. defined functional wrist motion as being flexion of 5 degrees, extension of 30 degrees, radial deviation of 15 degrees, and ulnar deviation of 10 degrees.[6] Patients lacking a functional arc of wrist motion who have failed a trial of dynamic/static progressive splinting are candidates for this procedure. Volar capsulotomies are less risky and are indicated to regain wrist extension. Dorsal capsulotomies are necessary to regain wrist flexion but they may require use of a volar arthroscopy portal and are technically more difficult.

Contraindications

Contraindications in this case include all of those general to wrist arthroscopy, including active infection, large capsular tears (which can lead to extravasation of irrigation fluid), bleeding disorders, neurovascular compromise, marked swelling (which distorts the anatomy), inadequate or marginal soft-tissue coverage of the wrist, and the inability to withstand anesthesia. Division of the radioscaphocapitate (RSC), long radiolunate (LRL), and short radiolunate (SRL) ligaments should be performed with caution in patients who are at risk for ulnar translocation (such as those patients with rheumatoid arthritis and those who have undergone previous radial styloidectomies).[7,8] A frank carpal volar or dorsal carpal instability pattern is another contraindication because release of the volar and/or dorsal extrinsic ligaments would likely exacerbate this condition.

Relative contraindications include an unfamiliarity with the regional anatomy as well as abnormal bony anatomy due to a distal radius mal-union. Patients who cannot comply with postoperative dynamic/static progressive splinting due to low pain threshold or psychological disorder are not appropriate candidates.

Equipment

A 2.7-mm 30-degree angled scope along with a camera attachment is used, although a 1.9-mm scope is useful in tight wrists. A 3-mm hook probe and Freer elevator are needed for palpation of intracarpal structures and for release of adhesions. An overhead traction tower greatly facilitates instrumentation. The use of a motorized shaver is needed for debridement, along with a selection of suction punches and arthroscopic straight and curved knives. Some type of diathermy unit may be useful if cautery is desired for lysis of adhesions.

Surgical Technique

Volar Capsulotomy

The procedure is done under tourniquet control. A 3-/,4 portal and 4-/,5 portal are established as described in Chapter 1. Inflow through the scope with outflow through a cannula in the 6-R portal is standard, although it may be necessary to switch in cases where adhesions block the flow. The radiocarpal joint space is identified with a 22-gauge needle and the joint is inflated with saline. A contracted joint may accept only a small amount of fluid.

A blunt trocar and cannula are initially inserted in the 3-/,4 portal and used in a sweeping fashion to clear a path for the arthroscope and the instrumentation in cases of severe arthrofibrosis. Clearing the intra-articular adhesions is tedious but essential in order to adequately visualize the capsular ligaments. Midcarpal arthroscopy should be performed to assess the scapholunate and lunotriquetral joints. Evidence of dynamic instability will affect the decision making with regard to which volar and dorsal ligaments may be released.

A suction punch and full-radius resector are used to clear adhesions off the volar capsule until the RSC, LRL, radioscapholunate ligament (RSL), and SRL are well defined. While viewing through the 3-/,4 portal, an arthroscopic knife is introduced through a cannula placed in the 4-/,5 portal (Figure 19.1). The cannula is necessary in order to protect the extensor tendons from inadvertent laceration during insertion and removal of the knife. The tip of the blade should be visualized at all times to prevent inadvertent perforation of the capsule or chondral damage. The RSC ligament is gently sectioned until the volar capsular fat and/or the flexor carpi radialis tendon is seen. Anatomical and MRI studies by Verhellen and Bain established that the radial artery was closest to the joint capsule at an average distance of 5.2 mm, the median nerve 6.9 mm, and the ulnar nerve 6.7 mm.[5]

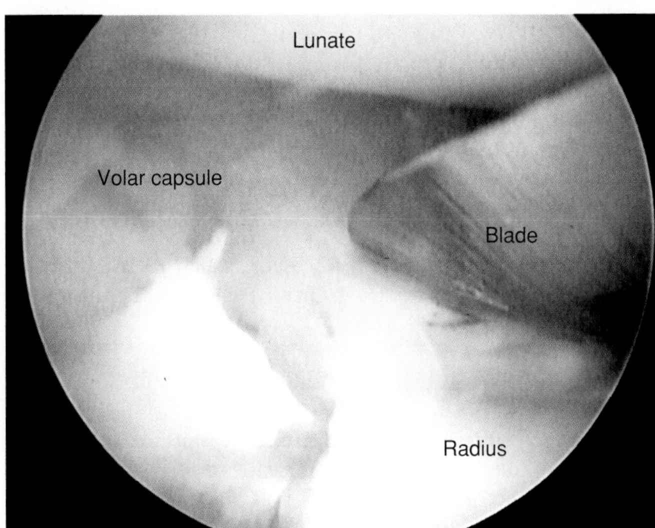

FIGURE 19.1. Volar capsulotomy. Arthroscopic knife is inserted through the 4-/,5 portal while viewing from the 3-/,4 portal.

In order to section the ulnolunate (UL) and ulnolunotriquetral (ULT) ligaments, it is often necessary to establish a 6-R portal because instrumentation and viewing across the radiocarpal joint are often limited due to scarring. The 6-U portal may be used interchangeably for instrumentation. The UL and ULT ligaments should not be released in the presence of a lunotriquetral ligament tear because the combination of these results in a volar intercalated segmental instability pattern in sectioning studies, especially when the dorsal radiocarpal ligament is also released.[9]

Dorsal Capsulotomy

It is the author's preference to use a volar radial (VR) portal (as previously described), although the 1-/,2 portal may be substituted or added. If both volar and dorsal capsulotomies are performed, it is preferable to release the dorsal capsule first because prior release of the volar capsule will make establishment of the VR portal more difficult. A 2-cm longitudinal incision is made in the proximal wrist crease, exposing the flexor carpi radialis (FCR) tendon sheath. The sheath is divided and the FCR tendon retracted ulnarly. The radiocarpal joint space is identified with a 22-gauge needle and the joint is inflated with saline.

A blunt trocar and cannula are introduced through the floor of the FCR sheath, which overlies the interligamentous sulcus between the radioscaphocapitate ligament and the long radiolunate ligament. The trocar is again used in a sweeping fashion to clear a path for the arthroscope. The arthroscope is then inserted through the cannula. A hook probe is inserted in the 3-/,4 portal. A suction punch and full-radius resector is exchanged with the probe or inserted through the 1-/,2 portal to clear adhesions until the dorsal capsule and the DRCL are seen. In patients with a partial or complete scapholunate ligament tear, sectioning the DRCL should be done with caution because it may exacerbate any preexisting scapholunate instability.[10–12]

While visualizing through the VR portal, an arthroscopic knife is then introduced through a cannula placed in the 3-/,4 portal (Figure 19.2a and b). The dorsal capsule and the DRCL are gently sectioned until the dorsal capsular fat and/or the extensor tendons can be seen. The wrist should be taken out of traction and the amount of extension assessed. If it is desirable to release the dorsoulnar capsule it is necessary to establish a volar ulnar (VU) portal (see Chapter 1) or to view through the 6-U portal. The adhesions are cleared through use of the 4-/,5 and 6-R portals and then a capsulotomy is performed in a similar fashion.

Postoperative Management

Bleeding may be quite brisk, and hence postoperative hematomas are minimized by the use of a compressive

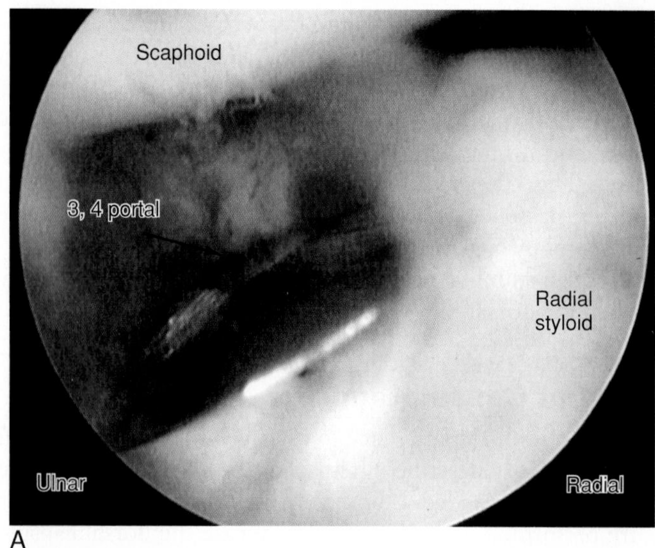

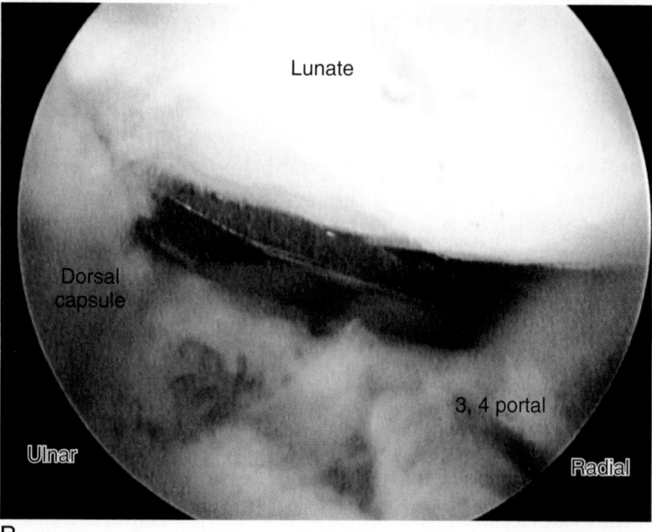

FIGURE 19.2. Dorsal capsulotomy. (A) Knife is inserted from the 3-/,4 portal while viewing from the volar radial portal. (B) Dorsal capsule is sectioned by sweeping the blade in an ulnar direction.

dressing. A below-elbow volar splint may be added for comfort. It is the author's custom to inject 5 mg of Duramorph into the radiocarpal joint in addition to 0.25% Marcaine infiltration of the portals for postoperative pain management. Excessive bleeding requires insertion of a hemovac drain for the first 24 to 48 hours. Immediate finger motion is instituted. Protected wrist motion is started within the first week, followed by dynamic and/or static progressive wrist flexion and/or extension splinting as soon as the patient's comfort allows in order to maintain any gains in wrist motion achieved at the time of surgery.

Complications

Potential complications abound and are largely related to judgment and technique. Complications include extensor tendon lacerations with dorsal capsulotomies and flexor tendon lacerations with volar capsulotomies. Overzealous release of the strong volar radiocarpal and ulnocarpal ligaments may lead to carpal dislocation or ulnar translocation. Release of the DRCL may exacerbate any preexisting or dynamic carpal instability. Penetration of the joint capsule also carries the risk of radial artery perforation as well as ulnar or median nerve lacerations.

Results

There are few series on arthroscopic release of contracture. Osterman initially advised against releasing the volar capsular ligaments due to the risk of destabilizing the carpus,[3] but did not report this complication in a later presentation of the results of combined volar and dorsal capsulotomies.[4] Verhellen and Bain reported a series of two patients.[5] They performed a release of the RSC, LRL, and SRL but recommended preserving the ULL and ULT ligaments. In light of the evidence from sectioning studies, however, the surgeon should strive to release as few of the volar and dorsal capsular structures as possible in order to achieve the desired result.

References

1. Watson HK, Dhillon SD. Stiff joints. In DP Green, WC Pederson (eds.), *Green's Operative Hand Surgery*. Philadelphia: Churchill Livingstone 1993:549–62.
2. Kleinman WB, Graham TJ. The distal radioulnar joint capsule: Clinical anatomy and role in posttraumatic limitation of forearm rotation. J Hand Surg [Am] 1998;23:588–99.
3. Osterman A. Wrist arthroscopy: Operative procedures. In DP Green, WC Pederson (eds.), *Green's Operative Hand Surgery, Fourth Edition*. Philadelphia: Churchill Livingstone 1999: 207–22.
4. Osterman A, Bednar JM. The Arthroscopic Release of Wrist Contracture. Presented at the American Society for Surgery of the Hand, 55th Annual Meeting. Seattle, WA. October 5–7, 2000.
5. Verhellen R, Bain GI. Arthroscopic capsular release for contracture of the wrist: A new technique. Arthroscopy 2000;16:106–10.
6. Palmer AK, Werner FW, Murphy D, Glisson R. Functional wrist motion: A biomechanical study. J Hand Surg [Am] 1985;10:39–46.
7. Siegel DB, Gelberman RH. Radial styloidectomy: An anatomical study with special reference to radiocarpal intracapsular ligamentous morphology. J Hand Surg [Am] 1991; 16:40–4.
8. Nakamura T, Cooney WP III, Lui WH, et al. Radial styloidectomy: A biomechanical study on stability of the wrist joint. J Hand Surg [Am] 2001;26:85–93.

9. Viegas SF, Patterson RM, Peterson PD, et al. Ulnar-sided perilunate instability: An anatomic and biomechanic study. J Hand Surg [Am] 1990;15:268–78.
10. Viegas SF, Yamaguchi S, Boyd NL, Patterson RM. The dorsal ligaments of the wrist: Anatomy, mechanical properties, and function. J Hand Surg [Am] 1999;24:456–68.
11. Slutsky DJ. Arthroscopic repair of dorsal radiocarpal ligament tears. Arthroscopy 2002;18:E49.
12. Slutsky DJ. Management of dorsoradiocarpal ligament repairs. Journal of the American Society for Surgery of the Hand 2005;5:167–74.

Kevin D. Plancher and César J. Bruno

CHAPTER 20

Arthroscopic Synovectomy and Abrasion Chondroplasty of the Wrist

Introduction: Rationale and Basic Science

The wrist is a crucial anatomical link between the hand and forearm, with multiple articular surfaces. When it is afflicted by arthritis and conditions that limit motion, it greatly affects the lives of our patients. The advent of arthroscopy has revolutionized the practice of orthopedic surgery, as well as the practice of hand surgery. Many pioneers have contributed newer techniques, and they have fueled the significant growth in wrist and small-joint arthroscopy.[1,2]

Wrist arthroscopy has provided a means of examining and treating intra-articular abnormalities. Early reports on arthroscopic wrist synovectomy have noted reduced pain, reduced swelling, and improvement of joint function.[3–6] The effects, either transitory or permanent, depend mainly on the activities of the patient and the underlying cause of arthritis. Abrasion chondroplasty of the wrist has not been described at length, but what is known is that in canine models "repair cartilage" (fibrocartilage) is formed in place of articular cartilage.[7] Excitingly, abrasion chondroplasty appears to have a role specifically in the treatment of patients with proximal pole hamate arthrosis as well as radiocarpal arthrosis. Preliminary results of this method of treatment have been excellent.[8–10] This chapter discusses the indications and techniques for arthroscopic synovectomy and abrasion chondroplasty.

Indications

Arthroscopic synovectomy is an effective modality for the treatment of patients with rheumatoid arthritis, juvenile arthritis (JRA), systemic lupus erythematosus (SLE), and postinfectious arthritis.[3–5] Patients who have developed post-traumatic joint contractures and patients with persistent septic arthritis of the wrist despite systemic antibiotics and lavage benefit from arthroscopic synovectomy as well. In the rheumatoid patient, we follow the protocol established by Adolfsson et al.[5] We treat those patients who present with radiographic changes of grades 0 through II (and who have failed to respond to pharmacologic treatment and who have a persistent joint synovitis for more than six months) according to the staging system by Larsen, Dale, and Eek.[4,11] In nonrheumatoid patients, the radiographic classification system used to evaluate the progression of the disease is the Outerbridge classification system (originally developed for chondromalacia patellae).[12]

Those patients with early presentation of SLE or reactive arthritis (bacterial or viral), and those patients with osteoarthritis with nominal radiographic changes and florid synovitis, are also considered candidates for wrist synovectomy. Furthermore, those patients who have sustained intra-articular fractures of the distal radius or who have undergone multiple previous wrist interventions also benefit from capsular release, removal of adhesions, and synovectomy (Figure 20.1).

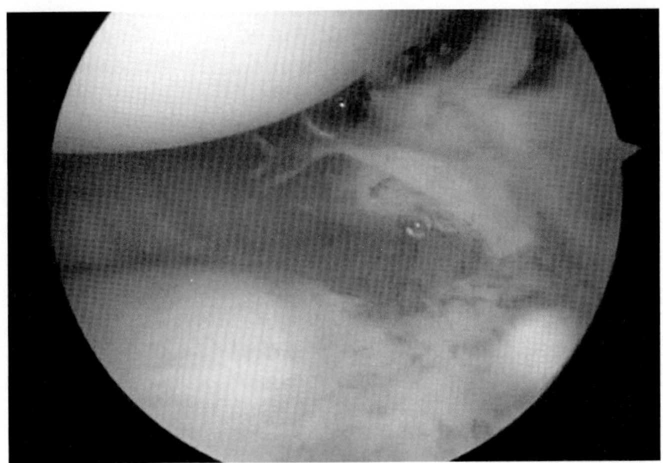

FIGURE 20.1. Wrist with dorsal hypertrophic synovitis viewed from the 3-4 portal.

Abrasion chondroplasty is very effective in patients with proximal pole hamate arthritis, specifically those patients with type II lunates (Figure 20.2). This condition causes ulnar-sided pain that occurs when those patients load their wrists in ulnar deviation. When the arthrosis in this area is advanced with exposure of subchondral bone (Outerbridge grade IV), we follow the recommendation of Yao et al. and proceed with an excision of the proximal pole.[13] The lunate morphology plays a key role in this condition.

The type II lunate and its medial facet can lead to arthritis with contact loading of the proximal pole of the hamate. This has been reported in up to 44% of type II lunates versus 2% in type I lunates.[9,13–19] Patients with this condition may also have concomitant wrist pathology that can be treated simultaneously, such as triangular fibrocartilage complex (TFCC) tears, lunotriquetral interosseous ligament (LTIL) tear (i.e., hamate arthrosis lunotriquetral ligament tear, or HALT),[9] ulnar impaction, and radial-sided, pathology. The presence of a TFCC injury can almost be assured when synovitis along the ulnar side of the wrist is seen during arthroscopy in the absence of any other structural problem.

Contraindications

Those patients who require extensive open wrist procedures are not candidates for arthroscopic synovectomy. Magnetic resonance imaging (MRI) in conjunction with clinical assessment of the patient aids in our decision planning. Patients with active rheumatoid disease, those medically unfit, and patients with active infections aside from the wrist are considered contraindications.

Radiographic Evaluation

The radiographic evaluation system of Larsen et al. is used for staging the wrist arthritis. We have found that along with an appropriate clinical history dedicated MRI coils and special imaging sequences of the articular cartilage improve the sensitivity and specificity of these studies for detecting chondral defects. This has been a great tool for correlating the clinical and expected arthroscopic findings. Others do not share this viewpoint. In a study of 41 indirect MR arthrograms and 45 unenhanced (nonarthrographic) MR images that were compared to the arthrographic findings, Haims et al. concluded that MRI of the wrist is not adequately sensitive nor accurate in the diagnosis of cartilage defects in the distal radius, scaphoid, lunate, or triquetrum.[20]

MRI is, however, a good predictor of cases of synovitis and ulnar-sided pathology. Arthroscopic abrasion arthroplasty, subchondral drilling, and microfracture can be

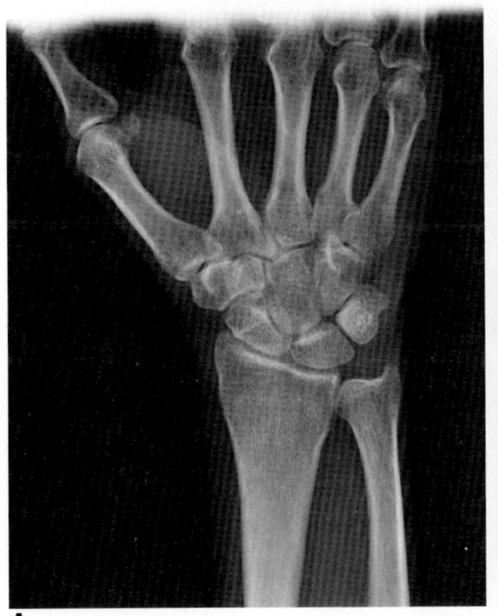

A

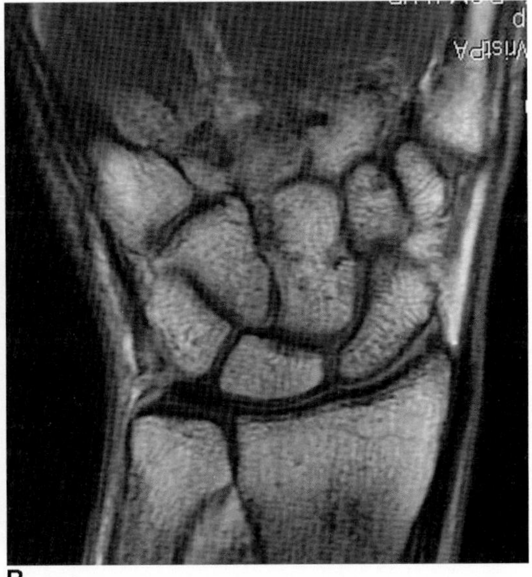

B

FIGURE 20.2. (A) Plain radiograph AP of a type II lunate. (B) MRI of type II lunate with proximal pole arthrosis.

performed for the treatment of focal chondral defects in patients with moderate degenerative wrist arthritis or when plain radiographs are suggestive of avascular necrosis. The MRI has been shown to be a sensitive modality that may be used to exclude avascular necrosis as well as to evaluate the extent to which fibrocartilaginous repair tissue has formed postoperatively. This has been demonstrated in the knee, and we have incorporated an MRI evaluation as a part of our postoperative protocol.[20,21]

Surgical Technique

The arthroscopic synovectomy can be carried out under general or regional anesthesia with the forearm suspended in a traction tower device with finger traps. We tend to use the long and index finger, but in rheumatoid patients with delicate skin it is often recommended that one should place all of the digits in the finger traps to distribute the traction load. Ten to 15 pounds of traction is used. Passive infusion of saline solution is accomplished by gravity traction through a separate inflow cannula or through the scope itself. A 2.7-mm 30-degree arthroscope is inserted through our working portals (which are the 3-, 4, 4-, 5, and 6-R portals for the radiocarpal joint). Outflow is through the 6-U portal. The radial and ulnar midcarpal portals are used to access the midcarpal joint (Figure 20.3).

Efficiency and speed are important to minimize wrist swelling. In cases with severe scaphotrapeziotrapezoidal (STT) joint arthritis, a separate portal can be established. All of the inflamed synovial tissue is removed using a motorized shaver system with a 3.5-mm synovial resector blade and 3.5-mm flexible shaver. We have also had good

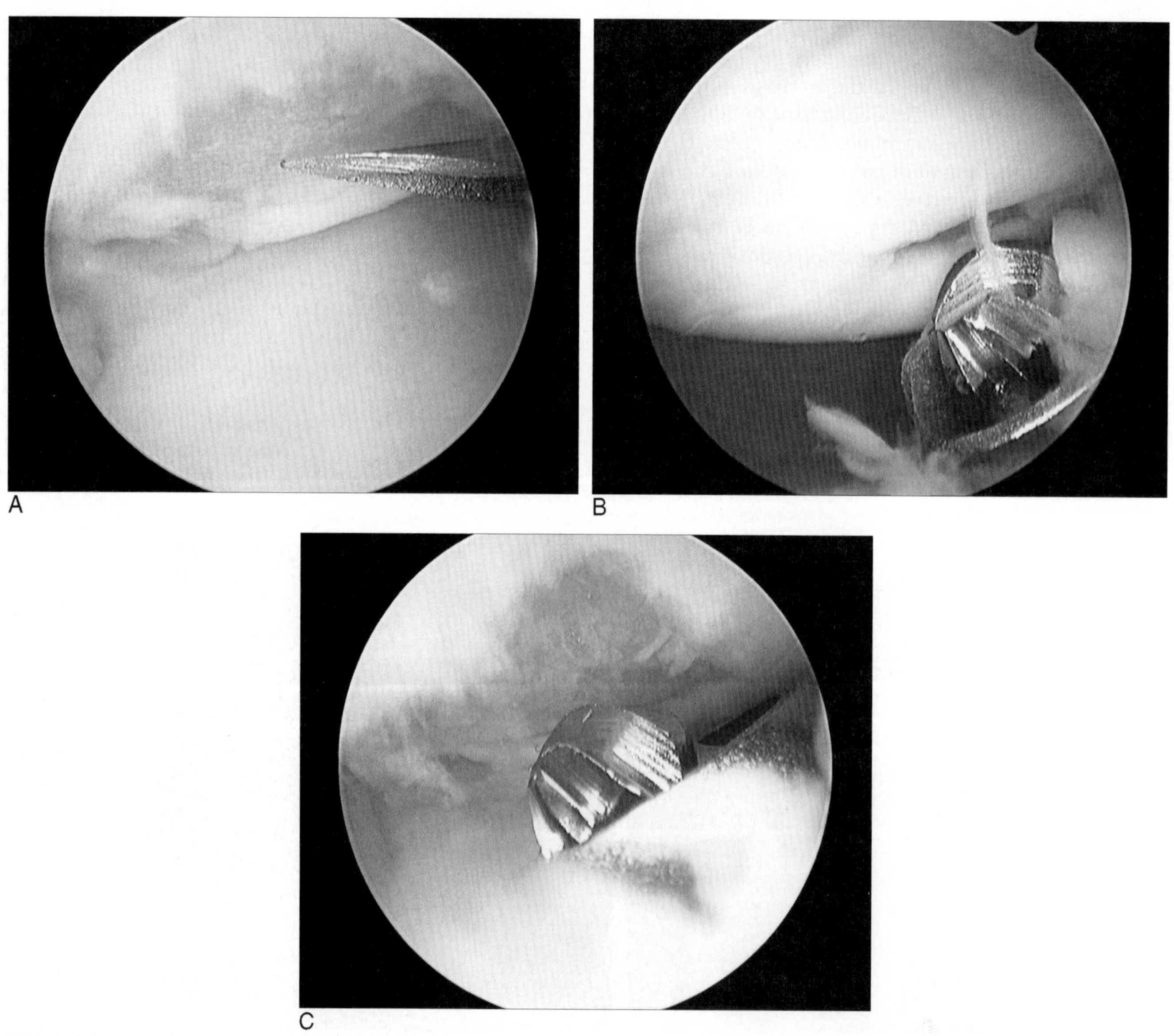

FIGURE 20.3. (A) Cartilage defect identified in the radiocarpal joint. (B) Motorized burr utilized for abrasion arthroplasty of the radiocarpal joint. (C) Widening of the defect during abrasion arthroplasty.

results with the use of thermal ablation, which also decreases bleeding (Figure 20.4). It is essential to maintain adequate irrigation of the wrist when using a thermal probe to avoid heat buildup. It is important to inspect the radial styloid, the radioscapholunate ligament, the ulnar prestyloid recess, and the dorsoulnar region beneath the extensor carpi ulnaris (ECU) subsheath.

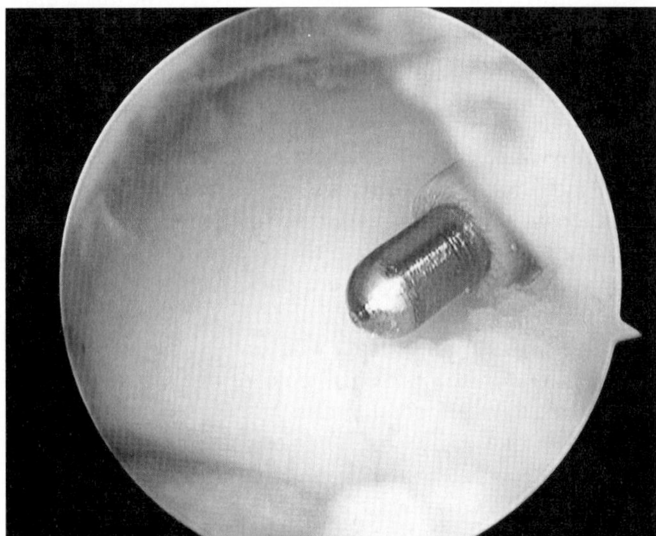

FIGURE 20.4. Ablator removing synovitis with good outflow and inflow being maintained to avoid heating the tissues.

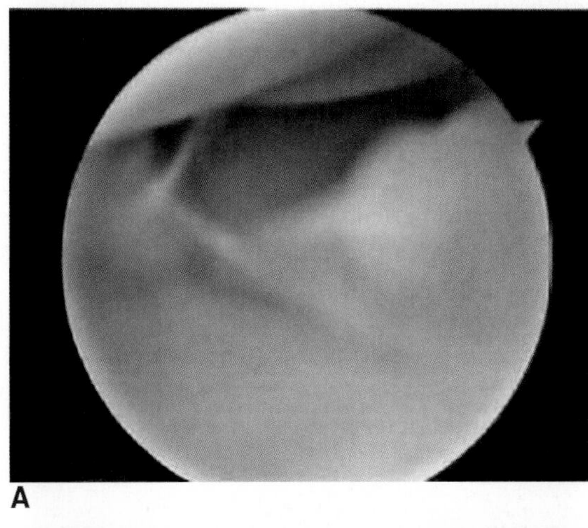

A

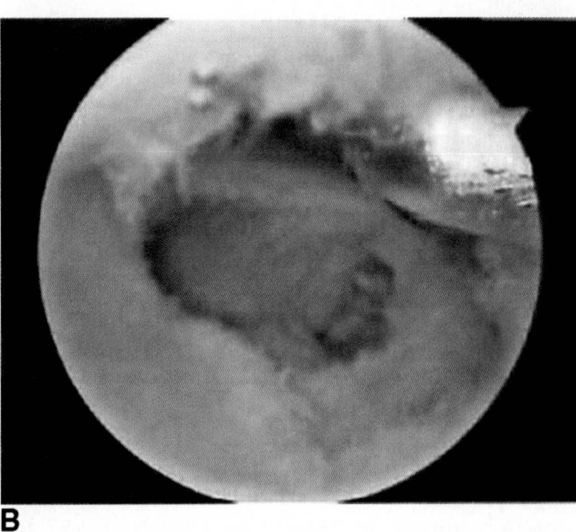

B

FIGURE 20.5. (A) Synovitis in the wrist with underlying TFCC tear. (B) Exposed ulnar-sided TFCC tear seen after shaving of hypertrophic synovitis.

Midcarpal synovitis is often found along the dorsoulnar region, volarly beneath the capitohamate joint, and in the STT joint. The distal radioulnar joint (DRUJ) is then inspected. This can often be performed through a central defect in the horizontal portion of the TFCC. A synovectomy can be carried out through the 6-R portal. A separate DRUJ portal immediately proximal to the TFCC can be used for debridement if a TFCC tear is not present. Meticulous and great care must be used at all times to avoid chondral damage to the articular surfaces. Incisions are closed with Dermabond and augmented with Steri-Strips or alternatively with subcuticular Monocril. Care is taken when establishing the 6-U portal to avoid laceration or painful neuroma of the dorsal sensory branch of the ulnar nerve. A light dressing is placed postoperatively, and range-of-motion exercises are carried out immediately under the supervision of a hand therapist.

The previously described traction setup is similarly used for abrasion chondroplasty of the proximal pole of the hamate. Once the radial midcarpal portal is established, a 2.9-mm bur is inserted into the ulnar midcarpal portal. An average of 2.4 mm of the proximal pole should be excised to fully unload the hamatolunate articulation. This amount of bony resection does not affect the loading characteristics of the triquetrohamate articulation.[9] The radial and ulnar midcarpal portals are used interchangeably in order to completely debride the proximal pole. The diameter of the 2.4-mm bur is used as a guide to the depth of resection. The postoperative dressing and protocol are similar to that following an arthroscopic wrist synovectomy.

Radiocarpal arthritis is treated with abrasion arthroplasty in a manner similar to that described by Steadman et al. for the knee (Figures 20.6 through 20.8).[10] The standard working portals are established as previously

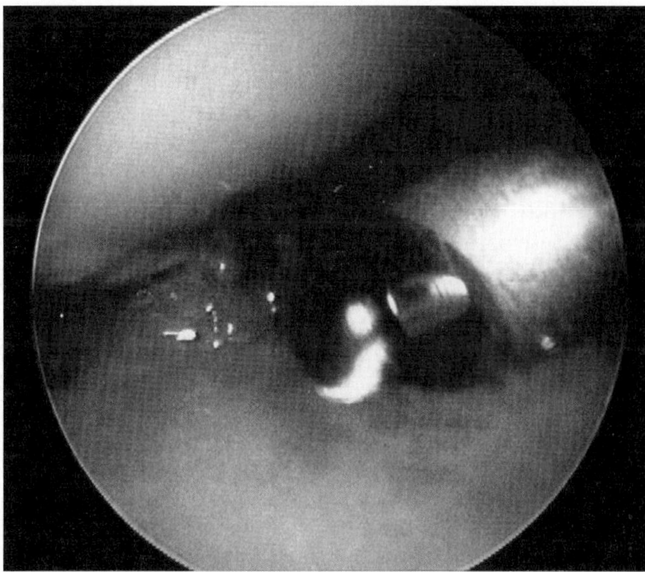

FIGURE 20.6. Bone-on-bone defect identified in the radiocarpal joint.

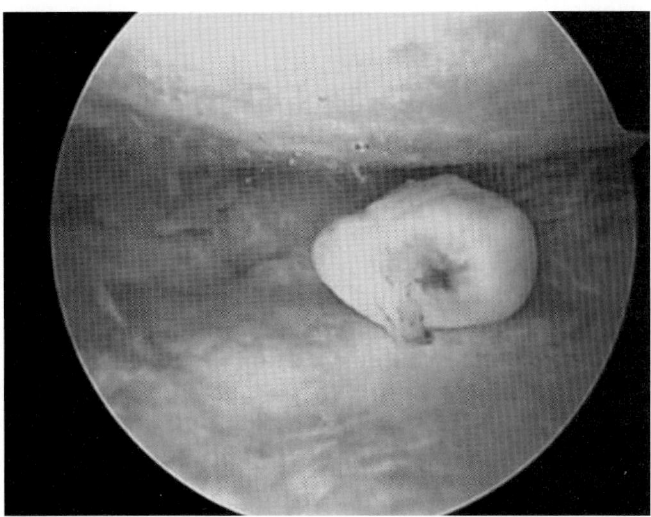

FIGURE 20.7. Loose body located in radiocarpal joint.

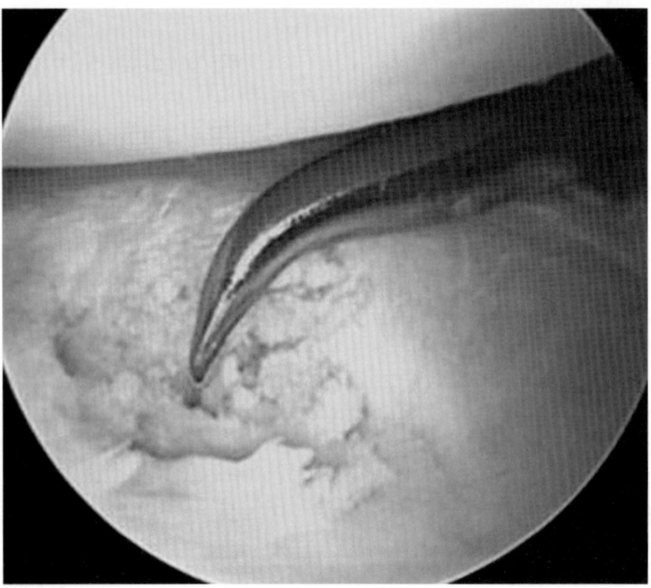

FIGURE 20.8. Microfracture of the radiocarpal joint.

described. Any loose bodies are removed during the initial diagnostic survey. Once a focal area of chondral damage is identified, specially designed Linvatec awls (Linvatec, Key Largo, FL) (2.5 mm, 3.5 mm) are used to make multiple perforations (microfractures) in the subchondral bone plate. These perforations are made as close together as possible while maintaining an adequate bony bridge. They are typically 1 to 2 mm apart. The integrity of the subchondral bone plate should be maintained.

A shaver is not used on the articular cartilage. The released marrow elements (mesenchymal stem cells, growth factors, and other healing proteins) form a surgically induced super-clot that provides an enriched environment for new tissue formation.[10] Marcaine and Kenalog are injected under direct visualization at the conclusion of the procedure. The rehabilitation program is crucial in optimizing the results of the surgery, and early range of motion is key. Dressings and closure are carried out as previously described.

Results

Wrist arthroscopy allows one to effectively perform a synovectomy, debride a torn TFCC, treat chondral defects and osteoarthritis, remove loose bodies, and resect the distal ulna and carpal bones. The surgeon should adhere to the anatomical principles that have been developed for open surgical procedures. "Ectomy" procedures of the wrist require a higher level of expertise from the surgeon, but when mastered provide considerable benefit to the patient.[22] We have found that these procedures are an excellent adjunct in the multifaceted treatment of patients with rheumatoid arthritis. They may also be of benefit in the treatment of other forms of arthritis. Superior results are obtained when it is combined with the treatment of the underlying cause.

In a review of 18 patients who underwent an abrasion arthroplasty for the proximal pole of the hamate, there were 10 excellent, 4 good, 3 fair, and 1 poor result—with a follow-up of 1 to 3 years. The poor result had associated radial carpal arthrosis and rheumatoid arthritis. The three fair results all had an associated lunotriquetral instability. The results following an arthroscopic chondroplasty have been variable. The durability of the fibrocartilage repair tissue that forms following microfracture is questionable, and the possibility of thermal damage to the subchondral bone and the adjacent normal articular cartilage following a laser/thermal chondroplasty exists.[23]

The senior author has had three of the patients return for unrelated reasons (distal radius extra-articular fracture) and took this opportunity to place the arthroscope in their wrists and noted hypertrophic synovitis and a small amount of fibrocartilage present. These three patients had no complaints of wrist pain and had returned to tennis, skiing, and lifting light weights prior to their new injury. A full analysis needs to be done to determine whether a microfracture can produce similar results in the wrist compared to the experience with chondral defects in the knee.

Summary

Although recent prospective, randomized, double-blind studies have demonstrated that the outcomes after arthroscopic lavage or debridement for knee osteoarthritis were no better than a placebo procedure, controversy still exists. The literature is scarce on the use of these procedures in the wrist.[24] Reports of abrasion chondroplasty for the treatment of advanced wrist arthritis have been anecdotal in nature, but it has been quite successful in our hands.

References

1. Ekman EF, Poehling GG. Principles of arthroscopy and wrist arthroscopy equipment. Hand Clin 1994;10(4):557–66.
2. Gupta R, Bozentka DJ, Osterman AL. Wrist arthroscopy: Principles and clinical applications. J Am Acad Orthop Surg 2001;9(3):200–09.

3. Adolfsson L, Nylander G. Arthroscopic synovectomy of the rheumatoid wrist. J Hand Surg [Br] 1993;18(1):92–6.
4. Adolfsson L, Frisen M. Arthroscopic synovectomy of the rheumatoid wrist: A 3.8 year follow-up. J Hand Surg [Br] 1997;22(6):711–13.
5. Adolfsson L. Arthroscopic synovectomy in wrist arthritis. Hand Clin 2005;21(4):527–30.
6. Roth JH, Poehling GG. Arthroscopic "-ectomy" surgery of the wrist. Arthroscopy 1990;6(2):141–47.
7. Altman RD, Kates J, Chun LE, Dean DD, Eyre D. Preliminary observations of chondral abrasion in a canine model. Ann Rheum Dis 1992;51(9):1056–62.
8. Steadman JR, Briggs KK, Rodrigo JJ, Kocher MS, Gill TJ, Rodkey WG. Outcomes of microfracture for traumatic chondral defects of the knee: Average 11-year follow-up. Arthroscopy 2003;19(5):477–84.
9. Harley BJ, Werner FW, Boles SD, Palmer AK. Arthroscopic resection of arthrosis of the proximal hamate: A clinical and biomechanical study. J Hand Surg [Am] 2004;29(4):661–67.
10. Steadman JR, Rodkey WG, Rodrigo JJ. Microfracture: Surgical technique and rehabilitation to treat chondral defects. Clin Orthop Relat Res 2001;391:S362–69.
11. Larsen A, Dale K, Eek M. Radiographic evaluation of rheumatoid arthritis and related conditions by standard reference films. Acta Radiol Diagn (Stockh) 1977;18(4):481–91.
12. Outerbridge RE. The etiology of chondromalacia patellae. J Bone Joint Surg Br 1961;43-B:752–57.
13. Yao J, Osterman AL. Arthroscopic techniques for wrist arthritis (radial styloidectomy and proximal pole hamate excisions). Hand Clin 2005;21(4):519–26.
14. Nakamura K, Patterson RM, Moritomo H, Viegas SF. Type I versus type II lunates: Ligament anatomy and presence of arthrosis. J Hand Surg [Am] 2001;26(3):428–36.
15. Nakamura K, Beppu M, Patterson RM, Hanson CA, Hume PJ, Viegas SF. Motion analysis in two dimensions of radial-ulnar deviation of type I versus type II lunates. J Hand Surg [Am] 2000;25(5):877–88.
16. Malik AM, Schweitzer ME, Culp RW, Osterman LA, Manton G. MR imaging of the type II lunate bone: Frequency, extent, and associated findings. AJR Am J Roentgenol 1999;173(2):335–38.
17. Dautel G, Merle M. Chondral lesions of the midcarpal joint. Arthroscopy 1997;13(1):97–102.
18. Viegas SF, Wagner K, Patterson R, Peterson P. Medial (hamate) facet of the lunate. J Hand Surg [Am] 1990;15 (4):564–71.
19. Viegas SF. The lunatohamate articulation of the midcarpal joint. Arthroscopy 1990;6(1):5–10.
20. Haims AH, Moore AE, Schweitzer ME, et al. MRI in the diagnosis of cartilage injury in the wrist. AJR Am J Roentgenol 2004;182(5):1267–70.
21. Amrami KK, Askari KS, Pagnano MW, Sundaram M. Radiologic case study: Abrasion chondroplasty mimicking avascular necrosis. Orthopedics 2002;25(10):1018, 1107–08.
22. Bain GI, Roth JH. The role of arthroscopy in arthritis. "Ectomy" procedures. Hand Clin 1995;11(1):51–8.
23. Hunt SA, Jazrawi LM, Sherman OH. Arthroscopic management of osteoarthritis of the knee. J Am Acad Orthop Surg 2002;10(5):356–63.
24. Smith MD, Wetherall M, Darby T, et al. A randomized placebo-controlled trial of arthroscopic lavage versus lavage plus intra-articular corticosteroids in the management of symptomatic osteoarthritis of the knee. Rheumatology (Oxford) 2003;42(12):1477–85.

Randy R. Bindra

CHAPTER 21

To Lisa and James for making everything worthwhile.

Arthroscopic Wrist Ganglionectomy

Rationale and Basic Science

Dorsal wrist ganglions are the most common type of soft-tissue swellings that present around the wrist. They usually originate from the dorsal portion of the scapholunate ligament, at or just distal to the dorsal folds of the radiocarpal capsule.[1] The dorsal wrist ganglion originates from the scapholunate joint. The cyst pedicle lies at the junction of the dorsal capsule and the distal-most part of the dorsal scapholunate interosseous ligament. From here, the ganglion swells into a sac lying along the dorsal capsule—from where it protrudes as a clinically obvious swelling. The intracapsular portion of the ganglion overlies the scapholunate joint, but the large extra-articular fundus of the cyst may vary in location (although it still remains in close vicinity of the joint).

The swelling is benign but can be painful, and surgical excision by an open procedure is recognized as the most effective method of treatment of this condition. Unfortunately, recurrence is possible even after open surgery and is likely related to removal of the externally visible cyst without addressing the intra-articular pedicle. Management of the "occult" ganglion that remains intracapsular and is not clinically visible provides an even further treatment challenge. As the swelling cannot be seen outside the wrist joint, open surgery consists of an almost empirical excision of a 1.5-cm diameter of dorsal wrist capsule overlying the scapholunate joint.

Wrist arthroscopy offers an excellent view of the wrist joint, and with modern mechanized shavers intra-articular pathology can be effectively debrided. In the case of a ganglion, the intra-articular portion is easy to see because it lies against the dorsal capsule. The pedicle of the ganglion at the scapholunate ligament can be visualized in the majority of cases, and can be resected effectively along with the intra-articular portion with minimal surgical incisions. This may reduce the incidence of recurrence after surgery. In addition, arthroscopy allows a thorough visual examination and palpation by probe of the radiocarpal and midcarpal joints to exclude other sources of wrist pain. The use of wrist arthroscopy to effectively treat dorsal wrist ganglia is not new and was first proposed by Osterman in 1995.[2]

The "occult" ganglion is entirely intracapsular and cannot the visualized during open surgery. Arthroscopy, however, allows visualization and resection of the entire ganglion. In the author's opinion, arthroscopy is the treatment of choice for an occult ganglion.

Routine wrist arthroscopy commences with joint inspection through the 3-4 radiocarpal portal. The ganglion overlies this portal and the intra-articular portion of the ganglion obscures visualization. If arthroscopic ganglionectomy is planned, the 6-R portal is used to gain initial entry to the wrist joint. When the scope is directed to the radial side, it is possible to obtain a tangential view of the ganglion adherent to the wrist capsule on one side and the scapholunate joint on the other. A shaver introduced through the 3-4 portal enters the joint through the ganglion. The perforated ganglion is then resected by running the shaver along the surface of the capsule.

Clinical Features and Indications

Most ganglia present in females in the second, third, or fourth decades of life. Spontaneous resolution is common but can take several years, with 50% of untreated patients "ganglion free" when assessed at six years.[3]

The most common presenting complaint is the cosmetic concern relating to a lump present on the back of the wrist. The other less common complaints are discomfort localized to the area of the swelling or fear of possible malignancy. Although the diagnosis is usually quite obvious in the majority of cases, other causes of wrist pain must be excluded by a thorough clinical examination and routine radiography. The ganglion is a soft cystic swelling that has no inflammatory signs. Transillumination by a penlight and fluctuation are two key clinical signs that demonstrate the clear fluid nature of the lump and exclude other soft-tissue tumors. If the patient seeks absolute confirmation, ultrasound examination is diagnostic. MR imaging is more expensive, but is indicated if Kienbock's disease is to be excluded.

The patient with an occult wrist ganglion will complain of wrist discomfort over the area of the scapholunate joint and may or may not notice intermittent swelling in the area. As the swelling is not visible clinically, confirmation by MR imaging or ultrasound is mandatory. Ultrasound is the most cost effective and will demonstrate the ganglion as a hypoechoic mass overlying the scapholunate joint and deep to the wrist capsule (Figure 21.1).[4]

Management options include reassurance that the swelling is harmless, and spontaneous resolution is possible if one is prepared to wait for a reasonable length of time. This holds true especially in the pediatric population, where cysts around the wrist are likely to resolve spontaneously in up to 80% of cases.[5] A brief period of rest in a splint may help to reduce pain. Needle aspiration does provide immediate symptom relief, with resolution of the swelling, but the reported recurrence rate is about 60%.[6,7] The injection of steroid after aspiration does not seem to affect the high recurrence rates, and with risk of subcutaneous atrophy and skin depigmentation is not routinely recommended.[8]

Surgery is indicated if there is failure to respond to conservative treatment or if the patient declines injection. Open surgical excision has long been considered the definitive treatment of choice, but even surgery cannot prevent the risk of recurrence that can occur in as many as 25% of cases. Open surgical excision also has complications of scar tenderness or hypertrophy, keloid formation, and stiffness if prolonged postoperative immobilization is used.

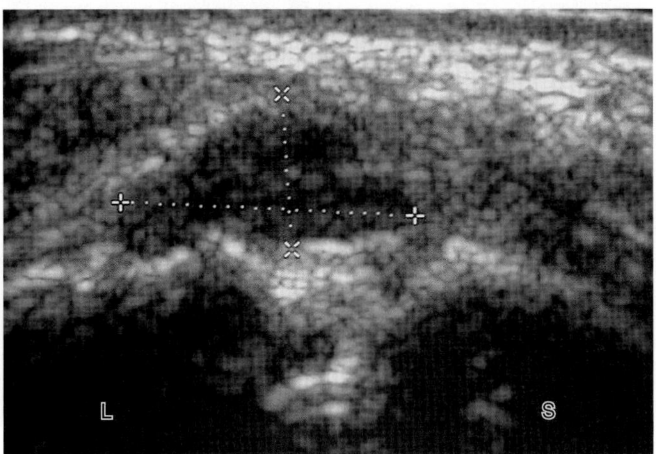

FIGURE 21.1. Ultrasound appearance of an occult ganglion on an axial view of the wrist. The 5-mm x 3-mm ganglion (marked by crosshairs) is seen overlying the interosseous ligament between the scaphoid (S) and the lunate (L).

Arthroscopic excision may be undertaken if the surgeon is familiar with arthroscopic techniques in the wrist. The patient who desires surgery must understand that surgery is one of the better options but spontaneous resolution is possible. The swelling itself is harmless. Pain arising from the wrist itself due to other pathology will not improve after ganglion excision. Patients who wish to have the swelling removed for cosmetic reasons must be informed that scar formation, even after arthroscopy, can be noticeable.

Contraindications

Absolute

There are no absolute contraindications to the surgery. If the patient's primary concern is the cosmetic appearance of the swelling, he or she has to be advised about scars of surgery. Although arthroscopic scars are smaller, they can hypertrophy.

Relative

Previous scarring in the area due to previous injury or surgery for recurrence may make identification of portals and development of portals difficult. Conversion to open surgery may have to be considered in these cases.

Surgical Technique

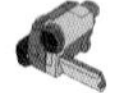

The technique for arthroscopic ganglionectomy includes the standard wrist arthroscopy instrumentation and setup. The upper extremity is prepped and draped and an exsanguinating tourniquet is applied. Finger traps are applied to the index and long fingers and the hand and wrist are placed in a distraction tower with 10 to 15 pounds of traction. The arm must be secured firmly to the table with sterile straps in order to provide countertraction. The 3-4 and 6-R portals are identified and the tourniquet is inflated. The ganglion is marked out because it may become less apparent during the surgical procedure.

Whereas it is routine to inflate the joint with saline prior to insertion of the arthroscope, in this procedure saline insufflation is avoided initially to allow identification of the ganglion and its stalk. A 1.9- or 2.7-mm arthroscope is used according to the size of the wrist.

Contrary to traditional wrist arthroscopy that commences on the radial side with initial visualization through the 3-4 portal, for ganglionectomy the author prefers to start from the ulnar side of the wrist from the 6-R portal for the following reasons. Introduction of the scope through the 3-4 portal may actually enter through the ganglion, causing it to rupture and making it less distinct. The intra-articular portion of the ganglion impairs visibility and examination of the joint is not possible. Furthermore, the 3-4 portal will be used for instrumentation to debride the ganglion. The author therefore recommends using the 3-4 portal for diagnostic arthroscopy only after the ganglion has been debrided.

An 18-gauge needle is inserted into the 6-R portal first to localize the level of the ulnocarpal articulation and to ensure that the triangular fibrocartilagenous disc is not violated. A 4-mm transverse incision is made in the skin and a small hemostat is introduced into the joint and spread gently. The blunt trocar and cannula are inserted and then the trocar is exchanged for the scope (Figure 21.2).

By directing the scope radially, it is possible to see the scapholunate articulation in profile. The ganglion can be seen lying against the dorsal capsule. Tracking the ganglion as the scope is tilted dorsally, the stalk of the ganglion can be seen running to the distal part of the dorsal scapholunate interosseous ligament along the capsular reflection. When the inflow of saline is commenced, the ganglion is compressed against the dorsal capsule and becomes less distinct (Figure 21.3). Fluid outflow may be provided by an 18-gauge needle inserted into the 1-2 portal. This, however, is not always necessary because adequate outflow will be provided during insertion of the shaver.

An 18-gauge needle is introduced through the ganglion and into the 3-4 arthroscopic portal. As landmarks may be obscured by the swelling, the portal is made in line with the radial border of the long finger. The needle is inserted into the joint under arthroscopic vision and is directed into the radiocarpal space (Figure 21.4).

The 3-4 portal is then developed by making a transverse incision through the skin and spreading the capsular entry with a small hemostat. A 2.3-mm full-radius shaver is introduced into the joint and the ganglion is then systematically resected, starting with the capsular portion (Figure 21.5).

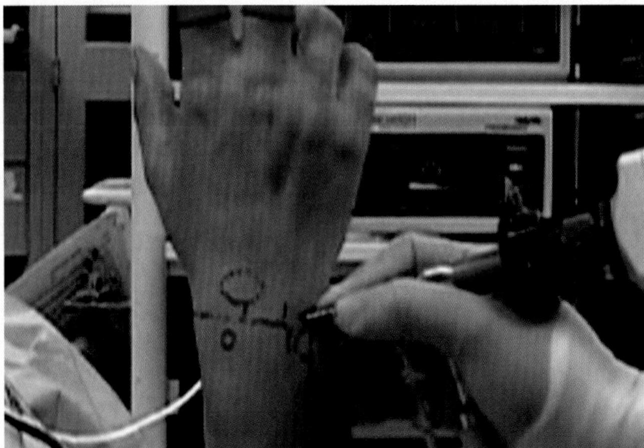

FIGURE 21.2. With the right arm suspended in traction, the arthroscope has been introduced from the 6-R portal. The ganglion has been marked and is seen to overlie the 3-4 portal.

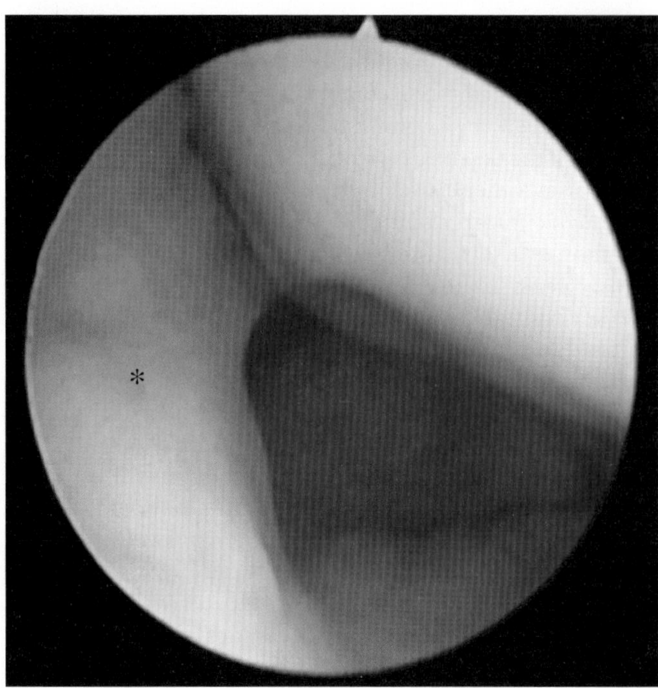

FIGURE 21.3. Arthroscopic view from the 6-R portal. The ganglion (*) is seen to the left, overlying the dorsal wrist capsule. The lunate, in profile, is seen to the right. The ganglion comes into contact with the lunate at the level of the dorsal part of the scapholunate interosseous ligament.

Resection requires working at a very steep angle, with the shaver at times almost parallel to the forearm as the surgeon resects the capsular portion of the ganglion. An aggressive shaver may be used for this purpose. The use of the 1-2 portal has been recommended for better visualization and ease of resection.[9,10] In the author's experience, however, this has not been necessary. The

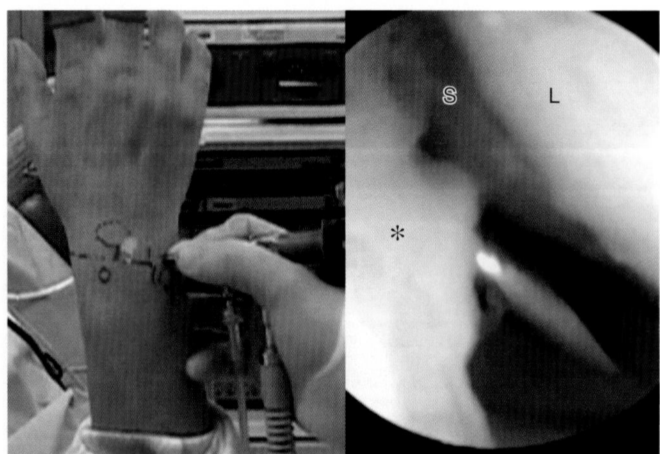

FIGURE 21.4. Arthroscopic view of the right wrist from the 6-R portal after a needle is inserted through the 3-4 portal (left). The needle has perforated the ganglion (*), which appears more flattened due to saline inflow through the joint. The scaphoid (S) and lunate (L) are seen in profile.

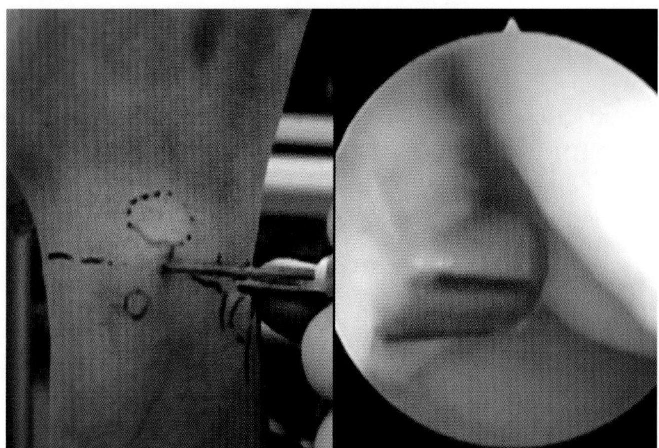

FIGURE 21.5. A 2.5-mm shaver is introduced through the 3-4 portal (left). When viewed from the 6-R portal, the scope enters the joint through the base of the ganglion itself (right).

author recommends avoiding this portal because of the risk of radial sensory nerve complications.

Attention is then turned to the pedicle that runs along the distal capsular reflection to the distal-most part of the dorsal SLIL. Using a nonaggressive shaver angled distally, the pedicle is debrided with gentle pressure against the SLIL. Caution must be exercised when using an aggressive shaver for this purpose because it may disrupt part of the ligament (Figure 21.6).

Some patients may demonstrate additional synovitis along the rim of the dorsal radius. This may be a manifestation of underlying scapholunate instability and needs to be evaluated with a midcarpal arthroscopy.[11] The red fragile fronds of synovitis are distinct from the well-localized and avascular ganglion. The synovitis can also be debrided using a shaver, or lesser amounts can be vaporized using a thermal probe. By this time, the intra-articular ganglion is completely debrided, there is a visible defect in the dorsal capsule, and the extra-articular portion of the ganglion should have been decompressed (Figure 21.7).

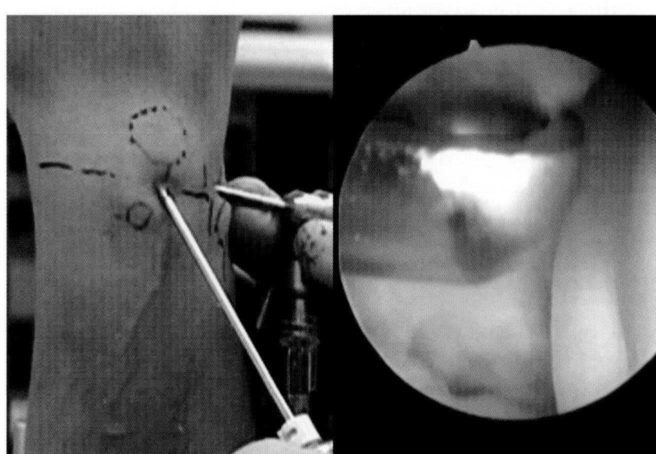

FIGURE 21.6. After debriding the capsular portion of the ganglion, the shaver is angled distally to the pedicle at the reflection of the dorsal capsule from the scapholunate joint.

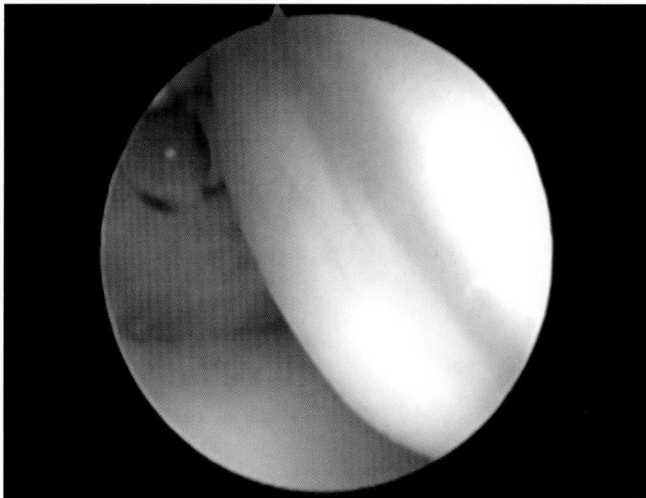

FIGURE 21.7. Arthroscopic view from the 6-R portal after completion of ganglion excision.

If the external ganglion mass is still tense, the capsular window needs to be widened to allow the ganglion to discharge into the joint. Using an arthroscopic punch forceps, the portal hole in the capsule is widened. This may help to minimize possibilities of recurrence by removal of the one-way "capsular valve" that allows fluid to accumulate in the extra-articular portion of the ganglion.[12] Capsular window enlargement is not necessary for the treatment of occult ganglia that are totally intra-articular. Some authors recommend capsular resection only for cases when the ganglion or its stalk is not identifiable through the arthroscope. The author prefers to enlarge the opening using controlled removal of small portions with a forceps, rather than an aggressive shaver, because this method has less risk of injury to the radial wrist extensor tendons (Figure 21.8).

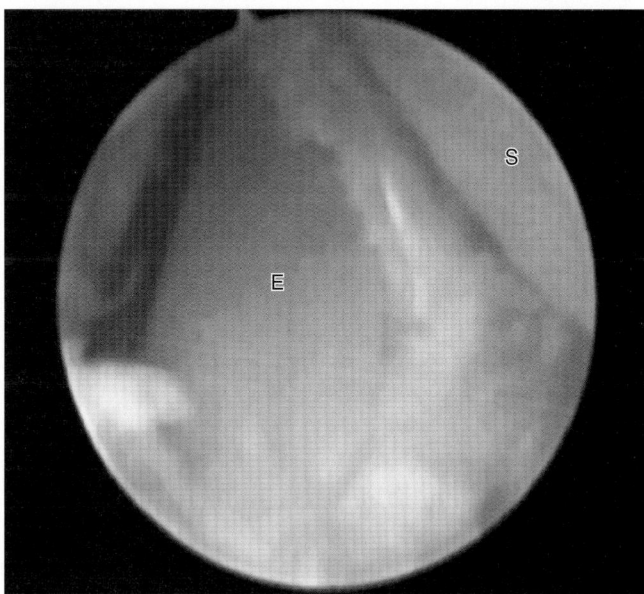

FIGURE 21.8. View from the 6-R portal. Widening of the capsular portal brings the wrist extensor tendon (E) into view.

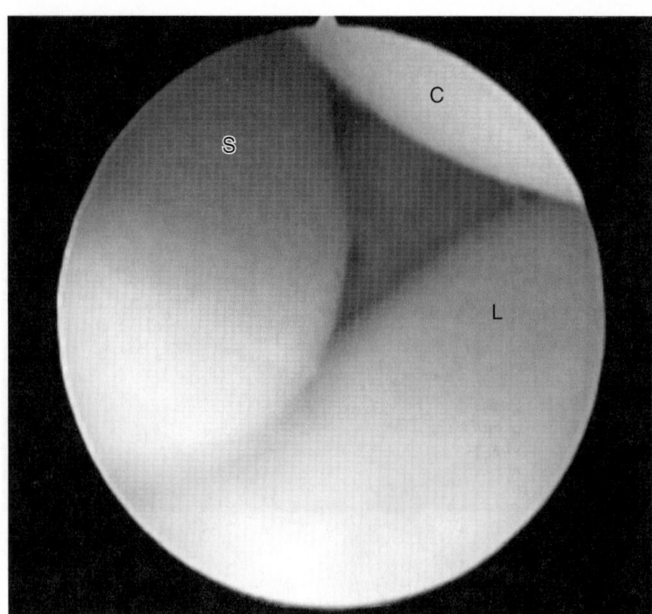

FIGURE 21.9. View of the midcarpal joint through the radial midcarpal portal, showing the scaphoid (S), lunate (L), and capitate (C). There is increased flexion of the scaphoid visible as a step-off at the scapholunate joint.

Once resection is complete, further examination of the radiocarpal joint is performed by inserting the arthroscope through the 3-4 portal. The appearance of articular surfaces is recorded and the integrity of the scapholunate ligament and the triangular fibrocartilage is confirmed with a probe.

Arthroscopic evaluation of the midcarpal joint is essential after resection of the ganglion. It is not uncommon to visualize a minor degree of scapholunate laxity with a step-off at the articulation. Less commonly, the ganglion extends into the midcarpal joint—obscuring visualization through the radial midcarpal portal. An ulnar midcarpal portal is then developed for the scope, and the ganglion is debrided with a shaver introduced through the radial midcarpal portal (Figure 21.9).

Upon completion, the scope is removed and the tourniquet is deflated. The skin edges of the portals are approximated with Steri-Strips. Postoperatively, the patient is splinted for comfort for a brief period of four to seven days. Active wrist motion is encouraged after this period of time, and the patient is allowed activities of daily living. Heavy lifting or strenuous work is not encouraged for the first six weeks.

Results

While providing the obvious result of removal of the soft-tissue mass, the additional benefits of arthroscopic ganglionectomy include improved pain scores and grip strength and an increase in wrist dorsiflexion. In the author's personal series, he reviewed 15 patients with occult dorsal wrist ganglia treated with arthroscopic resection with a mean follow-up of 18 months. All patients had tenderness over the scapholunate joint without clinically obvious swelling. The diagnosis was made by ultrasound or MRI in all cases. Although there was no radiographic evidence of carpal instability, six patients had clinical evidence of scapholunate instability. Twelve patients remained pain free at final follow-up, and three patients subsequently underwent dorsal capsulodesis for persistent scapholunate instability. Each of these patients did not show any recurrence of the ganglion on ultrasound scans.

The most common concern after surgery for ganglion removal is recurrence, with reported rates from less than 1 to 25% after open surgery. Recurrence rates after arthroscopic ganglionectomy appear to be much lower. Osterman[2] did not report any recurrences in 18 cases, whereas Fontes[13] reported recurrence in 1 of 32 cases, Luchetti in 2 of 34 cases, and Rizzo in 2 of 42 cases.[2,14,15] To prevent recurrence, it is essential to identify and effectively debride the pedicle. If the pedicle is not clearly visualized in the radiocarpal joint, the midcarpal joint must also be examined. A 1-cm section of dorsal capsular cuff must be resected if the pedicle is not well visualized or if the external ganglion remains tense even after the intra-articular portion is debrided.

Other complications (such as neuroma formation and scar hypertrophy) can occur with arthroscopic surgery (as they can with open surgery). Neuroma formation can be minimized by avoiding use of the 1-2 and 6-U portals and by developing portals by blunt dissection to the capsule after incising only the skin with a knife. Transverse skin incisions instead of the traditional longitudinal skin stabs for making portals may help minimize scar hypertrophy and keloid formation.

The author routinely recommends scar massage and silicone patch taping at night to minimize scar hypertrophy after all surgical procedures on the hand and wrist. Wrist stiffness is common after open ganglion surgery if the joint is immobilized after surgery. Arthroscopy has the advantage of smaller incisions with minimal soft-tissue dissection, allowing early postoperative rehabilitation. To avoid postoperative stiffness, joint mobilization is commenced as soon as three to four days after surgery (when the postoperative pain has settled).

Summary

Arthroscopic ganglionectomy offers a viable treatment option for management of dorsal wrist ganglia after nonoperative treatment fails to resolve symptoms. The procedure can be undertaken by any surgeon familiar with arthroscopic wrist surgery using standard wrist portals and instrumentation. Correct use of the 3-4 and 6-R portals is necessary to facilitate debridement. Longer-term studies are needed to demonstrate improved results over open surgery, but intuitively arthroscopic excision seems to be the preferred option because of the smaller scars, earlier rehabilitation, and lower recurrence rates.

References

1. Angelides AC, Wallace PF. The dorsal ganglion of the wrist: Its pathogenesis, gross and microscopic anatomy, and surgical treatment. J Hand Surg 1976;1(3):228–35.
2. Osterman AL, Raphael J. Arthroscopic resection of dorsal ganglion of the wrist. Hand Clin 1995;11:7–12.
3. Burke FD, Melikyan EY, Bradley MJ, Dias JJ. Primary care referral protocol for wrist ganglia. Postgraduate Medical Journal 2003;79(932):329–31.
4. Blam O, Bindra R, Middleton W, Gelberman R. The occult dorsal carpal ganglion: Usefulness of magnetic resonance imaging and ultrasound in diagnosis. American Journal of Orthopedics 1998;27(2):107–10.
5. Wang AA, Hutchinson DT. Longtitudinal observation of pediatric hand and wrist ganglia. J Hand Surg [Am] 2001; 26:599–602.
6. Nield DV, Evans DM. Aspiration of ganglia. J Hand Surg [Br] 1986;11:264.
7. Richman JA, Gelberman RH, Engber WD, et al. Ganglions of the wrist and digits: Results of treatment by aspiration and cyst wall puncture. J Hand Surg [Am] 1987;12:1041–43.
8. Varley GW, Needoff M, Davis TRC, et al. Conservative management of wrist ganglia. J Hand Surg [Br] 1997;22:636–37.
9. Nishikawa S, Toh S, Miura H, Arai K, Irie T. Arthroscopic diagnosis and treatment of dorsal wrist ganglion. J Hand Surg 2001;26B:547–49.
10. Luchetti R, Badia A, Alfarano M, Orbay J, Indriago I, Mustapha B. Arthroscopic resection of dorsal wrist ganglia and treatment of recurrences. J Hand Surg 2000;25B:38–40.
11. Watson HK, Rogers WD, Ashmead DIV. Reevaluation of the cause of the wrist ganglion. J Hand Surg [Am] 1989;14 (5):812–17.
12. Andren L, Eiken O. Arthrographic studies of wrist ganglions. J Bone Joint Surg Am 1971;53(2):299–302.
13. Fontes D. Ganglia treated by arthroscopy. In P Saar, PC Amadio, G Foucher (eds.), *Current Practice in Hand Surgery.* London: Martin Dunitz 1997: 283–90.
14. Pederzini L, Ghinelli L, Soragni O. Arthroscopic treatment of dorsal arthrogenic cysts of the wrist. Journal of Sports Traumatology and Related Research 1995;17:210–15.
15. Rizzo M, Berger RA, Steinmann SP, Bishop AT. Arthroscopic resection in the management of dorsal wrist ganglions: Results with a minimum 2-year follow-up period. J Hand Surg 2004;29(1):59–62.

Jeffrey A. Greenberg

CHAPTER 22

"Other things may change us, but we start and end with family."

—Anthony Brandt

To Nancy, Ryann, and Sawyer, who support and put up with me, constantly.

Arthroscopic Treatment of Volar Carpal Ganglion Cysts

Arthroscopic Resection of Volar Carpal Ganglia

The concept of using arthroscopy as a means for the management of intra-articular conditions of the wrist has evolved tremendously since Roth first described the technique.[1] Arthroscopy of the wrist has become an essential adjunctive tool not only for the diagnosis of multiple conditions but for their definitive treatment. Intra-articular lesions, including capsular lesions, can be assessed and treated arthroscopically.

In 1995, Osterman and Raphael presented a technique for the treatment of the dorsal carpal ganglion.[2] This cystic structure has a predictable origin from the dorsal distal third of the scapholunate ligament. The initial skepticism regarding treatment of this lesion (which is at the anatomical boundary for visualization with the arthroscope) has been quelled by experience and refinement of the technique. Arthroscopic treatment of dorsal ganglion cysts is now routine for the experienced arthroscopist.[3–5]

Volar ganglia occur less frequently than the more common dorsal carpal ganglion cyst, accounting for approximately 20% of wrist ganglia. They are sac-like structures (with no true cellular lining) filled with a thick viscous fluid consisting of glucosamine, albumen, globulin, and hyaluronic acid. The ganglion frequently presents externally as a mass in the interval between the flexor carpi radialis (FCR) tendon and radial artery, proximal to the wrist flexion crease (Figure 22.1). Usually, the ganglion presents as a visible and palpable mass—with symptoms that may include pain, numbness secondary to irritation of the palmar cutaneous branch of the median nerve (PcuBrMN), and cosmetic dissatisfaction.

Occult volar ganglia may also contribute to volar wrist pain without a visible or definitely palpable mass. These occult ganglia may be symptomatic due to capsular injury, inflammatory changes, or local pressure. The cause of ganglion cysts has been debated and has been attributed to synovial herniation, mucoid degeneration, degenerative arthritis, and stretch associated with trauma.[6,7]

The anatomical origin of the volar carpal ganglion (VCG) has not been as well defined as its dorsal counterpart. Current literature supports a radioscaphoid or scaphotrapezial joint origin.[7,8] They may occasionally originate from the FCR tendon or from aberrant locations.[6,9] When the ganglion originates from the radioscaphoid joint, it arises from the volar capsule in the relatively deficient area between the volar radioscaphocapitate (RSC) and long radiolunate (LRL) ligaments (Figure 22.2).[10]

Traditionally, these ganglions are excised through an open volar approach, developing the interval between the radial artery and FCR tendon. The ganglion is then excised along with a segment of volar capsule. Arthroscopic excision of volar ganglion cysts eliminates the need for extensive dissection, limits capsular damage, allows identification of associated intra-articular pathology, and facilitates recovery and return to activity. Arthroscopic treatment of these cysts is technically feasible and facile.[10] The volar capsular origin of these lesions is easily visualized, which allows excision of the ganglion stalk utilizing standard arthroscopic portals and instrumentation.

Technique

A standard arthroscopic technique and setup are utilized. Traction is essential, as with all wrist arthroscopy. The

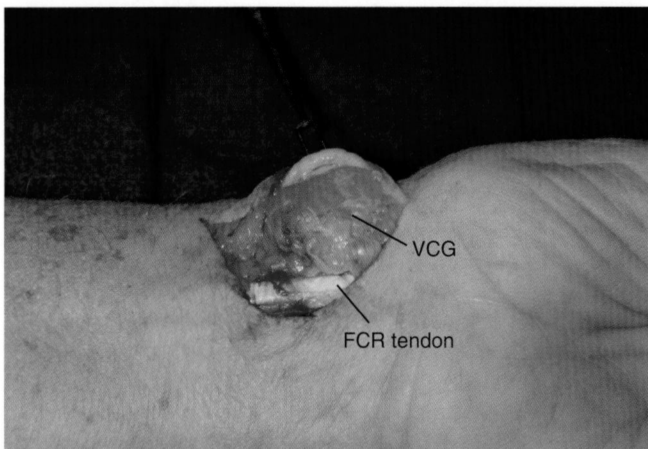

FIGURE 22.1. Clinical photo of a typical multilobular volar carpal ganglion located in the interval between the FCR tendon and radial artery.

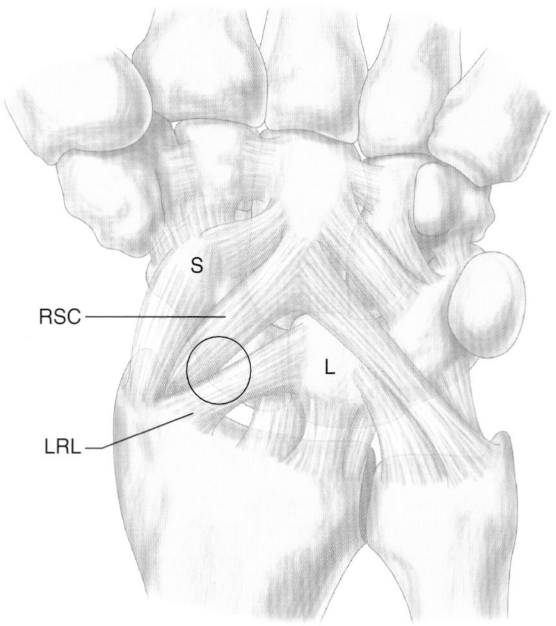

FIGURE 22.2. Diagrammatic representation of the volar extrinsic wrist ligaments demonstrating the interval (circle) between the radioscaphocapitate (RSC) and long radiolunate (LRL) ligaments.

portals are marked after the traction is applied. The joint is insufflated with saline via the 3-4 portal. The author has found it very useful, especially in the case of the occult VCG, to watch where the fluid accumulates as the wrist is insufflated. Frequently, an occult ganglion sac will develop an out-pouching that can be seen on the volar aspect of the wrist as the joint is injected.

The arthroscopic evaluation of the wrist begins with the arthroscope in the 3-4 portal, with instruments passed via the 4-5 portal. In the case of a VCG, significant redundancy of the capsule or an out-pouching can be visualized in the extrinsic ligament interval between RSC and LRL. This out-pouching and capsular redundancy can be exaggerated, and visualization can be facilitated by placing pressure on the wrist capsule from the volar side. In occult cases, the ganglion will usually become visible (Figure 22.3).

Once the lesion is identified and routine wrist arthroscopy is completed, attention is turned to resection of the mass. A high-speed full-radius resector is used to debride the lesion and resect the volar capsule between the two extrinsic ligaments. Frequently, during the capsular resection thick

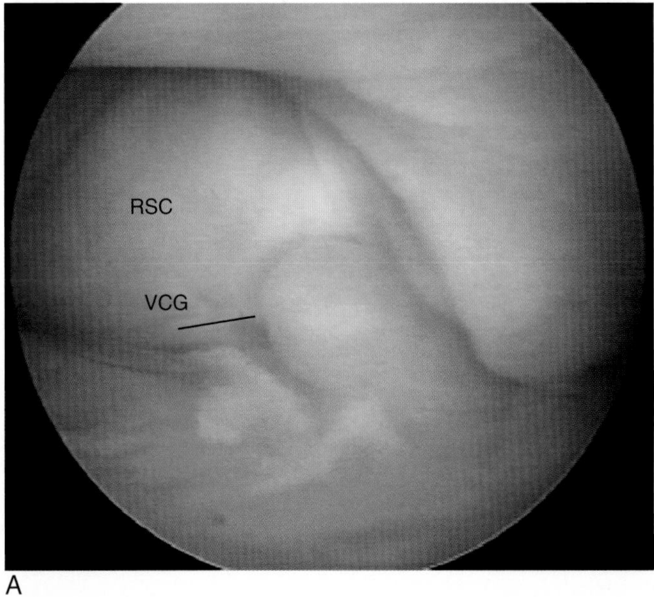

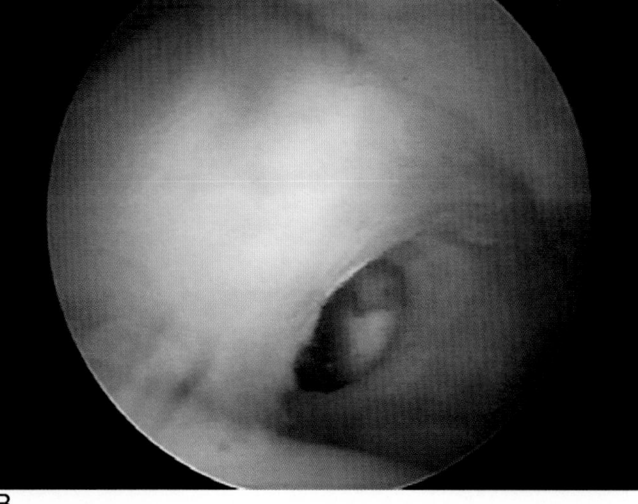

FIGURE 22.3. (A) Arthroscopic view of a volar carpal ganglion (VCG) located in the interval between the radioscaphocapitate (RSC) and long radiolunate ligaments. (B) The interval has been enlarged and the ganglion resected.

ganglion fluid will be encountered coincident with clinical resolution of the volar mass. In cases of very large ganglions, a blunt obturator can be passed from dorsal to volar through the capsular defect to facilitate intra-articular aspiration and mobilization of ganglion cyst fluid. Care should be taken to avoid plunging the resector too deeply (to avoid injury to volar neurovascular and tendinous structures). A volar portal[11] can be used with a cannula sheath to complete the debridement.

Preliminary Experience

This technique has been used to resect six volar ganglions. The initial case was in a patient who sustained a minor hyperextension injury to her wrist with a suspected occult volar ganglion coexisting with a possible volar capsular or extrinsic ligament tear. Wrist arthroscopy was performed as a confirmatory diagnostic maneuver. The occult mass was identified and resected with complete resolution of symptoms and rapid unrestricted return to all activities. One additional occult and four obvious ganglions have been resected using this technique. The location of the origin of the ganglion has been consistent in each case. There have been no recurrences or injuries to neurovascular structures.

Conclusions

New techniques and innovative uses of established techniques frequently meet with skepticism. Formerly skeptical surgeons now incorporate wrist arthroscopy as a routine diagnostic and therapeutic tool. Similar to our experience with resection of dorsal ganglia, experience, refinement of the technique, and practice have led to the routine use of arthroscopy for the resection of dorsal wrist ganglia.

We now understand that elimination of a dorsal ganglion is accomplished by excision of the stalk from its origin. Radical mass excision, dorsal capsulectomy, and posterior interosseous neurectomy are adjunctive procedures that are not essential to this technique. Similarly, the volar ganglion is a lesion of capsular origin. It arises in a predictable location and its removal is facilitated through the use of arthroscopic techniques. Experienced arthroscopists should be able to add this procedure to their armamentarium.

References

1. Roth JH, Poehling GG, Whipple TL. Hand instrumentation for small joint arthroscopy. Arthroscopy 1988;4:126–28.
2. Osterman AL, Raphael J. Arthroscopic resection of dorsal ganglia of the wrist. Hand Clinics 1995;11(1):7–12.
3. Gupta R, Bozentka DJ, Osterman AL. Wrist arthroscopy: Principles and clinical applications. J Am Acad Orth Surg 2001;9:200–09.
4. Osterman AL. Wrist arthroscopy: Operative procedures. In DP Green, RN Hotchkis,, WC Pederson (eds.), *Green's Operative Hand Surgery, Fourth Edition*. New York: Churchill Livingstone 1999: 207–22.
5. Rizzo M, Berger RA, Steinmann SP, Bishop AT. Arthroscopic resection in the management of dorsal wrist ganglions: Results with a minimum 2-year follow-up period. J Hand Surg 2004;29A:59–62.
6. Nahra ME, Bucchieri JA. Ganglion cysts and other tumor related conditions of the hand and wrist. Hand Clinics 2004;20(3):249–60.
7. Wright TW, Cooney WP, Ilstrup DM. Anterior wrist ganglia. J Hand Surg 1994;19A:954–58.
8. Greendyke SD, Wilson M, Shepler TR. Anterior wrist ganglia from the scaphotrapezial joint. J Hand Surg 1992;17A:487–90.
9. Shapiro PS, Seitz WH. Non-neoplastic tumors of the hand and upper extremity. Hand Clinics 1995;11(2):133–60.
10. Ho PC, Lo WN, Hung LK. Arthroscopic resection of volar ganglion of the wrist: a new technique. J Arthroscopic and Related Surgery 2003;19(2):218–21.
11. Abe Y, Doi K, Hattori Y, Ikeda K, Dhawan V. Arthroscopic assessment of the volar region of the scapholunate interosseous ligament through a volar portal. J Hand Surg 2003;28 (1):69–73.

N. Ashwood and G.I. Bain

CHAPTER 23

"Difficulties mastered are opportunities won."
—Winston Churchill

Arthroscopically Assisted Treatment of Intraosseous Ganglions of the Lunate

Introduction

Intraosseous ganglia of the carpal bones are an infrequent cause of chronic wrist pain. The pathogenesis remains obscure.[1,2] Bone scans and computerized tomography (CT) are used to distinguish these radiolucent carpal lesions from other pathologies, in particular degenerative cysts and osteoid osteomas.[1] Magnetic resonance imaging (MRI) will demonstrate the bony extent of the lesion and may help to delineate the presence of an extraosseous extension of the ganglion.[3]

Persistence and severity of symptoms rather than radiological findings determine the need for further management.[4] Curettage and bone grafting have been performed for patients with constant symptoms that have severely restricted their occupational or recreational activities.[1–6] Clinically, the patients improve. However in up to 40% symptoms persist that affect function.[1,2] The authors have published a minimally invasive technique of lunate ganglion grafting with the aim of reducing the morbidity that has been seen with open techniques.[7]

Pathology

Theories of pathogenesis of ganglia have included synovial herniation, neoplasia, metaplasia of mesenchymal precursor cells, proliferation of synovial rest cells, and traumatic mucoid degeneration of connective tissue.[1,2] The shear stresses concentrated at the scapholunate ligament insertion may predispose some individuals to developing the precursor cells that form the intraosseous ganglion.[8] Rather than proliferating dorsally from the scapholunate ligament, the cells head into the lunate itself.

Intraosseous ganglia are pathologically identical to the soft-tissue variety, with a thin wall of compressed collagen and fibroblasts containing a clear viscous fluid that has a high concentration of hyaluronic acid.[1–4,6,8–11] There is no endothelial or synovial lining. A thin sclerotic margin of bone often surrounds the ganglion. Some authors have suggested that this represents an attempt by the host bone to repair the defect within the lunate.[2] Bone scans invariably show increased uptake localized to the involved carpal bone. The advantages of arthroscopic surgery versus open techniques to treat lunate ganglion cysts include a lower morbidity and less risk of damaging the scapholunate ligament.

Indications

The patient presents with persistent dorsal wrist pain and swelling in the perilunate region that is exacerbated by activity and reduced grip strength. The decision to operate is based on the persistence and severity of the symptoms rather than on the outcome of the investigations, which help to localize the pathology. Preoperative symptoms often interfere with function at work or during recreation.[1,2,4]

Patients were not considered for surgery unless they had been symptomatic for at least six months and had failed a trial of activity, NSAIDs, and splints. Assessment included clinical examination for local tenderness and carpal stability.

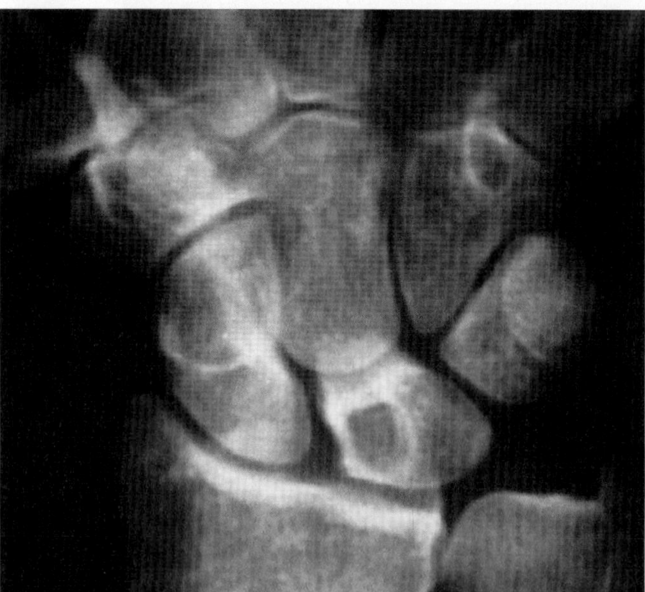

FIGURE 23.1. Radiographic appearances of an intraosseous ganglion of the lunate.

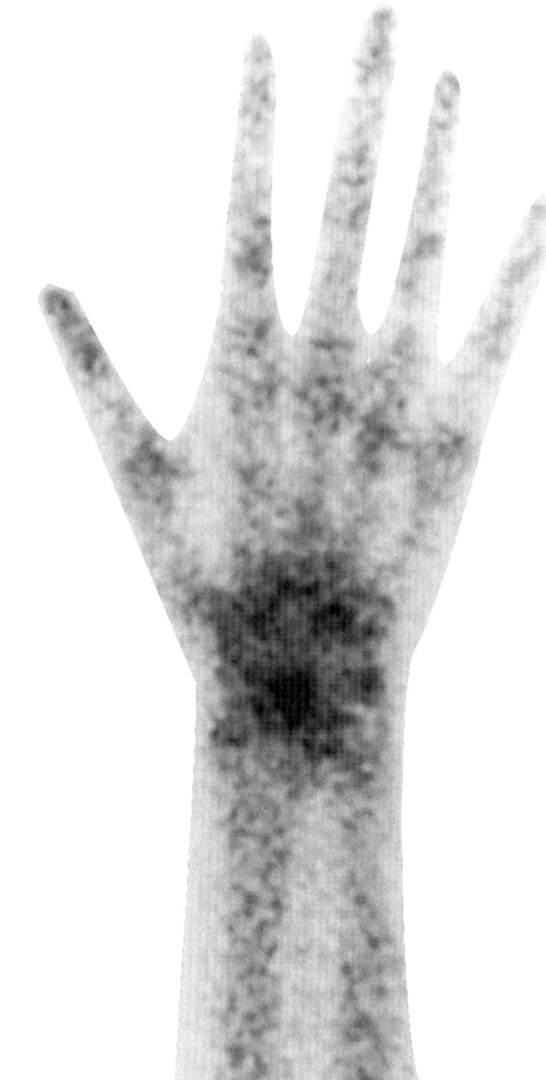

FIGURE 23.2. Technetium 99 radionuclide bone scan showing increased uptake in the lunate.

Radiographs usually revealed an eccentrically placed radiolucent lesion with a thin sclerotic margin contained within and not expanding the lunate (Figure 23.1).

All patients had a preoperative technetium 99 radionuclide bone scan demonstrating focal increased uptake within the lunate and no other site within the wrist (Figure 23.2). This investigation helped to confirm that the patients' symptoms were related to the intraosseous ganglion prior to any intervention. Patients who had a negative bone scan were not offered surgical treatment.

CT scans were used to define the location and extent of the lesion, which aided surgical planning. Localization of the cyst is particularly important with this technique, as the cyst may be volar or dorsal. Figure 23.3 shows a typical coronal CT scan in which the ganglion located close to the

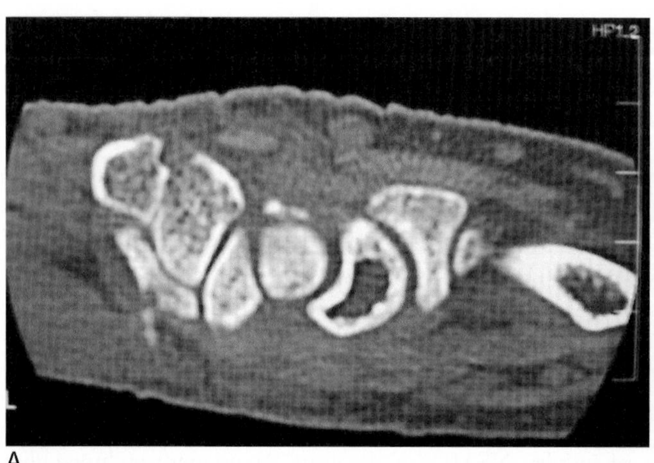

A

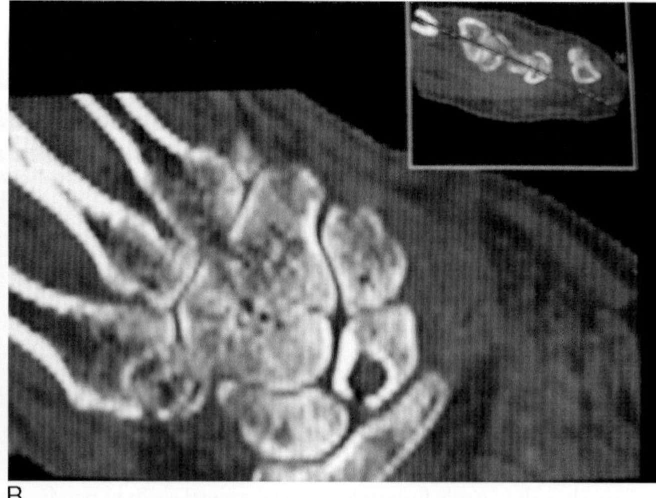

B

FIGURE 23.3. CT scan showing the extent of an intraosseous ganglion of the lunate. (A) Sagittal section. (B) Coronal section.

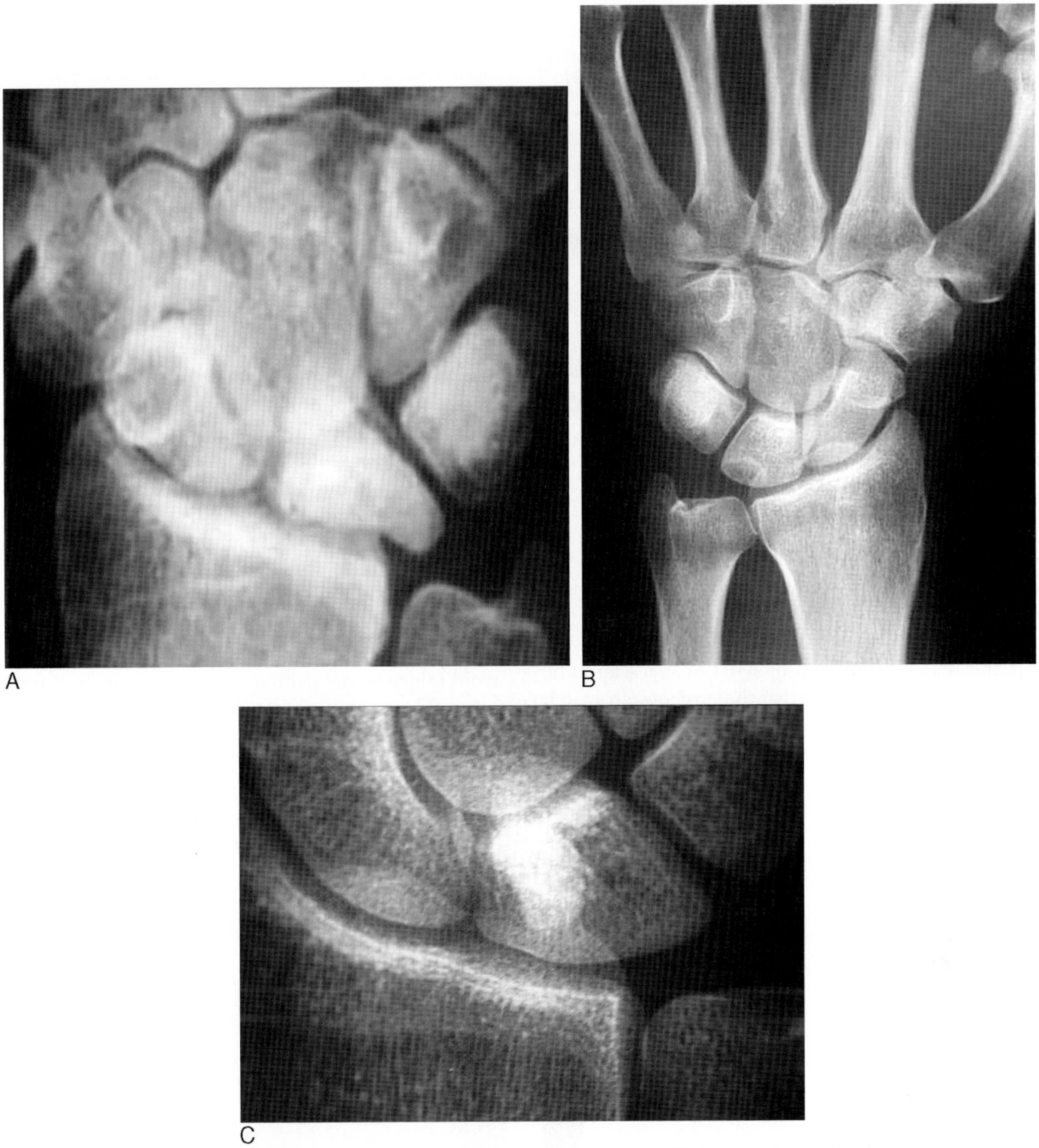

A

B

C

FIGURE 23.4. (A) Kienbock's avascular necrosis. (B) Ulnar carpal impaction. (C) Lunate bone island.

scapholunate ligament can be seen to perforate the cortex of the lunate at the site of attachment of the ligament. It is a common radiological finding, and confirms its origin as a ganglion from the scapholunate ligament. Some surgeons have previously interpreted this as a fracture.

Contraindications

Lesions with more sinister pathology of lesion need to be excluded. These are rare and can be differentiated with imaging. Other common pathological conditions that affect the lunate include Kienbock's diseases and avascular necrosis, which produces sclerosis and often collapse of the proximal convexity of the lunate 22 (Figure 23.4a). Ulnar carpal impaction is also common, but this affects only the ulnar side of the lunate and is often associated with a kissing lesion of the ulnar head (Figure 23.4b). Bone islands (Figure 23.4c), osteoid osteoma, and other lesions are rare. CT scans can help differentiate these lesions.

Surgical Technique

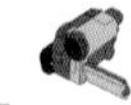

The arm is suspended on Chinese finger traps with 10 pounds of traction. Routine arthroscopy is performed via a

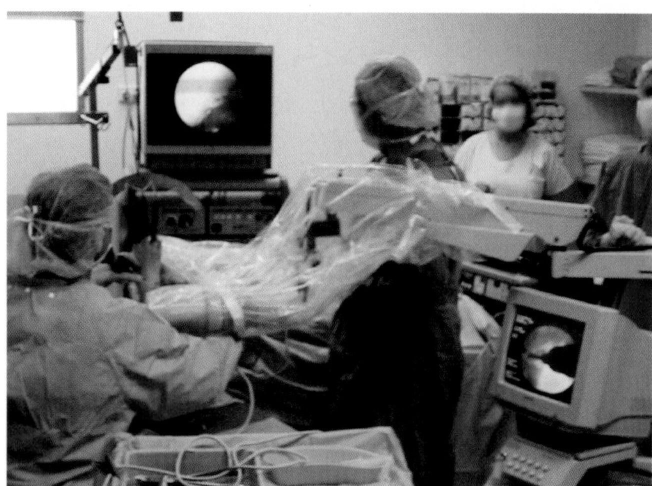

FIGURE 23.5. Setup for arthroscopy with portable fluoroscopy. Note that the C-arm is horizontal for easier working. The suspended hand can simply be rotated on the string.

3-/,4 portal and a 6-R portal created with trans-illumination and insertion of a needle.[12] It is not usually possible to visualize the ganglion through the arthroscope because the lesion is intraosseous. However, intra-articular extension can occur and may be predicted by MRI or CT scan. The fluoroscopy unit is positioned so that the surgeon can switch between assessment of the joint surface with arthroscopy and assessment of the skeletal anatomy with fluoroscopy (Figure 23.5).

A trocar and cannular are positioned on the lunate under arthroscopic vision and strategically positioned at the site of the lesion as determined by the preoperative imaging (Figure 23.6). A small-joint cannula is used as a drill guide to protect the adjacent soft tissue. The scapholunate ligament can often be used as an approximate guide to the position of the ganglion arthroscopically. Satisfactory positioning of the drill tip is then confirmed in the anteroposterior and lateral planes using fluoroscopy.[13]

The drill is then advanced into the body of the lunate corresponding to the site of the intraosseous ganglion as previously identified on the CT scan. If the lesion is on the volar aspect of the lunate on CT scan, a volar portal is used to drill the lunate (Figure 23.7). If it is on the dorsal aspect, the 3-/,4 portal is used—with the scope in the 6-R portal (Figure 23.6). Fluoroscopy is used to confirm the position of the drill.

The method of establishing the volar portal used by the senior author is an inside-out technique, which is created by placing the scope into the 3-/,4 portal. The scope is advanced into the interligamentous sulcus between the radioscaphocapitate (RSC) and long radiolunate (LRL) ligaments (Figure 23.8). The scope is withdrawn from the trocar and a small Wissinger rod is advanced through the sulcus into the volar wrist. With pressure on the Wissinger rod, the skin over the rod is incised. Care is taken to ensure that the rod passes to the radial side of the FCR tendon to avoid injury to the palmar cutaneous branch of the median nerve. The scope is then positioned over the Wissinger rod on the volar aspect of the wrist and advanced into the wrist. The senior author believes this technique is much simpler than other published techniques, which require an open approach or outside-in techniques.

Once an appropriate drill hole is made, a biopsy can be taken of the lesion using a curette or arthroscopic biopsy forceps (Figure 23.9). Usually the cavity is filled with a viscous gelatinous material. Histology should confirm

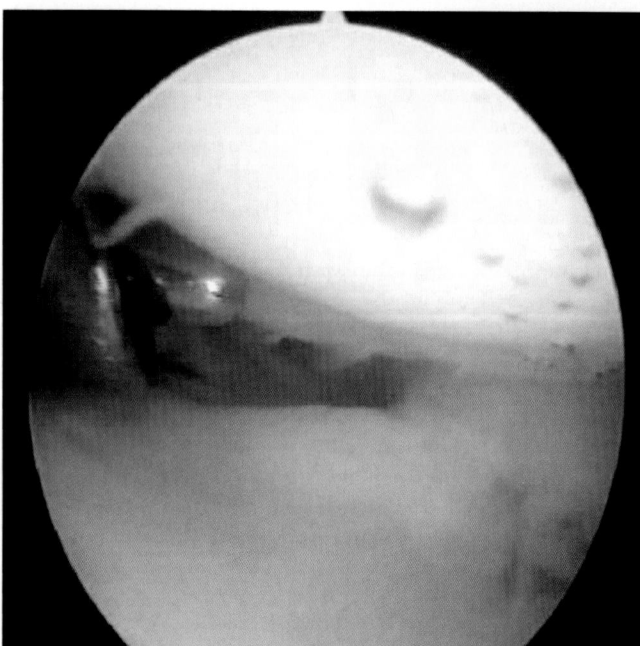

FIGURE 23.6. Arthroscopic view (6-R) with trocar and cannular being positioned from the 3-4 portal in preparation for drilling. The SL ligament assists in positioning of the instruments.

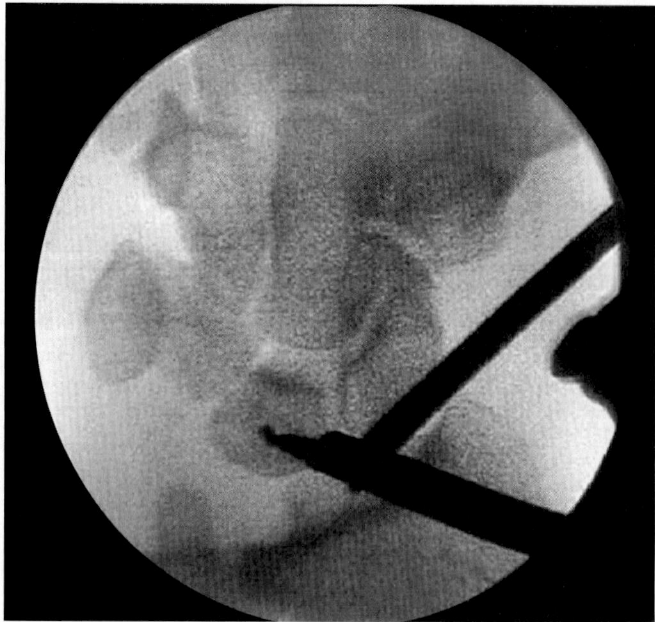

FIGURE 23.7. Fluoroscopic confirmation of drill placement within the lunate lesion. Arthroscope in 3-4 portal drill via volar portal.

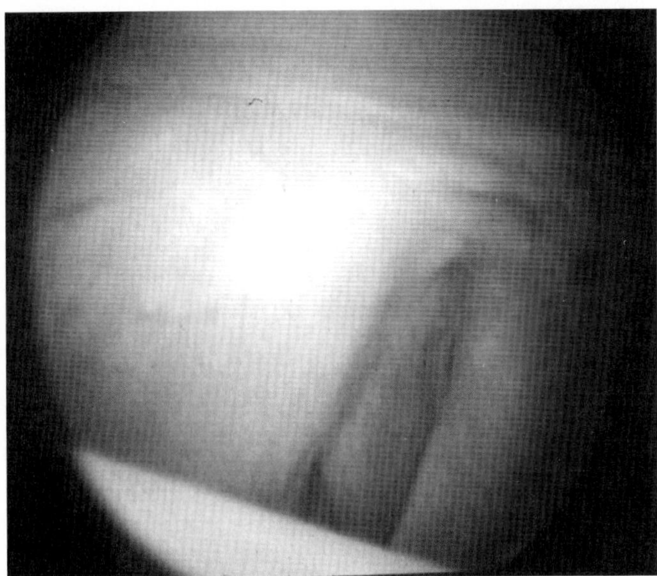

FIGURE 23.8. Interligamentous sulcus between RSC and RL ligaments.

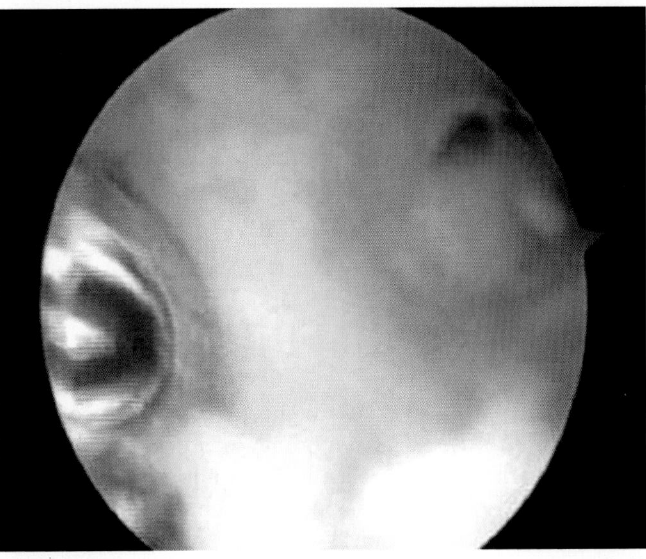

FIGURE 23.10. Arthroscopic view (6-R) of the lunate drill hole. Resector on left.

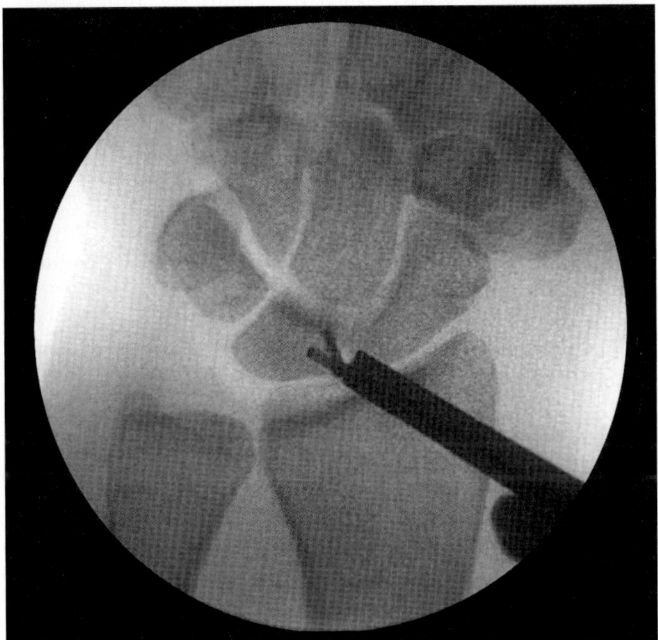

FIGURE 23.9. Biopsy forceps within lunate intraosseous ganglion.

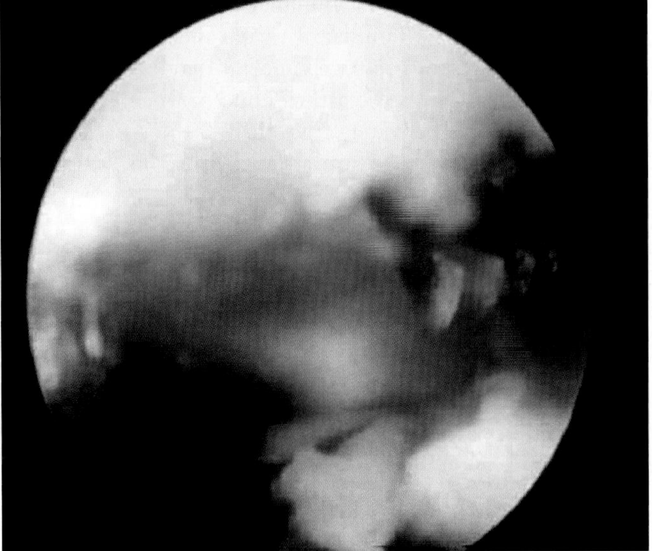

FIGURE 23.11. Resector advanced into the lunate for arthroscopic debridement of the ganglion.

a fibrous capsule of compressed collagen fibers, fibroblasts, and mesenchymal cells around a viscous clear mucinoid center. These features are consistent with an intraosseous ganglion.

A standard 3-mm arthroscopic motorized resector is introduced into the drill hole to enable debridement of the remaining soft tissue (Figures 23.10 and 23.11). Fluoroscopy is used intermittently to confirm position of the instruments during the procedure. To confirm the adequacy of the debridement, the arthroscope can be advanced to view the intraosseous cavity (osteoscopy!). This helps confirm that all soft tissue has been removed.

Bone grafting is performed to restore the normal architecture of the lunate and minimize the risk of lunate collapse. An incision is made over the dorsal aspect of the wrist proximal to Lister's tubercle. A small cortical window is made in the radius. Cancellous bone is then harvested. A 3-mm bore trocar can then be advanced directly into the hole in the lunate. Fluoroscopy is used to confirm that the trocar is well seated within the debrided lunate. The harvested bone graft is delivered through the trocar and impacted into the lunate by pushing the graft through the trocar using a small tamping rod. This reduces the risk of any graft falling into the wrist joint. The lesion is grafted up to the margin of the cortical bone rather than the articular cartilage. The lunate is finally assessed arthroscopically and fluoroscopically to ensure that the graft is suitably positioned. The joint is thoroughly irrigated prior to the wounds being sutured with an absorbable suture.

A volar plaster slab is applied for 10 days until the wounds have healed. Patients are advised not to return to light duties until six weeks, and heavy manual labor is avoided for a minimum of three months.

Potential Pitfalls

Patient selection is the key to the successful outcome of this procedure. Relief of symptoms in previous reports of curettage and grafting procedures was not uniform or predictable.[1,2,5,6] Symptoms appear to correlate uniformly with having a positive bone scan.[2] For this reason, patient recruitment should hinge on the presence of a bone scan with heightened activity in our opinion.

It is possible to have an extraosseous extension of the ganglion. Preoperative clinical radiographic and CT are therefore important. Fluoroscopic and arthroscopic assessments are important in this minimal-access technique. The surgeon needs to be familiar with advanced wrist arthroscopic techniques. A volar wrist portal may be required to enable visualization by the arthroscope or to act as a portal to introduce and advance the drill.[14] No patient has required a salvage procedure after arthroscopic treatment in the author's hands.

Results

In our published series there were 10 patients followed for a minimum of three years.[7] Following surgery, all patients had significant improvements in pain scores, grip strength, range of motion, and function. These have been represented as modified Green scores, which increased 34 points from 51 to 85 points ($p = 0.03$) by one year postoperatively.[10] The scores were maintained in all patients at last review.

Visual analog pain scores improved from an average preoperative level of 68 to 11 ($p = 0.01$). Grip strength averaged 12 (range 6 to 22) kg prior to surgery. This increased to 19 (range 14 to 34) kg following the procedure ($p = 0.04$), which compared well to the contralateral limb at 23 (range 12 to 36) kg ($p > 0.05$). The patients were all satisfied with the improvements in function and pain following surgery. There were no complications or re-operations in this series.

In summary, patients with IOG who were treated with this arthroscopic technique had significant improvements in pain scores and functional activity, which were well maintained. The results compare well with previous reports.[1,2,5]

References

1. Tham S, Ireland DC. Intraosseous ganglion cyst of the lunate: Diagnosis and management. J Hand Surg [Br] 1992;17(4):429–32.
2. Waizenegger M. Intraosseous ganglia of carpal bones. J Hand Surg [Br] 1993;18-33:350–55.
3. Sullivan PP, Berquist TH. Magnetic resonance imaging of the hand, wrist and forearm: Utility in patients with pain and dysfunction as a result of trauma. Mayo Clinic Proceedings 1991;66:1217–21.
4. Mogan JV, Newberg AH, Davis PH. Intraosseous ganglion of the lunate. J Hand Surg [Am] 1981;6(1):61–63.
5. Schajowicz F, Clavel Sainz M, Slullitel JA. Juxta-articular bone cysts (intra-osseous ganglia): A clinicopathological study of eighty-eight cases. J Bone Joint Surg Br 1979;61 (1):107–16.
6. Kambolis C, Bullough PG, Jaffe HI. Ganglionic cystic defects of bone. J Bone Joint Surg Am 1973;55(3):496–505.
7. Ashwood N, Bain GI. Arthroscopically assisted treatment of intraosseous ganglions of the lunate: A new technique. J Hand Surg [Am] 2003;28(1):62–68.
8. Gunther SF. Dorsal wrist pain and the occult scapholunate ganglion. J Hand Surg [Am] 1985;10(5):697–703.
9. Angelides AC, Wallace PF. The dorsal ganglion of the wrist: Its pathogenesis, gross and microscopic anatomy, and surgical treatment. J Hand Surg [Am] 1976;1(3):228–35.
10. Green DP, O'Brien ET. Open reduction of carpal dislocations: Indications and operative techniques. J Hand Surg [Am] 1978;3(3):250–65.
11. Young L, Bartell T, Logan SE. Ganglions of the hand and wrist. Southern Medical Journal 1988;81(6):697–703.
12. Bain GI, Richards RS, Roth JH. Wrist arthroscopy. In DM Lichtman, AH Alexander (eds.), *The Wrist and Its Disorders*. Second Edition, Philadelphia: W.B. Saunders 1997.
13. Bain GI, Hunt J, Mehta JA. Operative fluoroscopy in hand and upper limb surgery: One hundred cases. J Hand Surg [Br] 1997;22(5):656–58.
14. Tham S, Coleman S, Gilpin D. An anterior portal for wrist arthroscopy: Anatomical study and case reports. J Hand Surg [Br] 1999;24(4):445–47.

David J. Slutsky

CHAPTER 24

Arthroscopic Radial Styloidectomy

Introduction

Radial styloidectomy has typically been employed as a palliative procedure for any condition that results in painful impingement between the scaphoid and the radial styloid. It is most attractive to patients who wish minimal surgical intervention, but it does not address the underlying cause and hence may not be a long-term solution. Recommendations for the amount of bony resection have become more conservative with time due to several biomechanical studies that demonstrated increasing radial instability, with the risk of ulnar translocation and progressive loss of the strong volar radiocarpal ligaments.[1,2]

Osterman has written extensively on an arthroscopic technique that not only allows an assessment of the joint surfaces but allows one to visualize and preserve these crucial volar ligaments.[3–5] The arthroscopic procedure may carry less risk of injury to the superficial radial nerve branches, with less pain compared to an open procedure.

Indications

The indications for an arthroscopic radial styloidectomy are similar to the open procedure. Radial styloid impingement due to radioscaphoid arthritis is a common indication. This is often a consequence of long-standing scapholunate dissociation or end-stage Kienbock's disease. Culp et al. suggest that patients who have painful radial deviation and a positive Watson test but have preserved wrist motion and good grip strength are ideal candidates.[6] Chronic scaphoid nonunion, in which the hypertrophic distal scaphoid fragment impinges against the radial styloid during wrist radial deviation, is another common indication. If an attempt is made to internally fix the scaphoid, this impingement must be addressed. Resection of the distal scaphoid fragment will obviate the need for a radial styloidectomy.[7]

Secondary radial styloid impingement is a common sequella of a scaphotrapeziotrapezoidal (STT) fusion when it is used to treat rotary subluxation of the scaphoid or scaphotrapezialosteoarthritis (OA). Watson observed this in more than a third of his patients and now recommends a radial styloidectomy at the time of STT fusion.[8] Impingement may also occur following a capitolunate fusion, which should be checked for at the time of surgery.[9] Occasionally a limited styloidectomy is performed at the time of a proximal row carpectomy for treatment of radiocarpal OA.[10]

Contraindications

The main risk following a radial styloidectomy is ulnar translocation of the carpus. Siegal and Gelberman showed that short oblique osteotomies were the least destructive, whereas vertical oblique and horizontal osteotomies removed 92 to 95% of the radioscaphocapitate (RSC) ligament and 21 to 46% of the long radiolunate ligament (LRL).[2] Cooney and coauthors emphasized the importance of the RSC and LRL ligaments in preventing ulnar translocation. If too much of these ligaments is removed, the capitate is destabilized and no longer rests in the lunate fossa—resulting in radial instability. Biomechanical testing revealed a significant increase in radial translation under loading when $\geq$6 mm or the radial styloid was excised.

Some specimens demonstrated moderate to severe palmar and ulnar translation. They recommended limiting

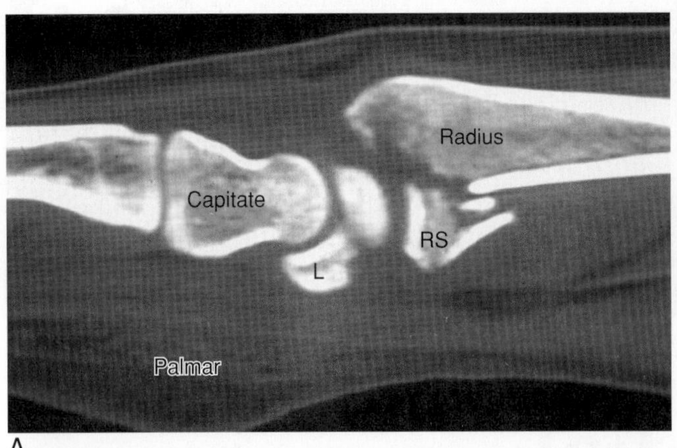

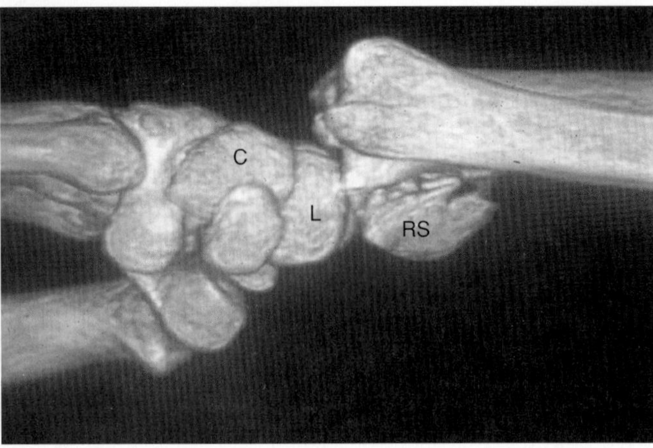

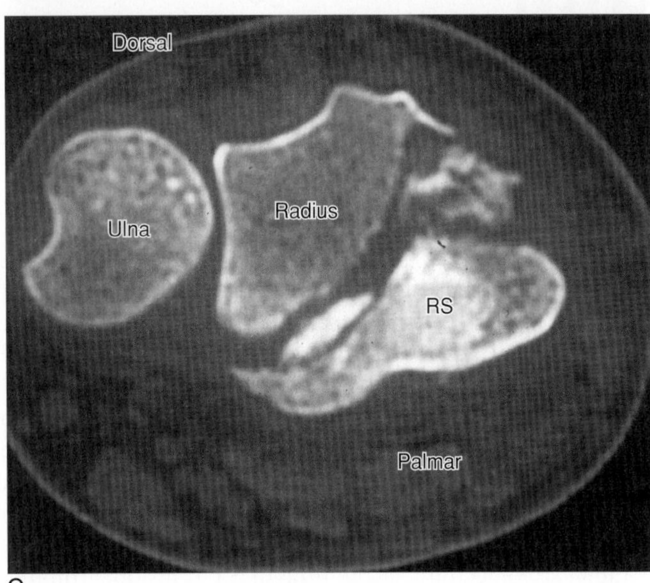

FIGURE 24.1. (A) CT scan of radial styloid fracture. Note the palmar dislocation of the carpus (L = lunate, RS = radial styloid). (B) 3D CT reconstruction (C = capitate). (C) Sagittal CT view showing large radial styloid fragment.

the bony resection to no more than 4 mm to minimize this risk.[1] Patients who do not have an intact RSC ligament due to distal radius fracture[11] (Figure 24.1a through c) or radiocarpal dislocation (Figure 24.2)[12–14] are at risk for ulnar translocation and are not candidates for this procedure, especially if a proximal row carpectomy is contemplated.[15] Ulnar translocation is a frequent sequella of long-standing rheumatoid disease. Hence, any patient with chronic wrist involvement is a poor candidate for this procedure.

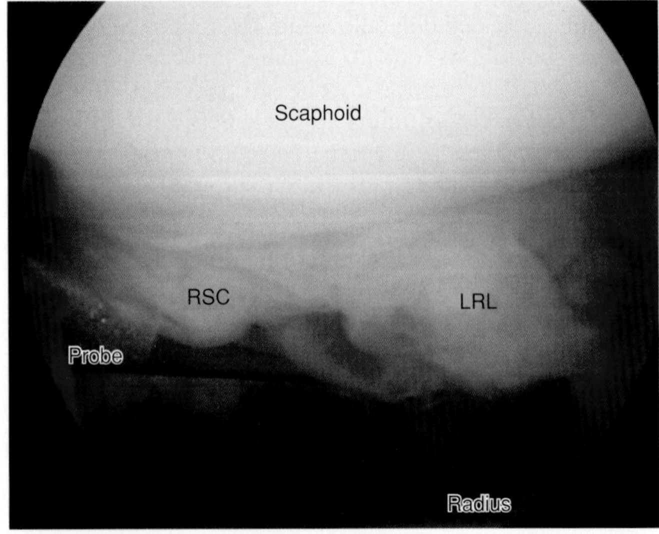

FIGURE 24.2. Traumatic avulsion of radioscaphocapitate (RSC) and long radiolunate (LRL) ligaments. View is from the 4-/,5 portal, probe in the 3-/,4 portal.

Equipment

A 2.7-mm 30-degree angled scope along with a camera attachment is used. A 2.9-mm bur and/or a 4.0-mm abrader is integral to the procedure. A small osteotome may also be useful. An overhead traction tower greatly facilitates instrumentation. The use of a motorized shaver is needed for debridement. Some type of diathermy unit may be useful, as well as arthroscopic straight and curved knives for lysis of adhesions. Intraoperative fluoroscopy is employed to assess the adequacy of bone resection.

Surgical Technique

This is one procedure in which the 1-/,2 portal is particularly helpful. The patient is positioned supine on the operating table, with the arm extended on a hand table. The fingers are suspended by Chinese finger traps with 10 to 15 pounds of countertraction. The relevant landmarks in the snuffbox are palpated and outlined, including the distal edge of the radial styloid, the abductor pollicis longus (APL), the extensor pollicis brevis (EPB) and extensor pollicis longus EPL tendons, and the radial artery in the snuffbox (Figure 24.3a through c). A tourniquet is elevated to 250 mmHg.

To minimize the risk of injury to branches of the superficial radial nerve and the radial artery, the 1-/,2 portal should be placed more palmar and proximal in the snuffbox. The entry site is outlined no more than 4.5 mm dorsal to the first extensor compartment and within 4.5 mm of the radial styloid.[16] A 22-gauge needle is used to identify the joint space, followed by a small superficial skin incision. The tissue is spread down to the capsule, which is pierced by

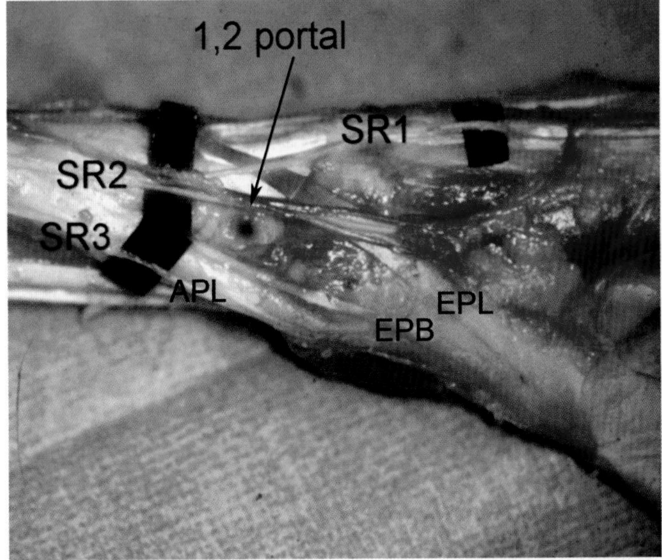

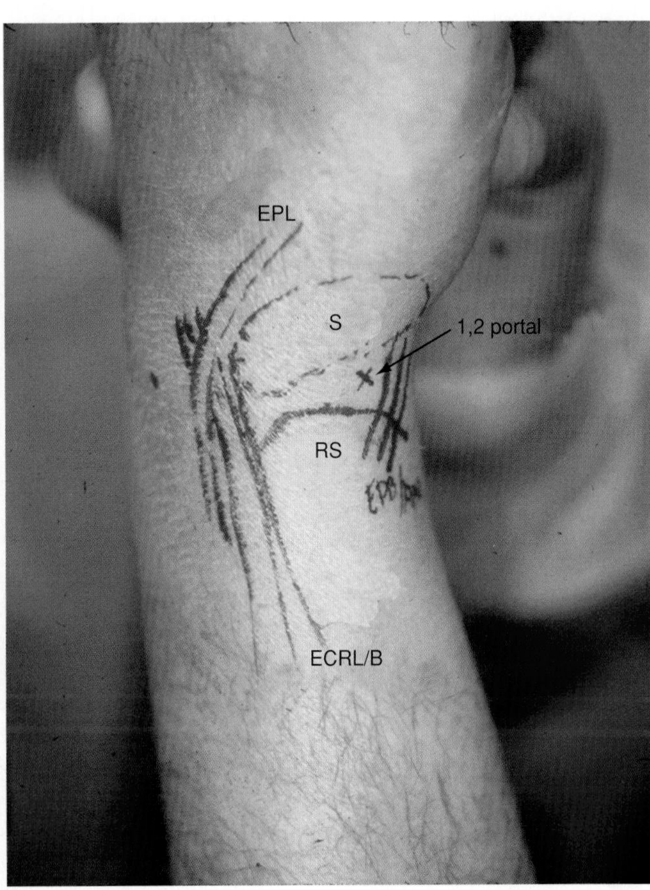

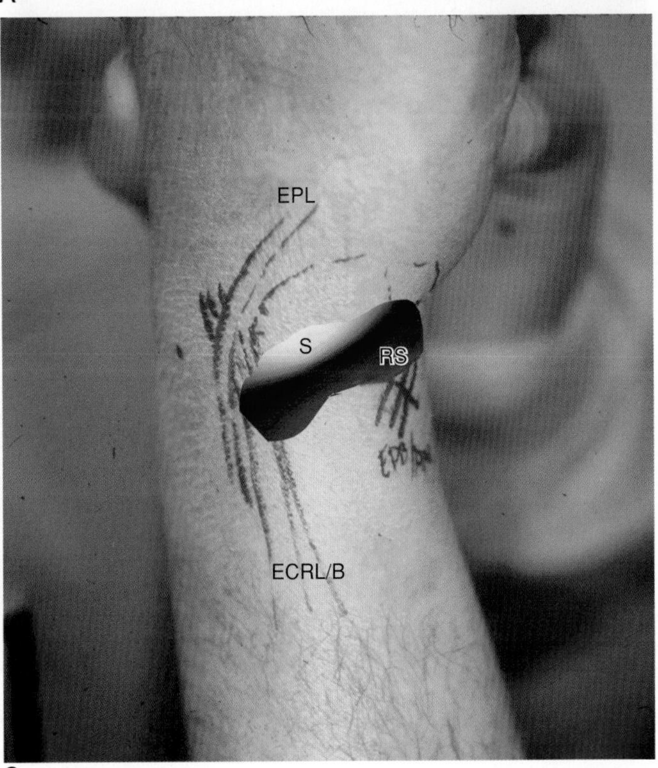

FIGURE 24.3. (A) Cadaver dissection of portal anatomy (SR1-3 = superficial radial nerve branches, EPL = extensor pollicis longus, EPB = extensor pollicis brevis, APL = abductor pollicis longus). (B) Surface landmarks for 1-/2 portal (ECRL/B = extensor carpi radialis longus/brevis, RS = radial styloid, S = scaphoid). (C) Superimposed field of view.

tenotomy scissors. A cannula and blunt trocar are inserted with the wrist in ulnar deviation to minimize damage to the proximal scaphoid, followed by a 3-mm hook probe.

A 3-/,4 working portal is established in a similar fashion. The author uses the volar radial (VR) portal interchangeably with the 3-/,4 portal for viewing and instrumentation in order to gain complete access to the dorsoradial aspect of the styloid (Figure 24.4a through d). A large-bore outflow cannula in the 4-/,5 or 6-U portal is desirable. A standard radiocarpal and midcarpal survey are performed, with debridement and synovectomy as necessary. With the arthroscope in the 3-/,4 portal, the origins of the RSC and LRL on the distal radius are noted—which mark the ulnar extent of the resection. The diameter of the bur will give a rough guide as to the amount of bony resection, but this needs to be confirmed fluoroscopically.

Various authors recommend from 4 to 7 mm of resection. The degree of bony resection should, however, be tailored to the individual and gauged at the time of surgery. Enough bone should be resected so that there is no residual impingement between the scaphoid and the radial styloid when the wrist is radially deviated with the traction released (Figure 24.5a and b). A small osteotome should be used judiciously because inadvertent penetration of the radial joint capsule carries the risk of radial artery perforation as it traverses the snuffbox.

Postoperative Management

The patient is placed in a removable below-elbow splint for comfort, and protected wrist motion is instituted after the

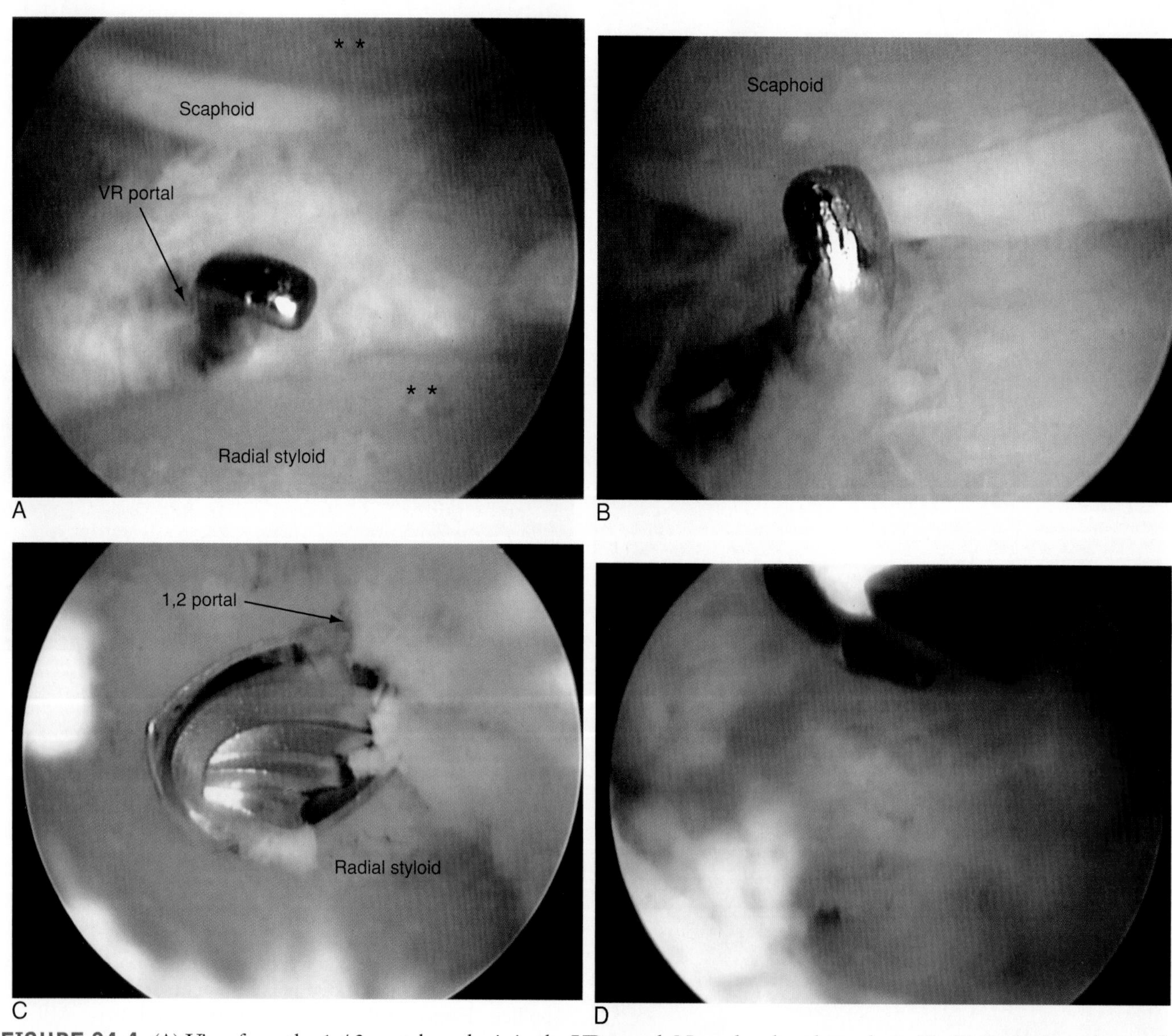

FIGURE 24.4. (A) View from the 1-/,2 portal, probe is in the VR portal. Note the chondromalacia (*). (B) Probe is exploring the bare area on the scaphoid. (C) Abrader introduced through 1-/,2 portal as seen from the VR portal. (D) View midway through the styloidectomy.

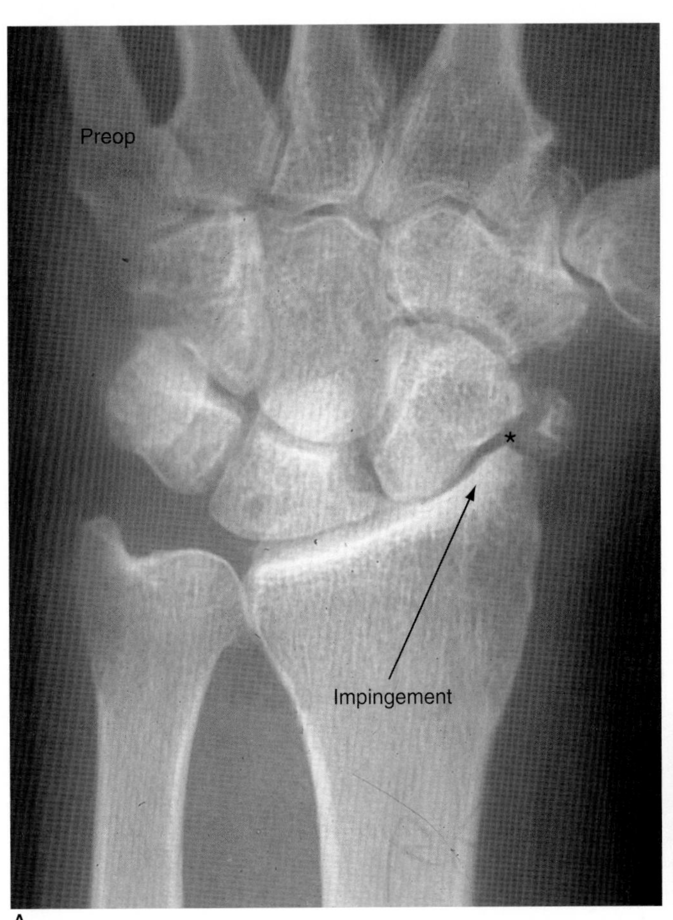

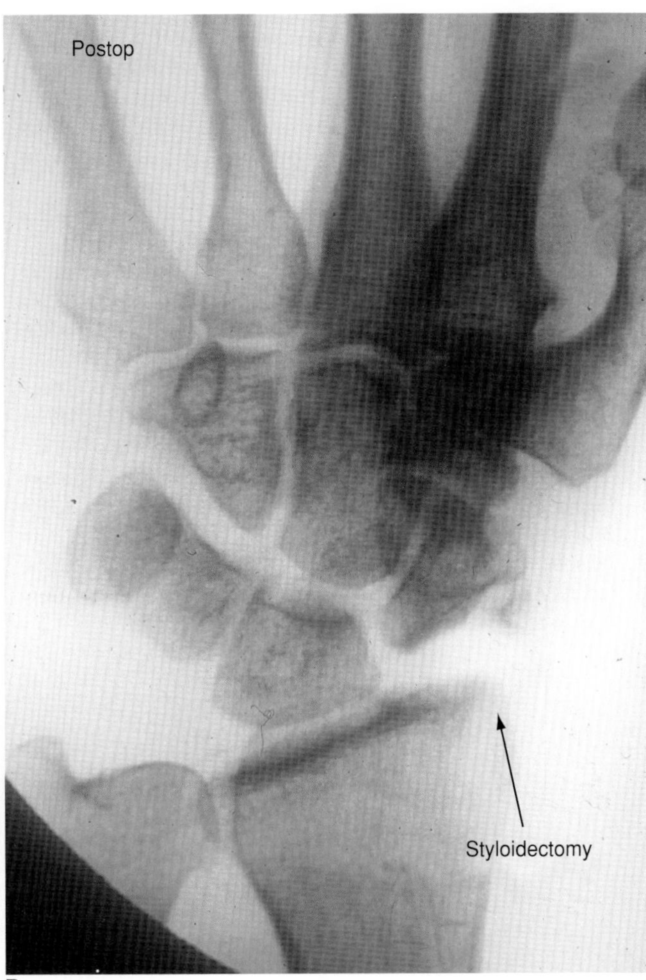

FIGURE 24.5. (A) Preoperative X-ray of chronic scapholunate dissociation. Note the radiocarpal narrowing (*). (B) After the arthroscopic styloidectomy, with no further impingement of the scaphoid and radial styloid.

first week. Gradual strengthening exercises are added as tolerated by the third to fourth week.

Complications

The most dire complication is ulnar translocation due to excessive resection of the radial styloid and radiocarpal ligaments. The superficial radial nerve and radial artery are perpetually at risk with use of the 1-/,2 portal.

Results

Open radial styloidectomies have been employed for more than 50 years. Arthroscopic techniques are more recent. Because it is often used in combination with other procedures, reports of isolated styloidectomies are scant. Similarly, there are no large series on arthroscopic resection. Some investigators have reported pain relief and improved wrist motion following internal fixation of scaphoid nonunions when combined with an open radial styloidectomy for arthritic changes.[17] Stark and coauthors found that the principal benefit obtained was pain relief rather than increased motion or grip strength.[18] Radial styloidectomy has been implicated as a causative factor in persistent scaphoid nonunion following internal fixation.[19]

References

1. Nakamura T, Cooney WP III, Lui WH, et al. Radial styloidectomy: A biomechanical study on stability of the wrist joint. J Hand Surg [Am] 2001;26:85–93.
2. Siegel DB, Gelberman RH. Radial styloidectomy: An anatomical study with special reference to radiocarpal intracapsular ligamentous morphology. J Hand Surg [Am] 1991;16:40–4.
3. Yao J, Osterman AL. Arthroscopic techniques for wrist arthritis (radial styloidectomy and proximal pole hamate excisions). Hand Clin 2005;21:519–26.
4. Gupta R, Bozentka DJ, Osterman AL. Wrist arthroscopy: Principles and clinical applications. J Am Acad Orthop Surg 2001;9:200–09.
5. Osterman A. Wrist arthroscopy: Operative procedures. In DP Green, WC Pederson (eds.), *Green's Operative Hand Surgery, Fourth Edition*. Philadelphia: Churchill Livingstone 1999:207–22.

6. Culp RW. Operative wrist arthroscopy. In DP Green, WC Pederson, SW Wolfe (eds.), *Green's Operative Hand Surgery, Fifth Edition*. Philadelphia: Churchill Livingstone 2005:798.
7. Ruch DS, Papadonikolakis A. Resection of the scaphoid distal pole for symptomatic scaphoid nonunion after failed previous surgical treatment. J Hand Surg [Am] 2006;31:588–93.
8. Rogers WD, Watson HK. Radial styloid impingement after triscaphe arthrodesis. J Hand Surg [Am] 1989;14:297–301.
9. Calandruccio JH, [name] GR. SLAC wrist: Capitolunate fusion with scaphoid and triquetrum excision. In R Gelberman (ed.), *Master Techniques in Orthopedic Surgery: The Wrist*. Philadelphia: Lippincott Williams & Wilkins 2002:234.
10. Van Heest AE HJ. Proximal row carpectomy. In R Gelberman (ed.), *Master Techniques in Orthopedic Surgery: The Wrist*. Philadelphia: Lippincott Williams & Wilkins 2002: 37–47.
11. Schoenecker PL, Gilula LA, Shively RA, Manske PR. Radiocarpal fracture: Dislocation. Clin Orthop Relat Res 1985: 237–44.
12. Jebson PJ, Adams BD, Meletiou SD. Ulnar translocation instability of the carpus after a dorsal radiocarpal dislocation: A case report. Am J Orthop 2000;29:462–64.
13. Howard RF, Slawski DP, Gilula LA. Isolated palmar radiocarpal dislocation and ulnar translocation: A case report and review of the literature. J Hand Surg [Am] 1997;22:78–82.
14. Dumontier C, Meyer zu Reckendorf G, Sautet A, et al. Radiocarpal dislocations: Classification and proposal for treatment. A review of twenty-seven cases. J Bone Joint Surg Am 2001;83-A:212–18.
15. van Kooten EO, Coster E, Segers MJ, Ritt MJ. Early proximal row carpectomy after severe carpal trauma. Injury 2005;36:1226–32.
16. Steinberg BD, Plancher KD, Idler RS. Percutaneous Kirschner wire fixation through the snuff box: An anatomic study. J Hand Surg [Am] 1995;20:57–62.
17. Herness D, Posner MA. Some aspects of bone grafting for non-union of the carpal navicular. Analysis of 41 cases. Acta Orthop Scand 1977;48:373–78.
18. Stark HH, Rickard TA, Zemel NP, Ashworth CR. Treatment of ununited fractures of the scaphoid by iliac bone grafts and Kirschner-wire fixation. J Bone Joint Surg Am 1988;70: 982–91.
19. Schuind F, Haentjens P, Van Innis F, et al. Prognostic factors in the treatment of carpal scaphoid nonunions. J Hand Surg [Am] 1999;24:761–76.

Brian J. Harley and Andrew K. Palmer

CHAPTER 25

Arthroscopic Resection of Arthrosis of the Proximal Hamate

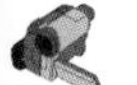

Rationale and Basic Science

Pain in the ulnar aspect of the wrist is a common symptom in the field of hand surgery. This presenting complaint has a large number of possible etiologies, however, and the treatment for any given etiology is largely dependent on the diagnosis. Although treatment options for isolated tears of the triangular fibrocartilage complex (TFCC) or the lunotriquetral (LT) ligament have been studied for many years, there is very little research on outcomes for patients with arthritic change of the proximal pole of the hamate. This is surprising, given that the proximal hamate is one of the most frequent sites of arthrosis in the wrist.[1,2]

In 1990, two unrelated anatomical studies closely characterized the lunate articular anatomy.[1,3] These descriptions referred to the distal joint morphology of the lunate in the midcarpal joint and two types were described (Figure 25.1). A type I lunate is one in which the distal lunate articulation makes contact with only the capitate. It was observed in approximately 30% of specimens. A type II lunate is one with an obvious distal lunate medial facet that articulates with the proximal pole of the hamate in addition to the regular facet that articulates with the capitate. The size of this medial facet ranges between 1 and 6 mm in width. This type II variant was observed in up to 70% of specimens. A type I lunate has no contact with the proximal pole of the hamate regardless of wrist position, whereas a type II lunate has a variable amount of contact between the hamate and medial lunate facet—primarily when the wrist is in an ulnarly deviated position.

Cadaver studies have revealed that cartilage erosion of the proximal pole of the hamate is the most common arthrotic condition within the wrist.[1,2] An increasing rate of degeneration is noted with increased age. When proximal hamate arthrosis is present, it is noted almost exclusively in specimens with type II lunates. This appears to be directly related to the increased midcarpal motion observed in patients with type II lunates during radioulnar hand movements, and is presumed to be a result of overloading of the proximal hamate over the long term.[4,5] Patients with symptomatic proximal hamate arthrosis typically complain of ulnar-sided wrist pain, especially with gripping. This appears to correlate with radiographic studies that clearly show increasing contact areas between the hamate and lunate with ulnar deviation. The larger the medial facet of the lunate the more likely arthrosis is to develop. The cartilage degeneration is most evident dorsally on the hamate, and matching degeneration on the medial facet of the lunate is observed up to 50% of the time.

Clinical and cadaveric studies have also demonstrated a strong association between arthrosis at the proximal hamate and tears in the lunotriquetral interosseous ligament (LTIL). Complete or partial disruption of the LTIL has been documented almost 90% of the time when arthrosis of the proximal hamate is identified. Because of this strong association, we have proposed the term *HALT* (hamate arthrosis lunotriquetral ligament tear) *wrist* to describe this common clinical condition. There has been little crossover of this anatomical and biomechanical data to the clinical arena, however. The role a torn LTIL may play in the development of hamate arthrosis has not been delineated. A prospective longitudinal study would be

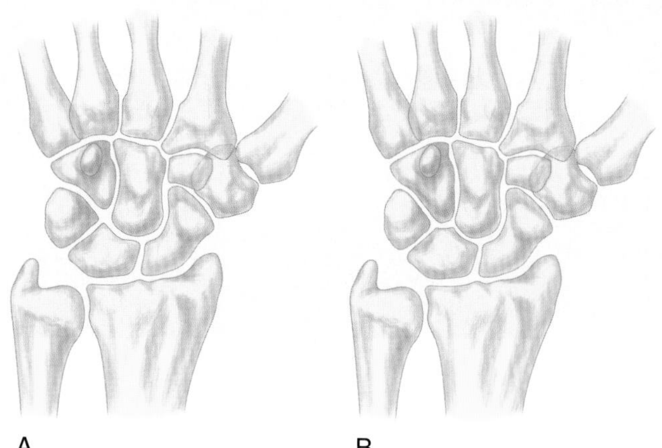

FIGURE 25.1. Lunate morphology. (A) Type I lunate: no contact between proximal hamate and medial lunate. (B) Type II lunate: contact between proximal hamate and medial facet of lunate.

required to delineate whether LT instability predisposes wrists with type II lunates to increased or earlier degeneration of the proximal hamate.

Published clinical studies examining the treatment regimens for hamate arthrosis are limited. Thurston and Stanley reported on four patients with arthrosis of the proximal pole of the hamate who were treated by proximal hamate excision. All of the patients were reported to have done well after surgery.[6] Harley et al. reviewed a much larger series of patients who were treated by arthroscopic excision of the proximal hamate and found favorable results in the majority of patients.[7] A biomechanical arm of this latter study evaluated the unloading effect of proximal hamate resection. Cadaver wrists with type II lunates were mounted on a custom vice and testing stand.

Pressure-sensitive film was inserted into the ulnar half of the midcarpal joint to measure the joint pressures in the hamatolunate and hamatotriquetral articulations with the wrist loaded in 25 degrees of ulnar deviation. The proximal pole of the hamate was then excised and the joint loading was repeated. These studies revealed that on average resecting 2.4 mm of the proximal pole of the hamate fully unloads the hamatolunate articulation. This amount of bony resection was not observed to alter the load across the triquetrohamate articulation. This biomechanical data supports our clinical observation that an arthroscopic resection of the proximal pole of the hamate for the treatment of arthrosis is a sound surgical procedure.

Indications

The typical patient with a HALT wrist presents with a long history of increasing ulnar-sided wrist pain. The patient frequently presents after an acute exacerbation from a lifting or twisting injury, or in some cases a fall on the affected wrist. The pain typically worsens over time and has the typical arthritic qualities: pain with activities, reduced motion, post-activity ache, and variable response to anti-inflammatory medicines or splinting.

On the physical examination the patient will typically have diffuse nonlocalizing ulnar-sided wrist tenderness. In that the spectrum of pathological findings seen in patients with a HALT wrist encompasses LTIL tears, ulnocarpal and midcarpal synovitis, and chondromalacia of the proximal hamate, it is not surprising that these patients frequently do not specifically localize their pain to the hamate. In most cases, the LT "shuck" test and deep palpation of the hamate elicit a withdrawal reflex. However, most patients have little or no radial-sided tenderness. TFCC tears are noted frequently in patients with proximal hamate arthrosis. Ulnar-sided wrist pain attributable to these tears can further diminish the specificity of the physical exam.

Plain radiographic studies of the affected wrist should be compared to the opposite asymptomatic wrist. Cystic change within the proximal hamate, or a sharp and sclerotic proximal hamate margin, can aid in the identification of this condition preoperatively. However, in most instances plain radiographic studies are noncontributory (Figure 25.2). Furthermore, it is important to realize that plain radiographs are not always diagnostic of a type II lunate morphology.[8] MRI scans of the wrist that demonstrate edema within the proximal hamate are suggestive of this condition. Likewise, a wrist CT-arthrogram study that outlines a thinned proximal hamate cartilage surface and/or reveals a sclerotic subchondral ridge can also assist in making the diagnosis preoperatively. Unfortunately, neither of these two expensive diagnostic modalities consistently identifies this condition.

Surgical intervention for the HALT wrist should generally not be entertained until all nonoperative measures have been tried and have failed. A motivated, healthy, active patient with persistent ulnar-sided wrist pain represents the ideal surgical candidate. In our experience, advanced patient age has not precluded a successful surgical outcome. The preoperative discussion with a patient undergoing wrist arthroscopy for ulnar-sided wrist pain should always include the possibility of excision of an arthritic proximal hamate. If advanced chondromalacia is identified at the time of midcarpal arthroscopy, the appropriate treatment can be rendered at that time.

Contraindications

Contraindications to arthroscopic resection of the proximal hamate are few. Any symptomatic patient with advanced chondromalaciac changes identified at the time of arthroscopy can derive significant benefits from a proximal pole resection. Proximal hamate arthrosis represents a spectrum of pathological changes. Resection of the proximal hamate in a patient with grade I or II change is usually contraindicated

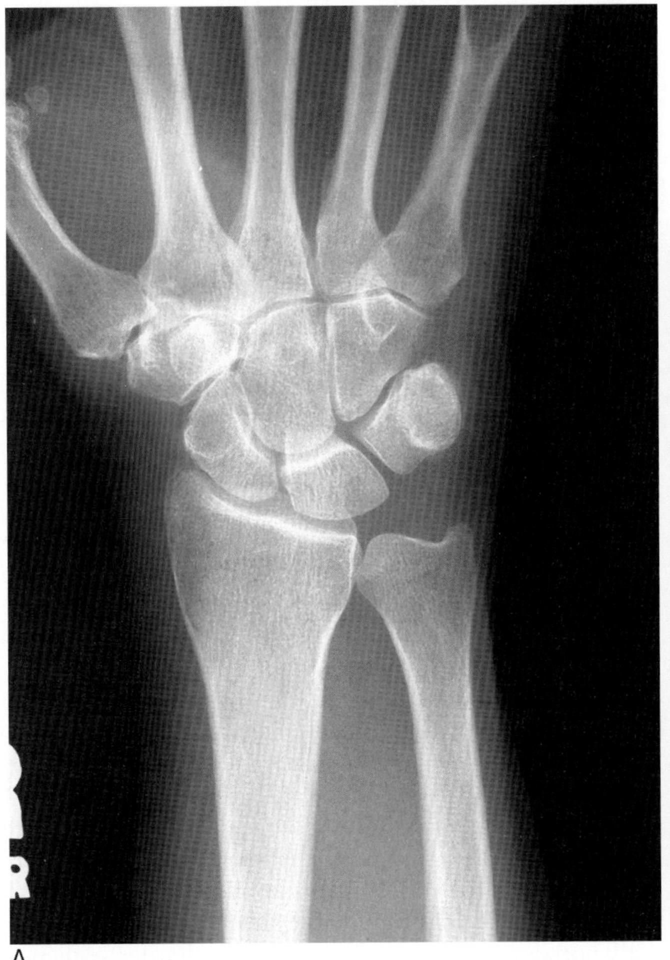

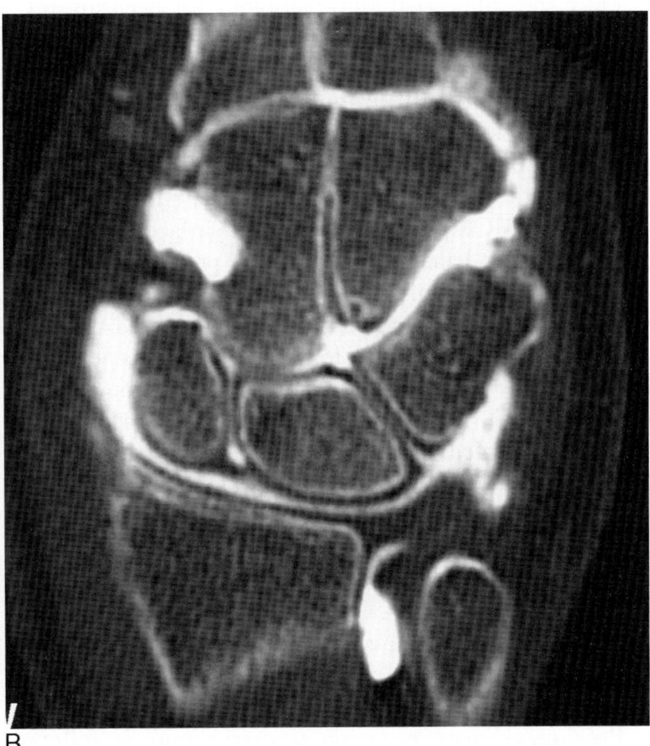

A B

FIGURE 25.2. (A) PA wrist radiograph of patient with proximal hamate arthrosis but no obvious changes on X-ray. (B) Same patient, for whom CT arthrogram reveals cyst in proximal hamate, loss of cartilage signal (absent black rim), and LTIL tear (contrast flow through LT articulation).

(Table 25.1). A gray area exists for those patients with limited or focal grade III or IV chondromalacia.

Although resection of the proximal hamate generally allows for marked symptom reduction in patients with isolated HALT wrist pathology, we have noted less impressive results from proximal pole resection in patients having multiple coincident interosseous ligament tears and/or cartilage surface degeneration elsewhere within the affected wrist. Similarly, proximal hamate excision in a patient with diffuse rheumatoid changes or an autoimmune disease that involves the wrist has a small likelihood of providing significant relief. A limited or total wrist fusion remains the treatment of choice in these more complex conditions.

Table 25.1.

Chondromalacia Classification

Type I	Localized softening, discoloration; no break in the surfaces
Type II	Softening, discoloration; small areas of fibrillation or irregular surface
Type III	Fibrillation and fissures extend to subchondral bone surface; "crabmeat" appearance
Type IV	Areas with complete loss of articular cartilage; exposed subchondral bone

Surgical Technique

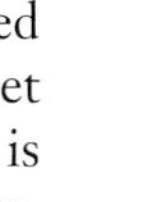

The involved wrist and forearm are prepped and draped and placed in some type of traction device. A tourniquet is elevated after exsanguination. Antibiotic prophylaxis is not required for an isolated proximal hamate resection. A standard arthroscopic survey of the radiocarpal and midcarpal joints is then performed, and all cartilage surfaces and ligamentous structures are assessed. The usual working portals include the 3-/,4 and 4-/,5 portals as well as midcarpal-radial (MCR) and midcarpal-ulnar (MCU) portals. In the radiocarpal joint, close attention must be paid to the articular surface of the lunate as well as to the TFCC. If a TFCC perforation is present, the distal ulnar chondral surface of the ulnar head can also be assessed. The LTIL is best seen through the 4-/,5 portal. The 6-U portal is frequently utilized for instrumentation to help probe or debride a torn LTIL.

Once the radiocarpal joint pathology has been inventoried, the cartilaginous surfaces of the midcarpal are inspected. A midcarpal synovectomy is performed as needed to enhance visualization. The proximal pole of the hamate is most clearly evaluated with the arthroscope in the MCU portal. Instability of the LT interval is best assessed with a probe in the MCU portal and the arthroscope in the MCR portal. The cartilage surface of the proximal pole of the hamate should also be probed at this time to define the extent of any chondromalacia present. Seemingly minimal chondromalaciac change observed with the arthroscope is often found to extend much deeper upon probing. After a complete diagnostic arthroscopy of the midcarpal and radiocarpal joints, one can proceed with definitive treatment.

The TFCC, LTIL, and/or scapholunate interosseous ligament (SLIL) can be debrided or repaired as indicated—based on the acuity and severity of the pathology and on the patient's preoperative symptoms. In our experience, the associated TFCC or LTIL pathology present in most patients with symptomatic arthrosis of the proximal hamate is chronic in nature and is hence usually treated with simple arthroscopic debridement.

Proximal hamate resection is carried out as follows. With the arthroscope in the MCR portal, a 2.7-mm full-radius resector and a 2.9-mm bur are placed alternately into the MCU portal. After the subchondral bone of the proximal hamate has been exposed with the shaver, 2 to 4 mm of the proximal pole of the hamate can be excised using the bur. Care must be taken to avoid damage to the cartilage surfaces of the proximal capitate or to the adjacent triquetrum. To allow adequate visualization during the procedure, frequent suctioning of the joint debris is required. The fat globules and bone debris arising from the resection must be adequately flushed out of the midcarpal joint to prevent leaving debris behind.

The most volar and distal portion of the proximal hamate resection is poorly visualized from the MCR portal. It is necessary to switch the arthroscope to the MCU portal to clearly visualize the full extent of the volar resection of the proximal hamate. Infrequently, the shaver or bur is placed into the MCR portal to complete the proximal hamate resection. The 2.9-mm bur can be used as a gauge to assess the adequacy of the bony resection. When placed in the area of resection, the exposed bur edge should lie nearly adjacent to the proximal capitate surface.

When the surgeon is satisfied with the arthroscopic decompression of the hamatolunate articulation, an intraoperative fluoroscopic assessment is performed to confirm the adequacy of the proximal hamate resection (Figure 25.3). Whereas this often requires some maneuvering of both the surgeon and the instruments, the fluoroscopic pictures provide an important secondary means of evaluation. If the radiographs confirm that the resection is satisfactory, all portals are closed with skin tapes, local anesthetic is infiltrated into the joint and the surrounding subcutaneous

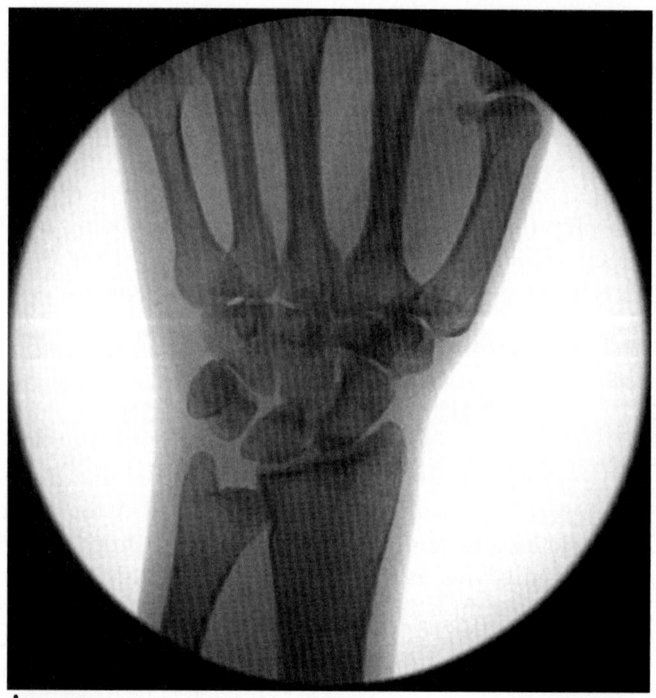

A

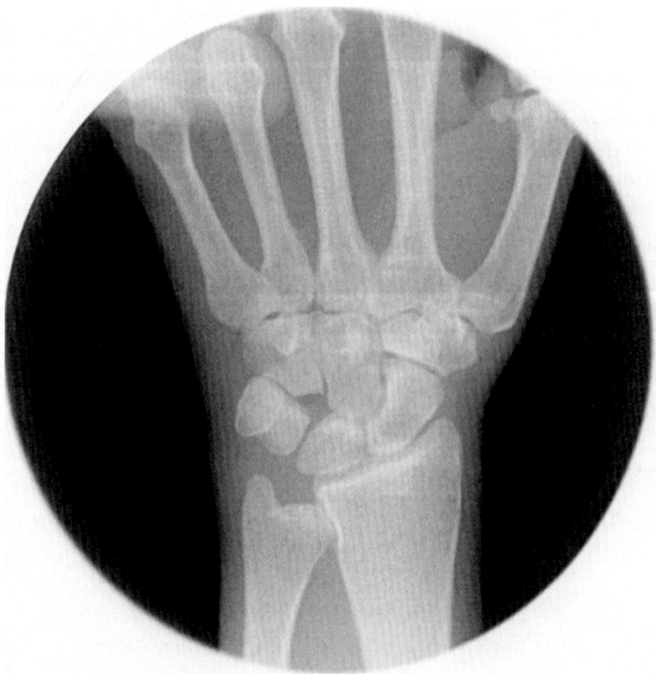

B

FIGURE 25.3. (A) Preoperative fluoroscopy of type II lunate with proximal hamate arthrosis. (B) Same patient, for whom post-operative fluoroscopy reveals adequate resection of proximal hamate.

tissues, and a light compressive bandage is applied for 10 days.

The postoperative regimen is determined primarily by the degree of intra-articular pathology and the amount of reconstructive work. In the setting of an isolated proximal hamate resection or a typical HALT wrist procedure (debridement of an LTIL tear followed by a proximal hamate resection), the patient is seen 10 days postoperatively and a hand therapy consultation is obtained. The therapist's instructions usually include an early active assisted-motion protocol as well as edema control.

Authors' Experience

A chart review of all patients undergoing wrist arthroscopy between 1991 and 2001 yielded 23 patients who had undergone arthroscopic resection of the proximal pole of the hamate. The mean age of the patients at the time of surgery was 43 years. Four patients were female and 19 were male. The symptomatic wrist was the patient's dominant wrist in 13 cases. Seventeen patients related a specific distant injury to their wrist (fall or twist). All patients consented to arthroscopic treatment because of wrist pain unresponsive to nonoperative treatment. Preoperative X-rays revealed that 20 patients had an obvious type II lunate. Eight radiographs were suggestive of an erosive lesion of the proximal pole of the hamate. None of the patients had a static LT or SL carpal instability pattern.

At the time of arthroscopy, all wrists were found to have a variable amount of midcarpal synovitis and diffuse grade III or IV chondromalacia of the proximal pole of the hamate. Twenty-one wrists had pathology of the LTIL, seven had a TFCC tear, three were noted to have early radiocarpal arthritis, and two had a tear of the SLIL. In addition to resection of the proximal pole of the hamate, six patients underwent debridement of the proximal portion of the LTIL, five had a concurrent TFCC debridement, one had an SLIL debridement, one had a TFCC repair, and one underwent an open LTIL repair. The average bone resection of the proximal pole of the hamate, as measured by postoperative X-ray, was 2.2 mm (range 1 to 4 mm).

At final follow-up at 4.7 years, 18 of 23 patients had good or excellent results according to the modified Mayo scoring system (and one had a fair result). Ten patients were able to return to work within two weeks of their surgery, and 78% of patients returned to their preoperative employment or recreational status at an average of nine weeks post-surgery. At final follow-up, 18 patients reported minimal to no change in work or recreational status—whereas 5 either were not working or had to change jobs because of persistent wrist problems.

All patients with isolated HALT pathology (hamate arthrosis, LTIL tear, and midcarpal synovitis) had good or excellent results from hamate resection. Two-thirds of the patients with TFCC perforations, LTIL tears, and midcarpal synovitis had good or excellent results—whereas only half of the patients with LTIL, TFCC, and SLIL tears achieved these outcomes. No patients with preexistent radiocarpal arthritis (scaphoid or lunate facet of distal radius) had good or excellent outcomes.

Four patients had salvage surgery for poor outcomes. Of these four, two had salvage procedures within 18 months (one wrist fusion and one STT arthrodesis) and one underwent a four-corner fusion three years after the index procedure. The last patient underwent a proximal row carpectomy seven years after hamate resection.

We found that the majority of patients did well after surgery, and that the good results were generally sustained at a mean of 4.7 years from surgery. As a result of this study, it has become our practice to ensure that we resect the proximal hamate to the level necessary to completely unload the medial facet of the lunate. Other important observations from this study include (1) patients with increasing associated wrist pathology do not do as well as patients with pathology limited to the HALT condition, which should be discussed with patients, and (2) patients that developed the onset of hamate arthrosis after prior wrist surgical procedures for unrelated lesions were also more likely to have poorer results.

We have found that in the treatment of HALT wrists a fairly conservative approach to the LT instability appears warranted. We believe that most patients we encounter with hamate arthrosis and LTIL tears can be treated by arthroscopic excision of the proximal pole of the hamate and (at most) by debridement of the LTIL. We did not find that reconstruction of the LTIL with pinning and/or casting is necessary for symptomatic improvement. Perhaps the biggest advantage from this simplified approach is the institution of early wrist motion postoperatively, which contributed to a rapid return to work in 78% of patients.

References

1. Viegas SF, Wagner K, Patterson R, Peterson P. Medial (hamate) facet of the lunate. J Hand Surg 1990;15A:564–71.
2. Viegas SF, Patterson RM, Hokanson JA, Davis J. Wrist anatomy: Incidence, distribution, and correlation of anatomic variations, tears, and arthrosis. J Hand Surg 1993;18A:463–75.
3. Burgess RC. Anatomic variations of the midcarpal joint. J Hand Surg 1990;15A:129–31.
4. Nakamura K, Beppu M, RM P, Hanson C, Hume P, Viegas S. Motion analysis in two dimensions of radial-ulnar deviation of type I versus type II lunates. J Hand Surg 2000;25A:877–88.
5. Nakamura K, Patterson R, Moritomo H, Viegas S. Type I versus type II lunates. J Hand Surg 2001;26A:428–36.
6. Thurston AJ, Stanley JK. Hamato-lunate impingement. Arthroscopy 2000;16:540–44.
7. Harley BJ, Palmer AK, Boles SD, Werner FW. Arthroscopic resection of arthrosis of the proximal hamate: A clinical and biomechanical study. J Hand Surg 2004;29A:661–67.
8. Sagerman SD, Hauck RM, Palmer AK. Lunate morphology: Can it be predicted with routine X-ray films? J Hand Surg 1995;20A:38–41.

Randall W. Culp and Eric S. Wroten

CHAPTER 26

Arthroscopic Proximal Row Carpectomy

Introduction

Proximal row carpectomy is a motion-sparing salvage procedure that consists of excising the scaphoid, lunate, and capitate—thus converting a complex link joint into a simple hinge.[1] Although the procedure has historically been criticized for loss of motion and strength, progressive radiocapitate arthritis, and unpredictability of outcome, much of this criticism has been anecdotal.[2] Recent studies, including three series with a minimum of nine years of follow-up, have demonstrated that proximal row carpectomy is as reliable a procedure as complex reconstructions and other salvage surgeries.[3–16] The advantages of proximal row carpectomy include preservation of a functional arc of motion, satisfactory strength, pain relief, and high patient satisfaction.

Wrist motion has been shown to be equal or slightly less than preoperative motion. Grip strength has been reported to range between 64 and 100% of the contralateral normal wrist.[4,7,11,12,17–21] In addition, patients may be converted to a wrist arthrodesis or arthroplasty if painful osteoarthritis develops. The disadvantages of proximal row carpectomy include loss of carpal height, an incongruous joint, and possible progression of radiocapitate arthrosis. Imbriglia et al. have shown that the radius of curvature of the capitate is approximately two-thirds of the lunate fossa of the distal radius. Using cineradiography, they demonstrated that the motion of the capitate on the distal radius is translational with a moving center of rotation.[21] Imbriglia reported that 12 of 27 patients in his long-term follow-up study developed radiographic evidence of cartilage space narrowing, although without clinical consequence.[13]

The role of wrist arthroscopy has vastly changed in the last decade. With advances in the development of smaller arthroscopes and instruments (as well as advances in arthroscopic surgery techniques), treatment of wrist pathology has significantly improved. The pathology the wrist arthroscopist can now treat includes but is not limited to triangular fibrocartilage complex (TFCC) tears, ganglion cysts, radiocarpal fractures, cartilage damage, loose bodies, and bony resections (including radial styloidectomy and proximal row carpectomy).

Literature regarding arthroscopic proximal row carpectomy is sparse. There are no long-term studies, although short-term results are promising. The majority of the literature mentions arthroscopy as an available technique for proximal row carpectomy without discussing clinical results.[5,22–25]

Indications and Contraindications

The indications for arthroscopic proximal row carpectomy are the same as those for the standard open technique. These indications include symptomatic arthritic disease secondary to scapholunate dissociation, scaphoid nonunion, and Kienbock's disease.

Proximal row carpectomy[26] has also been described in the treatment of failed carpal implants, cerebral palsy, spasticity, acute and chronic fractures and dislocations, and replantation. We do not currently recommend arthroscopic proximal row carpectomy in this latter subset of patients.

Other relative contraindications to proximal row carpectomy in general include degenerative changes of the capitate head or lunate fossa of the distal radius, multicystic carpal disease, and preexisting ulnar translocation of the carpus. Due to the high failure rate of open proximal row carpectomy in patients with inflammatory arthropathy (e.g., rheumatoid arthritis), both Culp et al. and Ferlic et al. do not recommend its use in these patients.[4,27]

Technique

The patient is positioned supine on the operating table, with the affected arm positioned on a radiolucent hand table. A well-padded arm tourniquet is placed proximal to the arm. The procedure can be carried out under general or regional anesthesia because operative times are generally less than two hours. The wrist is then suspended in a traction tower and 10 to 15 pounds of traction is applied (Figure 26.1). After distraction is obtained, landmarks are outlined on the dorsum of the wrist and the portals are made. The tourniquet is routinely inflated without additional exsanguination. Routinely, the 3-4 portal is the initial viewing portal.

After the 2.7-mm arthroscope is placed into the joint, outflow is established through the 6-R portal identified by triangulation and direct visualization upon entering the joint at the prestyloid recess. A mechanical pump is used to maintain a constant intra-articular pressure and flow rate. Initially, a routine evaluation of the joint is carried out. Particular attention is given to the lunate fossa of the distal radius. The radial volar extrinsic ligaments, particularly the radioscaphocapitate ligament, are identified and are preserved during the procedure. The arthroscope is then directed ulnarly, and the TFCC and extrinsic ulnar ligaments are identified.

Next, the midcarpal joint must be well visualized to ensure an adequate proximal capitate cartilaginous surface (Figure 26.2). If the status of the capitate joint is questionable, an alternative procedure is performed: four-corner fusion, capitolunate arthrodesis, proximal row carpectomy with interposition arthroplasty, or wrist arthrodesis. Assessment of the midcarpal articular surfaces is accomplished through the radial midcarpal portal, which is approximately 1 cm distal to the 3-4 portal. Arthroscopic instruments that will be needed to perform the proximal row carpectomy include a hook probe, a 2.9 shaver or radiofrequency device, a 4.0 bur, small sharp osteotomes, pituitary rongeurs, and an image intensifier.

The first step in performing the proximal row carpectomy, after one is satisfied with the cartilage status of the proximal pole of the capitate and the lunate fossa, is to remove the scapholunate and lunatotriquetral ligaments with a shaver or radiofrequency device. This is performed through the 4-5 and/or 6-R portal. Next, the core of the lunate is removed with a bur. Care is taken to avoid damaging the lunate fossa and proximal capitate by leaving an "eggshell" rim of lunate, which is morcellized with a pituitary rongeur under direct vision and/or with image intensification (Figure 26.3).

Next, using the 3-4 or 4-5 portal as a working portal the scaphoid and triquetrum are fragmented with an osteotome and bur under image intensification (Figures 26.4 and 26.5) and removed piecemeal with a pituitary rongeur. Coring out and fragmenting the carpal bones allows for easy removal

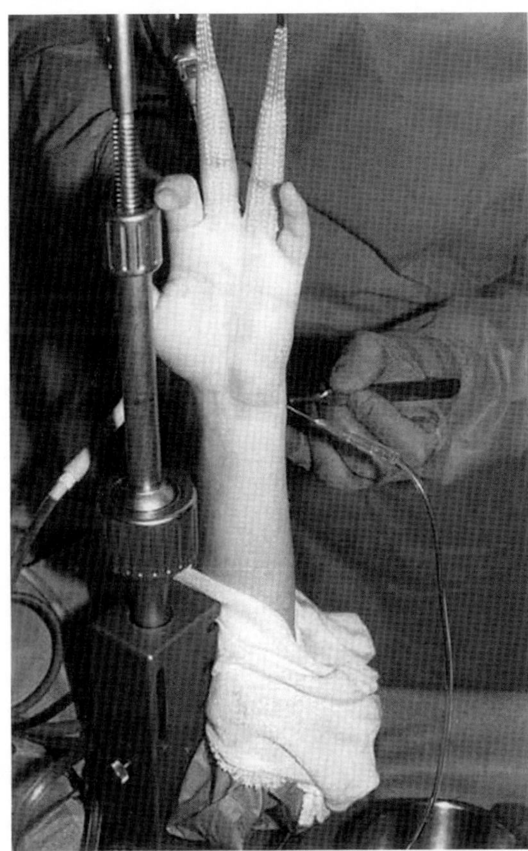

FIGURE 26.1. Standard traction tower with finger traps on the long and ring fingers. An 18-gauge needle in the 6-U portal to provide gravity drainage as outflow. *(Reproduced with permission from R.W. Culp et al, Tech in Hand and UE Surg 1997;(2):117).*

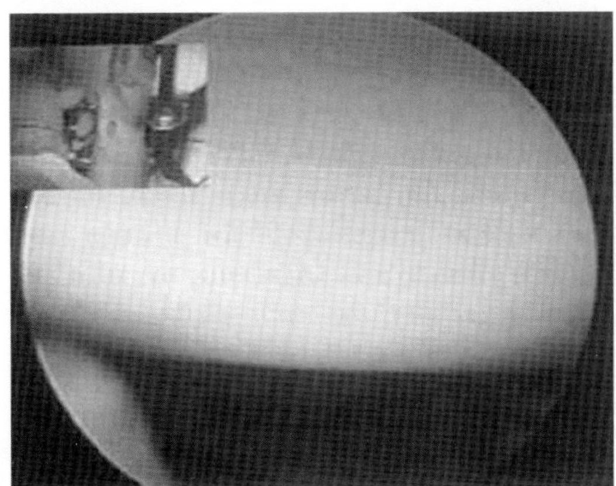

FIGURE 26.2. View from radial midcarpal portal demonstrating a healthy-appearing proximal capitate. *(Reproduced with permission from Culp RW, Osterman AL, Talsania JS. Arthroscopic proximal row carpectomy. Tech Hand and Upp Ext 1997;2(1):116–19).*

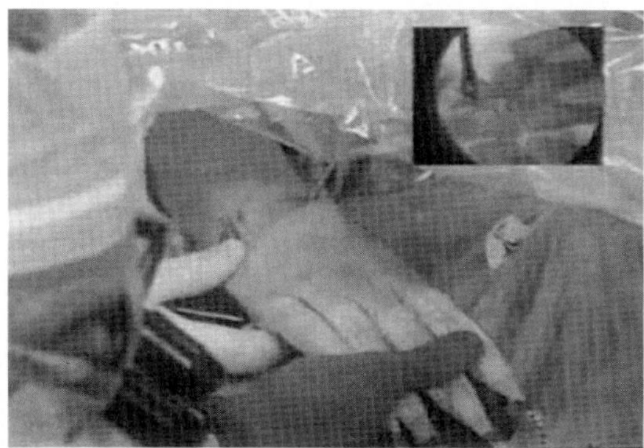

FIGURE 26.3. Creation of a central cavity within the lunate is performed with a large round bur. Care is taken to protect the lunate fossa and proximal capitate articular surfaces throughout the procedure. *(Reproduced with permission from Culp RW, Osterman AL, Talsania JS. Arthroscopic proximal row carpectomy. Tech Hand and Upp Ext 1997;2(1):116–19).*

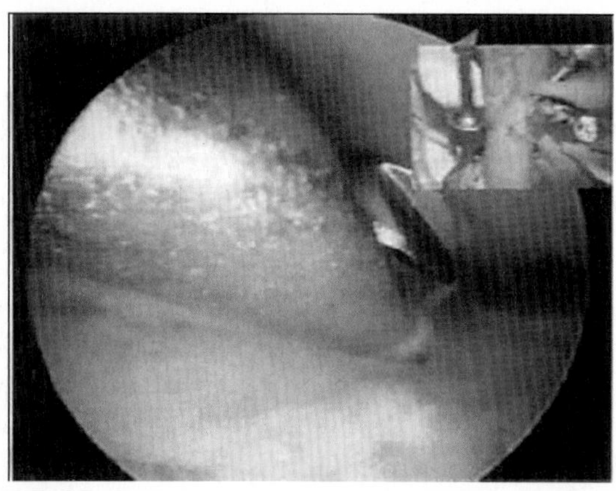

FIGURE 26.4. Fluoroscopic guidance is utilized to aid fragmentation of the scaphoid and triquetrum. *(Reproduced with permission from Culp RW, Osterman AL, Talsania JS. Arthroscopic proximal row carpectomy. Tech Hand and Upp Ext 1997;2(1): 116–19).*

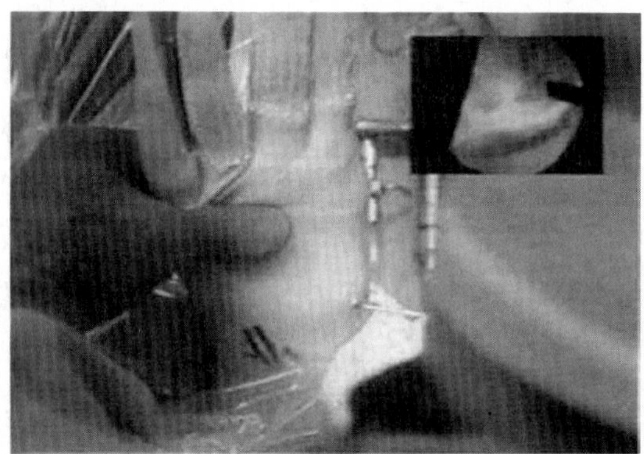

FIGURE 26.5. Pituitary rongeur, under fluoroscopic guidance, to remove the fragmented scaphoid. This may be performed in the traction tower or with the hand prone on the radiolucent hand table. *(Reproduced with permission from Culp RW, Osterman AL, Talsania JS. Arthroscopic proximal row carpectomy. Tech Hand and Upp Ext 1997;2(1):116–19).*

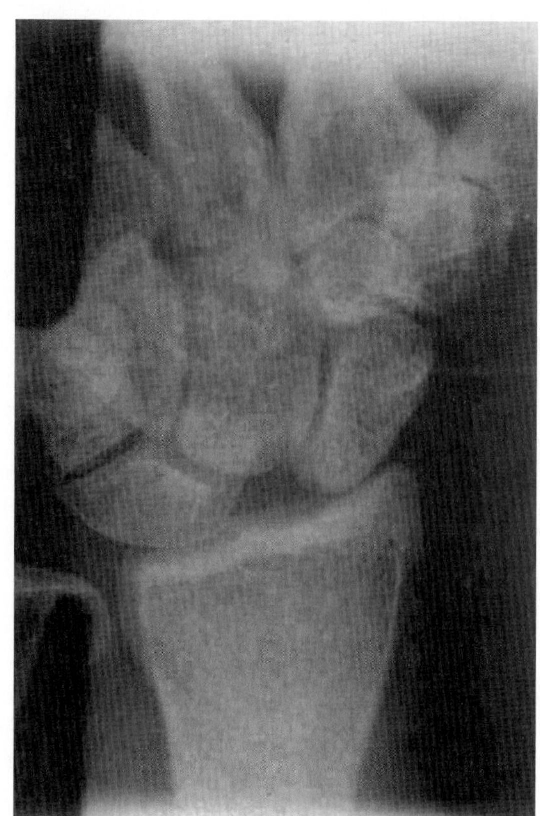

FIGURE 26.6. Preoperative radiograph demonstrating chronic scapholunate dissociation. *(Reproduced with permission from Culp RW, Osterman AL, Talsania JS. Arthroscopic proximal row carpectomy. Tech Hand and Upp Ext 1997;2(1):116–19).*

as well as protection of the articular cartilage. Great care is taken to avoid damaging the articular cartilage and to avoid damaging the volar extrinsic ligaments, especially the radioscaphocapitate—which will be responsible for maintaining the stability of the capitate in the lunate fossa.

After the entire proximal row is removed, the wrist is examined under radiographic image intensification (Figures 26.6 and 26.7). Care is taken to ensure that there is not impingement of the trapezium against the radial styloid. Some authors advocate a modest styloidectomy. Although we rarely perform this procedure, if necessary it can be done arthroscopically with the aid of image intensification.

Posterior interosseous neurectomy may be performed through a separate 1.5-cm longitudinal incision just ulnar to Lister's tubercle. The fourth compartment is partly opened on the radial side. One cm of the nerve is resected with bipolar electrocautery. The fourth compartment is then repaired with absorbable suture. All wounds are closed with 4-0 nylon monofilament suture.

Patients are initially placed in a short arm plaster splint. Sutures from the portals are removed at 7 to 10 days. The patients are then converted to a short arm thermoplastic splint for an additional three weeks. Gentle range-of-motion exercises are begun after splint removal at four weeks, and strengthening is begun approximately eight weeks postoperatively.

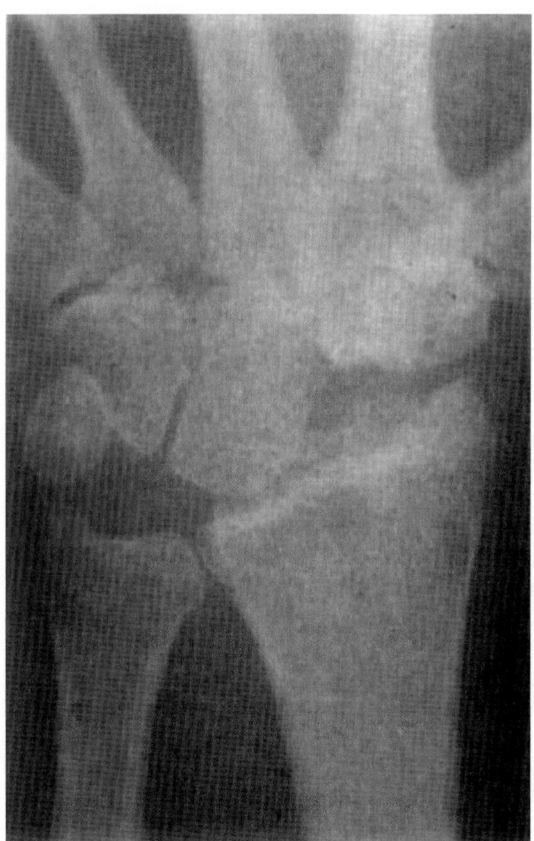

FIGURE 26.7. Postoperative radiograph, following arthroscopic proximal row carpectomy. *(Reproduced with permission from Culp RW, Osterman AL, Talsania JS. Arthroscopic proximal row carpectomy. Tech Hand and Upp Ext 1997;2(1):116–19).*

Complications

There are several potential complications associated with arthroscopic proximal row carpectomy that must be noted. Iatrogenic damage to articular cartilage must be avoided by careful instrument placement.

Care must be taken to avoid disrupting the volar extrinsic carpal ligaments, particularly the radioscaphocapitate ligament, during excision of the proximal carpal row (Figure 26.8). To avoid ligamentous injury, a thin shell of cortical bone may be left attached to the volar radiocarpal ligaments. In addition, there is also the potential to irritate nerves (particularly the dorsal ulnar sensory branch), and the possibility of damage to the median and ulnar nerves (particularly the ulnar nerve) while using the osteotomes.

Because the dorsal capsuloligamentous structures have been minimally disrupted during the procedure, there is a theoretical complication that dorsal instability may occur secondary to less dorsal scar formation. Although this complication has not occurred in our patients, should dorsal capsular laxity become evident concurrent or subsequent electrothermal capsulorrhaphy may be considered.

Advantages

Arthroscopic proximal row carpectomy involves less dissection, less postoperative pain, less stiffness, and a shorter recovery time. There is less damage to the dorsal ligaments, which are left almost completely intact, in contrast to standard proximal row carpectomy. The excellent visualization provided by arthroscopy allows for an increased likelihood of volar extrinsic preservation. Finally, patients are pleased with the smaller scars associated with arthroscopy.

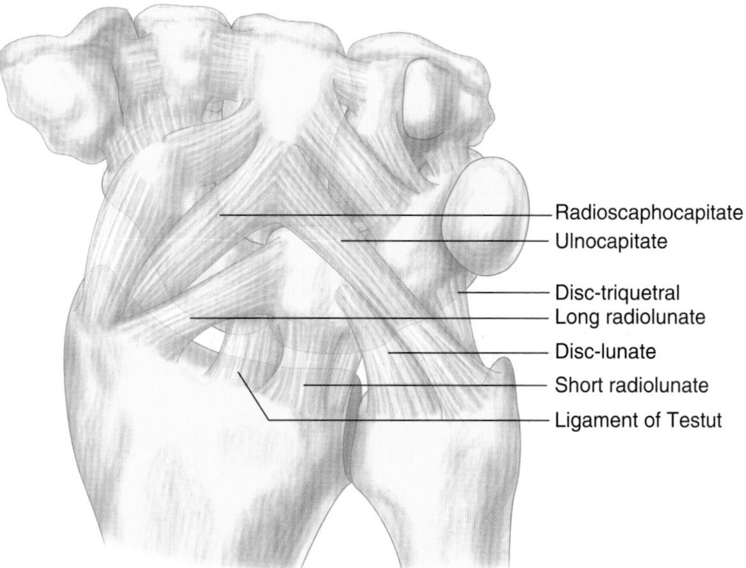

FIGURE 26.8. Diagram of the important stabilizing volar extrinsic radiocarpal and ulnocarpal ligaments. Note ulnocapitate ligament, important due to its position and contribution to the ulnar limb of the arcuate ligament and their attachment to the capitate.

Summary

This procedure involves minimal dissection and potentially less morbidity. As with any arthroscopic procedure, this technique requires a hand surgeon highly skilled in wrist arthroscopy. Overall patient satisfaction with this procedure has been excellent. Immediate postoperative pain has been less compared to those who have had an open technique. In our experience, patients who underwent arthroscopic proximal row carpectomy report satisfactory pain relief, functional range of motion, and effective grip strength.

References

1. Stamm TT. Excision of the proximal row of carpus. Proc Roy Soc Med 1944;38:74–5.
2. Lee RW, Hassan DM. Proximal row carpectomy. In HK Watson, J Weinzweig (eds.), *The Wrist*. Philadelphia: Lippincot Williams & Wilkins 2001: 545–54.
3. Culp RW. Proximal row carpectomy. Operat Tech Orthop 1996;2:69–71.
4. Culp RW, McGuigan FX, Turner MA, Lichtman DM, Osterman AL, McCarroll HR. Proximal row carpectomy: A multicenter study. J Hand Surg 1993;18A:19–25.
5. Roth JH, Poehling GG. Arthroscopic "-ectomy" surgery of the wrist. Arthroscopy J Arthroscop Relat Surg 1990;6(2): 141–47.
6. Siegel JM, Ruby LK. A critical look at intercarpal arthrodesis: Review of the literature. J Hand Surg 1996;21A:717–23.
7. Tomaino MM, Delsignore J, Burton RI. Long-term results following proximal row carpectomy. J Hand Surg 1994;19A: 694–703.
8. Wyrick JD, Stern PJ, Kiefhaber TR. Motion-preserving procedures in the treatment of scapholunate advance collapse wrist: Proximal row carpectomy versus four-corner arthrodesis. J Hand Surg 1995;20A:965–70.
9. Cohen MS, Kozin SH. Degenerative arthritis of the wrist: Proximal row carpectomy versus four corner arthrodesis. J Hand Surg 2001;26A:94–104.
10. Culp RW, Williams CS. Proximal row carpectomy for the treatment of scaphoid nonunion. Hand Clin 2001;17(4): 663–69.
11. Jebson PJL, Hayes EP, Engber WD. Proximal row carpectomy: A minimum 10-year follow-up study. J Hand Surg 2003;28A:561–69.
12. DiDonna ML, Kiefhaber TR, Stern PJ. Proximal row carpectomy: A study with a minimum of ten years of follow-up. J Bone Joint Surg [Am] 2004;86:2359–65.
13. Imbriglia JE. Proximal row carpectomy. Technique and long-term results. Atlas Hand Clin 2000;5:101–09.
14. van Kooten EO, Coster E, Segers MJM, Ritt MJPF. Early proximal row carpectomy after severe carpal trauma. Injury 2005;36:1226–32.
15. Thomas AA, Rodriguez E, Segalman K. Keinbock's disease in an elderly patient treated with proximal row carpectomy. J Hand Surg 2004;29A:685–88.
16. Diao E, Andrews A, Beall M. Proximal row carpectomy. Hand Clin 2005;21(4):553–59.
17. Begley BW, Engber WD. Proximal row carpectomy in advanced Kienbock's disease. J Hand Surg 1994;19A: 1016–18.
18. Nevaiser RJ. On resection of the proximal carpal row. Clin Orthop 1986;202:12–5.
19. Nevaiser RJ. Proximal row carpectomy for posttraumatic disorders of the carpus. J Hand Surg 1983;8A:301–05.
20. Clendenin MB, Green DP. Arthrodesis of the wrist: Complications and their management. J Hand Surg 1981;6A:253–57.
21. Imbriglia JE, Broudy AS, Hagberg WC, McKernan D. Proximal row carpectomy: Clinical evaluation. J Hand Surg 1990;15A:462–530.
22. Culp RW, Osterman AL, Talsania JS. Arthroscopic proximal row carpectomy. Tech Hand and Up Extrem Soc 1997;2 (1):116–19.
23. Gupta R, Bozentka DJ, Osterman AL. Wrist arthroscopy: Principles and clinical applications. J Am Acad Orthop Surg 2001;9(3):200–09.
24. Nagle DJ. Laser-assisted wrist arthroscopy. Hand Clin 1999;15(3):495–99, ix.
25. Atik TL, Baratz ME. The role of arthroscopy in wrist arthritis. Hand Clin 1999;15(3):489–94.
26. Calandruccio JH. Proximal row carpectomy. J Am Soc Surg Hand 2001;2(1):112–22.
27. Ferlic DC, Clayton ML, Mills MF. Proximal row carpectomy: Review of rheumatoid and non-rheumatoid wrists. J Hand Surg 1991;16A:420–24.

Richard A. Berger

CHAPTER 27

"Many of life's failures are people who did not realize how close they were to success when they gave up."

—Thomas Edison

Arthroscopy of the Small Joints of the Hand

Introduction

The past 25 years have been witness to a virtual explosion of interest and application of arthroscopy in the orthopedic surgeon's armamentarium. Beginning as a diagnostic tool, largely for conditions in large joints such as the knee and shoulder, the arthroscope soon developed into a therapeutic tool for a procedure with well-documented advantages over open procedures. Next, intermediate-size joints (such as the wrist and elbow) became amenable to arthroscopic procedures—due in large part to the reduction in size of arthroscopic tools. This, too, followed the pattern of diagnostic procedures followed by therapeutic applications. With further reduction in the dimensions of arthroscopic equipment, we now have the capability to enter very small joints—such as the carpometacarpal and metacarpophalangeal joints of the hand.[1–3] Although largely limited to diagnostic procedures, innovations are currently emerging in the use of the arthroscope for therapeutic intervention. Only time will tell if true advantages can be found in the application of arthroscopic technology to these small joints.

As a note of practicality, safety, and integrity, it must be emphasized that common sense must prevail with these techniques. Just because we have the capability to perform small-joint arthroscopy does not mean there is a universal indication that we *must* do so. In the large number of lectures and courses the author has participated in, and to each of the residents and fellows he has had the privilege to teach, he has stressed (1) how relatively seldom he actually employs arthroscopy in regard to these small joints and (2) the necessity of being convinced that there is a distinct advantage in performing arthroscopy over open procedures before considering using it.

These are decisions each surgeon must ask in an environment of personal honesty, resisting the urge to follow trends and to succumb to pressures from patients who have read about this procedure or the other on the Internet and want what is most modern. If a surgeon can get better results with an open procedure than with an arthroscopic procedure, they owe it to the patient to perform the procedure in the manner that gets the best results or to refer the patient to someone who is getting superior results with the other procedure.

First Carpometacarpal Joint

Arthroscopy of the first carpometacarpal (CMC) joint was developed and described nearly 10 years ago.[1,2] The first CMC joint is particularly attractive as a joint available for arthroscopic evaluation because of its relative depth, highly curved articular surfaces, and the nearly circumferential nature of the stabilizing ligaments. Each of these factors makes complete viewing of the joint difficult with arthrotomy, unless highly destructive capsulotomies are carried out through these vital ligaments. As such, the use of the arthroscope was initially proposed for a diagnostic joint evaluation (if nothing more).

Early on it became quite clear, however, that the arthroscope could be a useful tool to help visualize the adequacy of reduction of fractures involving the articular surfaces of the trapezium or the base of the first metacarpal (such as with a Bennett's fracture)—as well as for the debridement of an arthrotic joint. With miniaturization of thermocouple probes, a technique for an arthroscopically guided shrinkage of the joint capsule for the treatment of pain due to joint capsule laxity was developed—as well as arthroscopically guided arthroplasty for the treatment of end-stage arthrosis.

Indications

The principle indications for arthroscopy of the first CMC joint are, in general, the same as for other joints. These include the evaluation of a painful joint that is suspicious for arthrosis or ligament injury, the treatment of two-part fractures of the base of the first metacarpal, retrieval of floating loose bodies or foreign objects, and the irrigation of a septic joint. There has been a persistent interest in using the arthroscope as a means of performing a minimally invasive resection of arthritic joint surfaces and to facilitate the percutaneous interposition of tendon or other materials.[2]

Contraindications

The contraindications for arthroscopy of the first CMC joint are the same as for other joints, including poor soft-tissue coverage, active cellulites, and joint injury of such severity that it cannot be managed by percutaneous methods (such as a Rolando fracture).

Regional Anatomy

The skin overlying the first CMC joint is glabrous only on the palmar surface. Immediately deep to the skin and superficial to the deep fascia are numerous veins, including the principal tributaries forming the cephalic vein system. Within the periadventitial tissue of these tributaries are the major volar (S1) and major dorsal (S2) divisions of the superficial radial nerve, which are found just deep to the veins (Figure 27.1).

Several muscles and tendons cross the joint, beginning anteriorly with the abductor pollicis brevis—which originates from the anterior surface of the trapezium (Figure 27.1). Just lateral to this is the tendon of abductor pollicis longus, inserting into the posterior base of the first metacarpal. The tendon of extensor pollicis brevis passes distally just posterior to the abductor pollicis longus. Just superficial to the posterior joint capsule of the first CMC joint is the deep division of the radial artery, crossing the first CMC joint deep to the extensor pollicis longus tendon before coursing anteriorly between the proximal metaphases of the first and second metacarpals. Between the proximal epiphyses of the first and second metacarpals is the intermetacarpal ligament, which is entirely extracapsular.

Joint Anatomy

The first CMC joint is a bi-sellar—a double saddle joint formed by the distal articular surface of the trapezium and the base of the first metacarpal. The articular surface along the major axis of the trapezium is concave in the medial-lateral direction and the articular surface along the minor axis is convex in the antero-posterior direction.

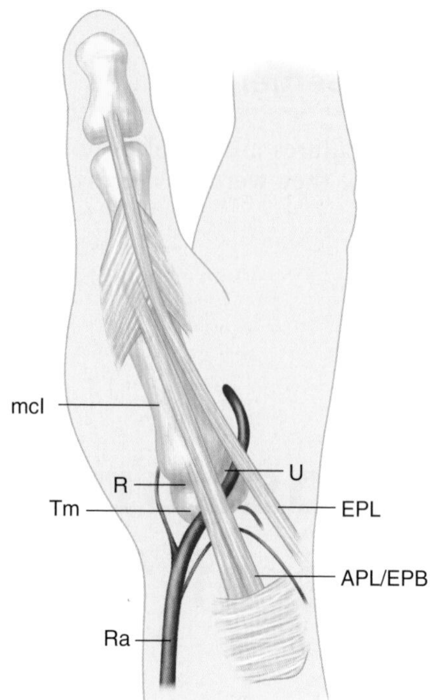

FIGURE 27.1. Drawing of the regional anatomy of the first carpometacarpal joint (mcl = first metacarpal, Tm = trapezium, Ra = radial artery, EPL = tendon of extensor pollicis longus, APL/EPB = tendons of abductor pollicis longus and extensor pollicis brevis, R and U = radial and ulnar arthroscopic portals, respectively).

The converse relationship is found with the base of the first metacarpal, where the articular surface is concave in the antero-posterior direction and convex in the medial-lateral direction. Although a joint capsule surrounds the entire joint, only 3/4 is reinforced by capsular ligaments.[4,5]

The anterior edge of the first CMC joint is reinforced by the anterior oblique ligament (AOL) complex, which is composed of superficial and deep divisions (Figure 27.2). The superficial division (AOLs) spans nearly the entire anterior edge of the joint and attaches to the anterior surface of the trapezium just proximal to the articular surface and just distal to the articular surface of the base of the fist metacarpal. The deep division (AOLd) is a well-demarcated thickening of the superficial band found just medial to the midline of the superficial division.

Often there is a distinct medial edge separating the AOLd from the AOLs. It is the deep division of the AOL that is often referred to as the "beak" ligament. The orientation of the fibers of the AOLs is slightly oblique, passing proximal to distal from lateral to medial. The fiber orientation of the AOLd is essentially proximal to distal. The extreme lateral (ulnar) surface of the joint is reinforced by the ulnar collateral ligament (UCL), which has fibers oriented in a proximal to distal direction (Figure 27.2). The lateral 30% of the posterior surface of the joint capsule is reinforced by the posterior oblique ligament (POL) (Figure 27.3). The fiber orientation of the POL is slightly oblique, passing from proximal and medial to distal and lateral.

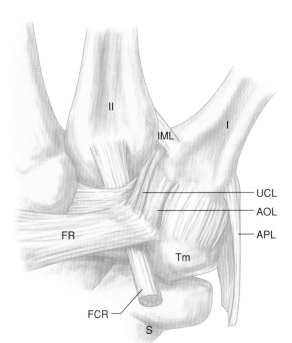

FIGURE 27.2. Drawing of the anterior surface of the first carpometacarpal joint capsule (I = first metacarpal, II = second metacarpal, Tm = trapezium, S = scaphoid, APL = tendon of abductor pollicis longus, FCR = tendon of flexor carpi radialis, FR = flexor retinaculum, AOL = anterior oblique ligament, UCL = ulnar collateral ligament, IML = intermetacarpal ligament).

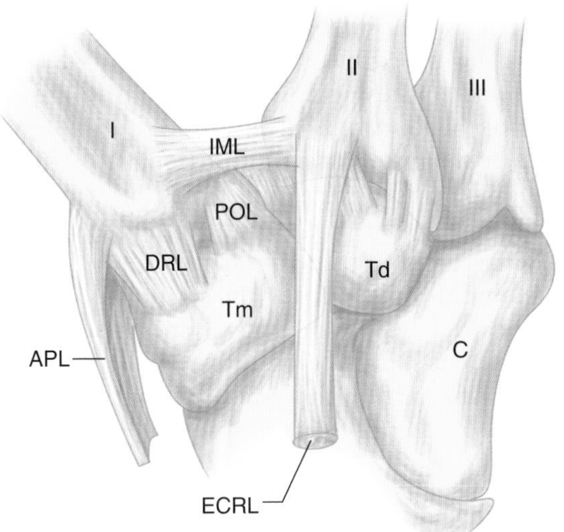

FIGURE 27.3. Drawing of the posterior surface of the first carpometacarpal joint capsule (I = first metacarpal, II = second metacarpal, III = third metacarpal, Tm = trapezium, Td = trapezoid, C = capitate, ECRL = tendon of extensor carpi radialis longus, APL = tendon of abductor pollicis longus, IML = intermetacarpal ligament, POL = posterior oblique ligament, DRL = dorsoradial ligament).

The remaining posterior joint capsule is reinforced by the dorsoradial ligament (DRL) (Figure 27.3). The fiber orientation of the DRL is generally proximal to distal. The joint capsule immediately deep to the tendon of abductor pollicis longus is not reinforced by a ligament. Although there is a distinct border between the AOLs and AOLd, there are no reliable demarcations between the remaining ligaments.

Portals

There are two recognized portals for arthroscopy of the first carpometacarpal joint. The naming of portals is related to their relationship with the extensor pollicis brevis and abductor pollicis longus tendons. The 1-R portal is established at the joint line just radial to the abductor pollicis longus tendon (Figure 27.1). The 1-U portal is established at the joint line just ulnar to the extensor pollicis brevis tendon (Figure 27.1).

Technique

The patient is positioned supine on the operating table, with either regional or general anesthesia. Parenteral antibiotics may be administered and a pneumatic tourniquet is typically applied to the arm. A single finger trap is secured to the thumb and between 5 and 8 pounds of longitudinal traction is applied. Using a 22-gauge hypodermic needle, the location of either the 1-R or 1-U portal is scouted by advancing the needle directly ulnarly. The needle should be angled approximately 20 to 30 degrees distally due to the curved nature of the joint surface. If there is any difficulty in passing the needle into the joint or if there is any concern about the proper identification of the joint, intraoperative radiographs or fluoroscopy may be used to verify the level of the needle prior to proceeding.

Once the proper level of the joint portals has been identified, small stab wounds are created with a scalpel—either transversely or longitudinally. The author advocates making the incisions for both portals at the beginning of the procedure. This facilitates switching portals during the operation without disturbing the cadence of the procedure. Subcutaneous tissues are dissected bluntly to the joint capsule level to be certain that underlying neurovascular tissues are displaced from harm's way. The arthroscope sheath is then introduced with a tapered trocar in one portal and a small probe is introduced in the other portal. It is rare that an outflow device is needed, particularly with judicious control of inflow fluid volume and rate. If an outflow tract is necessary, however, a large-bore hypodermic needle may be introduced—or a shaver may be used to evacuate excess or cloudy fluid. It may also be necessary to debride excess synovial tissue in order to visualize the joint surfaces and the ligaments. This may be accomplished with either a small shaver or a suction punch.

The author typically orients the camera and angles the arthroscope lens in a manner that places the image of the base of the first metacarpal at the top and the trapezium at the bottom. A comprehensive inspection of the articular surfaces is carried out. Next, the intra-articular appearance of the capsular ligaments is noted. It is best to use the probe to validate the integrity of these structures, rather than simply relying on their visual appearance.

The dorsoradial ligament, posterior oblique ligament, ulnar collateral ligament, and deep portion of the anterior oblique ligament can typically be visualized from the 1-R portal (Figure 27.4a through d). The superficial and deep portions of the anterior oblique ligament, ulnar collateral ligament, and posterior oblique ligament can be visualized through the 1-U portal (Figure 27.4a through d).

Procedures

The following procedures have been proposed, although largely based on personal communications and anecdotal experiences. This is by no means meant to be an all-inclusive list.

Synovectomy

A partial or radical synovectomy can be carried out arthroscopically using a shaver less than 3 mm in diameter, and thermocouple probe system or a small suction punch device. Care should be exercised when using the shaver or a punch to avoid iatrogenic compromise of the capsular ligaments themselves. Because of the small diameter of the shaver, the suction sheath frequently becomes clogged with debrided tissue. This requires frequent cleaning, which some surgeons may become frustrated with.

Capsular Shrinkage

It may be advantageous in some circumstances to be able to shrink, and hence stiffen, the joint capsule—such as in a substantially lax individual with early arthrosis of the first CMC joint. Commercially available thermocouple probe systems, in a diameter suitable for this joint, are available—but little experience has been gained in this specific joint at this time. Because of the proximity of overlying tissues to the joint capsule and the very real chance of thermal injury to nerves, tendons, and even skin, the author has not personally advocated the use of thermocouple capsular shrinkage in the first CMC joint.

Staging Arthritis

The precise staging of arthritic involvement of the articular surfaces of the first CMC joint is easily accomplished with the arthroscope. This is important in those patients with painful instability of the first CMC joint in whom one is considering performing an extra-articular ligament reconstruction.[6] If substantial arthrosis is present, but is not yet radiographically evident, a ligament reconstruction would be considered contraindicated. The most common locations for initial involvement of articular cartilage destruction in degenerative arthritis are the central aspect of the trapezial surface and the ulnar third of the metacarpal surface.

Resection of Joint Surface

There may be some indication for partially resecting either the base of the first metacarpal or the distal surface of the trapezium, although one would think that this would need to be accompanied by another procedure to either stabilize the joint or interpose some material (such as a section of tendon or fascia).[2] This was advocated by Menon, where a strip of flexor carpi radialis was interposed arthroscopically after arthroscopic resection of the arthritic joint surfaces.

Septic Arthritis

Although rarely encountered, the irrigation and debridement of a septic first CMC joint is easily accomplished with the arthroscope and a shaver. A large volume of normal saline can be passed through the joint by simply running the shaver in the middle of the joint space while connecting the inflow to a wide-open source of fluid. Cultures can be obtained by sampling the initial aspirate.

Reduction of Intra-Articular Fracture

The arthroscope may be a valuable adjunct to the treatment of simple intra-articular fractures involving the base of the first metacarpal. A Bennett's fracture consists of an intra-articular fracture through the ulnar condyle of the base of the first metacarpal. It may produce problems due to intra-articular step-off or to instability. The instability is generated by the uncompromised pull of the abductor pollicis longus on the thumb metacarpal, which results in a loss of contact with the ulnar collateral ligament. Because the first CMC joint is nearly circumferentially covered with stabilizing ligaments, any attempt to visualize the fracture line in a Bennett's fracture will necessarily compromise these ligaments. Accurate visualization of the adequacy of reduction by closed means using radiographic imaging is difficult due to the highly curved nature of the articular surfaces of the joint.

When contemplating an arthroscopically assisted fixation of a Bennett's fracture, it must first be determined that the fracture is mobile. It is important to remember that the arthroscope is not a reduction device per se. Rather, it is merely a means of visualizing the reduction carried out by other means. Regional or general anesthesia is required, and the patient should be prepared for the possibility that the procedure may be converted to an open reduction or aborted altogether if the arthroscopic procedure is not possible.

The easiest way to assess whether the fracture is mobile, and potentially amenable to closed reduction under arthroscopic assessment, is to distract the thumb on the operating table. Under fluoroscopy, the thumb metacarpal is manipulated while observing the fracture site. A typical manipulation maneuver is axial rotation, with the goal of reducing the thumb metacarpal (in the surgeon's grasp) to the small fragment (the ulnar condyle of the first metacarpal base). If the fracture moves close to what is considered an adequate reduction, one may proceed with arthroscopy.

Next, a 0.045 K-wire is advanced into the base of the first metacarpal under fluoroscopic guidance in a line that will either skewer the small fragment upon reduction or will penetrate an adjacent bone to stabilize the reduction.

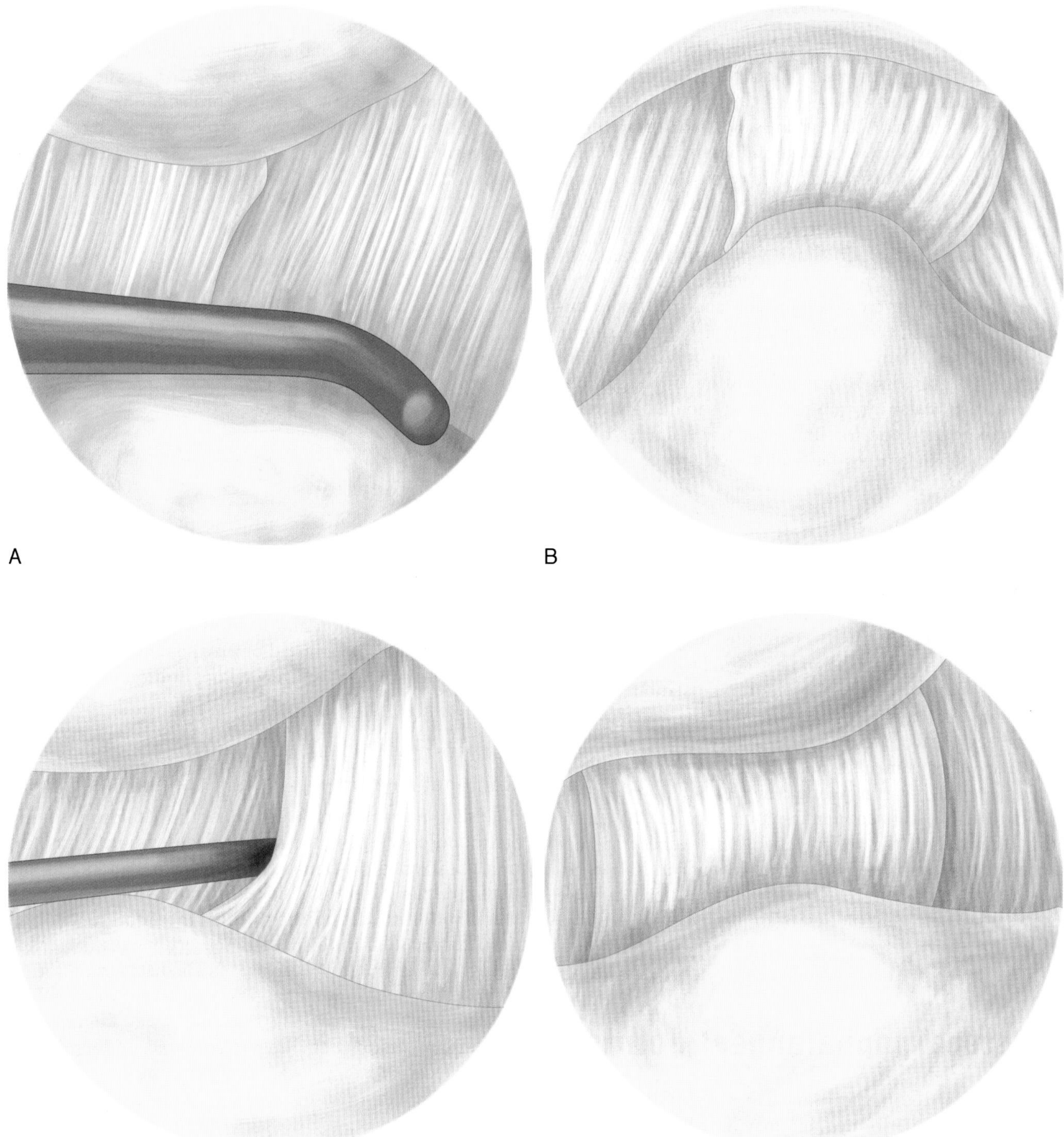

FIGURE 27.4. (A) Drawing of the posterior joint capsule viewed from the 1-R portal (MI = first metacarpal, Tm = trapezium, DRL = dorsoradial ligament, POL = posterior oblique ligament). (B) Drawing of the ulnar joint capsule viewed from the 1-R portal (MI = first metacarpal, Tm = trapezium, POL = posterior oblique ligament, UCL = ulnar collateral ligament, AOLd = deep portion of the anterior oblique ligament). (C) Drawing of the anterior joint capsule viewed from the 1-U portal (MI = first metacarpal, Tm = trapezium, AOLd = deep portion of the anterior oblique ligament, AOLs = superficial portion of the anterior oblique ligament). (D) Drawing of the anterior joint capsule viewed from the 1-U portal (MI = first metacarpal, Tm = trapezium, AOLd = deep portion of the anterior oblique ligament, AOLs = superficial portion of the anterior oblique ligament).

The arthroscope is introduced in the standard fashion, as is a small shaver. The shaver is used to evacuate the intra-articular hematoma universally present. A careful assessment of the articular surfaces and the capsular ligaments is made. Once clear visualization is possible, the fracture is manipulated into an acceptable reduction under arthroscopic guidance. Once an acceptable reduction is achieved, the assistant advances the previously placed K-wire for secure fixation of the fracture. Final radiographs are obtained, and external dressings with reinforcement are applied (as in an open reduction procedure).

Because of the severe comminution and soft tissue disrupted in a Rolando fracture, this fracture pattern should be viewed as a relative contraindication for arthroscopic reduction. There is no advantage to using an arthroscope for an extra-articular fracture pattern. It should be possible to use the arthroscope for intra-articular fractures of the trapezium, but the author has had no experience with this approach.

Complications

Few complications are encountered with careful application of standard arthroscopic principles. The most serious complications are injury to cutaneous nerves or to the radial artery, both of which can be avoided with careful dissection techniques based on a sound understanding of the underlying anatomy. Iatrogenic injury to the articular surfaces is easily encountered unless a very gentle approach to the use of instruments is maintained. It is important to remember that the arthroscope typically moves only a few millimeters in a telescoping fashion to cover the entire joint. Do not force the arthroscope where it does not want to go. Infection remains a risk, regardless of surgical procedure. Many surgeons prefer to administer a prophylactic dose of parenteral antibiotics prior to initiating a joint-related procedure.

Metacarpophalangeal Joints

Arthroscopy of the metacarpophalangeal (MCP) joints of the hand is rarely performed, but may have limited applications.[3] One must remember the advantages versus limitations of open versus arthroscopic procedures before deciding which technique to use. The advantages of open procedures typically hinge on the access to regions for procedural tasks, whereas the disadvantages include surgical scars, potential soft-tissue destabilization, and limitation of visualization in deep recesses. Arthroscopy offers the advantages of superior visualization of most regions of a joint that is otherwise difficult to access in an open procedure, through very small incisions with minimal impact on the status of contiguous tissues.

The major disadvantages of arthroscopic procedures lie in the limits of the procedural maneuvers possible through very small incisions. This dilemma is most evident in the MCP joint. Although a lengthy skin incision may be needed for an open exposure of the MCP joint, leaving largely a cosmetic effect, the disturbance of the soft tissues (extensor mechanism and joint capsule) probably has a minimal effect—especially with the proper postoperative rehabilitation protocol. However, there may be a case for which arthroscopy of the MCP joint may be an attractive option.

Indications

Indications for arthroscopy of the MCP joints are poorly worked out at this time, but may include assessment of arthritis, irrigation of a septic joint, retrieval of foreign bodies, and the identification and possible reapproximation of collateral ligaments avulsed from either the proximal phalanx or the metacarpal.[7]

Contraindications

The contraindications for arthroscopy of the MCP joints are the same as for other joints, including poor soft-tissue coverage, active cellulitis, and joint injuries not amenable to arthoscopic techniques. To this date, the techniques of arthroscopic reduction and fixation of intra-articular fractures of the metacarpal head or proximal phalanx base have not been worked out for general application.

Anatomy

Regional Anatomy

The skin over the dorsal surfaces of the MCP joints is typically loosely held to the subcutaneous tissue. Thus, care must be exercised when marking palpated landmarks such that stretching the skin location does not displace the marks prior to committing to an incision. Immediately deep to the skin are cutaneous sensory nerves (superficial radial and lateral antebrachial cutaneous nerves for the thumb, index, and long fingers; dorsal sensory branches of the ulnar nerve for the ring and small fingers). The major veins draining the fingers are typically found in the intermetacarpal valleys, well away from most arthroscopic approaches.

The tendons on the dorsal surfaces of the MCP joints share a common feature: the extensor hood (Figure 27.5). At the level of the joint, the extensor hood is composed of the extrinsic extensor tendon(s) and the sagittal fibers passing toward the volar plate. The extensor tendons for the thumb include the extensor pollicis brevis (radially) and longus (ulnarly). For the index through small fingers, the extensor digitorum communis tendon passes across the MCP joint as the radial-most tendon. Each finger also has an independent proprius tendon, although the extensor indicis proprius and extensor digiti minimi (quinti) tendons are the most widely recognized. These tendons do not insert directly into the proximal phalanx but are connected to the dorsal joint capsule and hence indirectly insert into the phalanx.

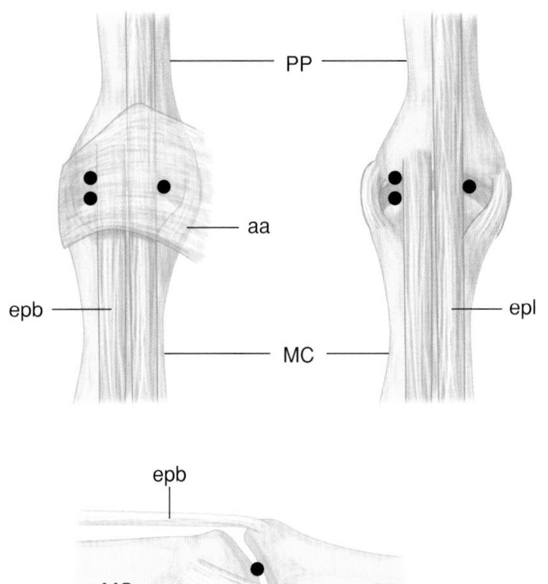

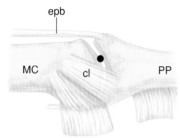

FIGURE 27.5. Drawings of the relevant anatomy for metacarpophalangeal (MP) joint arthroscopy. Top left: thumb MP joint showing the extensor hood formed in part by the adductor aponeurosis (aa) and the extrinsic extensor tendons (epb = extensor pollicis brevis). Top left: thumb MP anatomy after removal of the extensor hood, revealing the tendon of extensor pollicis longus (epl). Bottom: lateral view of the MP joint demonstrating the relationships among the metacarpal (MC), proximal phalanx (PP), tendon of extensor pollicis brevis (epb), and the collateral ligament system (cl). The black dots represent the location of recommended arthroscopic portals.

Intra-Articular Anatomy

The intra-articular anatomy of the first through fifth MCP joints is similar. The joint is described as a shallow glenoid-type joint. The articular surface of the second through fifth metacarpal heads is largely spherical, but widens palmarly in the transverse plane. The first metacarpal has little medial-lateral variance. The bases of the proximal phalanges have a shallow glenoid shape for articulation with the metacarpal head.

The lateral joint capsule is reinforced by the collateral ligament system. The true collateral ligaments span the distance from a depression on the lateral and medial surfaces of the head of the metacarpal to the palmar half of the proximal rim of the proximal phalanx. The accessory collateral ligaments are fan-shaped extensions of the true collateral ligaments, which attach to the lateral edges of the volar plate.

The volar plate forms the palmar surface of the MCP joint capsule. It has a poorly defined proximal attachment to the metacarpal, but has a definite attachment along the palmar rim of the base of the proximal phalanx. Often, there is a meniscal rim of the volar plate protruding into the joint space—biased toward the distal end of the volar plate. The dorsal joint capsule is thick and redundant, extending proximally to a line which is proximal to the level of collateral ligament attachment to the metacarpal head.

Portals

There are two recognized portals for arthroscopy of the MCP joints (Figure 27.5). The naming of the portals is related to the relationship with the extensor tendons. The radial portal is established at the joint line just radial to the extrinsic extensor tendons. The ulnar portal is established at the joint line just ulnar to the extrinsic extensor tendons.

Technique

The patient is positioned supine on the operating table, with either regional or general anesthesia. Parenteral antibiotics may be administered and a pneumatic tourniquet is typically applied to the arm. A single finger trap is secured to the thumb or finger to be evaluated and between 5 and 8 pounds of longitudinal traction is applied. Using a 22-gauge hypodermic needle, the location of either the 1-R or 1-U portal is scouted by advancing the needle directly palmarly. If there is any difficulty in passing the needle into the joint or if there is any concern about the proper identification of the joint, intraoperative radiographs or fluoroscopy may be used to verify the level of the needle prior to proceeding.

Once the proper level of the joint portals has been identified, small stab wounds are created with a scalpel—either transversely or longitudinally. I would advocate making the incisions for both portals at the beginning of the procedure. This facilitates switching portals during the operation without disturbing the cadence of the procedure. Subcutaneous tissues are dissected bluntly to the joint capsule level to be certain that underlying neurovascular tissues are displaced from harm's way. The arthroscope sheath is then introduced with a tapered trocar in one portal and a small probe is introduced in the other portal. It is rare that an outflow device is needed, particularly with judicious control of inflow fluid volume and rate. If an outflow tract is necessary, however, a large-bore hypodermic needle may be introduced—or a shaver may be used to evacuate excess or cloudy fluid. It may also be necessary to debride excess synovial tissue in order to visualize the joint surfaces and the ligaments. This may be accomplished with either a small shaver or a suction punch.

A comprehensive inspection of the articular surfaces is carried out. Next, an inspection of the intra-articular appearance of the collateral ligaments and volar plate may be completed. It is best to use the probe to validate the integrity of these structures, rather than simply relying on their visual appearance.

Procedures

The following procedures have been proposed, although largely based on personal communications and anecdotal experiences. This is by no means meant to be an all-inclusive list.

Septic Arthritis

Irrigation and debridement of a septic first CMC joint is easily accomplished with the arthroscope and a shaver. This may be considered particularly useful in the so-called "fight bites," where an open intrusion of the patient's MP joint has occurred during an altercation due to contact with an opponent's teeth—which creates a septic hazard for the joint. A large volume of normal saline can be passed through the joint by simply running the shaver in the middle of the joint space while connecting the inflow to a wide-open source of fluid. Cultures can be obtained by sampling the initial aspirate.

Diagnosis of Collateral Ligament Injury

Most ligament injuries about the MCP joints are treated well with closed means. However, the Stener-type lesion creates a situation that is less likely to result in successful closed management. In the Stener lesion, the distally avulsed collateral ligament is displaced and trapped under the free proximal edge of the extensor hood.[8] Although the ulnar collateral ligament of the thumb is the avulsion injury most commonly associated with a Stener lesion, it can occur in the fingers.[8–10] This is particularly so with the ulnar collateral ligament of the index finger MCP joint and the radial collateral ligament of the small finger MCP joint. The arthroscope provides a minimally invasive means of readily identifying the presence of a Stener-type lesion in any of the digits.

In a subacute setting of instability following injury, it may prove to be a difficult task to know whether the injury is due to involvement of either the proximal or distal attachment of a finger MCP collateral ligament. Because scar tissue has likely developed, the surgeon will have a difficult time knowing where the injury occurred—leading to potential complications of elevating the wrong end of the ligament during open repair. Again, the arthroscope offers a ready means of identifying the level of the injury prior to conversion to an open procedure.

Reapproximation of Collateral Ligament Avulsion Injury

Ryu has advocated arthroscopic techniques as the definitive treatment for thumb Stener lesion injuries of the ulnar collateral ligament.[7] After verifying the presence of the Stener lesion, the ligament is "hooked" by a probe and drawn back deep to the adductor apponeurosis—where it comes to rest adjacent to its normal attachment point on the ulnar rim of the base of the proximal phalanx. From here, it is treated as a nondisplaced collateral ligament injury. The author has no personal experience with this technique, but instead opts for an open procedure to stabilize all ulnar collateral ligament injuries with measurable instability.

Complications

Few complications are encountered with careful application of standard arthroscopic principles. The most serious complications are injury to cutaneous nerves, which can be avoided with careful dissection techniques based on a sound understanding of the underlying anatomy. Iatrogenic injury to the articular surfaces is easily encountered unless a very gentle approach to the use of instruments is maintained. It is important to remember that the arthroscope typically moves only a few millimeters in a telescoping fashion to cover the entire joint. Do not force the arthroscope where it does not want to go. Infection remains a risk, regardless of surgical procedure. Many surgeons prefer to administer a prophylactic dose of parenteral antibiotics prior to initiating a joint-related procedure.

Summary

Arthroscopy of the small joints of the hand has become a reliable clinical tool, although it is still somewhat limited to diagnostic applications. Therapeutic options are becoming increasingly available, but must be balanced against the efficacy of open procedures. Arthroscopy of these joints is safe, provided the surgeon thoroughly understands the relevant anatomy and is truly facile with the equipment and techniques. Again, the author would like to emphasize the need for restraint and honesty on the part of the surgeon to do what is truly best for the patient—not what is *in vogue*.

References

1. Berger RA. A technique for arthroscopic evaluation of the first carpometacarpal joint. J Hand Surg 1997;22(A):1077–80.
2. Menon J. Arthroscopic management of trapeziometacarpal arthritis of the thumb. Arthroscopy 1996;12:581–87.
3. Ryu J, Fegan R. Arthroscopic treatment of acute complete thumb metacarpophalangeal ulnar collateral ligament tears. J Hand Surg 1995;20(A):1037–42.
4. Bettinger PC, Linscheid RL, Berger RA, Cooney WP III, An K-N. An anatomic study of the stabilizing ligaments of the trapezium and trapeziometacarpal joint. J Hand Surg 1999; 24(A):786–98.
5. Bettinger PC, Berger RA. Functional ligamentous anatomy of the trapezium and trapeziometacarpal joint. Hand Clin 2001;17(2):151–68.
6. Eaton RG, Littler JW. Ligament reconstruction for the painful thumb carpometacarpal joint. J Bone Joint Surg 1973;55A:1655–66.
7. Ishizuki M. Injury to collateral ligament of the metacarpophalangeal ligament of a finger. J Hand Surg 1988;13A: 444–48.
8. Schubiner JM, Mass DP. Operation for collateral ligament ruptures of the metacarpophalangeal joints of the fingers. J Bone Joint Surg 1989;71B:388–89.
9. Stener B. Displacement of the ruptured ulnar collateral ligament of the metacarpo-phalangeal joint of the thumb: A clinical and anatomical study. J Bone Joint Surg 1962; 44B:869–79.
10. Wolf BA, Cervino AL. Rupture of the radial collateral ligament of the fifth metacarpophalangeal joint. Annals of Plas Surg 1988;21:382–87.

SECTION 6

Small-Joint Arthroscopy

David J. Slutsky

CHAPTER 28

Arthroscopic Treatment of Trapeziometacarpal Disease

Introduction

There are myriad techniques for open treatment of trapeziometacarpal (TM) osteoarthritis (OA). These have included partial and complete trapezium excision with or without ligament reconstruction and with or without interposition of tendon, fascia lata, gortex, artelon, or silicone. Instances of reactive synovitis have tempered the enthusiasm for interposition of foreign substances. Recent reports in the North American literature[1,2] of good results following complete trapeziectomy with hematoma arthroplasty have rejuvenated interest in this technique, which has been commonplace in Europe for some time.[3] Arthroscopic techniques for evaluating and treating trapeziometacarpal disease surfaced in 1994.[4,5]

The question of whether to interpose tendon is still a matter of debate. Proponents of the hematoma arthroplasty cite data that demonstrates no advantages in terms of pinch strength, thumb motion, and pain relief following an arthroplasty with tendon interposition compared to an isolated trapeziectomy.[6] The hematoma arthroplasty relies on the development of a stable pseudarthrosis that develops from the ingrowth of fibrous tissue, which replaces the blood that immediately fills the cavity following an excision of the trapezium. Pinning the thumb metacarpal base to the index for five to six weeks is integral to the procedure, but augmentation or reconstruction of the TM joint capsule is not. The good results that have been obtained with open trapeziectomy have provided the impetus for the development of arthroscopic techniques.

The scaphotrapezotrapezoidal (STT) joint is also commonly affected by OA. The STT fusion popularized by Watson has largely fallen out of favor. As an alternative to this, distal scaphoid resection has been shown to provide good symptomatic relief.[7]

Indications

The main indication for surgery is basilar thumb pain that is unresponsive to conservative treatment. This typically includes a trial of splinting with a forearm- or palmar-based thumb spica splint, NSAIDs, and activity modification. A TM joint cortisone injection may be used as a temporizing procedure. Although it is well known that X-ray findings do not always correlate with clinical symptoms, they are nevertheless instrumental in determining which patients may be appropriate candidates for an arthroscopic resection.

Littler and Eaton described a radiographic staging classification of TM OA.[8] Stage I comprises normal articular surfaces without joint space narrowing or sclerosis. There is less than 1/3 subluxation of the metacarpal base. Stage II reveals mild joint space narrowing, mild sclerosis, or osteophytes <2 mm in diameter. Instability is evident on stress views, with >1/3 subluxation. The STT joint is normal. In stage III there is significant joint space narrowing, subchondral sclerosis, and peripheral osteophytes >2 mm in diameter (but a normal STT joint).

In stage IV there is pantrapezial OA with narrowing, sclerosis, and osteophytes involving both the TM and STT joints. Burton modified this classification by incorporating the clinical findings.[9] Stage I includes ligamentous laxity and pain with forceful and/or repetitive pinching. The joint is hypermobile, which can be seen on stress views (but X-rays are normal). In stage II, crepitus and instability can be demonstrated clinically—whereas X-rays reveal a loss of the joint space. Stages III and IV are similar to Eaton's classification. Patients in stage I (and possibly early stage II) are appropriate candidates for arthroscopic debridement and capsular shrinkage.[10]

Badia proposed a more specific classification based on arthroscopic changes.[11] Stage I included intact articular cartilage, stage II included eburnation on the ulnar 1/3 of the metacarpal base and central trapezium, stage III comprised widespread full-thickness cartilage loss on both surfaces. Based on intraoperative findings, he recommended debridement for stage I, with thermal capsulorrhaphy in the presence of dorsal subluxation, extension/abduction osteotomy of the metacarpal base ∀ thermal shrinkage for stage II, and an arthroscopic interposition arthroplasty for stage III. He recommended an open arthroplasty in the presence of associated severe STT joint OA.

As a general rule, any patient who is an appropriate candidate for a hemiresection arthroplasty of the TM joint would also be suitable for an arthroscopic hemitrapeziectomy. This would typically include patients in stage II and stage III with unremitting pain despite appropriate conservative measures. This form of treatment does not preclude an open trapeziectomy and/or ligament reconstruction at a later date as a salvage procedure for failed arthroscopic surgery. The presence of Eaton stage IV disease is a relative contraindication to a hemitrapeziectomy, although an arthroscopic hemitrapeziectomy combined with an arthroscopic debridement or limited resection of the distal scaphoid is an option. The rationale for this would be similar to that of the double interposition arthroplasty described by Eaton and Barron, in which the TM and STT joints are resurfaced while the body of the trapezium is left intact in order to prevent a loss of height of the thumb ray.[12] Failing this, a complete arthroscopic (or open) trapeziectomy would be necessary.

Precautions

Any significant lateral subluxation of the thumb metacarpal base will not be corrected without some type of ligament reconstruction or capsular shrinkage, and may compromise the long-term result if not corrected. Metacarpophalangeal (MP) joint hyperextension must be treated concomitantly. Otherwise, the reconstruction may ultimately fail. MP hyperextension of 10 to 20 degrees may be treated by percutaneous fixation of the MP joint in flexion for four to six weeks, and/or transfer of the extensor pollicis brevis to the thumb metacarpal base. MP hyperextension of 20 to 40 degrees can be addressed with a volar plate advancement[13] or capsulodesis.[14] A sesamoidesis MP hyperextension >40 degrees is typically controlled by an MP fusion.

Contraindications

This would include any general contraindication to thumb arthroscopy, including distortion of the anatomy due to swelling, unstable or friable skin (which would preclude the use of traction), and recent infection. Ehler Danlos syndrome is a relative contraindication for this procedure, although a successful arthroscopic tendon arthroplasty has been reported.[15]

Equipment

A 1.9-mm 30-degree angled scope along with a camera attachment is used. A larger 2.7-mm scope may be substituted after the space has been partially decompressed. A 3-mm hook probe is needed for palpation of intracarpal structures. The use of an overhead traction tower greatly facilitates instrumentation. A motorized shaver is needed for debridement. Some type of diathermy unit is required if a capsular shrinkage is contemplated. Intraoperative fluoroscopy is employed to assess the adequacy of bone resection and for locating the portals as needed.

Surgical Technique

The patient is positioned supine on the operating table, with the arm extended on a hand table. The thumb is suspended by Chinese finger traps with 5 pounds of countertraction, which forces the wrist into ulnar deviation. The relevant landmarks are outlined, including the proximal and dorsal edge of the thumb metacarpal base, the tendons of the abductor pollicis longus (APL), the extensor pollicis longus (EPL), and the radial artery in the snuffbox (Figure 28.1). The procedure is performed with a tourniquet elevated to 250 mmHg. Saline inflow irrigation is provided through the arthroscope and a small-joint pump or pressure bag.

To establish the 1-R portal, the thumb metacarpal base is palpated and the joint is identified with a 22-gauge needle just radial to the APL, followed by injection of 2 cc of saline. This step may be facilitated by fluoroscopy. A small skin incision is made, followed by wound spread technique with tenotomy scissors. The capsule is pierced and a cannula and blunt trocar are inserted, followed by the arthroscope. An identical procedure is used to establish the 1-U portal, just ulnar to the EPB tendon, followed by insertion of a 3-mm hook probe. The portals are interchangeably used to systematically inspect the joint, which is facilitated by expedient use of a 2.0-mm synovial resector.

Access to medial trapezial osteophytes may sometimes be difficult. Hence, the author has found the use of a distal/dorsal (D-2) accessory portal to be of some value.[16] Its main utility is that it allows one to look down on the trapezium rather than across it, which facilitates resection of medial osteophytes (Figure 28.2a through e). This accessory portal allows views of the dorsal capsule with rotation of the scope and facilitates triangulation of the instrumentation. It is situated in the dorsal aspect of the first web space. An anatomical study of five cadaver hands revealed that the D-2 portal surface landmark is ulnar to the EPL tendon and 1 cm distal to V-shaped cleft at the juncture of the index and thumb metacarpal bases.

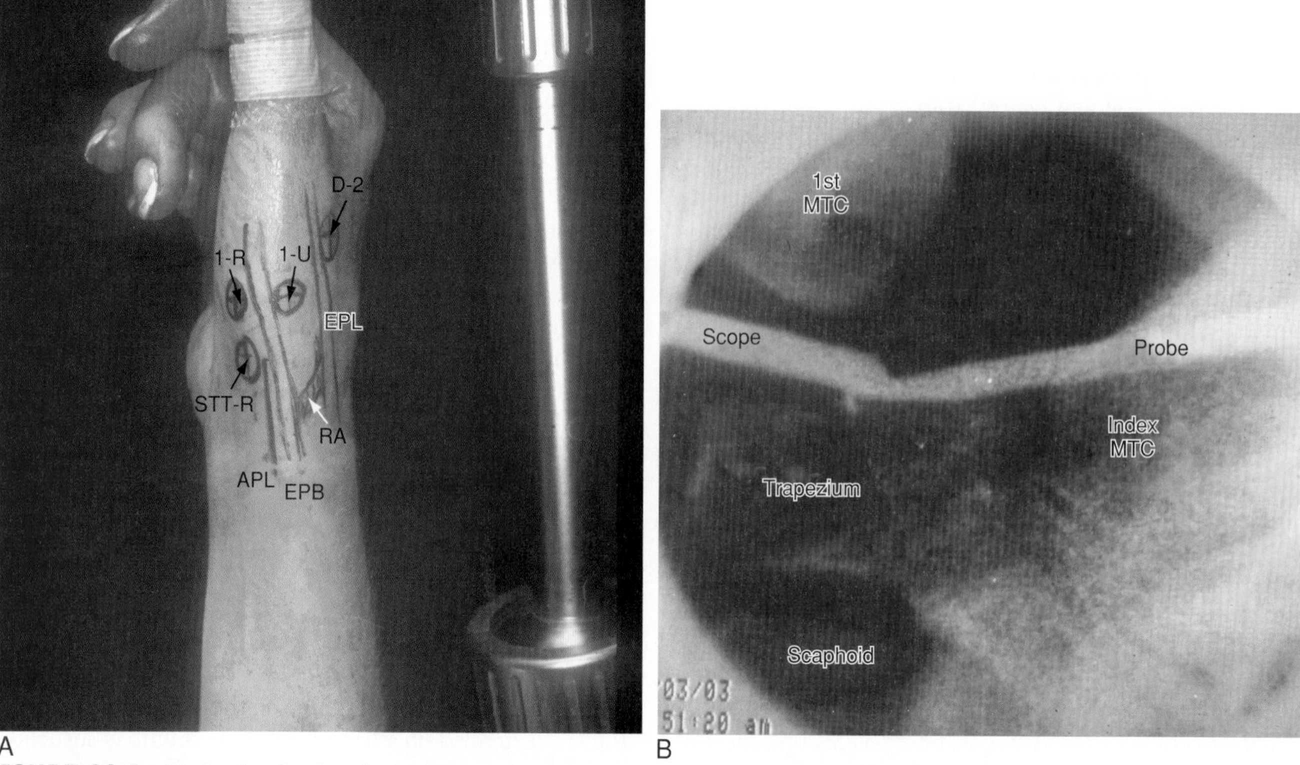

FIGURE 28.1. (A) Surface landmarks for TM and STT portals (APL = abductor pollicis longus, EPB = extensor pollicis brevis, EPL = extensor pollicis longus, RA = radial artery). (B) Intraoperative fluoroscopy used to check position of probe (in 1-U portal) and the scope (in 1-R portal) (MTC = metacarpal).

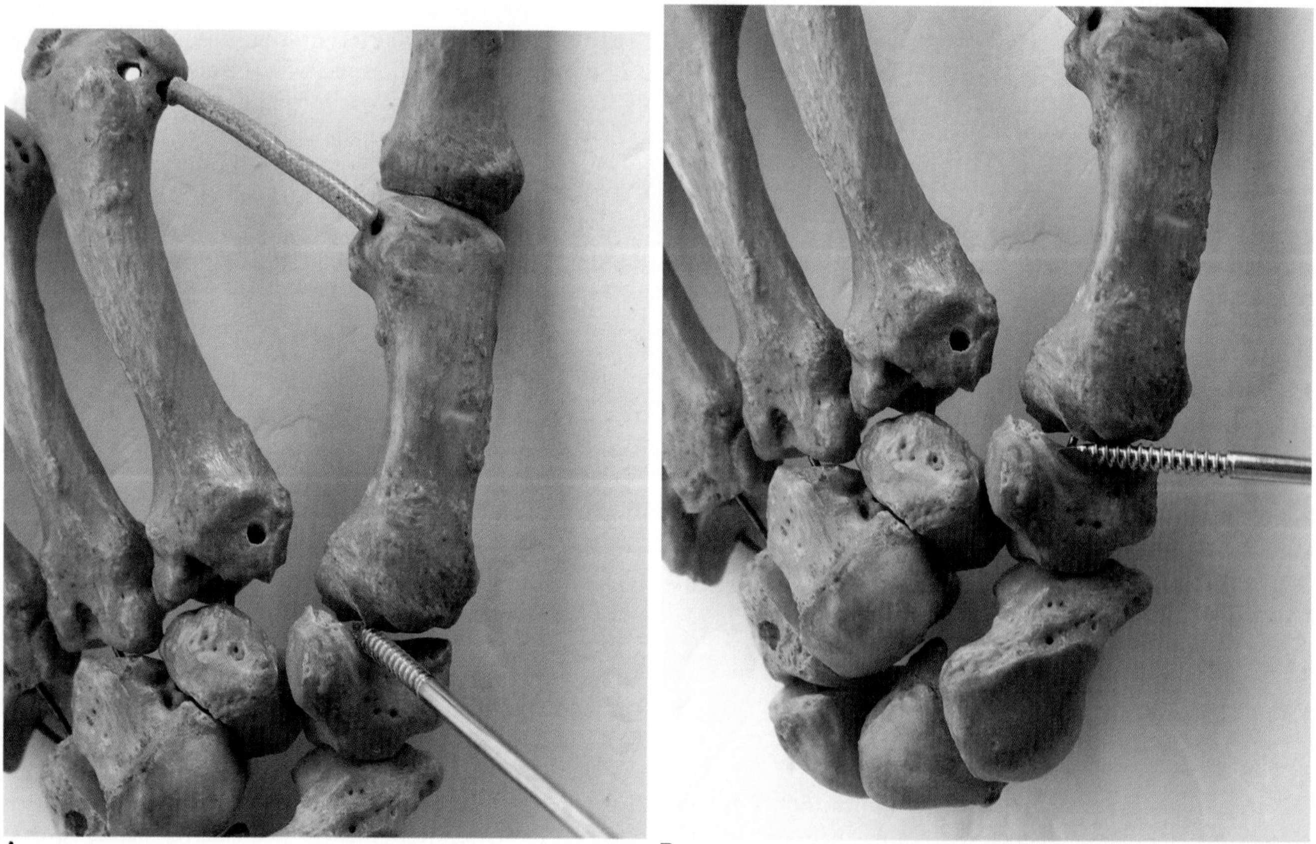

A B

FIGURE 28.2. (A) Direction scope in 1-U portal. Note that the angle of the scope runs parallel to the trapezial surface and the medial aspect of the trapezium. (B) Direction scope in 1-R portal. Note that the angle of the scope makes access to the medial ridge of the trapezium difficult.

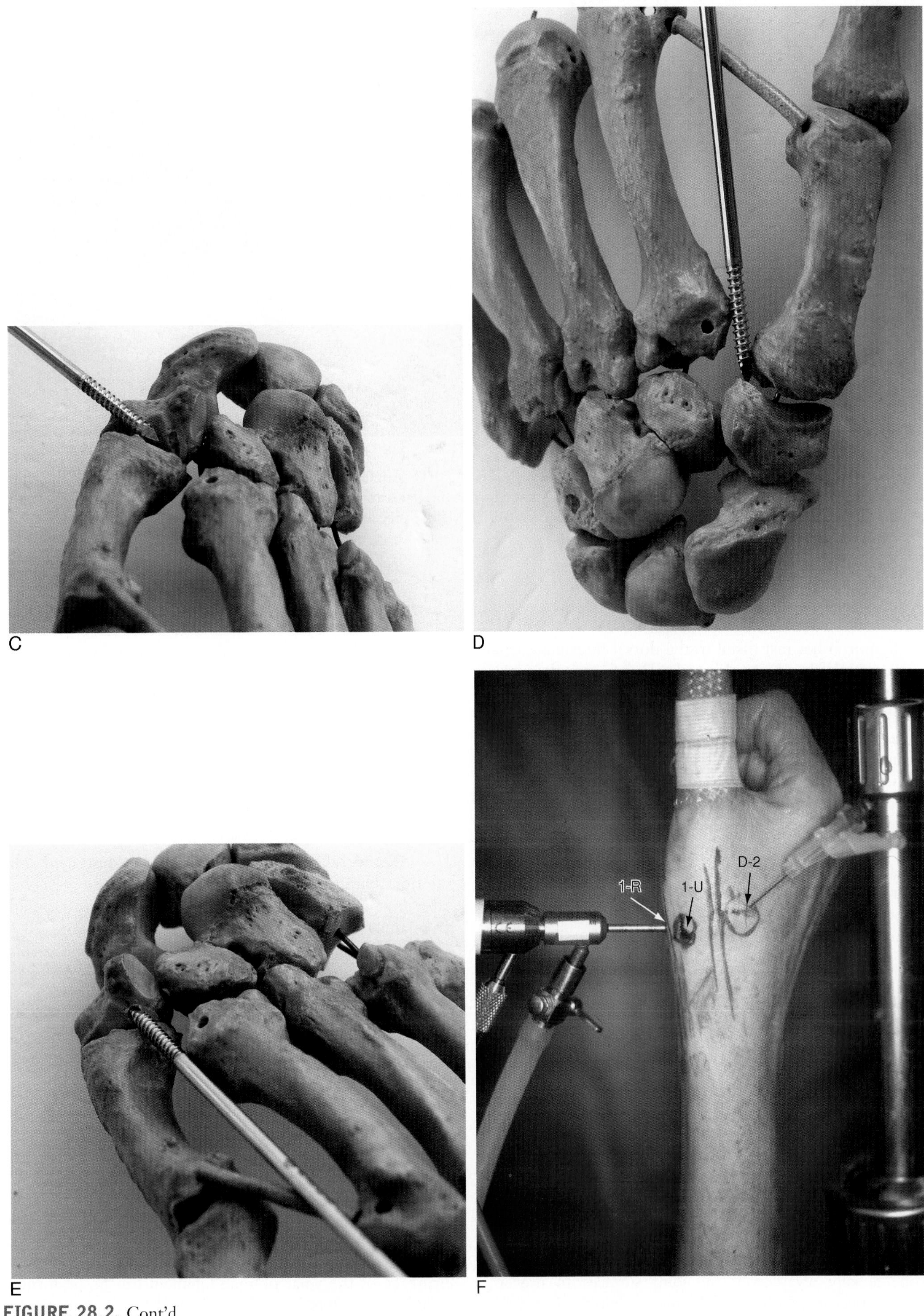

FIGURE 28.2. Cont'd

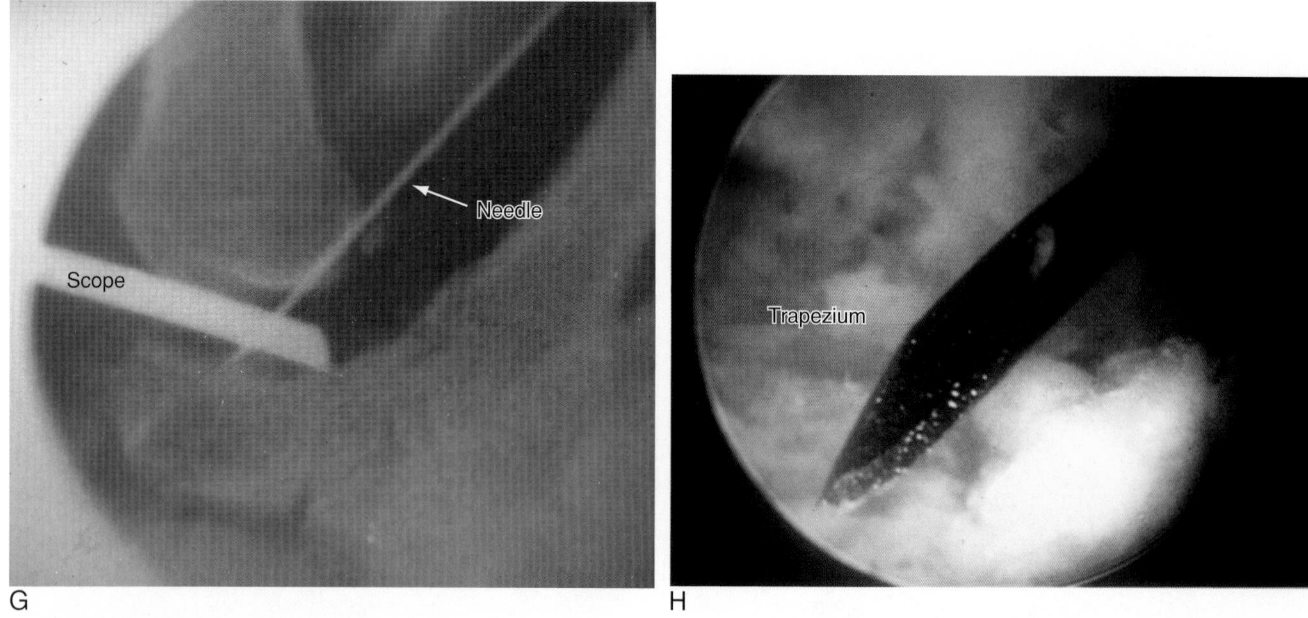

FIGURE 28.2. Cont'd (C) Top view of angle of scope in 1-R portal. (D) Angle of instruments in D-2 portal. Note that the angle looks down on the medial trapezium, which facilitates resection of medial osteophytes. (E) Top view of angle of scope/bur in the D-2 portal in relation to the medial ridge of the trapezium. (F) Needle placement for the D-2 portal. (G) Fluoroscopic view of scope and needle. (H) View from the 1-R portal.

The portal lies just distal to the dorsal intermetacarpal ligament (DIML). To establish the D-2 portal, the intersection of the base of the index and thumb metacarpal is identified just distal and ulnar to the extensor pollicis longus (EPL) tendon. The course of the radial artery is outlined by palpation or Doppler with the tourniquet down. A 22-gauge needle is inserted 1 cm distal to this juncture and angled in a proximal, radial, and palmar direction—hugging the thumb metacarpal while viewing from either the 1-R or 1-U portal (Figure 28.2f through h). A small skin incision is made, and tenotomy scissors are used to spread the soft tissue and pierce the joint capsule. This is followed by insertion of a blunt trocar and cannula and then the arthroscope or alternatively a hook probe, motorized shaver, or 2.9-mm bur.

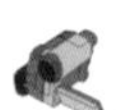

Arthroscopic Debridement and Capsular Shrinkage Interposition

The essence of arthroscopic capsular shrinkage is akin to that of a volar oblique ligament reconstruction. It relies on thermal heating of the collagenous fibers in the surrounding ligaments and capsule, followed by a period of joint immobilization in a reduced position. A motorized shaver is used to debride any synovitis and to expose the capsular ligaments. A diathermy probe is then employed to paint the volar oblique ligament and surrounding capsule, taking care to leave bands of tissue between. The probe is kept away from the joint surfaces to prevent cartilage necrosis. In light of the meager joint volume, the outflow fluid temperature is frequently monitored to prevent overheating. Use of an 18-gauge needle in an accessory portal enhances fluid circulation, which minimizes this risk.

Arthroscopic Partial or Complete Trapeziectomy Without Tendon Interposition

The 1-R and 1-U portals are established as described. The anterior oblique ligament (AOL) is identified and preserved. After joint debridement, a 2.9-mm bur is applied in a to-and-fro manner to resect the distal trapezium (Figure 28.3a through d). The diameter of the bur along with fluoroscopy provides a gauge as to the amount of bony resection. A larger bur may be substituted as the space between the metacarpal base and distal trapezium enlarges. It is crucial to remove any medial osteophytes, which will lead to impingement and possibly to persistent pain.

The D-2 portal is useful for this step because it allows one to debride the medial trapezium from above rather than from across the joint (Figure 28.4a). Culp recommends resecting at least half the distal trapezium,[10] although it is my experience that excising 4 to 5 mm is sufficient—provided that all of the medial osteophytes are removed (Figure 28.4b). After the bony resection is complete, the thumb is K-wired in a pronated and abducted position. If there is lateral subluxation of the metacarpal base, thermal shrinkage of the volar oblique ligament can be performed at this time (Figure 28.5a through i).

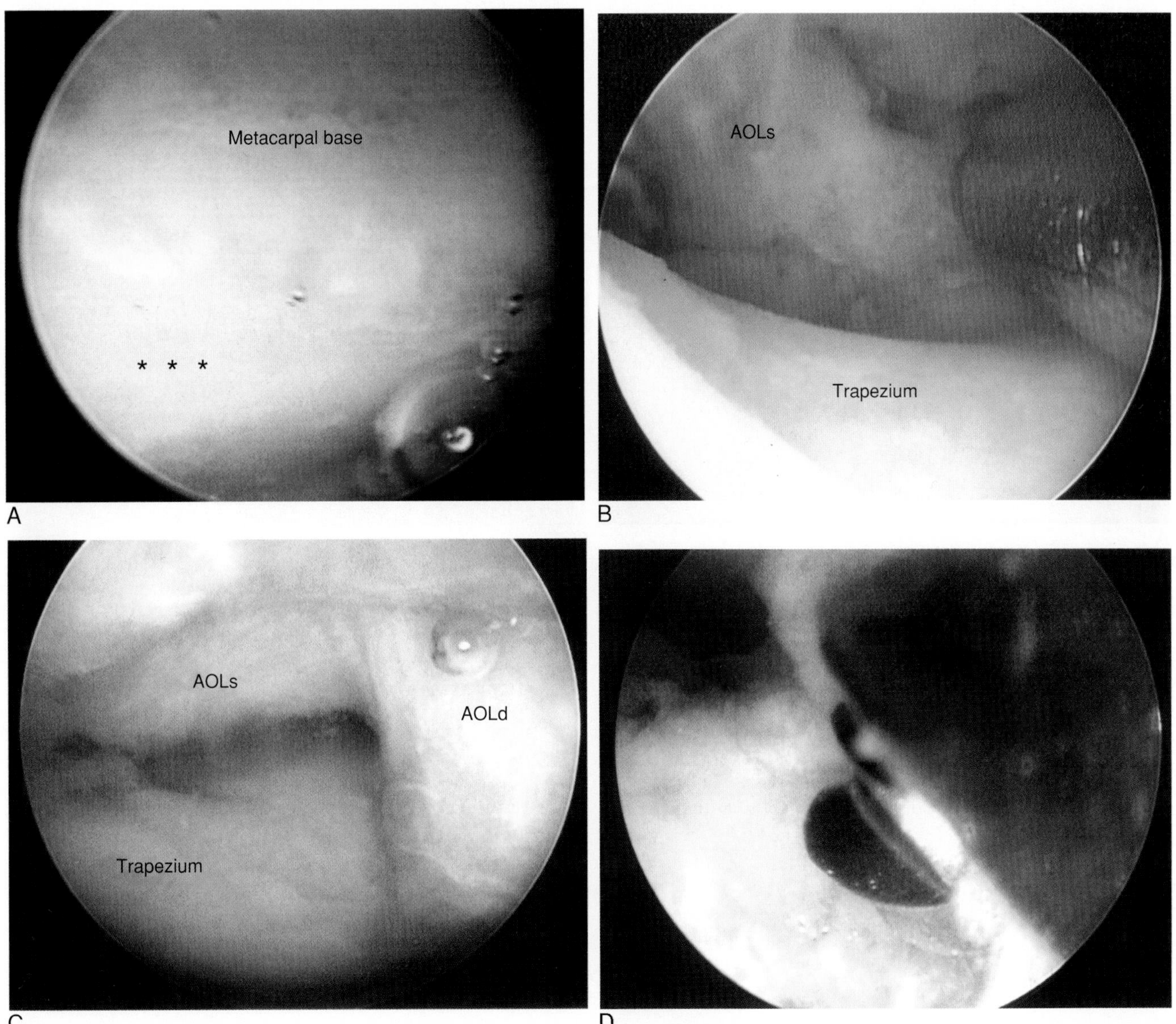

FIGURE 28.3. (A) View of the thumb metacarpal base from the 1-U portal. Note the exposed subchondral bone (*). (B) View of the distal trapezium from the 1-R portal. Probe is in the 1-U portal (AOLs = superficial anterior oblique ligament). (C) View of the superficial (AOLs) and deep (AOLd) anterior oblique ligament from the 1-U portal. (D) A 2.9-mm bur in the 1-U portal as seen from the 1-R portal.

Arthroscopic Partial or Complete Trapeziectomy with Interposition

After a partial or complete resection of the trapezium, autogenous tendon graft such as the palmaris longus, 1/2 of the flexor carpi radialis, or a slip of the APL is harvested through multiple transverse incisions. Alternatively, some other form of interposition material can be substituted. Menon reported a high incidence of cystic change following the use of Gortex, which is no longer recommended. An absorbable suture is placed in the leading end of the tendon graft and swaged onto a large curved needle, which is used to pass the graft through the joint. The needle is passed through the 1-U portal and brought out though the volar capsule and bulk of the thenar eminence. Traction on the suture pulls the graft into the joint. The remaining graft is packed in with forceps and the portals are closed. The thumb is K-wired in abduction for four weeks.

Arthroscopic Distal Scaphoid Resection

If there is significant STT OA, the joint can be debrided as described by Ashwood and Bains.[16] Alternatively, a minimal arthroscopic resection of the distal scaphoid can be performed. The STT joint can be viewed through the midcarpal radial portal (MCR) with the bur in the STT-U portal or STT-R portal (Figure 28.6a through j). The portals are likewise interchangeable. The volar and radial scaphotrapezial ligaments are preserved and the bony resection is confined to 2 to 4 mm to lessen the risk of a dorsal intercalated segmental instability (DISI) pattern.

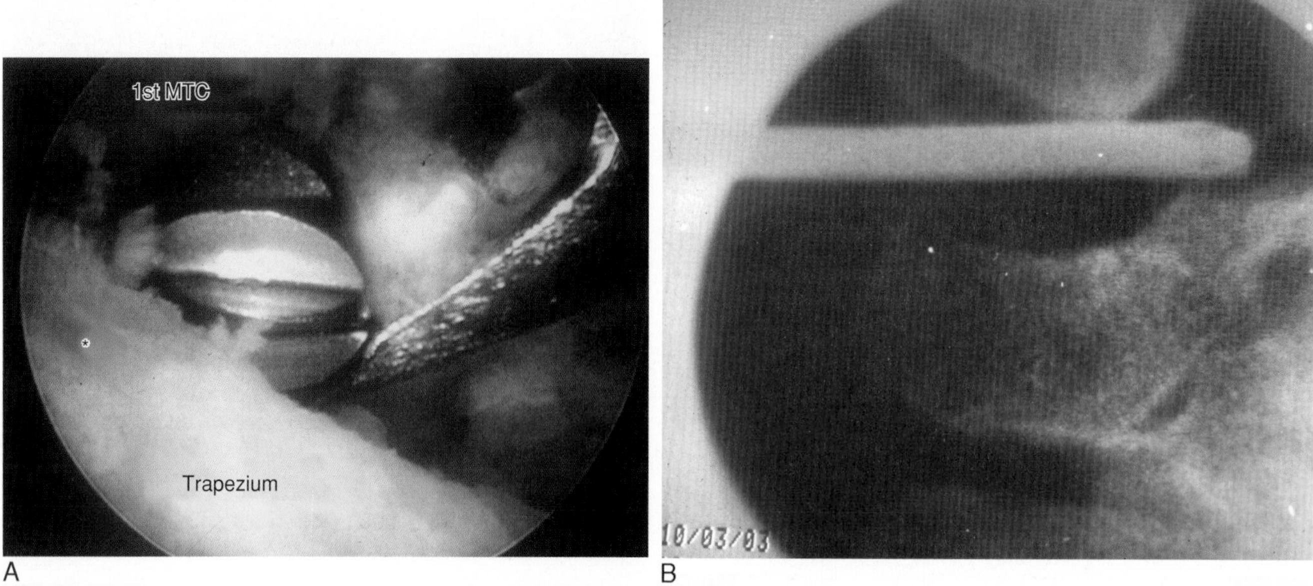

FIGURE 28.4. (A) View of a 2.9-mm bur in the D-2 portal. Note chondromalacia of the distal trapezium (*). (B) Scope placement to check resection of medial osteophytes.

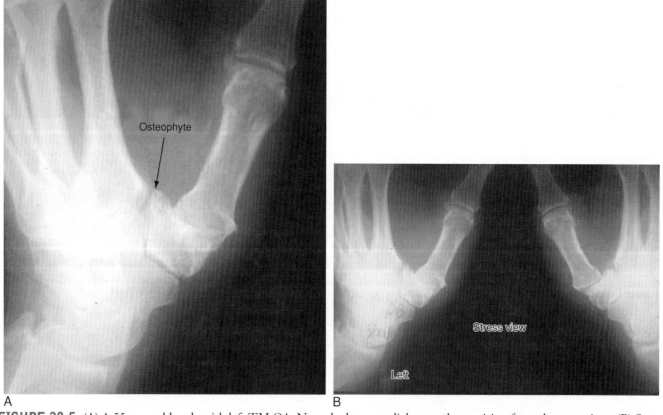

FIGURE 28.5. (A) A 55-year-old male with left TM OA. Note the large medial osteophyte arising from the trapezium. (B) Stress X-ray.

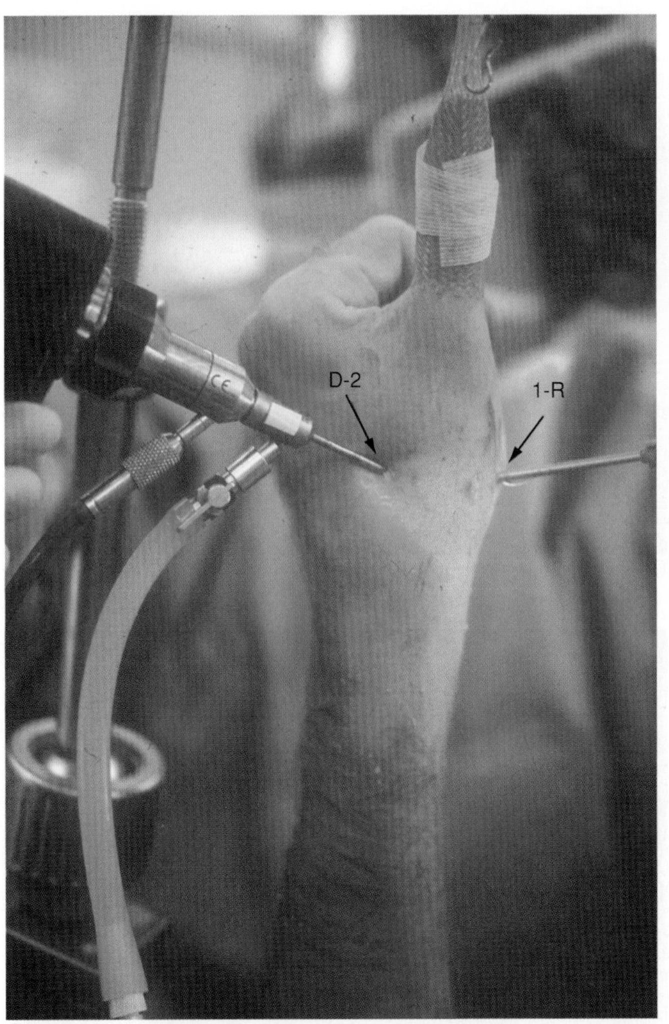

C

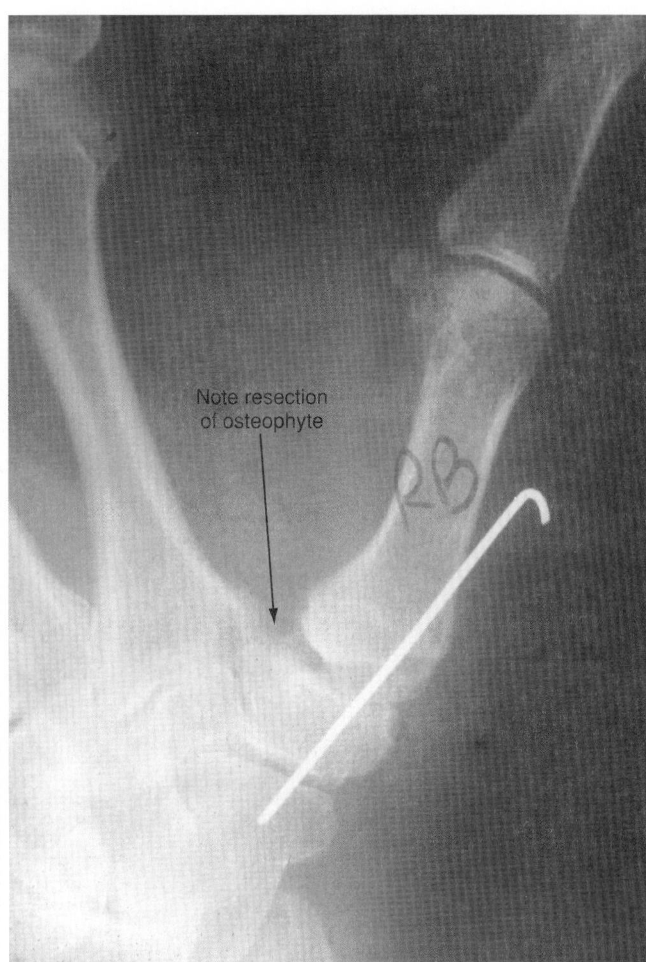

E

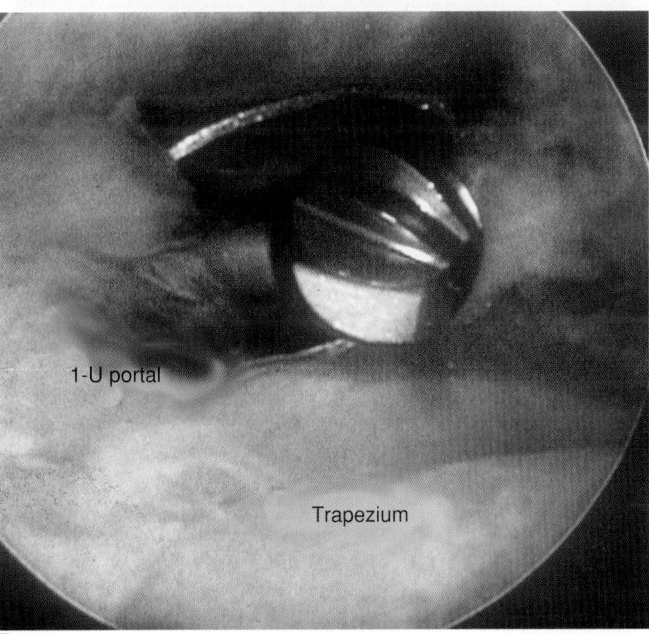

D

FIGURE 28.5. Cont'd (C) Arthroscopic TM arthroplasty. Scope in the D-2 portal, bur in the 1-R portal. (D) View from the D-2 portal with the bur in the 1-R portal. (E) X-ray after partial trapeziectomy.

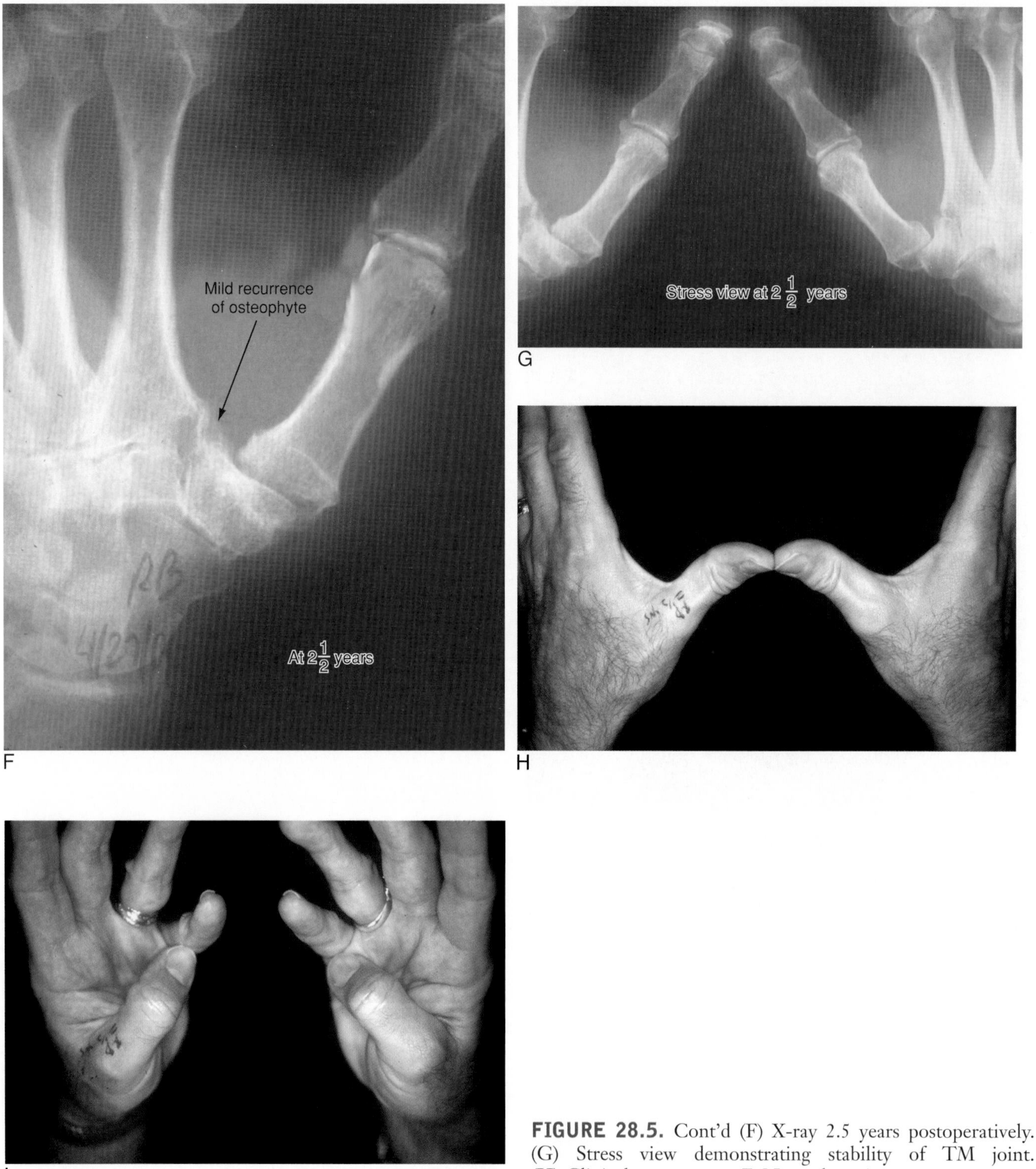

Mild recurrence of osteophyte

At $2\frac{1}{2}$ years

F

Stress view at $2\frac{1}{2}$ years

G

H

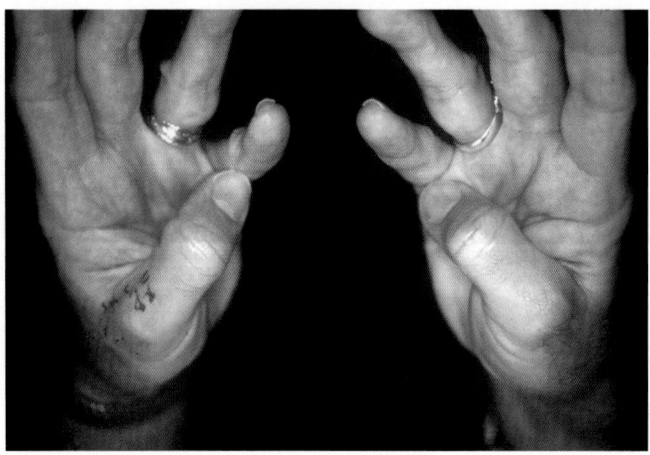

I

FIGURE 28.5. Cont'd (F) X-ray 2.5 years postoperatively. (G) Stress view demonstrating stability of TM joint. (H) Clinical appearance. (I) Normal motion.

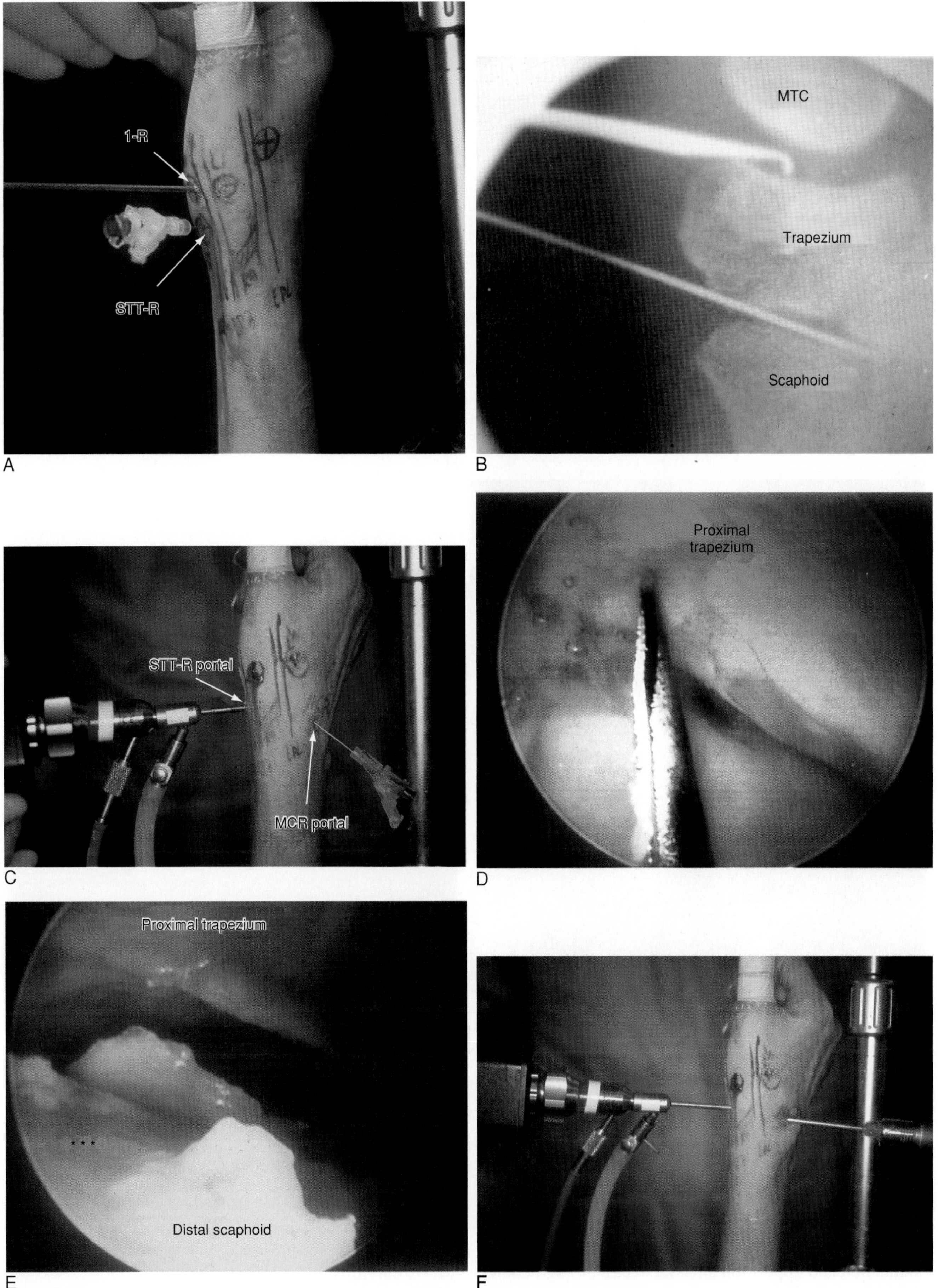

FIGURE 28.6. (A) Localizing the STT-R portal in relation to the 1-R portal. (B) Fluoroscopic view. (C) Scope in the STT-R portal with needle in the midcarpal radial (MCR) portal. (D) Arthroscopic view of the proximal surface of the trapezium. (E) View of the STT joint. Note the exposed subchondral bone (*). (F) Bur in MCR portal.

(Continued)

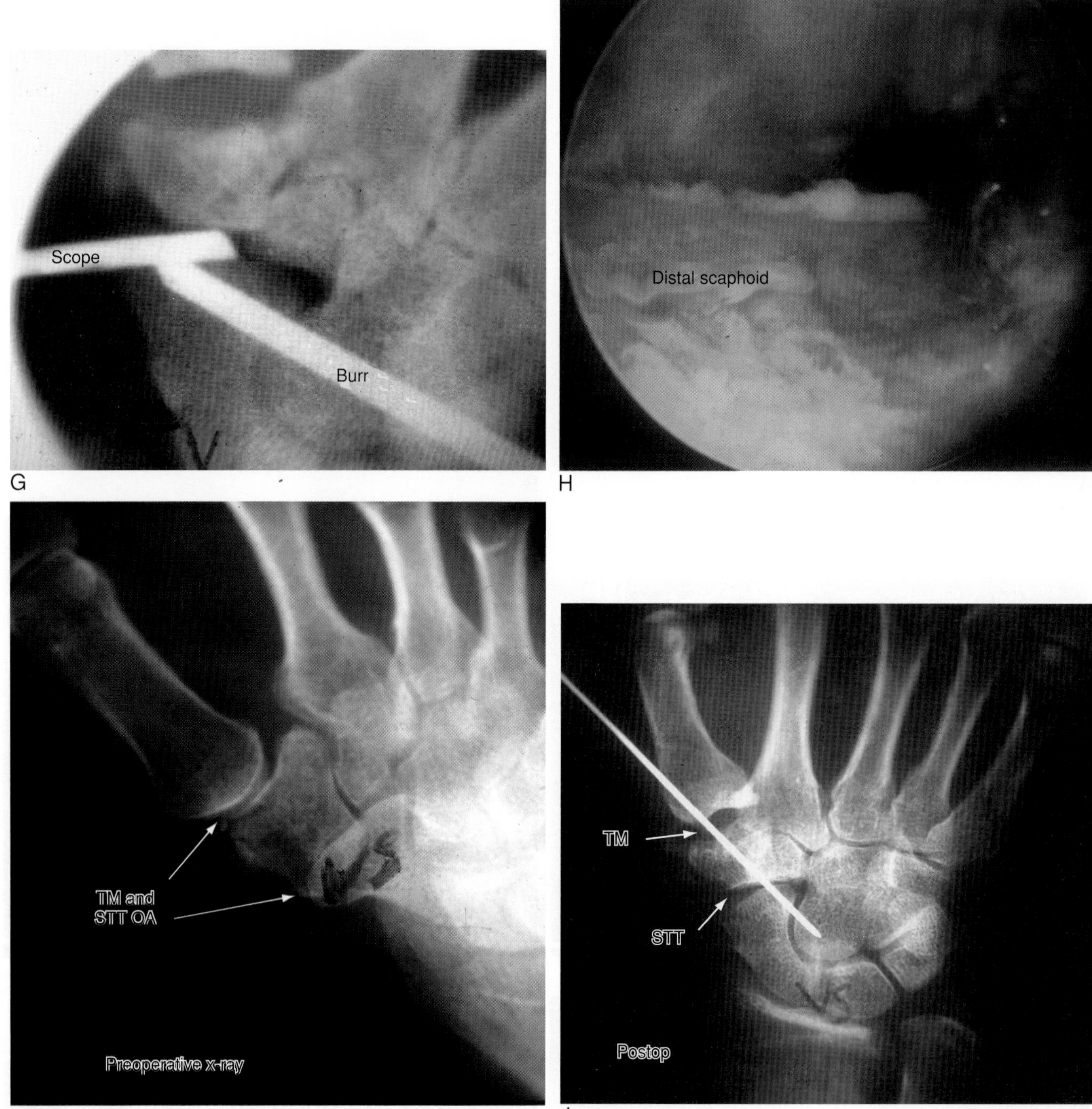

FIGURE 28.6. Cont'd (G) Fluoroscopic view. (H) After resection of distal scaphoid. (I) Preoperative X-ray. (J) Immediate postoperative X-ray following partial trapeziectomy and minimal distal scaphoid resection.

Postoperative Management

The thumb is immobilized in abduction by cast or splint for four weeks, after which the TM K-wire is removed. Thumb abduction and extension are instituted, followed by adduction and opposition after six weeks. Strengthening ensues once motion has been restored. The rehabilitation protocol is modified as necessary if concomitant surgery on the MP joint has been performed.

Results

Menon reported his results on performing a partial arthroscopic resection of the trapezium and an interposition arthroplasty in 31 patients (33 hands).[4] The mean age was 59 years (range 48 to 81 years), with an average follow-up of 37.6 months (range 24 to 48 months). Gortex was used in 19 patients and autogenous tendon or allograft in 14. Complete pain relief was obtained in 25 patients/hands (75.7%). Three patients had mild pain (four hands), and four patients had persistent pain that required conversion to an open trapeziectomy and ligament reconstruction. All patients maintained their preoperative motion. Pinch strength improved from 6 psi preoperatively to 11.1 psi postoperatively. Because of osteolysis in three patients (four hands), the use of Gortex as an interpositional substance was not recommended.

Culp and Rekant performed a partial or complete arthroscopic trapeziectomy in 22 patients (24 thumbs) with electrothermal shrinkage.[10] Detailed data is not available, but they reported 88% excellent or good outcome scores at a follow-up of 1.2 to 4 years. Subsidence of the thumb metacarpal was 2 to 4 mm, and pinch strength improved by 22%.

There are no clinical series on arthroscopic distal scaphoid resection at this time. Arthroscopic debridement of the scaphotrapezial joint without distal resection, however, has been shown to be beneficial.[17] There is always the worry that a distal scaphoid resection will worsen any preexisting scapholunate instability by weakening the scaphotrapezial ligaments. In a series of 21 patients who were treated with an open distal scaphoid resection, Garcia-Elias et al. demonstrated the alleviation of pain and discomfort in all cases.[7]

At a mean follow-up of 29 months, a dorsal intercalated segmental instability (DISI) carpal malalignment was evident in 12 patients—although this did not compromise the overall result. Interposition of FCR tendon or dorsal capsule resulted in less wrist flexion-extension compared to patients without fibrous interposition, especially when combined with arthroscopic resection of the trapezium. The author's experience with combined arthroscopic resection of the TM and STT joints is limited to two patients, with one excellent and one fair result. Hence, this technique requires further study.

Summary

Early results with this procedure are encouraging. It may have special application in the younger patient in whom a trapeziectomy is undesirable. The use of the arthroscopic procedure does not preclude a more formal procedure at a later date for recurrent symptoms or progression of the OA. Long-term follow-ups are as yet unavailable. Hence, this procedure should be viewed as a useful adjunctive treatment method for TM OA but unlikely to supplant the more time-tested open procedures.

References

1. Kuhns CA, Emerson ET, Meals RA. Hematoma and distraction arthroplasty for thumb basal joint osteoarthritis: A prospective, single-surgeon study including outcomes measures. J Hand Surg [Am] 2003;28:381–89.
2. Jones NF, Maser BM. Treatment of arthritis of the trapeziometacarpal joint with trapeziectomy and hematoma arthroplasty. Hand Clin 2001;17:237–43.
3. Gervis WH. Excision of the trapezium for osteoarthritis of the trapezio-metacarpal joint. J Bone Joint Surg Br 1949;31B: 537–39.
4. Menon J. Arthroscopic management of trapeziometacarpal joint arthritis of the thumb. Arthroscopy 1996;12:581–87.
5. Menon J. Arthroscopic evaluation of the first carpometacarpal joint. J Hand Surg [Am] 1998;23:757.
6. Davis TR, Brady O, Dias JJ. Excision of the trapezium for osteoarthritis of the trapeziometacarpal joint: A study of the benefit of ligament reconstruction or tendon interposition. J Hand Surg [Am] 2004;29:1069–77.
7. Garcia-Elias M, Lluch AL, Farreres A, Castillo F, Saffar P. Resection of the distal scaphoid for scaphotrapeziotrapezoid osteoarthritis. J Hand Surg [Br] 1999;24:448–52.
8. Eaton RG, Littler JW. Ligament reconstruction for the painful thumb carpometacarpal joint. J Bone Joint Surg Am 1973;55:1655–66.
9. Burton RI. Basal joint arthrosis of the thumb. Orthop Clin North Am 1973;4:347–48.
10. Culp RW, Rekant MS. The role of arthroscopy in evaluating and treating trapeziometacarpal disease. Hand Clin 2001; 17:315–19, x–xi.
11. Badia A. Trapeziometacarpal arthroscopy: A classification and treatment algorithm. Hand Clin 2006;22:153–63.
12. Barron OA, Eaton RG. Save the trapezium: Double interposition arthroplasty for the treatment of stage IV disease of the basal joint. J Hand Surg [Am] 1998;23:196–204.
13. Eaton RG, Floyd WE III. Thumb metacarpophalangeal capsulodesis: An adjunct procedure to basal joint arthroplasty for collapse deformity of the first ray. J Hand Surg [Am] 1988;13:449–53.
14. Kessler I. A simplified technique to correct hyperextension deformity of the metacarpophalangeal joint of the thumb. J Bone Joint Surg Am 1979;61:903–05.
15. Badia A, Riano F, Young LC. Bilateral arthroscopic tendon interposition arthroplasty of the thumb carpometacarpal joint in a patient with Ehlers-Danlos syndrome: A case report. J Hand Surg [Am] 2005;30:673–76.
16. Slutsky DJ. Use of the D-Z portal in trapeziometarpal arthroscopy. Arthroscopy. In press 2007.
17. Ashwood N, Bain GI, Fogg Q. Results of arthroscopic debridement for isolated scaphotrapeziotrapezoid arthritis. J Hand Surg [Am] 2003;28:729–32.

N. Ashwood and G.I. Bain

CHAPTER 29

"It is no use saying, 'We are doing our best.' You have got to succeed in doing what is necessary."
—Winston Churchill

Arthroscopic Debridement for Isolated Scaphotrapeziotrapezoid Arthritis

Introduction

Degenerative changes of the scaphotrapeziotrapezoid (STT) joint are seen in almost 40% of cadaveric wrists.[1] Clinical involvement of the triscaphe joint occurs in 15 to 30% of wrists.[2] Concomitant trapeziometacarpal arthritis occurs in the majority of patients, but isolated pathology is present in up to 20% of the population[3,4]—particularly in postmenopausal women.[5] Symptomatically isolated STT disease leads to tenderness over the palmar aspect of the thenar eminence and is an important differential diagnosis in radial wrist pain. Frequently, flexor carpi radialis tendinitis and radiopalmar ganglia are also noted upon examination.[6]

Previous reports of treatment for STT osteoarthritis (OA) following failed conservative treatment include excisional arthroplasty (with[7] or without[4] a silicone spacer) and limited wrist fusion, including STT fusion.[6] Pain relief is not uniform in these series, and morbidity due to postoperative complications has been noted. Wrist arthroscopy is a useful tool for visualizing articular damage, which can be a source of chronic wrist pain.[8] Arthroscopic debridement has proven to be an effective method of achieving pain relief in the knee in two-thirds of patients for up to two to five years and carries a low morbidity.[9,10] The authors have successfully used arthroscopic debridement of isolated STT arthritis to improve symptoms in selected patients.

The pain associated with STT arthritis can be surprisingly debilitating and leads to disability when axially loading the thumb during strong pinch and key turning. There are, however, other patients who have minimal symptoms. For example, the patient with a distal radius fracture will often have advanced STT joint arthritis on radiographs but will deny any symptoms. Watson and Ottoni[11] suggested rotatory subluxation of the scaphoid as a possible cause of isolated STT arthritis. They noted that early degenerative changes of the STT joint occurred when abnormal unilateral hypermobility of the scaphoid was present. STT arthrodesis has been the traditionally recommended procedure and is noted to give good function and excellent pain relief.[6] STT fusion, however, disturbs the usual wrist mechanics—which results in a high incidence of STT nonunion and secondary radial styloid arthritis due to impingement.

Arthroscopy in the Treatment of Arthritis

Arthroscopic debridement and washout remains a popular treatment method for degenerative arthritis in the knee.[9,10] Considerable pain relief is noted in a third of patients, lasting into the medium term. Further surgical intervention is required in only a small proportion of those treated. The use of arthroscopy allows for joint assessment and therapeutic interventions.

We had previously treated patients with STT OA with either an excisional arthroplasty consisting of a distal scaphoid pole resection as described by Garcia-Elias et al.[4] or STT joint arthrodesis using the technique reported by Watson and Hempton.[12] Two of the excisional arthroplasty patients complained of persistent symptoms, and plain radiographs demonstrated increased extension of the scaphoid and the lunate. Some of the patients treated with an STT joint arthrodesis had continuing pain at sites of nonunion. We therefore searched for alternative methods of achieving good pain relief and function without the potential morbidity ensuing from the traditional techniques used to treat STT arthritis. It was felt that the arthroscopy had potential use for joint debridement and joint excision.

It is the authors' experience that the degenerative changes noted at the time of arthroscopy are more advanced than those reported in recent cadaveric studies.[13] This is probably because all patients who require therapeutic intervention have significant pain associated with advanced degenerative osteoarthritis. Moritomo et al. have noted that the most common site of degenerative changes is on the ulnar side of the distal scaphoid and centrally on the trapezoid and trapezium.[1] Half of cases have involvement of the trapezoid alone, with the trapezium being involved in only a third.

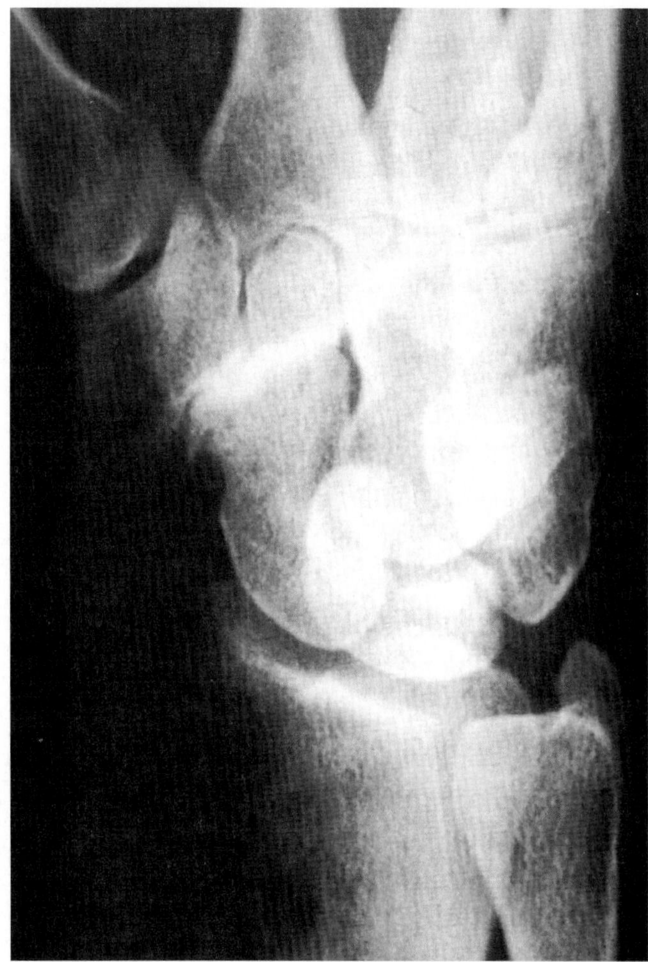

FIGURE 29.1. Radiograph showing isolated STT arthritis.

Patient Selection

Patients typically presented with persistent pain localized to the radial side of the wrist and base of the thumb. The persistent pain, swelling, restriction in motion, and loss of grip and pinch strength lead the patients to seek therapeutic intervention. Localized tenderness and pain accentuation with radial deviation of the wrist helped isolate the STT joint as the source.

Radiographs showed joint narrowing and osteophyte formation isolated to the STT joint (Figure 29.1). Longitudinal computer tomography (CT) scans were performed, particularly if thumb carpometacarpal (CMC) joint arthritis was suspected (Figure 29.2).[14] The thumb CMC joint pain can also be isolated with a diagnostic injection. Typically, the CT scans demonstrated complete loss of the joint space—which was often associated with osteophytes and degenerative cysts within the distal scaphoid. The scaphoid was always extended and the plain radiograph often showed dorsal instability of the lunate.

All patients should receive a minimum period of three months of conservative treatment, including resting splints, anti-inflammatory drugs, and physiotherapy. Persistence of the localized symptoms was an indication for surgical intervention. Patients should have a minimum of six months of symptoms and confirmatory investigations, and should have failed a three-month trial of conservative treatment with splints and hand therapy. In this group of patients, we perform a diagnostic injection into the STT joint.

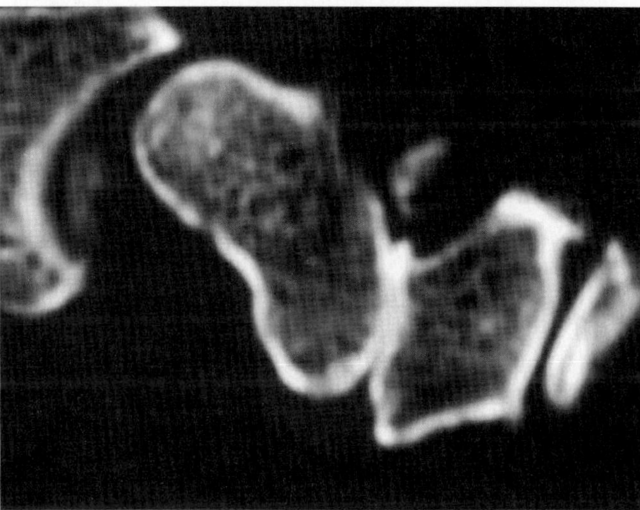

FIGURE 29.2. Longitudinal CT scan demonstrates the degenerative changes between the scaphotrapezium articulation and shows degenerative cysts within the scaphoid.

The patient should obtain significant symptomatic relief before surgery is offered. As the STT joint communicates with the midcarpal joint, false positives may occur. In our experience, patients who were actively pursing a worker's compensation claim tended to do poorly.

Contraindications

This would include any patient with ongoing active infection or local skin or neurovascular compromise.

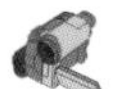

Surgical Technique

A standardized approach to the arthroscopic debridement is used. The arm is suspended on Chinese finger traps with 5 kilograms of traction.[15] No extra or special equipment is required to view the STT joint. Routine arthroscopy was performed with a 2.7-, 2.4-, or 1.9-mm arthroscope. The radial midcarpal arthroscopy (MCR) portal was used to evaluate the midcarpal joint—including the STT joint, which is just the radial extension of the midcarpal joints.[15]

STT Dorsal

This is the portal radial to the EPL tendon. The authors undertook a cadaveric study to assess the safe positioning of the STT joint portal.[13] Placement to the ulnar side of the extensor pollicis longus (EPL) tendon is safer for the radial artery, but the superficial branch of the radial nerve and the extensor carpi radialis longus (ECRL) tendon are still at risk. If the surgeon goes to the radial side of the EPL tendon, the radial artery and superficial branch of the radial nerve are both at risk (Figure 29.3). The radial artery is often tortuous within the "anatomical snuffbox." The authors recommend a "mini-open" approach with a 1.5-cm incision made in the skin to enable safe blunt dissection. This mini-open approach minimizes the risk to the neurovascular structures. The portal to the radial side of the EPL tendon provides a wider span from the radial midcarpal portal, facilitating triangulation.

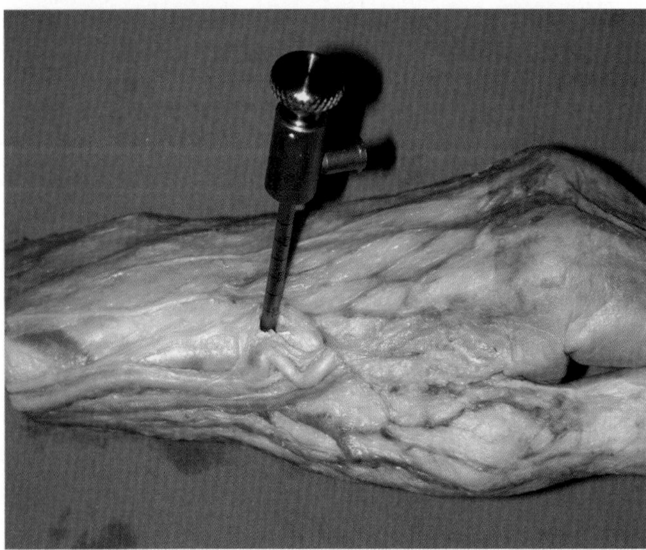

FIGURE 29.3. Cadaveric specimen with EPL, radial artery (RA), and superficial branch of the radial nerve at risk.

STT Volar Portal

This is the volar to abductor pollicis longus.[16] Bare describes an alternative palmar portal to facilitate the visualization of the dorsal rim of the STT joint.[16] This portal is located 3 mm ulnar to the abductor pollicis tendon, 6 mm radial to the scaphoid tubercle, and midway between the radial styloid and the base of the thumb metacarpal.

STT Radial Portal

This accessory portal is radial to the abductor pollicis longus tendon.

STT Ulnar Portal

This accessory portal is just ulnar to the EPL tendon.[17] In difficult cases, portable operative fluoroscopy can assist in identifying the joint. The presence of eburnated bone on the distal scaphoid and proximal trapezium and trapezoid was recorded (Figure 29.4). Synovitis in the joint is usually present (Figure 29.5). The eburnated bone was not removed, but any synovitis, chondral flaps, or rim osteophytes were debrided with an arthroscopic bur and resector. Any synovitis on the volar aspect of the joint was removed.

A 3- to 5-mm resector (Figure 29.6) can be introduced in most patients to perform the synovectomy. Monopolar cautery can be of assistance (Figure 29.7). The scope and resector are moved among the three portals to provide adequate debridement. Care is taken not to disturb the main ligaments connecting the scaphoid, trapezium, and trapezoid.

Patients with crystalline deposition should be biopsied. The STT joint is a not an uncommon site for CPPD deposition. It is common to have synovitis and chondral changes on the dorsal aspect of the lunate in the midcarpal row. This is a secondary area of degeneration that can also be debrided. The joint was then thoroughly irrigated and the

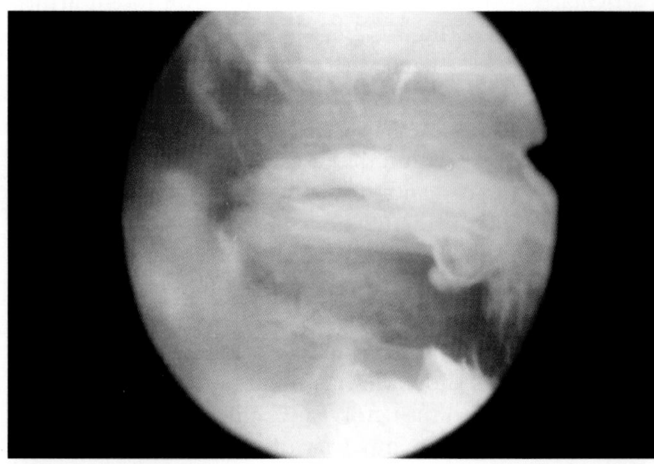

FIGURE 29.4. Arthroscopic view of the trapezium (foreground) and the trapezoid (background) with eburnated bone.

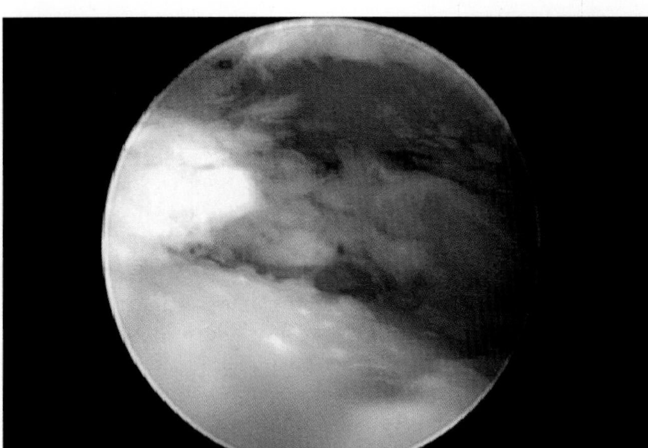

FIGURE 29.5. Photo of STT joint eburnated bone and synovitis.

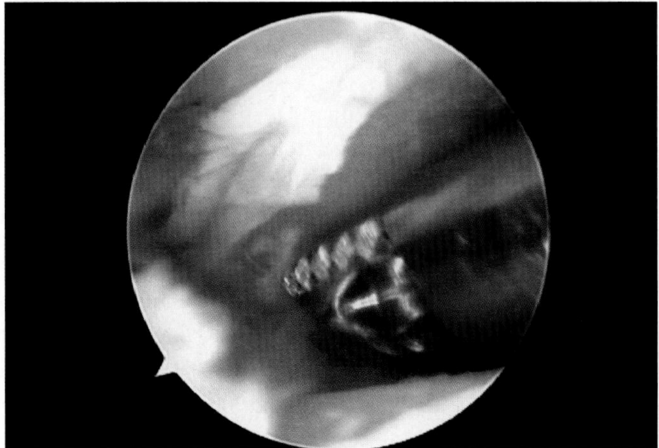

FIGURE 29.6. A 3- to 5-mm motorized resection to debride synovium.

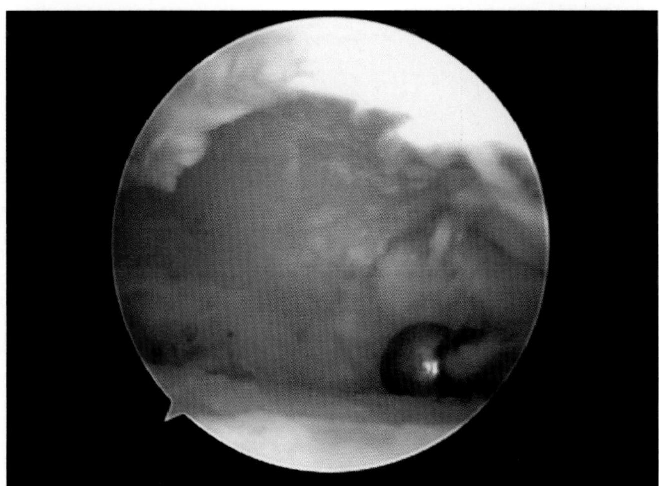

FIGURE 29.7. Monopolar cautery of synovitis.

wounds were sutured using an absorbable suture. A light bandage was applied. Following surgery, gentle mobilization was permitted within the patient's pain tolerance. Return to light duties was recommended from six weeks, and heavy manual labor was avoided for a minimum of three months.

Results

We have previously reported our results in a series of 12 consecutive patients with symptomatic isolated STT arthritis who underwent an arthroscopic debridement.[13] Prior to surgery, four patients could be categorized as having fair wrist function (and six poor) based on the modified Green and O'Brien[18] wrist scores. All patients had a minimum follow-up of one year, with an average of 36 (range 12 to 80) months. The results are summarized in Table 29.1. The average wrist score following surgery increased by 28 points at the one-year review, with patients now fitting into good[4] or excellent[6] categories.

Eleven patients were satisfied with the outcome and would have repeated the surgery. One patient—although content with the improvement of function, pain levels, and grip strength—was not satisfied with the level of wrist motion compared to the other arm. No significant deterioration in the scapholunate or capitolunate first angle was noted following surgery.

Summary

Typically, arthroscopic debridement of the STT joint is a minimally invasive procedure with low morbidity. It does not require immobilization and allows early return to work. Our cadaveric studies have demonstrated that caution should be exercised when placing the STT portals because of the risk to branches of the radial artery and the superficial branch of the radial nerve. Using a mini-open approach, with soft-tissue dissection to the capsule, minimizes the risk of neurovascular complication. *We continue*

Table 29.1.

Summary of Results Used to Calculate Wrist Scores[13]

	Preoperative Score	Most Recent Postoperative Score
Pain (visual analog score)	90 (65–95)	12 (0–25)
Grip strength (kilograms)	20 (18–36)	45 (24–52)
Green + O'Brien scores (points)	63 (45–75)	93 (80–95)

to use this procedure, which carries a low morbidity and has generally good results. In the authors' opinion it avoids the high complication rate associated with an STT fusion.

Results for excisional arthroplasty have been less satisfactory in our hands because of synovitis and dorsal instability of the proximal carpal row. Carro et al. reported their results with STT joint debridement, including distal scaphoid excision.[19] We have not included the distal scaphoid excision, as it is likely to produce further carpal collapse (as occurs in open distal scaphoid excision).

Arthroscopic debridement alone achieved good pain relief and range of motion following surgery, without a deterioration of the carpal angles. It does not further destabilize the wrist and does not prevent the use of future reconstructive or salvage procedures. The debridement removed synovitis, rim osteophytes, and unstable cartilage flaps but still left denuded articular surfaces. Arthroscopic debridement is simple, safe, and effective when compared with other treatment modalities. It achieves excellent pain relief and restoration of function in patients with isolated idiopathic STT arthritis. Longer-term follow-up is no doubt required.

References

1. Moritomo H, Viegas SF, Nakamura K, et al. The scaphotrapeziotrapezoidal joint. Part 1: An anatomic and radiographic study. JHS 2000;25A:899–910.
2. Rogers WD, Watson KH. Degenerative arthritis at the triscaphe joint. JHS 1990;15A:232–35.
3. Chamay A, Piaget-Morerod F. Arthrodesis of the trapeziometacarpal joint. JHS 1994;19A:489–97.
4. Garcia-Elias M, Lluch AL, Farreres A, Castillo F, Saffar P. Resection of the distal scaphoid for scaphotrapeziotrapezoid osteoarthritis. JHS 1999;24A:448–52.
5. Armstrong AL, Hunter JB, Davis TRC. The prevalence of degenerative arthritis of the base of the thumb in postmenopausal women. JHS 1994;19A:340–41.
6. Srinivasan VB, Matthews JP. Results of scaphotrapeziotrapezoid fusion for isolated idiopathic arthritis. JHS 1996; 21B:378–80.
7. Eiken O. Implant arthroplasty of the scapho-trapezial joint. Scandinavian Journal of Plastic and Reconstructive Surgery 1979;13:461–68.
8. Poehling GG, Roth JH. Articular cartilage lesions of the wrist.. In RN McGinty (ed.), *Operative Arthroscopy*. New York: Raven Press 1991: 635–39.
9. Bert JM, Maschka K. The arthroscopic treatment of unicompartmental gonarthrosis: A five year follow-up study of abrasion arthroplasty plus arthroscopic debridement and arthroscopic debridement alone. Arthroscopy 1989;5:25–32.
10. Dandy DJ. Arthroscopic debridement of the knee. JBJS 1991;73:877–78.
11. Watson HK, Ottoni L, Pitts EC, Handal AG. Rotatory subluxation of scaphoid: A spectrum of instability. Journal of Hand Surgery [Br] 1993;18:62–68.
12. Watson HK, Hempton RF. Limited wrist arthrodeses. I. The triscaphoid joint. J Hand Surg 1980;5(4):320–27.
13. Ashwood N, Bain GI, Fogg Q. Results of arthroscopic debridement for isolated scaphotrapeziotrapezoid arthritis. J Hand Surg [Am] 2003;28(5):729–32.
14. Bain GI, Bennett JD, Richards RS, Slethaug GP, Roth JH. Longitudinal computed tomography of the scaphoid: A new technique. Skeletal Radiology 1995;24:271–73.
15. Bain GI, Richards RS, Roth JH. Wrist arthroscopy. In DM McGinty, AH Alexander (eds.), *The Wrist and Its Disorders. Second Edition*. Philadelphia: W.B. Saunders 1997: 151–68.
16. Carro LP, Golano P, Farinas O, Cerezal L, Hidalgo C. The radial portal for scaphotrapeziotrapezoid arthroscopy. Arthroscopy 2003;19(5):547–53.
17. Bare J, Graham AJ, Tham SK. Scaphotrapezial joint arthroscopy: A palmar portal. J Hand Surg 2003;28(4):605–09.
18. Green DP, O'Brien ET. Open reduction of carpal dislocations: Indications and operative technique. Hand 1978;3A:250–56.
19. Whipple TL. *The Wrist. Arthroscopic Surgery*, Philadelphia: Lippincott 1992.

SECTION 7

Extra-Articular Procedures

David J. Slutsky

CHAPTER 30

Agee Endoscopic Carpal Tunnel Release

Introduction

In 1989, Chow et al. described a two-portal endoscopic carpal tunnel release (ECTR) technique.[1] This method has undergone a number of modifications since that time and is described in a separate chapter. Agee et al. published a prospective randomized clinical trial on his uniportal technique in 1992.[2] Other investigators have published their preferred technique of using a one- or two-portal approach. The decision as to which technique to use is largely based on personal preference and comfort with the procedure. This chapter discusses the uniportal technique using the Agee endoscope.

Indications

The indications for ECTR are the same as for an open carpal tunnel release (CTR). The patient should have the appropriate symptoms and signs of carpal tunnel syndrome and should have failed a trial of conservative treatment with splinting, NSAIDs, and activity modification. Positive electrodiagnostic studies are not a requirement but may be useful in ruling out associated neuropathies.

Contraindications

Absolute contraindications include any distortion of the carpal canal due to tumor, previous surgery, carpal fracture/dislocation, or mal-union of the radius. A loss of wrist extension of 20 to 30 degrees either from bony fusion or wrist contracture would hamper this procedure by impeding the correct placement of the endosocope. Unfamiliarity with the regional anatomy is another contraindication. Due to the high learning curve, it is recommended that anyone contemplating this procedure should take a cadaver training course prior to attempting it clinically—unless training has been provided in a teaching environment.[3]

Relative contraindications abound and are not universally agreed upon. Flexor tendon thickening due to synovial hyperplasia or adhesions from previous flexor tendon repairs will complicate the procedure. Recurrent or persistent carpal tunnel syndrome following a previous release often includes a component of traction neuropathy due to scar, which may thwart attempts at ECTR. However, successful cases have been reported.[4] Any suspicion of separate entrapment of the recurrent motor branch mandates an open procedure.

Equipment

The use of the Agee endoscope (3M, Orthopedic Products, St. Paul, MN) is integral to this procedure. A 2.7-mm 30-degree angle arthroscope along with a fiberoptic light source and camera setup are interfaced with the Agee system. The instrumentation includes two dilators and a soft-tissue elevator.

Relevant Anatomy

The flexor retinaculum (FR) consists of three distinct and continuous segments that extend from the distal radius to the base of the long finger metacarpal.[5] The proximal segment is continuous with the deep forearm fascia and is inseparable from the thickened antebrachial fascia. The transverse carpal ligament (TCL) makes up the second part of the FR. The TCL arises from the scaphoid tuberosity and trapezial beak radially, and from the pisiform and hook of the hamate ulnarly. The distal segment of the FR consists of the aponeurosis between the thenar and hypothenar muscles. The median nerve becomes superficial in the forearm approximately 5 cm proximal to the wrist. It lies between the tendons of the flexor digitorum superficialis (FDS) and the flexor carpi radialis (FCR), and is dorsal or dorsoradial to the palmaris longus (PL).

It passes under the FR in the radiopalmar portion of the carpal tunnel at a level that corresponds to the volar flexion crease of the wrist. At the distal edge of the retinaculum, the nerve normally divides into six branches: the recurrent motor branch, three proper digital nerves, and two common digital nerves. The motor branch typically passes through a separate fascial tunnel immediately before entering the thenar muscles. The palmar cutaneous branch (PCN) originates 5 cm proximal to the proximal wrist crease. It travels with the median nerve for 1 to 2 cm and then separates and enters a short tunnel medial to the FCR tendon to innervate the skin of the thenar eminence.

Anatomically, two areas of the carpal tunnel may cause median nerve compression. The first is at the proximal edge of the TCL, where compression may be produced by acute flexion of the wrist—which is the basis for a positive Phalen's test. The second is adjacent to the hook of the hamate, which is the usual location for any hourglass deformity of the median nerve.

Surgical Considerations

The position of the ulnar nerve and artery are of particular significance for endoscopic carpal tunnel release. Most endoscopic devices are designed to divide the flexor retinaculum just to the radial aspect of the hamate hook. In an anatomical study of the boundaries of Guyon's canal, however, Cobb et al. showed that the confines of this space do not extend from the pisiform to the hook of the hamate (as previously accepted).[6] The fascial roof extends radial to the hook of the hamate, which allows the ulnar neurovascular bundle to course radial to the hamate hook. Utilizing cross-sectional analysis of nine cadaver specimens, they found the ulnar artery to course radial to the hamate hook in five and palmar to it in four. Therefore, the ulnar artery may be at greater risk of injury during endoscopic procedures than previously recognized.

The safest path for release of the TCL has been studied extensively. Rotman and Manske investigated the anatomical relationships of an endoscopic carpal tunnel device to surrounding soft-tissue structures along the ring finger and the long-ring interspace axis.[7] The average distance from the center of the device to the median nerve in the carpal tunnel averaged 3.3 mm in the ring finger axis and 2.5 mm in the long-ring interspace axis. The average distance from the distal edge of the transverse carpal ligament to the superficial palmar arch was 4.8 mm in the ring finger axis and 5.5 mm in the long-ring interspace axis. These and other more subtle anatomical observations indicate the greater safety of using the ring finger axis for endoscopic carpal tunnel release.

Surgical Technique

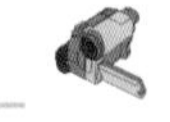

The patient is positioned in the supine position, with the arm abducted and lying on an arm board. The procedure is performed under tourniquet control after limb exsanguination. The author's preference is to use a general anesthetic due to the not-infrequent difficulties with instrumentation, including fogging of the camera lens. However, regional anesthesia will also suffice.

The landmarks to localize the hook of the hamate are as follows.[8,9] First, the pisiform is palpated and marked. A second mark is placed on the proximal palmar skin crease, in line with the mid portion of the index finger. These two points are then connected, forming the index-pisiform line. A second line is drawn from the midpoint of the base of the ring finger, proximally to the wrist crease at the junction of its middle and ulnar third—forming the fourth metacarpal line. The intersection of the index-pisiform line and the fourth metacarpal line directly overlies the hook of the hamate (Figure 30.1). The palmar longus tendon (if present) is traced. The dissection should stay medial to the PL, which protects the median nerve.

A 2-cm transverse incision is placed in the proximal wrist crease between the PL and pisiform. As the surgeon's comfort level increases, this incision can be placed in the distal wrist crease—although there is more subcutaneous fat to contend with (Figure 30.2). The plane between the subcutaneous fat and the deep forearm fascia or flexor retinaculum is identified and developed. A distally based U-shaped flap of the flexor retinaculum is elevated by making two parallel incisions approximately 1 cm apart and 1 to 2 cm long through the deep fascia between the FCU and PL/median nerve (Figure 30.3A). The incisions are then connected by a proximal transverse cut. Care is taken to avoid penetration of the underlying flexor synovium to lessen inadvertent tendon laceration. The distally based flap is elevated (Figure 30.3b) while developing the plane between the FDS tendons and the undersurface of the TCL. Establishing this plane is integral to proper scope placement.

The wrist is then hyperextended over two folded towels. A small dilator is gently inserted, superficial to the plane of the flexor tendons but underneath the TCL—keeping it aligned with the ring metacarpal line and radial to the hamate hook. With proper placement, the dilator will abut against the hook of the hamate when sweeping it in an

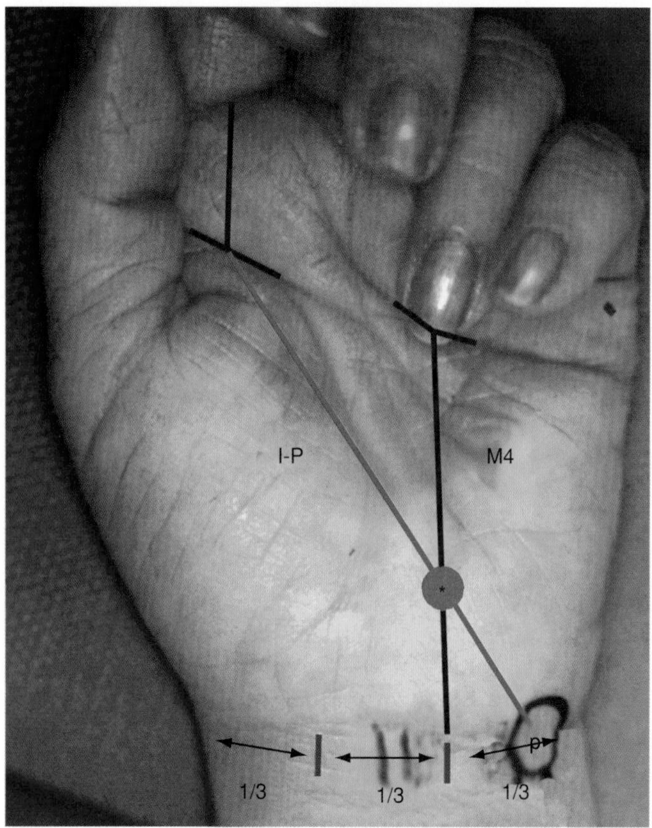

FIGURE 30.1. Landmarks for locating the hamate hook (*) (p = pisiform, M4 = fourth metacarpal line, I-P = index pisiform line).

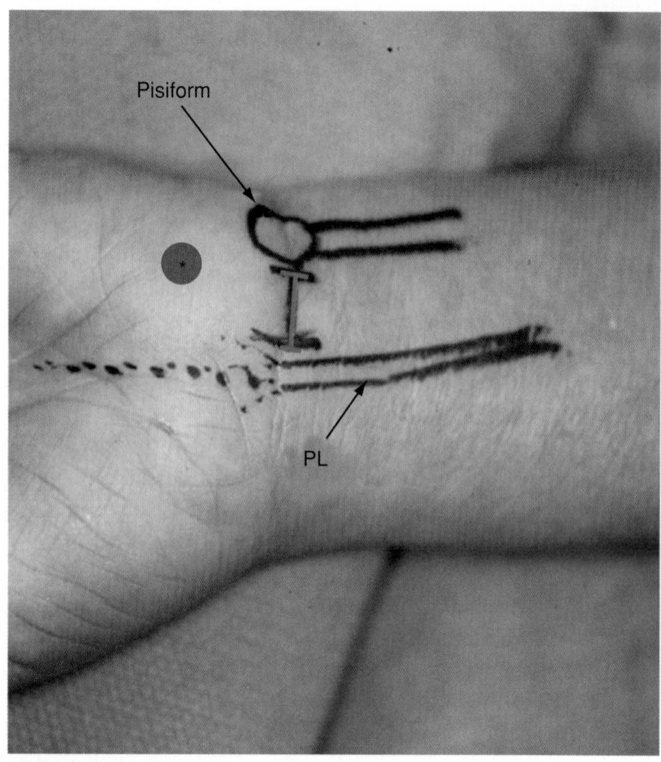

FIGURE 30.2. Skin incision at distal wrist crease (in red).

ulnar direction. If there is an obstruction to ulnar passage of the dilator, it should be removed and reinserted. Otherwise, there is a risk of grievous injury to the ulnar nerve and artery.

A larger dilator is next inserted to enlarge the gliding path for the scope. The distal tip of the dilators can be easily palpated in the midpalm by levering the tip anteriorly. Multiple passes of the dilators increases the risk of a median neuropraxia, especially in small wrists, and should be avoided. The soft-tissue elevator is then inserted and used to gently scrape any synovium from the undersurface of the TCL. While keeping the wrist hyperextended, the tip of the Agee endoscope is then gently inserted into the canal. The surface line marking the axis of the ring finger is used as a guide (Figure 30.4 and b).

At this point, the shiny transverse fibers of the undersurface of the TCL should be visualized. Often, fogging of the scope, fluid from fatty tissue, or synovial remnants will

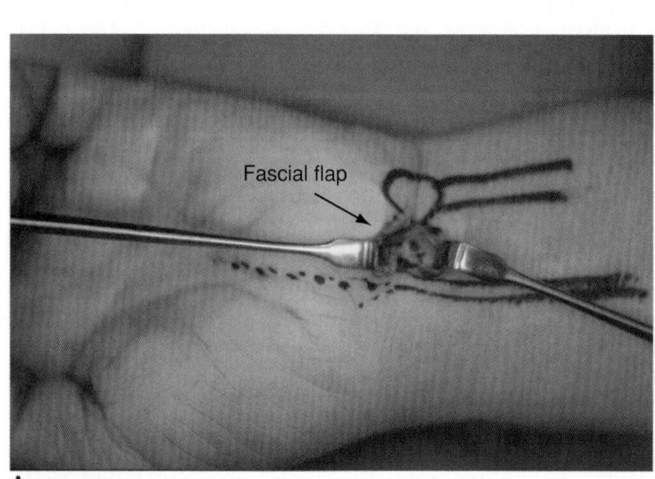

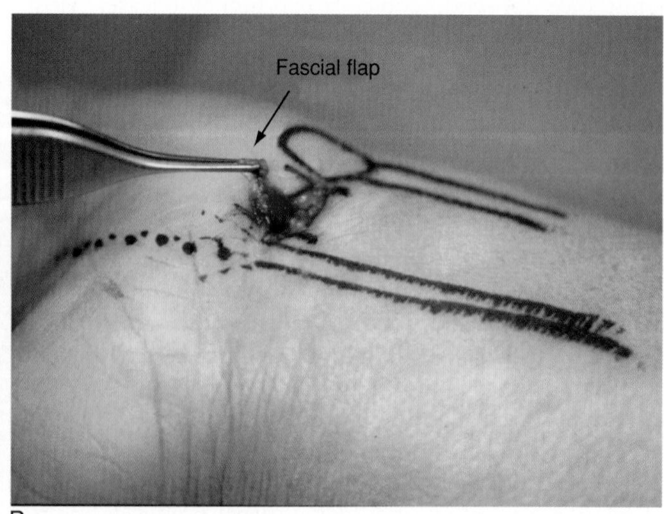

FIGURE 30.3. (A) Outlining a distally based fascial flap. (B) Elevation of the fascial flap.

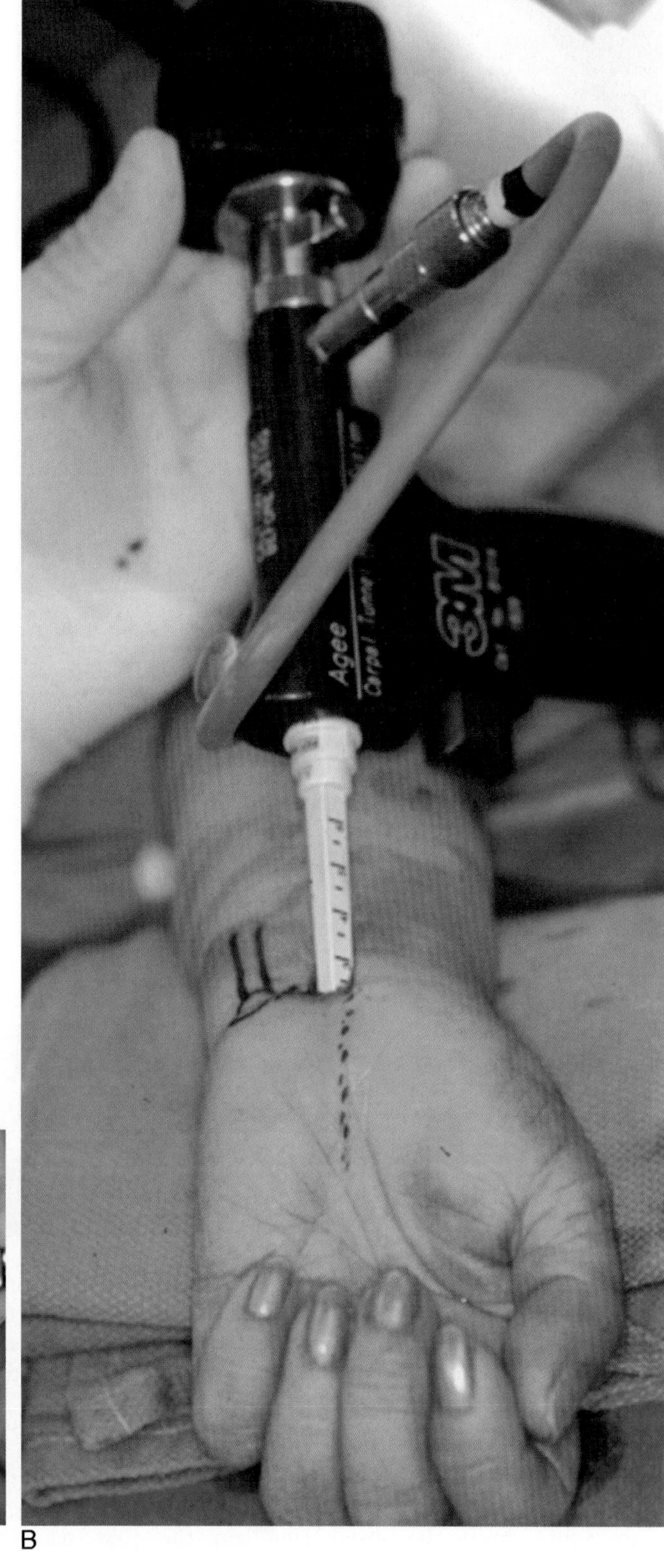

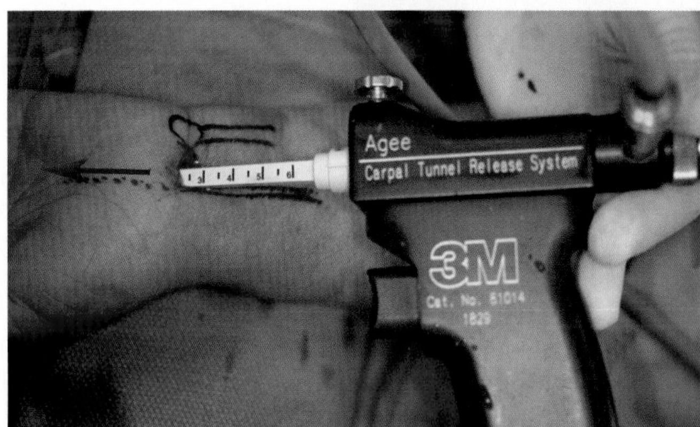

A B

FIGURE 30.4. (A) Insertion of the Agee endoscope, which is aligned with the ring finger axis. (B) End on view of proper scope placement.

block the view. In this event, the scope should be removed and defogged and the synovial elevator used once more. Because the scope is often colder than the carpal canal, keeping the scope in warm water until just before use may minimize the fogging. The distal edge of the TCL must be completely visualized (Figure 30.5a). This can be identified by a change of the transverse fibers to an ill-defined fat pad, which contains the superficial palmar arch and the common digital branch to the third web space.

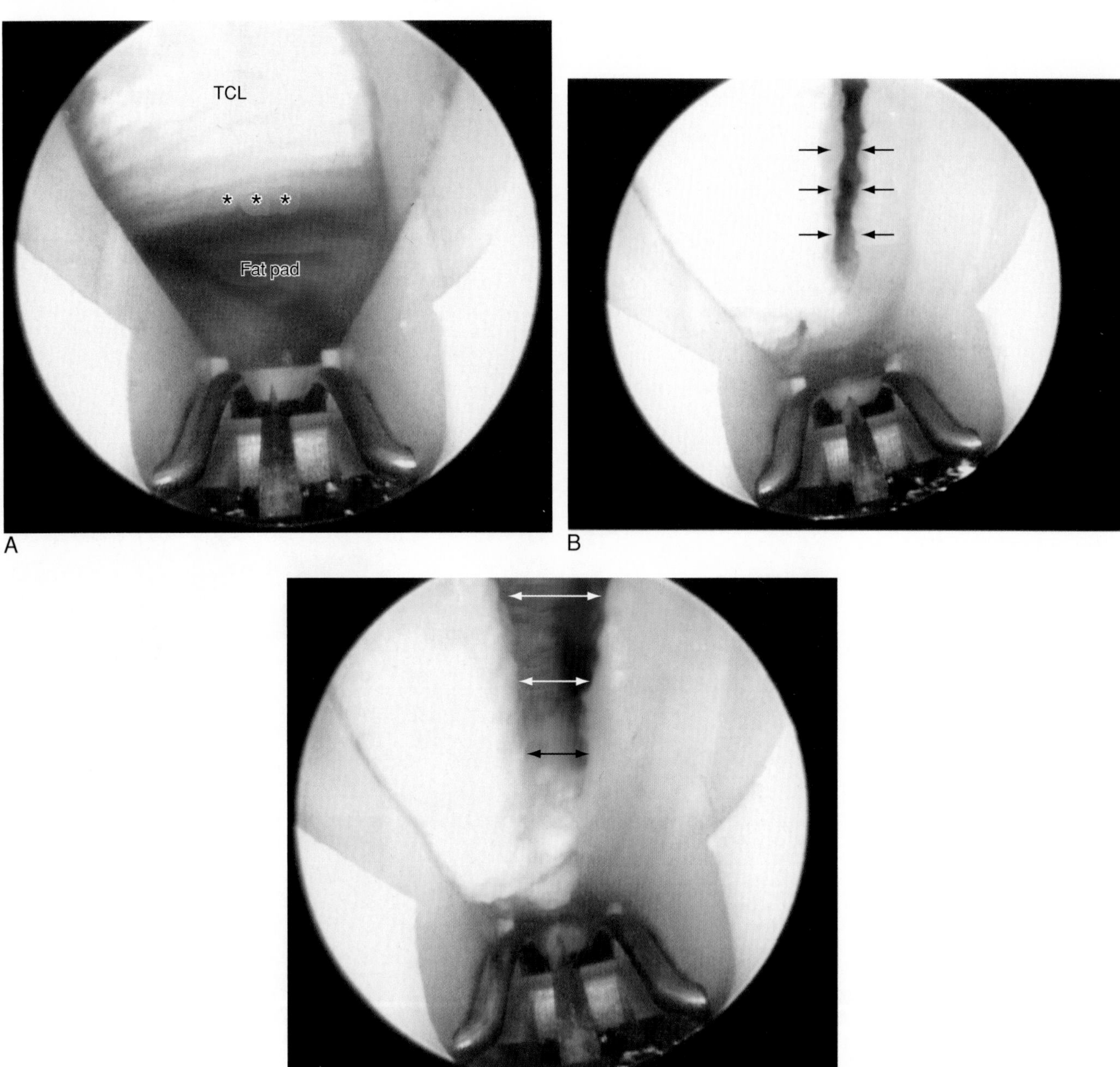

FIGURE 30.5. (A) View through the endoscope of the white undersurface of the transverse carpal ligament (TCL). The appearance of the midpalmar fat pad demarcates the distal edge of the TCL (*). (B) Partial release of the TCL results in a minor separation of the ligament edges (arrows). (C) After complete release of the TCL. Note the increased separation of the ligament edges (arrows) with exposure of the palmar brevis, which denotes a complete ligament release.

Ballottement of the fat pad can aid in the demarcation zone. The hook blade should not be engaged until the distal edge is well seen. It is prudent to start the blade 2 to 3 mm from the distal edge on the first pass (Figure 30.5b). The hook blade is then maintained upright while the scope is slowly withdrawn proximally, keeping the blade in sight at all times. The scope is then reinserted to visualize the cut. The TCL is under tension and will usually split apart, allowing identification of the muscle fibers of the overlying palmar brevis or the longitudinally oriented fibers of the palmar aponeurosis. A second pass may be made at this point to release the distal-most fibers of the TCL (Figure 30.5c). The scope is then removed.

The proximal skin flap is next retracted to allow visualization of the deep flexor retinaculum. Tenotomy scissors are used to divide the retinaculum for an additional 2 cm. The scope is then reinserted into the carpal canal, and the tourniquet is deflated. Pulsatile bleeding is suggestive of an injury to the superficial palmar arch, which is explored through an open incision. Digital nerve injury cannot be recognized by any means, but a high level of suspicion and due diligence will dictate the need for exploration.

It is possible for the mesoneural tissue surrounding the median nerve to become interposed between the scope and the undersurface of the TCL. It will not have the appearance of nerve tissue and can be drawn in by the hook blade, which may lead to a partial or complete median nerve laceration. If there is any doubt, the scope should be removed and the field cleared. If the view cannot be improved, conversion to an open procedure is necessary. The wound is infiltrated with Marcaine and closed with an absorbable subcuticular suture and Steri-Strips.

Postoperative

The patient is placed in a large bulky hand dressing with a volar wrist splint for comfort. Finger motion begins immediately, which also accomplishes some nerve gliding. The splint is removed at one week, and the patient is started on a wrist range-of-motion program. The sutures are removed at two weeks, followed by gradual strengthening.

Complications

There have been significant and devastating complications reported, which are often related to poor scope placement or inadequate visualization of the TCL. This includes partial and complete median nerve lacerations, common digital nerve lacerations, and injuries to the superficial palmar arch.[10] The author has noted a neurapraxia of the third common digital nerve branch in small women patients with small carpal canals that has lasted up to six months. Flexor tendon lacerations have also been reported. If there is anything less than complete visualization, the procedure should be converted to an open CTR. Placing the scope in Guyon's canal due to inadequate identification of the hook of the hamate has resulted in ulnar nerve and artery lacerations.[11] Incomplete release of the TCL is commonly reported and is a major criticism of this technique.[12,13]

Results

Controversy continues to dog any method of ECTR. Advocates proclaim less postoperative pain, quicker recovery of grip strength, and a faster return to work.[14–16] Critics cite the higher occurrence of incomplete release of the transverse carpal ligament, disturbing reports of neurovascular injury, and a similar incidence of pillar pain.[10,17–22] Agee et al. carried out a 10-center randomized prospective multicenter study of endoscopic release using his technique. There were 122 patients in the study. Twenty-five had carpal tunnel surgery on both hands and 97 had surgery on one hand. Of the surgical procedures, 65 were in the control group and 82 were in the device group.

For patients in the device group with one affected hand, the median time for return to work was 21.5 days less than that for the control group. Another large multicenter prospective study of 192 cases demonstrated at least in the short term that the patients treated with the endoscopic method had significantly greater grip strength, pinch strength, and hand dexterity. The open technique resulted in greater scar tenderness during the first three months after surgery, as well as a longer time until the patients could return to work.[23]

Everyone is not in agreement on this point, though. In a small study of 25 patients with bilateral carpal tunnel syndrome who underwent an endoscopic release by the Agee technique on one hand and open release on the other, the investigators found no significant advantages in terms of return of grip strength, manual dexterity, or sensation.[22] Foucher et al. examined his initial experience with this technique in 95 hands at 4.5 years.[24] Seventy-two percent of hands were free of symptoms and 94% were described by the patients as functionally normal. Seventeen hands (out of 27) with residual or recurrent symptoms were examined. Nine hands (nine patients) were only partially improved (mean 6.7 on a 10-point scale) and in eight hands (seven patients) some symptoms had recurred after a mean delay of 3.8 years.

One utility of the endoscopic method is the ability to perform simultaneous bilateral CTR without significantly increasing patient morbidity.[25] This, however, has been replicated with simultaneous bilateral open release as well.[26,27]

References

1. Chow JC. Endoscopic release of the carpal ligament: A new technique for carpal tunnel syndrome. Arthroscopy 1989;5:19–24.
2. Agee JM, McCarroll HR Jr., Tortosa RD, et al. Endoscopic release of the carpal tunnel: A randomized prospective multicenter study. J Hand Surg [Am] 1992;17:987–95.
3. Wheatley MJ, Hall JW, Pratt D, Faringer PD. Is training in endoscopic carpal tunnel release appropriate for residents? Ann Plast Surg 1996;37:254–57.
4. Teoh LC, Tan PL. Endoscopic carpal tunnel release for recurrent carpal tunnel syndrome after previous open release. Hand Surg 2004;9:235–39.
5. Cobb TK, Dalley BK, Posteraro RH, Lewis RC. Anatomy of the flexor retinaculum. J Hand Surg [Am] 1993;18:91–9.
6. Cobb TK, Carmichael SW, Cooney WP. The ulnar neurovascular bundle at the wrist: A technical note on endoscopic carpal tunnel release. J Hand Surg [Br] 1994;19:24–6.
7. Rotman MB, Manske PR. Anatomic relationships of an endoscopic carpal tunnel device to surrounding structures. J Hand Surg [Am] 1993;18:442–50.
8. Cobb TK, Cooney WP, An KN. Clinical location of hook of hamate: A technical note for endoscopic carpal tunnel release. J Hand Surg [Am] 1994;19:516–18.
9. Cobb TK, Knudson GA, Cooney WP. The use of topographical landmarks to improve the outcome of Agee endoscopic carpal tunnel release. Arthroscopy 1995;11:165–72.
10. Murphy RX Jr., Jennings JF, Wukich DK. Major neurovascular complications of endoscopic carpal tunnel release. J Hand Surg [Am] 1994;19:114–18.
11. Luallin SR, Toby EB. Incidental Guyon's canal release during attempted endoscopic carpal tunnel release: An anatomical

study and report of two cases. Arthroscopy 1993;9:382–86; discussion 81.
12. Varitimidis SE, Herndon JH, Sotereanos DG. Failed endoscopic carpal tunnel release: Operative findings and results of open revision surgery. J Hand Surg [Br] 1999;24:465–67.
13. Hulsizer DL, Staebler MP, Weiss AP, Akelman E. The results of revision carpal tunnel release following previous open versus endoscopic surgery. J Hand Surg [Am] 1998;23:865–69.
14. Atroshi I, Larsson GU, Ornstein E, et al. Outcomes of endoscopic surgery compared with open surgery for carpal tunnel syndrome among employed patients: Randomised controlled trial. BMJ 2006;332(7556):1473.
15. Futami T. Surgery for bilateral carpal tunnel syndrome: Endoscopic and open release compared in 10 patients. Acta Orthop Scand 1995;66:153–55.
16. Jimenez DF, Gibbs SR, Clapper AT. Endoscopic treatment of carpal tunnel syndrome: A critical review. J Neurosurg 1998;88:817–26.
17. Ecker HA Jr. Persistent or recurrent carpal tunnel surgery following prior endoscopic carpal tunnel release. J Hand Surg [Am] 1999;24:647–48.
18. Forman DL, Watson HK, Caulfield KA, et al. Persistent or recurrent carpal tunnel syndrome following prior endoscopic carpal tunnel release. J Hand Surg [Am] 1998;23:1010–14.
19. Ludlow KS, Merla JL, Cox JA, Hurst LN. Pillar pain as a postoperative complication of carpal tunnel release: A review of the literature. J Hand Ther 1997;10:277–82.
20. Nath RK, Mackinnon SE, Weeks PM. Ulnar nerve transection as a complication of two-portal endoscopic carpal tunnel release: A case report. J Hand Surg [Am] 1993; 18:896–98.
21. Wheatley MJ, Kaul MP. Recurrent carpal tunnel syndrome following endoscopic carpal tunnel release: A preliminary report. Ann Plast Surg 1997;39:469–71.
22. Schonauer F, Varma S, Belcher HJ. Endoscopic carpal tunnel release: Practice in evolution. Scand J Plast Reconstr Surg Hand Surg 2003;37:360–64.
23. Trumble TE, Diao E, Abrams RA, Gilbert-Anderson MM. Single-portal endoscopic carpal tunnel release compared with open release: A prospective, randomized trial. J Bone Joint Surg Am 2002;84-A:1107–15.
24. Erhard L, Ozalp T, Citron N, Foucher G. Carpal tunnel release by the Agee endoscopic technique: Results at 4 year follow-up. J Hand Surg [Br] 1999;24:583–85.
25. Fehringer EV, Tiedeman JJ, Dobler K, McCarthy JA. Bilateral endoscopic carpal tunnel releases: Simultaneous versus staged operative intervention. Arthroscopy 2002; 18:316–21.
26. Wang AA, Hutchinson DT, Vanderhooft JE. Bilateral simultaneous open carpal tunnel release: A prospective study of postoperative activities of daily living and patient satisfaction. J Hand Surg [Am] 2003;28:845–48.
27. Weber RA, Boyer KM. Consecutive versus simultaneous bilateral carpal tunnel release. Ann Plast Surg 2005;54:15–9.

Daniel J. Nagle

CHAPTER 31

To Jan

Endoscopic Carpal Tunnel Release: The Chow Dual-Portal Technique

Rationale and Basic Science

James C. Y. Chow published his dual-portal technique in 1989[1] and reported his clinical results in 1990.[2] The rationale for developing an endoscopic carpal tunnel release is similar to that used in the development of other endoscopic techniques such as laparoscopic cholecystectomy and arthroscopy. A minimal incision approach to carpal tunnel release leads to a decrease in postoperative pain and an earlier return to daily activities. The dual-portal system has the advantage of creating a fixed space in which to operate. The cannula is fixed at the proximal and distal portals. The cannula creates an operative field into which instruments can be easily moved (Figure 31.1).

Indications and Contraindications

The indications for endoscopic and open carpal tunnel release are similar. There are, however, certain situations in which endoscopic carpal tunnel release may not be helpful. One such situation is that of the patient who has undergone a previous carpal tunnel release. The patient's history must be carefully reviewed. If the patient had a successful carpal tunnel release and presents with a recurrent carpal tunnel syndrome some years later without intervening trauma, an endoscopic carpal tunnel release could be considered. If, however, only transient relief after an ECTR is noted it would make sense to perform an open exploration of the carpal tunnel—assuming that a structure not seen during the ECTR continues to compress the median nerve.

A fused wrist constitutes a contraindication for ECTR. The inability to extend the wrist on the hand holder precludes the safe placement of the cannula. In addition, if one suspects the presence of proliferative tenosynovitis an open carpal tunnel release would be preferable. Of course, any suspicion of the presence of a mass within the carpal tunnel would be an indication for an open carpal tunnel release rather than an endoscopic carpal tunnel release.

Technique

Anesthesia

The anesthetic used is a matter of personal preference. Chow feels very strongly that local anesthesia be used because this allows instant feedback from the patient if the median or ulnar nerve is touched. Local anesthetic also allows the surgeon to assess the neurovascular status of the patient immediately after completion of the carpal tunnel release while the patient's hand is still prepped. Should there be signs of a nerve, tendon, or arterial injury, immediate exploration could be carried out. It should be understood that the "local" anesthetic is supplemented with IV fentanyl and midazolam just prior to the cannula being passed into the carpal tunnel. Local anesthesia is particularly well suited to performing bilateral ECTR in one sitting.

IV regional anesthesia (Bier block) can also be used. It does not allow the instant feedback of local anesthesia, but once the tourniquet is released the patient's neurological status returns quickly to preoperative levels such that a complete neuromuscular exam can be performed prior to breaking the sterile field. The Bier block eliminates the need to give fentanyl and midazolam in the doses needed during the "pure" local anesthesia as the patient does not feel the cannula pass into the carpal tunnel. Axillary block and general anesthesia have been used but eliminate the patient feedback noted with the local techniques.

Surgical technique

The dual-portal endoscopic carpal tunnel release, as described by Chow and modified by others, uses a proximal portal that is established 1 cm proximal to the wrist flexion crease just ulnar to the palmaris longus. The distal portal is established just distal to the distal edge of the transverse carpal ligament along the long axis of the ring finger. The volar antebrachial fascia is carefully entered, and a curved dissector is passed into the carpal tunnel—taking care to hug the hook of the hamate.

A "washboard" sensation is felt as the tip of the dissector passes over the ridges in the dorsal surface of the transverse carpal ligament (TCL). If this washboard sensation is not felt, the dissector is either palmar to the TCL or in Guyon's canal. The distal edge of the transverse carpal ligament is able to be palpated using the curved dissector and the position of the distal edge of the transverse carpal ligament is marked on the overlying palmar skin (Figure 31.1).

The curved dissector is removed and the slotted cannula/obturator is placed into the carpal tunnel. The operator's hand is placed on the palmar aspect of the hand between the thenar and hypothenar eminences and the cannula system is lifted (the *lift* test). The examiner's palpating fingers should not be able to feel the cannula. If the cannula is palpable, it is either palmar to the TCL or in Guyon's canal and must be removed and repositioned. Once the cannula is safely placed, taking care to stay close to the hook of the hamate and keeping the cannula system parallel to the long axis of the arm, the wrist and fingers are extended and the hand is placed on the hand holder. The tip of the cannula system is palpated just distal to the distal edge of the TCL. The cannula system is then passed through the distal portal while pushing the superficial palmar arch dorsally with the palmar arch depressor (Figure 31.2).

The distal portal is established approximately 4 to 5 mm distal to the distal edge of the transverse carpal ligament along the long axis of the ring finger. This effectively allows the cannula system to pass between the common digital nerves of the third and fourth web spaces, distal and palmar to the superficial palmar arch and palmar to the communicating branch sensory branch between the median and ulnar nerves.[3] Once the cannula system passes out through this distal portal, the system is fixed in position. The elastic band is placed across the fingers to hold the hand in position. The assistant extends the thumb, thus placing tension on the TCL (Figure 31.3).

The endoscope is then passed into the proximal portal. A 30-degree 4-mm scope is used. Often, a layer of synovial-like tissue lining the dorsal aspect of the transverse carpal ligament must be cleared. A "nerve hook" or commercially available rasp can be used for this. *It is of paramount importance the surgeon clearly identify the transverse carpal ligament and that there be no intervening soft tissues!* The transverse carpal ligament has a very characteristic feel and morphology. Its transverse fibers are visible and palpable (the washboard feeling). Proximally, the transverse carpal ligament is whiter and distally is more yellowish in color. The distal edge of the transverse carpal ligament should be clearly identifiable. Just distal to the distal edge of the transverse carpal ligament, one will notice a fat pad falling into the cannula system (Figure 31.5).

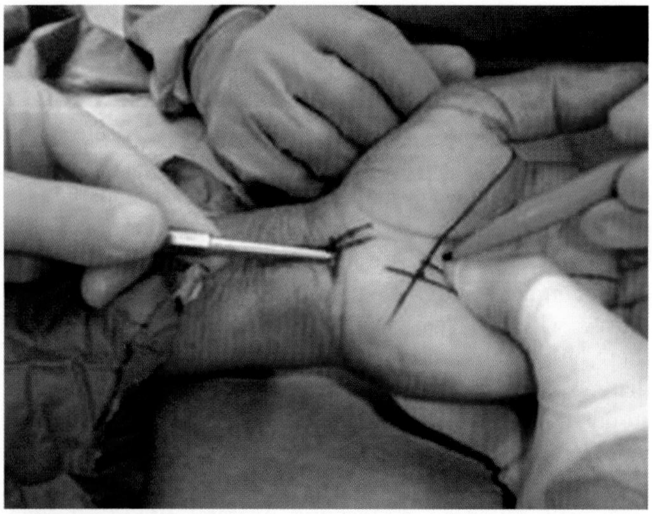

FIGURE 31.1. Palpation and marking of distal edge of transverse carpal ligament.

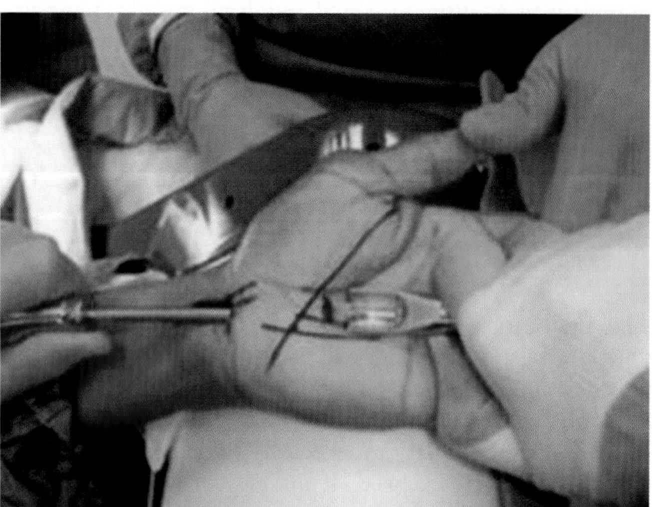

FIGURE 31.2. Passage of the cannula system out the distal portal while applying dorsally directed pressure with the arch depressor to displace the superficial palmar arch dorsal to the cannular system.

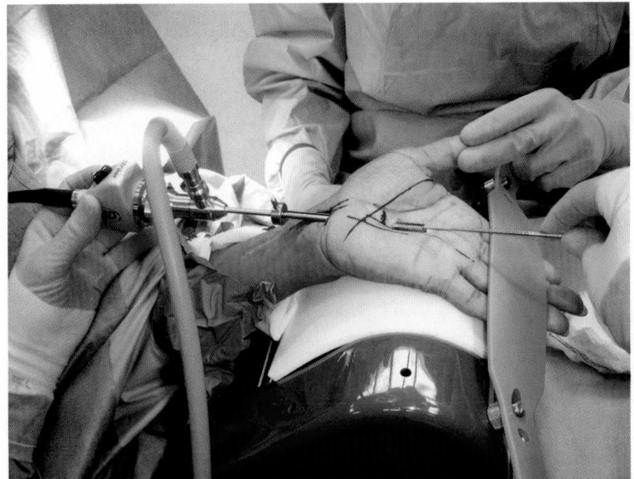

FIGURE 31.3. Chow dual-portal endoscopic carpal tunnel release setup. Cannular in position while assistant palmarly adducts the thumb.

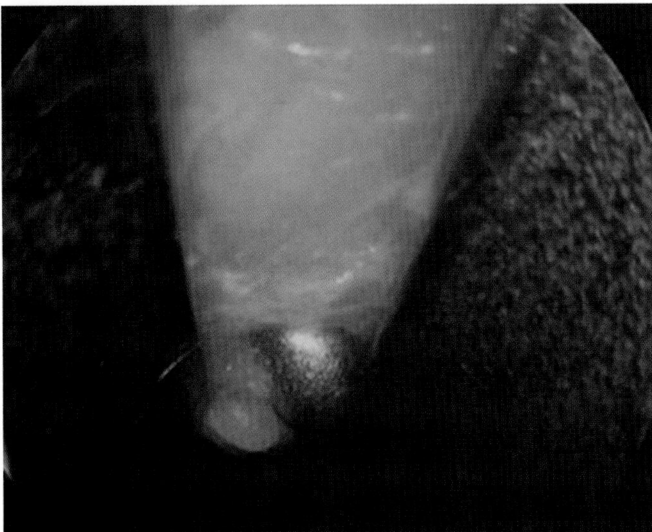

FIGURE 31.4. Fat pad and probe at the distal edge of the transverse carpal ligament.

The cannula system, when placed as described, is extrabursal; that is, it lies palmar to the flexor tendon bursa. The median nerve is also extrabursal and can occasionally be seen in the cannula system. If this is the case, the cannula system can be rotated radially 350 degrees. This will push the median nerve out of the cannula. If this does not clear the cannula system, it should be reinserted, and if clear visualization of the transverse carpal ligament without obstruction is not able to be achieved an open carpal tunnel release should be carried out.

Once one is absolutely certain there is no obstruction and no intervening structures (such as the median nerve, flexor tendon, or superficial palmar arch), the probe blade is inserted. This is a blade designed to cut forward and is blunt except at its axilla. It resembles a meniscotome. The probe blade is passed into the cannula system under direct vision and then withdrawn from proximal to distal until it slips palmarly and its axilla engages the distal edge of the transverse carpal ligament (Figure 31.5a and b).

This maneuver allows the surgeon to retract any structures that may have been in the area of the distal edge of the transverse carpal ligament, such as a communicating branch of the median and ulnar nerves or the superficial palmar arch. The probe blade is then advanced 1 cm from distal to proximal, cutting the distal edge of the TCL. The initial cut (that is, the cut with the probe blade) cuts the distal edge of the transverse carpal ligament and creates a safety zone into which the retrograde blade can be drawn. The probe blade is usually not sharp enough to completely cut the distal edge of the transverse carpal ligament because the distal edge of the transverse carpal ligament can be as thick as 7 to 10 mm.

The probe blade is then removed and the triangular blade is inserted approximately 1.5 cm proximal to the distal edge of the transverse carpal ligament. An incision is made into the transverse carpal ligament. This incision is large enough to accept the retrograde blade, and deep enough to penetrate the full thickness of the TCL

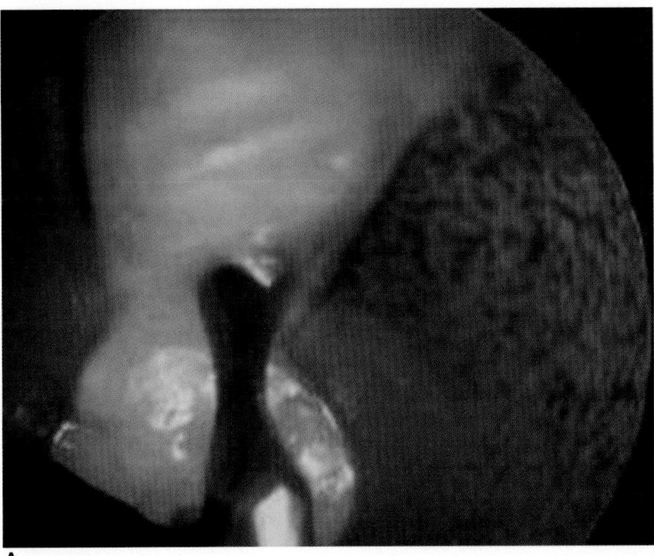

A

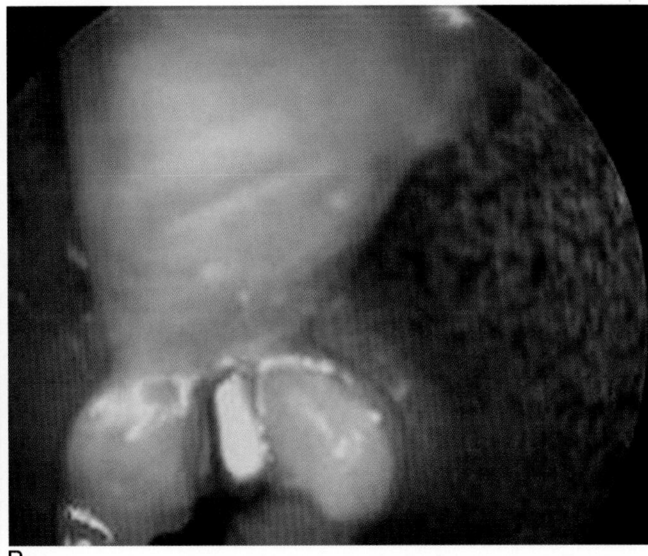

B

FIGURE 31.5. (A) Probe blade being withdrawn to distal edge of the transverse carpal ligament (TCL). (B) Probe blade engaging distal edge of the TCL at distal edge.

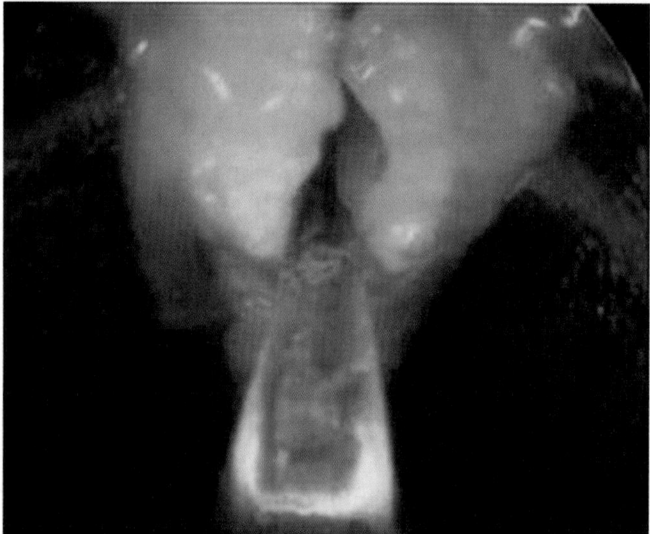

FIGURE 31.6. Incision of the central TCL with the triangular blade.

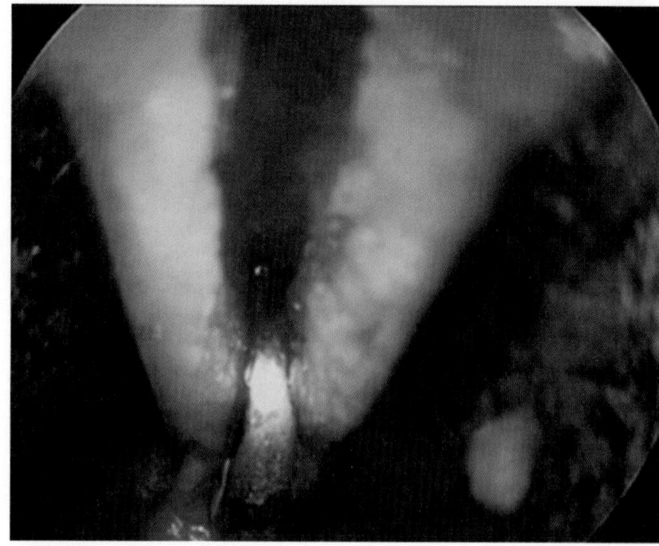

FIGURE 31.7. Completion of the distal TCL release using the retrograde "hook" knife.

(Figure 31.6). The triangular blade should not be used to cut the distal edge of the TCL because it has a tendency to cut too deeply and cause more bleeding as it enters the palmar fascia and fat.

The triangular blade is then removed and the retrograde blade is passed into the cannula system and into the defect created by the triangular blade. The retrograde blade is then used to cut the rest of the distal edge of the transverse carpal ligament from proximal to distal (Figure 31.7). This technique is safe as long as the surgeon has full control of the retrograde blade. The surgeon should hold the handle of the retrograde knife in his/her palm with the small and ring fingers. The shank of the blade is held between the long finger and the thumb while the index finger controls the cut by pushing off the cannula system.

Once the distal edge of the transverse carpal ligament is released, the retrograde blade is placed proximally and the scope distally. The proximal edge of the transverse carpal ligament is released under direct vision from distal to proximal. Occasionally, there are attachments between the palmar fascia and the transverse carpal ligament that need to be released—which can be done accurately using the triangular blade.

Once the release is complete, the proximal subfascial fat should cascade into the cannula system. In the rest of the cannula system, one should see the palmar fascia. The cut edges of the transverse carpal ligament will retract out of the field of view such that the cannula system must be rotated to see them (Figures 31.8 and 31.9). If this is not the case, the transverse carpal ligament has not been completely released and further release is needed. Once a complete release has been performed, the obturator is reinserted into the cannula and the cannula system is removed. A subcuticular stitch is used at the wrist, and a simple stitch

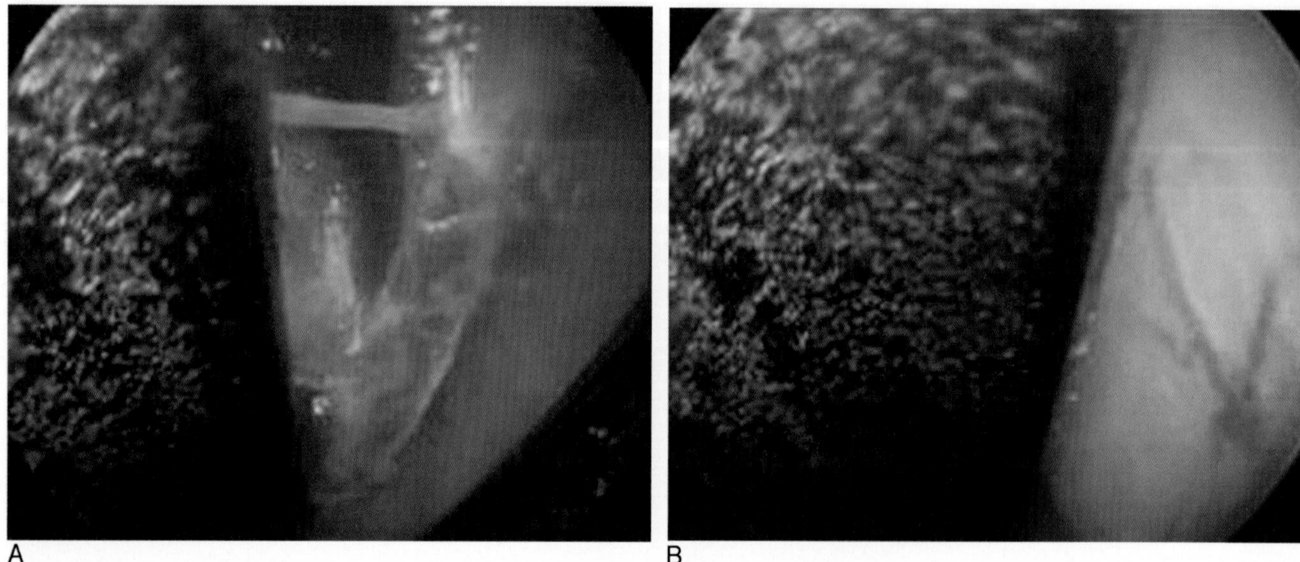

FIGURE 31.8. (A) Radial aspect of the cut edge of the TCL. (B) Median nerve.

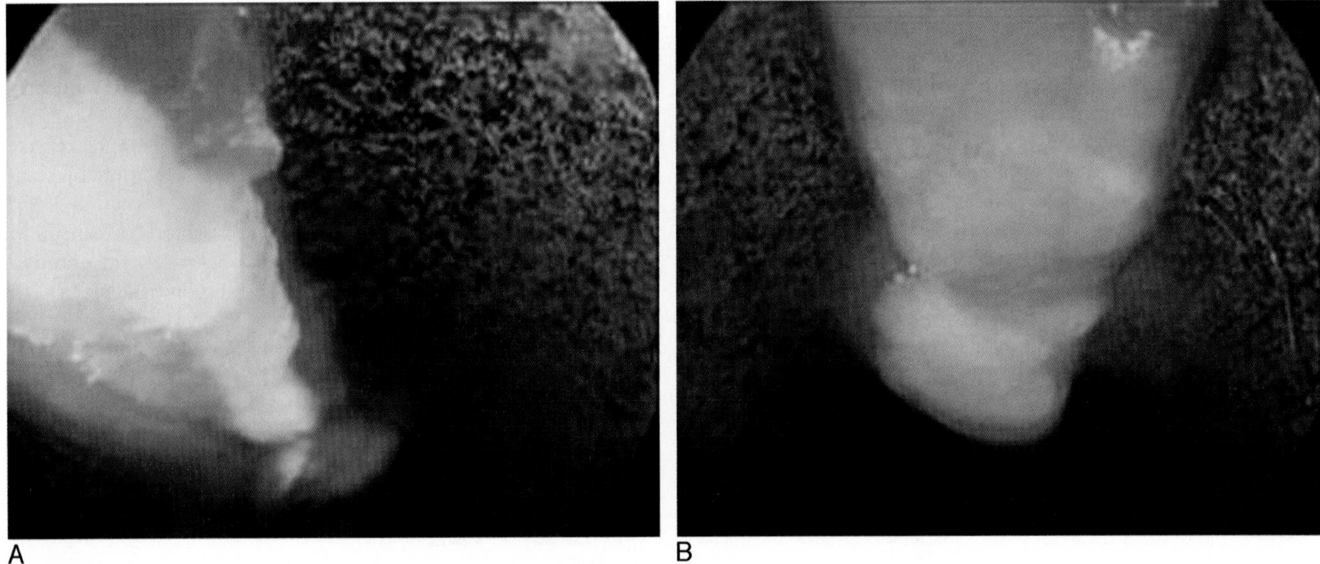

FIGURE 31.9. (A) Ulnar edge of cut TCL. (B) Palmar fat in cannula.

at the palm, and a bulky dressing is applied. No splint is needed. The patient's circulation, sensation, and motor function are then tested, and the patient is discharged from the operating room.

Our postoperative regime includes a visit to the office the next day for removal of the bulky dressing and application of a light dressing. The patient is encouraged to use the hand for light daily activities and to maintain the range of motion of the wrist, fingers, and thumb. The patient is asked to keep the wounds clean and dry.

No splint is needed. We remove the sutures two weeks after the surgery. We discovered that early aggressive therapy such as strengthening exercises produces a reactive tenosynovitis. If a patient is engaged in heavy manual labor and needs to work on endurance and strength, we begin a graded strengthening and endurance program after six weeks. The immediate resolution of nocturnal paresthesias is very consistent with this procedure. If the patient states that the nocturnal paresthesias have not resolved, this may be a sign that the nerve has not been completely decompressed.

Results

We published our early results in the early 1990s.[4,5] Since then, hundreds of studies have been published. These studies have confirmed the efficacy of ECTR. It is, however, beyond the scope of this chapter to present a detailed review of that literature. A relatively recent study by Trumble, Diao, Abrams, and Gilbert-Anderson is of note in that it compares ECTR to OCTR within the context of a randomized prospective study. The study attests to the fact that ECTR reliably and safely relieves patients of their carpal tunnel syndrome symptoms.[6]

The relative safety of ECTR has been looked at by Aaron Barr and his coauthors at our institutions. Dr. Barr and his colleagues performed a meta-analysis of the world's literature, specifically looking at the complication rate of ECTR versus OCTR. They collected data on 15,787 endoscopic carpal tunnel releases and 5,669 open carpal tunnel releases. The complication rate (including nerve, tendon, and artery injury) was 0.49% for OCTR and 0.20% for ECTR. The frequency of major nerve injury was 0.11% for OCTR and 0.14% for ECTR.[7] Their results compare well to those of Boeckstyns et al., who performed a similar meta-analysis of the outcomes of ECTR and OCTR.[8] Jim Chow has looked at his long-term results in 2,402 patients (average follow-up of six years ten months) and has reported a recurrence rate of 0.5%.[9]

Summary

The first ECTR was reported 19 years ago by Okutsu.[10] Some predicted endoscopic carpal tunnel release would be a passing fad. It would appear that endoscopic carpal tunnel release has withstood the test of time. Indeed, the Medicare data indicates that the frequency of endoscopic carpal tunnel release continues to increase.[11]

References

1. Chow JCY. Endoscopic release of the carpal ligament, a new technique for carpal tunnel syndrome. Arthroscopy 1989; 5:19–24.
2. Chow JCY. Endoscopic release of the carpal ligament for carpal tunnel syndrome: 22 month clinical result. Arthroscopy 1990;6:288–96.
3. Meals RA, Shaner M. Variations in digital sensory patterns: A study of the ulnar nerve-median nerve palmar communicating branch. J Hand Surg [Am] 1983;8:411–14.
4. Nagle DJ, Fischer TJ, Harris GD, Hastings H II, Osterman AL, Palmer AK, et al. A multicenter prospective review of 640

endoscopic Carpal tunnel releases using the transbursal and extrabursal Chow techniques. Arthroscopy 1996;12(2):139–43.
5. Nagle D, Harris G, Foley M. Prospective review of 278 endoscopic carpal tunnel releases using the modified Chow technique. Arthroscopy 1994;10(3):259–65.
6. Trumble TE, Diao E, Abrams RA, Gilbert-Anderson MM. Single-portal endoscopic carpal tunnel release compared with open release: A prospective, randomized trial. J Bone Joint Surg [Am] 2002;84-A(7):1107–15.
7. Aaron A, Bare LS, Benson CS, Williams JL, Visotsky D, Nagle J, Harder V. Complications of carpal tunnel surgery: An analysis of open and endoscopic techniques. Arthroscopy, 2006;22(9):919-24.
8. Boeckstyns ME, Sorensen AI. Does endoscopic carpal tunnel release have a higher rate of complications than open carpal tunnel release? An analysis of published series. J Hand Surg [Br] 1999;24(1):9–15.
9. Chow JC, Hantes ME. Endoscopic carpal tunnel release: Thirteen years' experience with the Chow technique. J Hand Surg [Am] 2002;27(6):1011–18.
10. Okutsu I, Ninomiya S, Natsuyama M, Takatori Y, Inanami H, Kuroshima N, et al. Subcutaneous operation and examination under the universal endoscope. Nippon Seikeigeka Gakkai Zasshi 1987;61(5):491–98.
11. Centers for Medicare and Medicaid Services.

Joseph F. Slade III and Greg Merrell

CHAPTER 32

Endoscopic Release of the First Dorsal Extensor Tendon Compartment

Rationale

One might ask if arthroscopic first dorsal compartment release is a triumph of technology over reason, given that the open release is usually considered straightforward and effective. However, upon closer examination there are several reasons to consider this approach. First, although traditional open release gives generally good results complications (due to the approach) do occur and are most likely underreported. One study by Harvey et al. documented scar adherence to the underlying tendon in 2 of 20 surgical patients, 1 minor wound infection, and temporary parathesias of the radial sensory nerve in 3 patients.[1] Another study by Arons et al. documents in 16 consecutive patients 14 complications, including 2 neuromas, 3 adhesions, 1 tendon subluxation, and 3 hypertrophic painful scars.[2] A study by Ta et al. documented a 5% recurrence rate, 2% sensory nerve injury, and 2% with severe scar tenderness out of 43 patients.[3] There have been other case reports of palmar subluxation of the tendon following operative release.[4] Clearly, although an open release of the first extensor compartment is perceived as a safe, simple, and effective surgical procedure when examined closely there is room for improvement.

Second, the 45 patients in our initial series experienced a faster return to pain-free activity. Third, when considering treatment one must fully understand the pathophysiology of the disease process. We believe that not only is there mechanical constriction from the restrictive tendon sheath but an element of peripheral nerve hypersensitivity.

We hypothesize that an arthroscopic approach allows for an extensive neurectomy of the tiny branches of the superficial radial nerve, which may innervate the first dorsal compartment. In addition, the endoscopic approach allows us to keep our incisions outside the hypersensitized zone of injury. Therefore, the minimally invasive approach along with this neurectomy may result in faster and more complete pain relief—with less risk for painful scar development. Last, with the proper training we believe this to be a safe technique. We must be clear that at this point the neurectomy component of the procedure is strictly a working hypothesis and not yet substantiated by substantial basic science and clinical research.

Indications and Contraindications

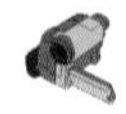

Surgical indications include any patient who has failed conservative treatment of splinting and/or injections. The diagnosis of De Quervain's tenosynovitis should be confirmed by examination. Alternative causes of radial-sided wrist pain (e.g., first carpometacarpal arthritis) should be excluded. There are no contraindications for the arthroscopic release that would differ from the open procedure. We have not yet performed an arthroscopic release on a patient with recurrent symptoms that failed previous open surgery. This would be a relative contraindication due to potential scarring and the displaced anatomy.

Surgical Technique

The patient is placed supine. The arm is elevated and exsanguinated, and a tourniquet inflated. The wrist is placed over a towel roll in a neutral position. A distal portal is established by making a 5-mm superficial transverse incision just distal to the thumb carpometacarpal (CMC) joint. The incision is placed in line with the first dorsal compartment at the insertion of the abductor pollicis longus (APL) tendon, 2 to 3 cm distal to the end of the radial styloid (Figure 32.1). Blunt dissection with a small hemostat is used to clear the overlying subcutaneous tissue from the fascia enveloping the thumb CMC joint, which is then elevated off the tendons of the first dorsal compartment with a small right-angle retractor.

A narrow and long hemostat snap is next used to bluntly create a working space between the skin and subcutaneous tissue (Figure 32.2). A small-joint arthroscopic cannula and trocar are inserted above the fibrous fascial sheath of the first dorsal compartment, proximal to the radial styloid and the extensor tendon retinaculum. A proximal portal is established by making a second 5-mm transverse incision over the trocar tip approximately 4 to 6 cm proximal to the radial styloid (Figure 32.3). The trocar is removed and a 2.7-mm 30-degree angled scope is inserted into the cannula through the proximal portal (Figure 32.4).

The scope is fully inserted into the cannula until the tip of the scope is visible through the distal portal. The cannula is then removed. A small right-angled retractor is placed in the proximal portal to maintain a working space, and a dry endoscopic inspection of the fascia overlying the first dorsal compartment is performed starting distally over the CMC joint (Figure 32.5). The superficial radial nerve (SRN) is easily identified in the subcutaneous tissue above as it sweeps downward, crossing the fascia below (Figure 32.6). Long thin cardiovascular Mueller scissors are introduced into the distal portal and used to bluntly and carefully dissect the overlying subcutaneous tissue from the fascia (Figure 32.7).

This is a key step because we hypothesize that there are small neurofibrils extending from the major branches of the SRN down to the underlying fascia, which are divided off the fascia and swept aside. We believe this procedure serves as a neurectomy, separating these terminal branches from

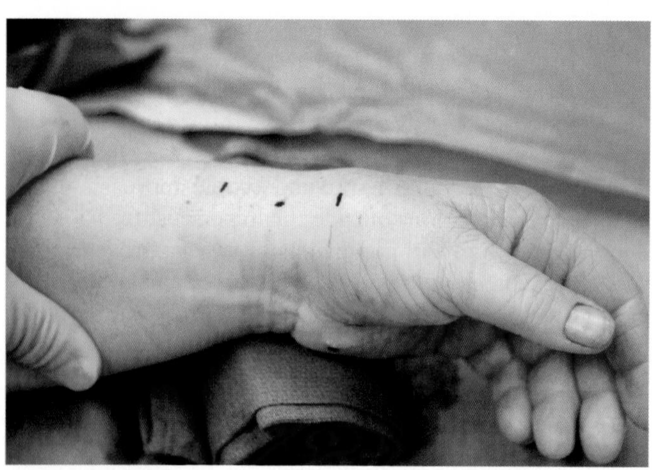

FIGURE 32.1. Incisions for endoscopic De Quervain's release.

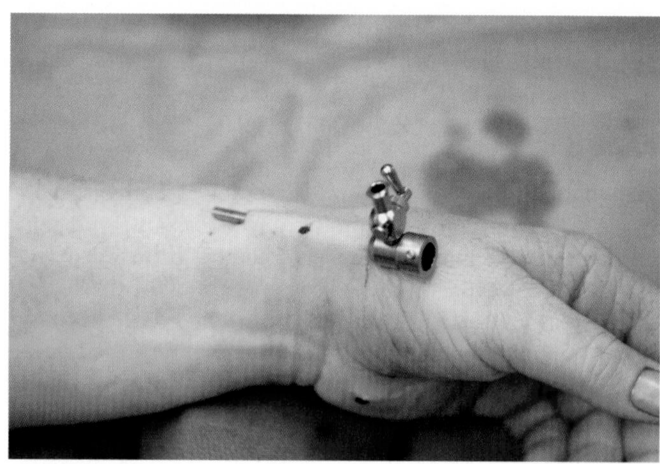

FIGURE 32.3. Cannula inserted to create appropriate path for endoscope.

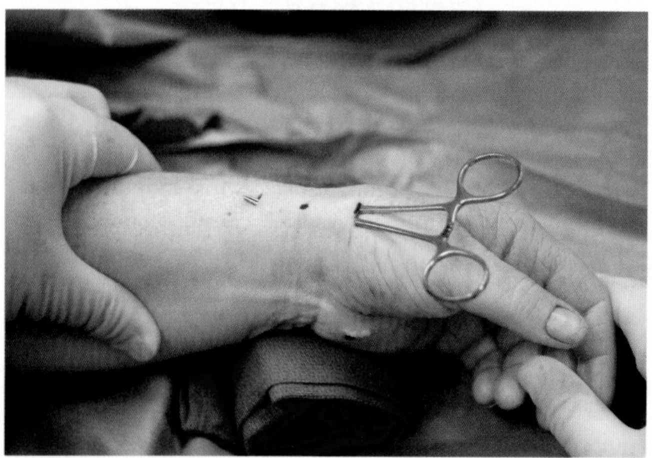

FIGURE 32.2. Hemostat inserted to clear path for trocar.

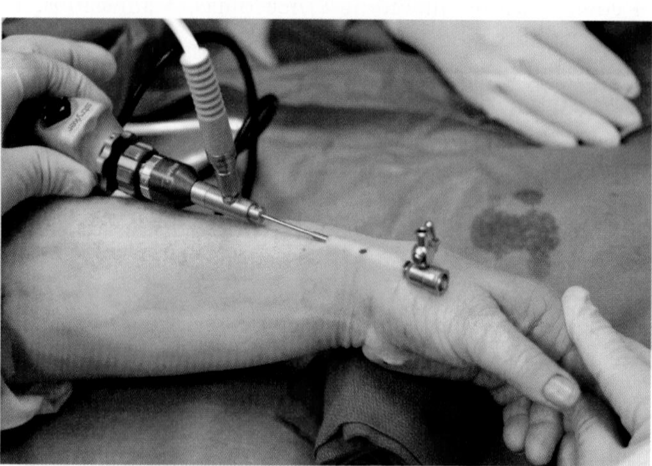

FIGURE 32.4. Endoscope inserted into cannula in reverse fashion through proximal portal.

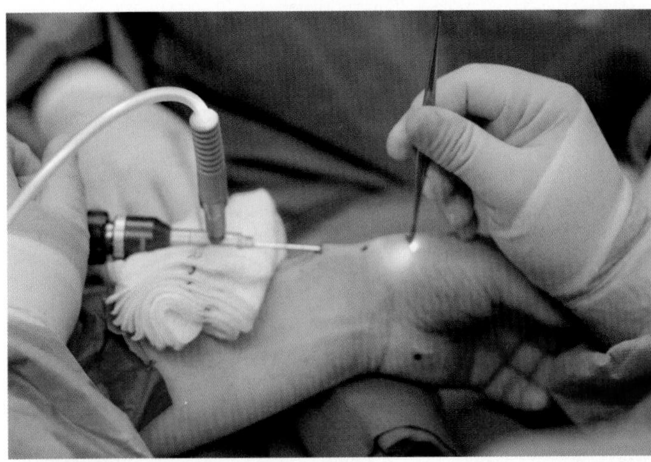

FIGURE 32.5. Dry scope technique with right-angle retractor to increase working space.

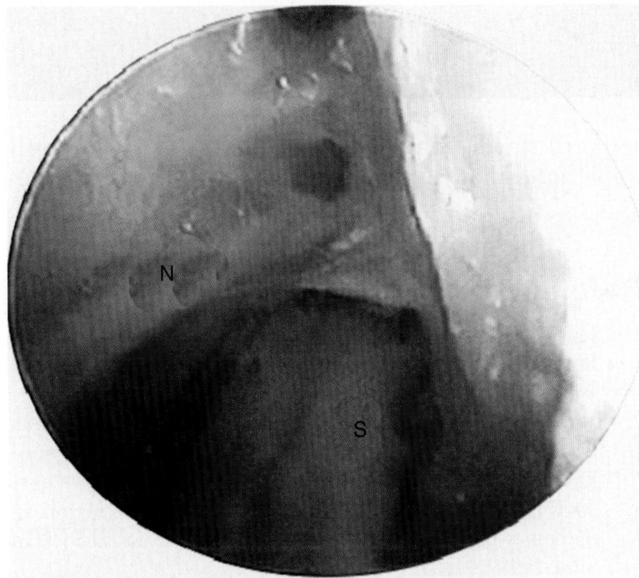

FIGURE 32.6. Endoscopic visualization of superficial radial nerve (N) and first dorsal compartment sheath (S) below.

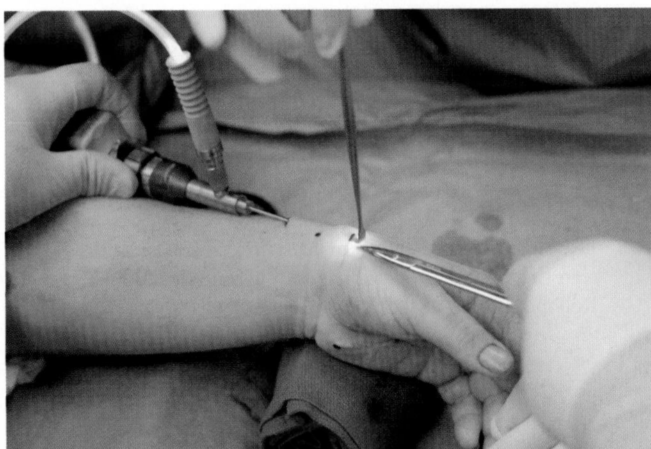

FIGURE 32.7. Mueller scissors used to dissect soft tissue and microscopic innervations to the first dorsal compartment sheath from the superficial radial nerve under direct vision.

their sensory receptors on the fascia. Although there are some corroborating anatomical studies published, much of this needs further substantiation. One might suggest that the open procedure also provides for some subcutaneous dissection that has an element of neurectomy. However, an open procedure is addressing only a centimeter or so around the sheath. In the endoscopic procedure, we are providing a subcutaneous dissection/neurectomy of 6 to 8 cm. We believe that this step may be responsible for the immediate and profound relief in symptoms.

Next, the fascia of the first dorsal compartment is incised—starting proximal to the radial styloid and moving distally. The tendon slips of the APL and extensor pollicis brevis (EPB) are identified (Figure 32.8a and b). The EPB is often in a separate compartment and must be released. This tendon can be easily identified by stabilizing the first metacarpal and manually flexing and extending the metacarpal phalangeal joint. Through the endoscope, the EPB tendon can be visualized gliding proximally and distally (whereas the APL tendons remain stationary). As necessary, the camera and working instruments can be switched to evaluate the adequacy of the release or to improve access to different parts of the sheath. The wound is irrigated, the skin is closed with nylon suture, and a sterile dressing and volar spica splint are applied. The tourniquet is deflated. The typical tourniquet time is approximately 10 minutes.

The technique achieves two goals by addressing two possible sources of pain. The first goal is to perform a neurectomy of the small SRN branches to the first dorsal extensor compartment. Lin et al. demonstrated that the ligaments of the dorsal wrist capsule have an extensive array of sensory nerve endings.[5] We surmise that a similar arrangement may exist in the first extensor compartment and may help explain the severe pain that occurs in De Quervain's from the mechanical constriction of the thumb extensor tendons.

Berger and Weinstein have shown that partial wrist denervation by ablation of the terminal portions of the anterior and posterior interosseous nerves (which supply proprioceptive fibers to the wrist capsule) can be an effective treatment for a variety of chronic unreconstructable pathologies.[6,7] Our surgical technique for De Quervain's may provide pain relief through a similar denervation of the first extensor compartment. Additional support for the neurectomy hypothesis is found in the pattern of referred pain from the APL. It has been shown to resemble the C6, 7, and 8 dermatomes. This parallels the superficial radial sensory nerve distribution, and is very similar to the radiation of pain experienced in de Quervain's tenosynovitis.[8]

The second goal is the reversal of increase in friction, which results in a restriction of tendon gliding. This is accomplished by release of the unyielding fascial compartment overlying the thumb extensor tendons. This fascial release facilitates tendon gliding by decreasing friction, allowing for a gradual reduction in tendon irritation. Over time, swelling decreases and the tissues recover. We postulate that the sheath will likely be eventually reinnervated,

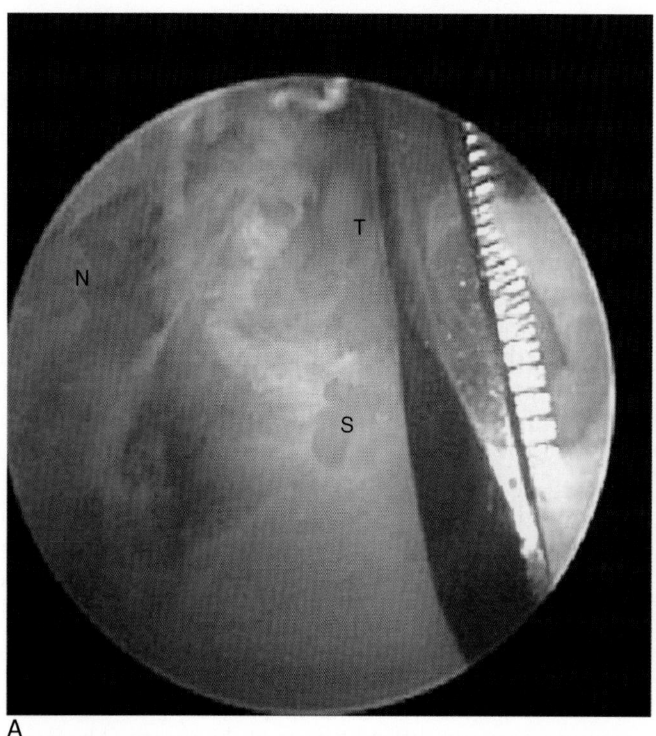

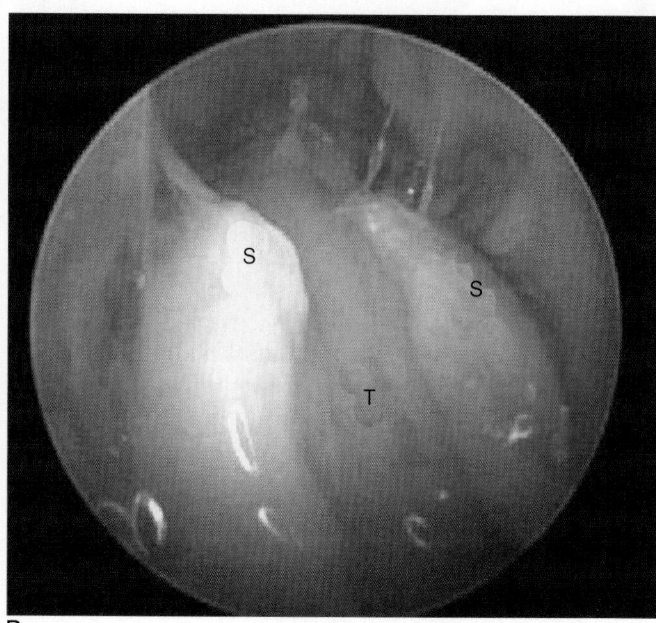

FIGURE 32.8. (A) Endooscopic image showing beginning of the fascial sheath (S) release of the first dorsal compartment, underlying tendons (T), and superficial radial nerve (N). (B) Arthroscopic image showing complete release of first dorsal compartment sheath (S) with underlying tendons (T).

but only after the tendon pathology has resolved—which breaks the cycle of local nerve irritation.

Postoperative Management

Dressings and stitches are removed after seven days, and the patient is allowed to resume activities of daily living without restrictions.

Complications

In our initial series of 45 patients, there have been no infections, neuromas, or significant scar tenderness. There have been no injuries to the superficial radial nerve. No patient had to be converted to the open procedure for failure of visualization or inability to achieve appropriate release. There has been good subjective patient satisfaction, and none were considered treatment failures. As with any arthroscopic surgery, it is imperative that the surgeon be comfortable with arthroscopic equipment and technique and that the relevant anatomy is fully understood.

References

1. Harvey FJ, Harvey PM, Horsely MW. De Quervain's disease: Surgical or nonsurgical treatment. J Hand Surg 1990; 15A:83–7.
2. Arons MS. De Quervain's release in working women: A report of failure, complications and associated diagnoses. J Hand Surg 1987;12A:540–44.
3. Ta KT, Eidelmen D, Thomson JG. Patient satisfaction and outcomes of surgery for de Quervain's tenosynovitis. J Hand Surg 1999;24A:1071–77.
4. White GM, Weiland AJ. Symptomatic palmar tendon subluxation after surgical release for de Quervain's disease. J Hand Surg 1984;9A:704–06.
5. Lin YT, Berger RA, Berger EJ, Tomita K, Jew JY, Yang C, et al. Nerve endings of the wrist joint: A preliminary report of the dorsal radiocarpal ligament. J Orthop Res 2006;24 (6):1225–30.
6. Berger RA. Partial denervation of the wrist: A new approach. Tech Hand Up Extrem Surg 1998;2(1):25–35.
7. Weinstein LP, Berger RA. Analgesic benefit, functional outcome, and patient satisfaction after partial wrist denervation. J Hand Surg [Am] 2002;27(5):833–39.
8. Hwang M, Kang YK, Shin JY, Kim DH. Referred pain pattern of the abductor pollicis longus muscle. Am J Phys Med Rehabil 2005;84(8):593–97.

Index

I

J

K

L

M

N

O

P

R

S